# MOLECULAR CONSIDERATIONS AND EVOLVING SURGICAL MANAGEMENT ISSUES IN THE TREATMENT OF PATIENTS WITH A BRAIN TUMOR

Edited by **Terry Lichtor**

**Molecular Considerations and Evolving Surgical Management Issues in the Treatment of Patients with a Brain Tumor**

http://dx.doi.org/10.5772/58501

Edited by Terry Lichtor

**Contributors**

Jafri Malin Abdullah, Abdul Aziz Mohamed Yusoff, Farizan Ahmad, Zamzuri Idris, Hasnan Jaafar, Ryuya Yamanaka, Yasushi Shibata, Hassan Mahmoud Fathallah-Shaykh, Caroline Agha, Hannah C. Machemehl, Daniela Parolaro, Jun Liu, Shoumin Bai, Zhihua Yang, Beibei Gu, Liao Wang, Shuling Peng, Davide Schiffer, Rui Manuel Reis, Fátima Baltazar, Vera Gonçalves, Mehdi H. Shahi, Mohammad Mobarak Hossain, Javier S Castresana, Bárbara Meléndez, Juan Rey, Todd Vitaz, Jarosław Markowski, Krzysztof Siemianowicz, Wirginia Likus, Michael Graner, Justin Hellwinkel, Helen Madsen, Soliman Oushy, Mike Fay, Stephen Rose, Chris Bell, Nicholas Dowson, Simon Puttick, Adrianna Ranger, David Diosy

**Published by InTech**

Janeza Trdine 9, 51000 Rijeka, Croatia



**Publishing Process Manager** Iva Lipovic

**Technical Editor** InTech DTP team

**Cover** InTech Design team

First published March, 2015

Printed in Croatia

Additional hard copies can be obtained from orders@intechopen.com

Molecular Considerations and Evolving Surgical Management Issues in the Treatment of Patients with a Brain Tumor, Edited by Terry Lichtor

p. cm.

ISBN 978-953-51-2031-5

For EU product safety concerns:
IN TECH d.o.o., Prolaz Marije Krucifikse Kozulić 3, 51000 Rijeka, Croatia,
info@intechopen.com or visit our website at intechopen.com.

# Meet the editor

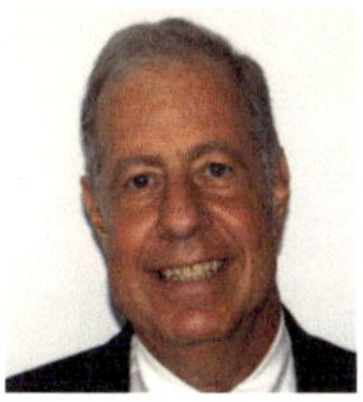

Terry Lichtor is a practicing neurosurgeon. He has a number of research interests, and his brain tumor work is largely focused on the development of a DNA vaccine for treatment of primary and metastatic intracerebral tumors. In particular Dr. Lichtor has shown that vaccines prepared by transfer of DNA from the tumor into a highly immunogenic cell line encompass the array of tumor antigens that characterize the patient's population. Poorly immunogenic tumor antigens, characteristic of malignant cells, can become strongly antigenic if they are expressed by highly immunogenic cells. The introduction of the vaccine directly into the tumor bed of animals with an intracerebral tumor stimulates a systemic cellular anti-tumor immune response associated with a prolongation of survival. It is hopeful that this vaccine strategy will be efficacious in the treatments of patients with brain tumors. Dr. Lichtor is a member of the neurosurgery faculty at Rush University Medical Center in Chicago, Illinois, USA.

# Contents

# Preface

Although technical advances have resulted in marked improvements in the ability to diagnose and surgically treat primary and metastatic brain tumors, the incidence and mortality rates of these tumors are increasing. Particularly affected are young adults and the elderly. The present standard treatment modalities following surgical resection, including cranial irradiation and systemic or local chemotherapy, each have limited efficacy and serious adverse side effects. Furthermore, the relatively few long-term survivors are inevitably left with cognitive deficits and other disabilities. The difficulties in treating malignant gliomas can be attributed to several factors. Glial tumors are inherently resistant to radiation and standard cytotoxic chemotherapies. The existence of blood-brain and blood-tumor barriers impede drug delivery to the tumor and adjacent brain infiltrated with tumor. In addition, the low therapeutic index between tumor sensitivity and toxicity to normal brain severely limits the ability to systemically deliver therapeutic doses of drugs or radiation therapy to the tumor. New treatment strategies for the management of patients with these tumors are urgently needed.

In this book, a review of the important features involving the clinical management of patients with these tumors is outlined. In particular, advances in the molecular biology of brain tumors including the evolution of microRNAs along with angiogenesis and tumor invasion patterns are reviewed. In addition, advances in radiology both for pre-operative diagnostic purposes along with surgical planning are described. A discussion of the particular resistance to radiation therapy and the long-term consequences of radiation therapy treatments is provided.

An important emerging strategy in the treatment of patients with brain tumors involving the stimulation of an immunologic response against the neoplastic cells is outlined in this book. Although in most instances proliferating tumors do not provoke anti-tumor cellular immune responses, the hope is that the immune system can be called into play to destroy malignant cells. Hopefully this information coupled with advances in the understanding of the molecular biology of brain tumors, which are also outlined in this book, will translate into additional novel therapeutic treatment strategies that should lead to the prolongation of survival without a decline in cognitive functions or other side effects in patients with brain tumors.

**Terry Lichtor, MD, PhD**
Department of Neurosurgery
Rush University Medical Center
USA

Section 1

# Molecular Biology of Tumors

Chapter 1

# Understanding Mitochondrial DNA in Brain Tumorigenesis

Abdul Aziz Mohamed Yusoff, Farizan Ahmad,
Zamzuri Idris, Hasnan Jaafar and
Jafri Malin Abdullah

Additional information is available at the end of the chapter

http://dx.doi.org/10.5772/58965

## 1. Introduction

In developed countries, most studies reveal that the number of people who develop brain tumors and die from them has increased. Brain tumor, one of the most devastating central nervous system pathologies, is the leading cause of solid tumor death in children under the age of 15, and the second leading cause of cancer death in male adults ages 20-39. So far, researches on genesis and development of tumor are intensively focused and studied on alteration of the gene in nucleus and brain tumors is the one where most were reported arise as the result of progressive nuclear genetic alterations. Multiple genetic events have been identified in brain tumor cells involving some well-known susceptibility genes such as tumor suppressor and oncogenes that are encoded by the nuclear DNA (nDNA). For instance, the p53 tumor suppressor gene is frequently mutated and often detected altered or lost early in brain tumor mainly in astrocytic tumors formation [1-3]. Similarly, mutations or loss of PTEN (phosphatase and tensin homolog), p16, RB (retinoblastoma) and amplification of EGFR (epidermal growth factor receptor), MDM2, CDK4, CDK6 (cyclin-dependent kinase) are also involved in the pathogenesis of brain tumor [4,5].

Although, it is well established that multiple alterations in the nuclear-encoded genes are associated with tumor development, it is reasonable to consider and postulate that there is another factor or genome yet to be investigated. The involvement of the mitochondrial genome in tumorigenesis and cancer progression remains controversial to date. Mitochondria are cytoplasmic organelles in eukaryotic cell and recognized as "the power houses of the cell", thus one of their principal functions is providing cellular energy, adenosine triphosphate

(ATP) through the oxidative phosphorylation (OXPHOS) [6]. OXPHOS can be defined as the oxidation of electron transfer chain by oxygen and the concomitant transduction of this energy into ATP. The OXPHOS system is composed of five protein complexes: NADH-ubiquinone oxidoreductase as complex I, succinate-ubiquinone oxidoreductase as complex II, ubiquinone-cytochrome *c* oxidoreductase as complex III, cytochrome *c* oxidase as complex IV and ATP synthase as complex V.

In addition to energy production, mitochondria are also key components in calcium signalling, regulation of cellular metabolism, haem synthesis, steroid synthesis and, perhaps most importantly, the initiation and execution of apoptosis [7,8]. Over the last 25 years, mitochondrial abnormalities that associated with mitochondrial DNA (mtDNA) alterations, has been identified in human disease, including seizure, ataxia, ophthalmoplegia, optic atrophy, short stature, sensorineural hearing loss, cardiomyopathy, diabetes mellitus and kidney failure [9,10]. Accumulation of altered mtDNA has also been widely believed to play the pivotal role in aging and the development of various age-related degenerative diseases [11]. In recent years, more attention has been directed towards the role of mitochondrial dysfunction in various cancer due to genetic defects of OXPHOS system [12-17]. Proteins that take part in the proper functioning of the OXPHOS system are encoded by both nDNA and mtDNA. Similar to nDNA, mtDNA mutations and deletions have been identified in a wide variety of cancers including brain tumor [18-26], although it is unclear whether these are causal or a consequence of the neoplastic process.

This chapter begins with a general overview of basic mitochondrial structure and OXPHOS system functions and then outlines more specifically the link between mitochondrial reactive oxygen spices (ROS) and apoptosis with tumorigenesis and genetic alterations in mitochondria associated with human cancers mainly brain tumor.

## 2. Mitochondrial structure

Mitochondria are seen by electron microscopy to be intracellular oblong or ovoid shaped organelles with a transverse diameter of 0.1-0.5 μm and a variable length [27]. The structure of mitochondria is shown in Figure 1. Most eukaryotic cells contain many mitochondria, which cover up to 25% of the volume of the cytoplasm. The number of mitochondria within a cell increases with the amount of substrate and oxygen. Mitochondria are large enough to be observed under a light microscope, but the detail of their structure can be viewed only with the electron microscope.

Initial studies based on electron microscopy investigations by two researchers Palade and Sjöstrand, revealed that mitochondria contain more than one membrane system with the existence of an outer membrane and of a highly folded inner membrane [28,29]. The baffle model which was coined by Palade has been accepted and currently depicted as a model of mitochondria structure in all the textbooks [28]. The baffle model describes mitochondria as having four compartments (Figure 1). The first compartment is termed the outer membrane. This smooth membrane surrounds with a very convoluted or folded inner membrane. The

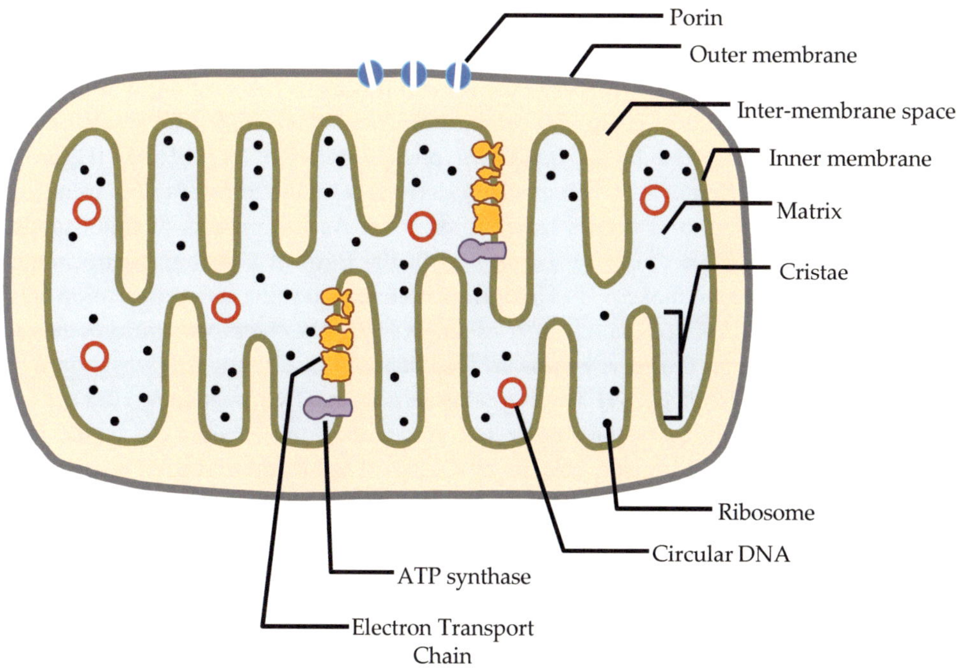


**Figure 1.** The structure of a mitochondrion

inner membrane is folded to create cristae. The outer and inner membranes have very different properties. Together they create two compartments, namely the intermembrane space (the space between the outer and inner membranes), and the matrix (closed by the inner membrane-the very interior of the mitochondria).

Nowadays, the baffle model has been shown to be inaccurate. Based on the investigations of 3-D structure of mitochondrial morphology by electron microscope tomography, the inner membrane is believed to be further divided into two distinct domains: an inner boundary membrane and cristae membranes [27, 30-32]. The inner boundary membrane is located close to the outer membrane and makes close contact with it at numerous positions. Cristae membranes protrude into the matrix compartment and are connected to the inner boundary membrane by narrow tubular structures called cristae junctions.

The outer bilayer lipid membrane contains channels made of voltage dependent anion channels called porins and are permeable to molecules < 10,000 Da. It is composed of approximately 50% lipids and 50% proteins. The inner bilayer lipid membrane is folded and impermeable to most molecules and protons. It is built up of 70% protein. The inner membrane is also the site of the electron transport chain and contains transport proteins for OXPHOS system. Within the matrix a large number of enzymes and other proteins and peptides, including DNA-polymerase, chaperones (heat shock proteins), ribosomes, mRNAs, tRNAs, and the mtDNA are located.

## 3. Mitochondrial function: OXPHOS system

Mitochondria play a central role in energy conversion processes (respiration) within the cell through the electron transport chain, the primary function of which is ATP synthesis via a complex mechanism referred to as "oxidative phosphorylation" (OXPHOS) (Figure 2). OXPHOS is the production of ATP using energy derived from the transfer of electrons in an electron transport system and occurs by chemiosmosis. As the process of mitochondrial electron transport takes place, energy is released in the form of a proton electrochemical gradient that can be used to make ATP. Though, the details regarding the conservation of this released energy are still being debated, most scientists accept the chemiosmotic hypothesis as the general mechanism for the energy transfer. The chemiosmotic hypothesis was formulated in the 1960s by Peter Mitchell [33,34]. This hypothesis states that hydrogen ions ($H^+$or protons) are transferred from mitochondrial matrix out across the inner membrane to the inter-membrane space as electron transport occurs by a series of reduction-oxidation reactions that establish an electrochemical gradient. The membrane is impermeable to protons, which flow back down the proton gradient through a large enzyme called ATP synthase or complex V, the energy from which is subsequently used to produce ATP.

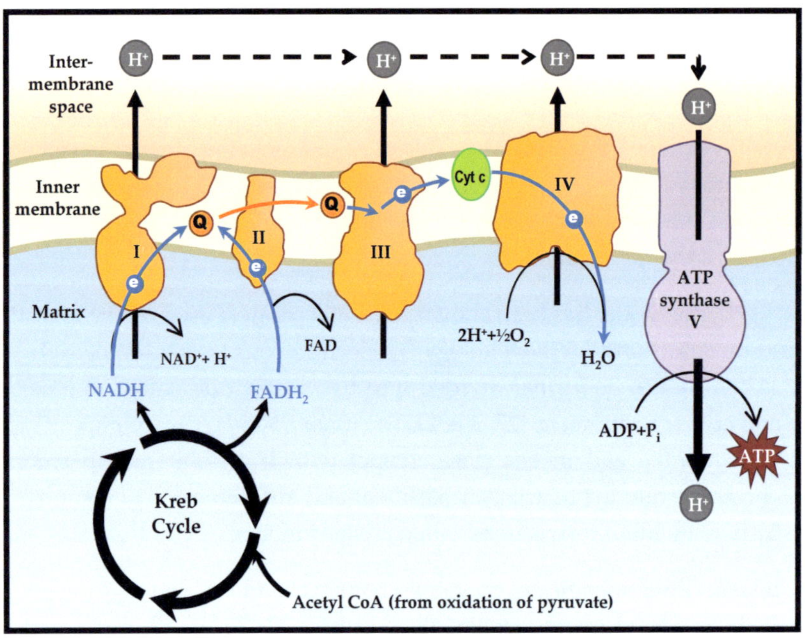


**Figure 2.** A schematic representation of the mitochondrial OXPHOS system

For achieving the whole process, in first stage pyruvate, which is generated in the cytosol during glycolysis, is transported across the double mitochondrial membranes and enters the matrix. The pyruvate molecules are produced by the breakdown of glucose molecules from carbohydrates via glycolysis. Once inside the matrix, pyruvate molecules are converted to the two carbon compound acetyl coenzyme A (acetyl CoA). This oxidative decarboxylation reaction is catalyzed by the pyruvate dehydrogenase complex. The acetyl CoA is then taken into a sequence of enzymatically catalyzed reactions known as the citric acid cycle which completes the oxidation of carbon and regenerates an electron acceptor to keep the cycle going. The oxidation of acetyl CoA in the citric acid cycle (which is also called the Krebs cycle or tricarboxylic acid cycle) is catalyzed by a set of enzymes localized in the mitochondrial matrix. During this process, the released electrons are transferred to co-enzymes, $NAD^+$and FAD to form the reduced molecules NADH and $FADH_2$. Later, NADH and $FADH_2$ transfer electrons to acceptor molecules in the electron transport chain, in the inner mitochondrial membrane. Coenzyme Q (ubiquinone) and cytochrome c are also involved in mitochondrial respiration, serving as 'electron shuttles' or mobile electron carriers between the complexes.

Electrons donated from NADH to Complex I or from $FADH_2$ to Complex II are passed to coenzyme Q. Electrons then flow from coenzyme Q to Complex III which transfers the electrons to cytochrome c. From cytochrome c the electrons move to Complex IV and finally to ½ $O_2$ to produce $H_2O$ [35]. As electrons pass through these complexes in a series of oxidation-reduction reactions, the energy that is released by this electron transport chain is used to pump protons out from the mitochondrial matrix to the inter membrane space via Complexes I, III and IV creating the electrochemical gradient. The electrochemical gradient allows protons to drive back into the matrix through a pore in Complex V (ATP synthase), using the released energy to catalyze the synthesis of ATP from ADP and phosphate.

## 4. Mitochondrial genome

Mitochondria have a genetic system of their own, separate from the nuclear one, with all the machinery necessary for its expression; that is, to replicate, transcribe and translate the genetic information they contain. The mitochondrial deoxyribonucleic acid (mtDNA) was discovered in 1963 [36] and the near complete sequence for human mtDNA was available in 1981 [37] and was minimally revised in 1999 [38]. Human mtDNA is mostly a double-stranded, closed circular molecule composed of 16,569 base pairs.

Figure 3 shows the human mitochondrial genome. It is very compact, containing little non-coding sequence, essentially just the 1.1 kb D-loop (displacement loop or non-coding) region, and having even some overlapping genes. The non-coding region that includes the D-loop is located between genes encoding tRNA phenylalanine (F) and proline (P). The two strands of mtDNA have been named light strand (L-strand, rich in cytosines) and heavy strand (H-strand, rich in guanines) according to their buoyancy through a denaturing caesium chloride gradient [39].

The D-loop region of mtDNA contains the origin of replication for H-strand synthesis as well as both mitochondrial transcription promoters (the light strand promoter, LPS and two heavy strand promoters, HSP1 and HSP2), and serves as the main site for mitochondrial genomic replication and transcription [40,41]. Between different mammalian species, the mtDNA is about the same size and has the similar organization and content of genes [42-44]. The mitochondrial genome has been sequenced and mapped for many species yet the regulation of its expression is poorly understood.

The human mtDNA contains 37 genes coding mRNAs for 13 polypeptides that are part of four of the five multi-enzymatic complexes in the OXPHOS system, 22 tRNAs (that are able to decode all open reading frames) and 2 rRNAs (components of the specific mitochondrial ribosomes) necessary for synthesis of the polypeptides. Unlike nuclear DNA, mtDNA coding sequences have no introns. Seven of those polypeptides, ND1 to ND6 and ND4L are subunits of Complex I; one, cytochrome *b*, is part of Complex III; three, COX I, COX II and COX III, are the catalytic subunits of Complex IV, and ATPase 6 and 8 are subunits of Complex V ($F_0F_1$ ATP synthase). The heavy strand is the main coding strand, and codes for 2 rRNAs, 14 tRNAs and 12 polypeptides. The light strand codes for remaining 8 tRNAs and only one polypeptide, the ND6 subunit (NADH-dehydrogenase) [6].

Mammalian mitochondria are not self-supporting entities in the cell. Replication and transcription depend upon *trans*-acting nuclear-encoded factors. All proteins of mitochondrial ribosomes and their associated translation factors and, indeed, all other mitochondrial proteins including the components of the mitochondrial import machinery are encoded by the nuclear DNA. For instance, mitochondrial tRNAs are charged by imported aminoacyl-tRNA synthetases from nuclear genes.

There are approximately hundreds or thousands copies of mitochondrial genome in each somatic cell. Normally, all of the mitochondrial DNAs within the cells of an individual are identical, which is termed homoplasmy. However, in the presence of a mitochondrial DNA mutation, the affected individual cells will usually harbour a mixture of mutated and wild-type mitochondrial DNA. The condition of these two populations of mitochondrial DNA molecules is called heteroplasmy [45]. As cells divide, the mutant and wild-type mitochondrial DNA are randomly distributed to the daughter cells, so the proportion of mutant to wild-type mitochondrial DNA may increase or decrease with each subsequent generation of the cell line. If that proportion increases past a certain level, the cellular energy capacity will decline, and clinical signs appear. This is referred to as the threshold effect. The threshold may vary from tissue to tissue because the percent of mutant mitochondrial DNA needed to cause cell dysfunction varies according to the oxidative requirements of the tissue and the severity of the mutation. It has often been claimed that tissues with high requirements for oxidative energy metabolism, such as muscle and brain, have relatively low thresholds and are particularly vulnerable to mitochondrial DNA mutation.

Human mitochondrial DNA is a 16,569 base pair circle of double-stranded DNA that encodes 13 essential respiratory chain subunits. ND1–ND6 and ND4L encode seven complex I (NADH–ubiquinone oxidoreductase) subunits, CYT b encodes one subunit of complex III (ubiquinol:cytochrome *c* oxidoreductase), COX I–COX III encode the three major catalytic subunits of complex IV, and ATPase6 and ATPase8 encode two subunits of complex V (ATP synthase). Also shown are the two ribosomal RNA (12S rRNA and 16S rRNA) genes and the 22 transfer RNA genes (red spheres, depicted by single letter amino acid code abbreviation) required for mitochondrial protein synthesis. tRNAs are F, Phenylalanine; V, Valine; L, Leucine; I, Isoleucine; Q, Glutamine; M, Methionine; W, Tryptophan; A, Alanine; N, Asparagine; C, Cysteine;

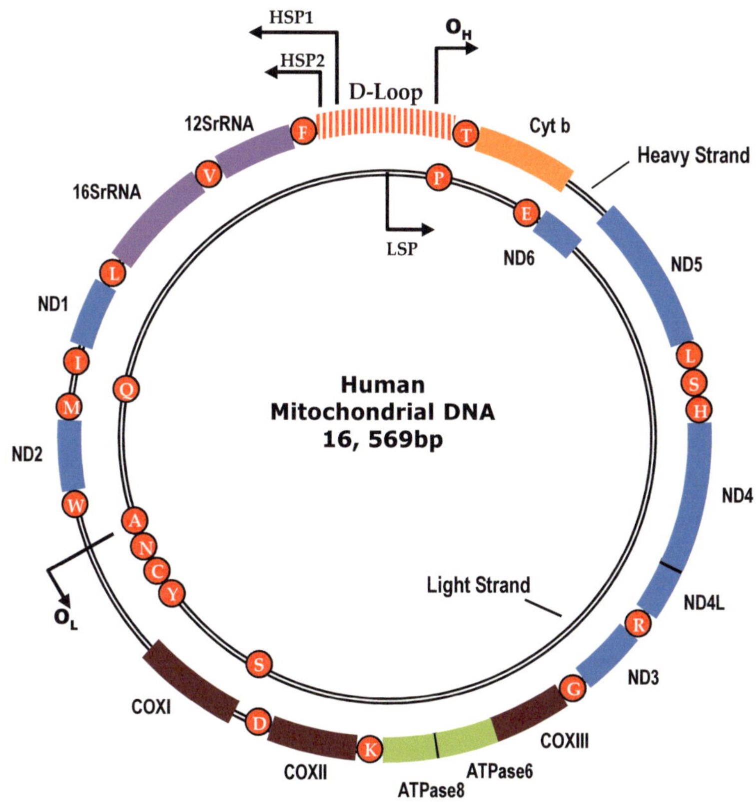


**Figure 3.** The human mitochondrial genome

Y, Tyrosine; S, Serine; D, Aspartic acid; K, Lysine; G, Glycine; R, Arginine; H, Histidine; E, Glutamic acid; T, Threonine; P, Proline. The genome is highly organised and shows little redundancy of its coding sequence. The displacement loop (D-loop), or non-coding control region contains the promoters for transcription of the L (LSP) and H strands (HSP1 and HS2) and the origin of replication of the H strand ($O_H$). The origin of light-strand replication is shown as $O_L$.

## 5. Warburg theory and mitochondrial dysfunction in cancer cells

In the 1930s, the German scientist, Dr. Otto H. Warburg pioneered the research specifically targeted to the alterations of mitochondrial respiration in the aspect of cancer. He reported that cancer cells exhibited a high glycolysis rate even in the presence of abundant oxygen. This phenomenon was known as the "Warburg effect". Cancer cells had to depend on anaerobic glycolysis rather than respiration to generate ATP [46]. He further proposed that defects in energy metabolism, especially due to mitochondrial malfunction, are involved in the initiation or progression of cancer. Dr. Warburg's discovery encouraged many scientists to realize the potential role of mitochondria in cancer cells.

Since then, alterations of mitochondria in the number, shape and function have been reported in various cancers [47]. The conversion of ATP production from mitochondrial OXPHOS to glycolysis has been suggested to be the bioenergetic hallmark of cancer cells [48]. Furthermore, it has been shown that mitochondrial dysfunction is able to initiate critical signaling pathways that modulate cell proliferation or growth [49,50]. A study done by Pelicano's group found that mitochondrial respiration defects promoted to increased level of NADH, which could inactivate PTEN via a redox modification mechanism [51]. PTEN deactivation could lead to activation of the protein kinase B (Akt) survival pathway [51]. Akt was show to stimulate glycolysis and also trigger an increase in cell survival of cancer cells [52,53]. In addition, Lopez-Rios and colleagues showed that inhibition of OXPHOS activity by incubation of lung cancer cells with oligomycin could trigger a rapid increase in aerobic glycolysis [54]. This finding demonstrates that suppression of mitochondrial energy production can lead tumor cells become glycolytic [54]. However, when glycolysis was inhibited, tumor cells were unable to sufficiently upregulate mitochondrial OXPHOS and this indicating was due to partial mitochondrial impairment [55].

## 6. Reactive Oxygen Spices (ROS) and tumorigenesis

ROS such as superoxide anion radical ($O_2^-$), hydrogen peroxide ($H_2O_2$) and hydroxyl radical (OH ) are constantly generated during metabolic process in all living species [56]. Mitochondrial respiratory chain is a major intracellular source or producer of ROS generation, as some of the electrons passing to molecular oxygen are instead leaked out of the chain. Under normal physiological conditions, cellular ROS generation is counterbalanced by the action of the endogenous systems include mainly antioxidant enzymes for instance superoxide dismutases (SODs), cytosolic copper/zinc SOD (CuZnSOD) and mitochondrial manganese SOD (MnSOD). Low levels of ROS regulate cellular signaling and are essential in proliferation of normal cell. However, overproduction of ROS will lead to various cellular components injury, such as damage to DNA, proteins and lipids. Recent studies have demonstrated a role of ROS in promoting tumor development. The exposure of normal cells to ROS led to an increase in proliferation [57] and expression of growth-related genes [58-60]. Furthermore, cancer cells are commonly known to generate more ROS than normal cells [61,62]. These observations suggest that the stimulation of ROS may be an important contributing factor in the initiation, maintenance and development of cancer *in vivo*.

ROS are highly active and can also cause damage to mitochondrial genome [63,64]. It has been proposed that damage to mtDNA, if not repaired properly, could initiate tumorigenesis and promote cancer development [65,66]. Mutations in mtDNA may lead to a decreased efficiency of the OXPHOS system and increased leakage electrons as well as enhanced more mitochondrial and cellular ROS production. This situation may result in creating oxidative stress which will further accumulate more total damage to mtDNA because the location of mtDNA is in close proximity to the ROS-generating electron transport system. Thus, it is possible that persistent oxidative stress on cells may favour the neoplastic process through induction of mtDNA damage which leads to mutations [67].

Moreover, in contrast to nDNA, mtDNA does not contain intronic sequences and not cover up with protective proteins such as histones. Due to these reasons, it has been suggested that most mtDNA mutations occur in coding sequences. However, more recent data shows that mtDNA can be almost completely covered by the DNA binding protein Tfam (mitochondrial transcription factor A) [68]. In addition, mtDNA also harbors limited effective DNA repair mechanisms. All these conditions are believed may contribute to the increased sensitivity of mitochondrial genome to damage, and ultimately leads to mutations. Whether mutations in mtDNA are a cause or a consequence of cancer is still debatable and need to be worked out. However, it is proven that mutations of mtDNA induced by oxidative damage could contribute significantly to OXPHOS defects and genetic instability in tumours and thereby promoting a higher propensity for tumour cell growth and progression [69]. This can be suggested that mutation of mtDNA may worsen oxidative stress or vice versa.

## 7. Apoptosis and tumorigenesis

Apoptosis, also called programmed cell death, is a crucial physiological process in the development and homeostasis of multicellular organisms which requires the involvement of mitochondria. Mitochondria have long been recognized for their essential role in regulating apoptotic signaling pathways [70,71]. Defects in apoptotic cell-death pathways are believed to contribute to genomic instability and tumorigenesis [72]. Study recently conducted shows that the mitochondrial respiratory chain has the ability to modulate apoptosis [73]. Respiratory chain dysfunction has been shown to either promote or suppress apoptotic cell death, relying on the specific alteration of electron flux [73]. Stimulation of ROS production can initiate apoptosis in the mitochondria. Mitochondrial defects normally can lead to reduced phosphorylation with low ATP generation and high cytosolic calcium and theses situations become a signal which triggers the apoptotic cell death [74]. Mitochondrial respiration defects in cancer cells can lead to activation of the Akt survival pathway which promotes cell death resistance. As mentioned earlier, this activation of Akt was suggested to result from increased level of NADH and inactivation of PTEN through a redox modification mechanism [51]. More interestingly, another study has elucidated the role of mitochondrial chaperones in modulating mitochondrial function for the survival of cancer cells [75,76]. Molecular chaperone heat shock protein 60 (Hsp60) was shown to orchestrate a broad cell survival program centered on stabilization of mitochondria and also to restrain p53 function [75]. Another chaperone, Hsp90 and its mitochondrial-related molecule, TRAP-1, were suggested to interact with cyclophilin D to suppress cell death [76].

## 8. Mitochondrial DNA mutations in cancer

Over 300 mtDNA mutations and even more mtDNA deletions have been reported that are associated with human diseases, since the first diseases caused by mtDNA damage were described 25 years ago [77-79]. Diseases that have been shown to be linked with mitochondrial dysfunction are diabetes mellitus, Parkinson's disease, Alzheimer's disease, epilepsy, sensorineural deafness and a variety of syndromes involving muscles and the central nervous system as well as a variety of forms of cancer [80-83]. The same mutation or different mutations in the same mtDNA gene may present with very different clinical manifestations, while the same clinical phenotype may be caused by different mutations (DiMauro and Schon, 2003). A large number of mtDNA mutations have been associated to a wide variety of clinical manifestations/ phenotypes of mitochondrial diseases include mitochondria encephalomyopathy, lactic acidosis and stroke-like syndrome (MELAS), myoclonic epilepsy and ragged red fiber disease (MERRF), Lebers hereditary optic neuropathy (LHON), Leigh's syndrome, Kearns-Sayre syndrome, chronic progressive external ophthalmoplegia (CPEO), neuropathy, ataxia, retinitis pigmentosa (NARP).

Although the role of nDNA mutations in carcinogenesis is well established, the importance of mtDNA alterations in the development and maintenance of cancers is only now beginning to be focused by researchers. Alterations in mtDNA which may lead to OXPHOS system destabilization seem to be particularly crucial because 13 proteins encoded by mtDNA are essential for complex I, and III–V respiratory chain assembly and these enzymatic complexes defects have been reported in human solid tumours [85]. There is considerable evidence suggesting that mitochondria may serve as potential contributors to carcinogenesis even though the exact mechanism of how mitochondria involved is still debatable and is not well-documented. Thus, mtDNA is now being targeted organelle by an increasing number of laboratories in order to investigate its potential role as biomarker for tumorigenesis in various types of tissues [86,87].

DNA alterations in mitochondria are believed to become fast hotspots of cancer research. Indeed, numerous mutations in mtDNA has now been observed in multiple cancer types (88-90] since the first somatic mtDNA mutation was detected 15 years ago by Bert Vogelstein's group in human colorectal cancer cells [91]. After these initial findings, mtDNA mutations or alterations have also been identified in bladder cancer [92], breast cancer [93-96], esophageal cancer [97-99], head and neck cancer [100], hepatocellular carcinoma [101-103], lung cancer [104-106], ovarian cancer [107,108], prostate cancer [109-111], renal cancer [112], thyroid cancer [113] and a number of blood cancers [114,115]. More recently, various types of molecular abberations in mtDNA such as point mutations, polymorphisms, depletion, insertions, microsatellite instability and changes in mtDNA copy number have been characterized throughout the mitochondrial genome in human cancers [89,90,116].

## 9. Somatic mitochondrial DNA alterations and brain tumors

Although there have been studies reporting about the association of mtDNA mutations with brain tumors, it is still no clear evidence whether mitochondrial abnormalities are contributing factors in brain tumorigenesis. Several types of somatic mtDNA alterations have been identified in brain tumors. These mtDNA alterations include point mutations, deletions, insertions, mtMSI (mitochondrial microsatellite instability) and copy number changes.

### 9.1. Point mutations

A number of studies have detected mtDNA point mutations in cancer of the brain and other central nervous system, including gliomas, astrocytomas, gliomatosis cerebri, medulloblastoma, meningiomas, schwannomas, and neurofibromas [19,20,117-120]. Mitochondrial genome somatic point mutations were most frequently found in the D-loop region, especially in a polycytosine (poly-C) mononucleotide repeat tract located between 303 and 315 nucleotides known as D310. This location has been identified as a hot spot region for somatic mtDNA mutations in various human cancers, including in brain cancer. In 2005, Montanini's groups analyzed the D-loop region of mtDNA in 42 patients affected by malignant gliomas and found sequence alterations in 36% of the patients including 16 somatic mutations, mostly in the D310 area. The authors suggested that mtDNA mutations were easily amplified from post-surgical tumor cavities and could be used for the clinical follow-up of malignant gliomas [121].

Instead of focusing on D-loop region, the complete of mitochondrial genome was also examined by various researchers in brain cancer patients. In a study that involved the entire mtDNA mutation scanning by temporal temperature gel electrophoresis (TTGE) in medulloblastomas, 40% of the cases (6/15) were found to have at least one somatic mutation [20]. Seven matched cerebrospinal fluid (CSF) samples were also analyzed to detect mtDNA mutations, where some of them were harbored mtDNA mutations in the tumors. This study suggests that somatic mtDNA mutations in CSF shows some promise as potentially useful biomarkers for disease prognosis. On the other hand, Lueth's group (2010) also reported the existence of somatic mtDNA mutations in 6 of 15 medulloblastoma patients. These results are in support of their previous findings on frequency of somatic mitochondrial mutations in medulloblastoma [23]. Before investigation on medulloblastoma patients, Lueth and colleagues have sequenced entire mitochondrial genome of tumor tissue and matched blood samples from 19 pilocytic astrocytomas patients and identified somatic mutations in as many as 16 (84%) cases [22].

In the cases of neurofibromas, Kurtz and team (2004) analyzed the whole mitochondrial genome in 37 neurofibromatosis type 1 patients and found somatic mutations in 7 individuals with cutaneous neurofibromas (37%) and 9 patients with plexiform neurofibromas (50%) [119]. All of the mtDNA somatic mutations detected in this study occurred in the D-loop region. The reason of most genetic mutations to occur in non-coding regions of the mitochondrial genome is currently unknown. However, mutations in the D-loop are believed to influence the origin of replication and promoter region and thus may lead to impair mitochondrial biogenesis and defective transcription and protein expression [122,123].

### 9.2. Deletion

Amongst the large-scale deletions identified in the mitochondrial genome, the 4977-bp deletion is the most common mtDNA deletion detected in various types of cancers including thyroid tumors, esophageal carcinoma, hepatocellular carcinoma, gastric cancer, and breast cancer [124-128]. This deletion recognized as "common deletion" removes all 5 tRNA genes and 7 genes encoding 4 complex I subunits, 1 complex IV subunit, 2 complex V subunits, which are essential for maintaining normal mitochondrial OXPHOS function. The consequence of this deletion could cause a complete failure of ATP production and abnormal ROS generation [129]. Although the 4977-bp deletion has been implicated in the process of carcinogenesis, the involvement or role of this deletion in brain tumors has not yet been investigated. Besides no study to date on the brain tumors, Wallace's group examined the existence of 4977-bp deletion in the aging process using brain normal individuals [130]. They found a significant increase in the 4977-bp deletion from young to old individuals, in different regions of the brain between cortex, putamen and cerebellum. Therefore, it was suggested that this mtDNA deletion might contribute to the neurological impairment associated with ageing. The 4977-bp deletion was also detected in the autopsied brains of patients with bipolar disorder [131].

### 9.3. Mitochondrial microsatellite instability

In 1999, Kirches and colleagues revealed high mtDNA sequence variants in 12 astrocytic tumors [117]. Two years later, the same group extended the study by examining 55 gliomas specimens for mtDNA instability in the poly-C tract of mitochondrial D-loop using a combination of laser microdissection and PCR technique [19]. They found a lower frequency of 9% of specimens with the poly-C tract alterations. In addition, they also sequenced the entire D-loop in 17 frozen glioblastoma samples and corresponding blood samples for detecting somatic mutation. In 2003, a follow up study of mitochondrial genome instability was carried out and the author later determined that poly-C tract of the hypervariable region (HVR2) as a clonal marker in gliomatosis cerebri patients [118].

Most recently, Yeung's team investigated the contribution of mitochondrial genome variants in glioblastoma multiforme (GBM) [132]. In this study, mtDNA variants were analysed in a series of GBM cell lines using a combination of next generation sequencing and high resolution melt (HRM) analysis. They reported a greatest frequency of mtDNA variants in the D-loop and origin of light strand replication in non-coding regions. Moreover, in coding region, ND4 and ND6 were the most affected genes to mutation which both of them encode subunits of complex I of the electron transport chain. The author concluded that these novel variants at the mitochondrial genome offer an advantage to cells for promoting GBM tumorigenesis [132].

### 9.4. Copy number changes

In addition to mtDNA mutations and deletion, changes in the mtDNA copy number have been studied in gliomas [133,134]. As first previously reported by Liang (1996), 15 of low-grade were assessed with cDNA homologous to mtDNA at position 1,679-1,946 and 2,017-2,057 and the results revealed that these tumors had increased mtDNA copy number when compared to normal brain tissue controls [133]. In a separate study done by Liang and Hays (1999), 39 out of 45 (87%) examined gliomas, both low-grade and high-grade specimens, had increased up to 25-fold in mtDNA copy numbers [134]. They claimed that this frequency was much higher than erb-b gene amplification which was present in only 18% of these tumors.

### 9.5. Mitochondrial gene expression changes

In 2005, Dmitrenko's group screened cDNA libraries of human fetal glioblastoma and normal human brain samples and revealed 80 differentially expressed genes [135]. They identified 30 were corresponded to mitochondrial genes for ATP6, COXII, COXIII, ND1, ND4 and 12S rRNA. According to their data, all these mitochondrial transcripts were expressed at lower level in glioblastomas as compared to tumor-adjacent histologically normal brain [135].

## 10. Conclusion

The role of mtDNA mutations in cancer remains largely unclear and therefore more studies and attentions should been given before a clear conclusion could be achieved. There is a lot of evidence suggesting that some mtDNA mutations do play a role in certain stages of cancer development and progression, but further research is needed to clarify this possible link. There are still multiple potential experimental pitfalls and weaknesses, thus relevant caution and basic guidelines in research should be followed in order to obtain the best results [136,137]. Based on our ongoing research and previous studies from other researchers, it could be suggested that mtDNA mutations could be a genetic aberration target in cancer development, instead of nuclear oncogenes and tumor suppressor genes. Cancer cells are very mutagenic in the early stage either due to exposure to high levels of carcinogenic substances or conditions or because of lack of repair mechanism. Thus, mtDNA simply seem to be more prone to mutation at this stage and has a limited ability to repair itself.

Mitochondria produce energy and their genome is responsible for regulating OXPHOS function. Aberrations in mtDNA may interrupt this process and ultimately lead to abnormal function of the cell. The unique properties of mtDNA, including its high copy number, high susceptibility to mutations, and quantitative and qualitative changes in cancer, stimulate researchers to closely be involved in the clinical relevance investigation of mtDNA alterations in cancers. In addition, the screening of mtDNA mutations is more easy and cost-effective than nDNA analysis, due to several advantages that mtDNA have such as a simple circular structure with a short sequence length. It has been shown that the existence of mtDNA mutations in cancer cells is particularly consistent with the intrinsic sensitivity of mtDNA to accumulate oxidative damage. Impairment of mitochondrial OXPHOS activity and mtDNA damage seem to be a common feature of malignant cells. Instability and abnormality in DNA and protein of mitochondria have been identified in various solid tumors and hematologic malignancies. However, up to now many studies have been directed toward identifying and characterizing the altered mtDNA. There have been only limited studies, mainly in relation to its functional consequences and clinical relevance. The functional aspects of mtDNA mutations in cancer development will provide a mechanistic link between mitochondria and carcinogenesis and also will translate into some useful prevention and therapeutic strategies of cancer in the future research.

Although to date mutations, polymorphisms, and variants of mtDNA have been described in brain tumors, there are more studies that need to be done to fully understand the role of mtDNA in these tumor cells. Further studies which include the assessment of the different types and stages of brain tumor need to be carried out. It is very crucial because perhaps that only certain stages and types will be sensitive to the effects of mtDNA mutations. Based on available evidence suggests that mtDNA may play a key role in the development and modulation of different steps of carcinogenesis. They could be used in the future as new potential target markers for rapid and effective early detection of brain tumorigenesis.

## Acknowledgements

This work was supported in part by the Research University Grant for Individual (RUI) from Universiti Sains Malaysia 1001/PPSP/812110.

## Author details

Abdul Aziz Mohamed Yusoff[1*], Farizan Ahmad[1], Zamzuri Idris[1], Hasnan Jaafar[2] and Jafri Malin Abdullah[1,3]

*Address all correspondence to: azizmdy@yahoo.com

1 Department of Neurosciences, School of Medical Sciences, Universiti Sains Malaysia, Health Campus, Kubang Kerian, Kelantan, Malaysia

2 Department of Pathology, School of Medical Sciences, Universiti Sains Malaysia, Health Campus, Kubang Kerian, Kelantan, Malaysia

3 Center for Neuroscience Services and Research, Universiti Sains Malaysia, Health Campus, Kubang Kerian, Kelantan, Malaysia

## References

[1] Louis DN. The p53 gene and protein in human brain tumors. Journal of Neuropathology & Experimental Neurology 1994;53(1) 11-21.

[2] Nozaki M, Tada M, Kobayashi H, Zhang CL, Sawamura Y, Abe H, Ishii N, Van Meir EG. Roles of the functional loss of p53 and other genes in astrocytoma tumorigenesis and progression. Neuro-Oncology 1999;1(2) 124-137.

[3] Yusoff AA, Abdullah J, Abdullah MR, Mohd Ariff AR, Isa MN. Association of p53 tumor suppressor gene with paraclinical and clinical modalities of gliomas patients in Malaysia. Acta Neurochirurgica (Wien). 2004;146(6) 595-601.

[4] Louis DN. Molecular pathology of malignant gliomas. Annual Review of Pathology. 2006;1 97-117.

[5] Ohgaki H, Kleihues P. Genetic pathways to primary and secondary glioblastoma. American Journal of Pathology 2007;170(5) 1445-1453.

[6] Attardi G, Schatz G. Biogenesis of mitochondria. Annual Review of Cell Biology 1988;4 289-333.

[7] Galluzzi L, Kepp O, Kroemer G. Mitochondria: master regulators of danger signalling. Nature Reviews Molecular Cell Biology 2012;13(12) 780-788.

[8] Wallace DC. Mitochondria and cancer. Nature Reviews Cancer 2012;12(10) 685-698.

[9] Wallace DC. Mitochondrial DNA in aging and disease. Scientific American 1997;277(2) 40-47.

[10] DiMauro S, Schon EA. Mitochondrial DNA mutations in human disease. American Journal of Medical Genetics 2001;106(1) 18-26.

[11] Wallace DC. A mitochondrial paradigm for degenerative diseases and ageing. Novartis Foundation Symposia 2001;235 247-263; discussion 263-246

[12] Kaipparettu BA, Ma Y, Wong LJ. Functional effects of cancer mitochondria on energy metabolism and tumorigenesis: utility of transmitochondrial cybrids. Annals of the New York Academy of Sciences 2010;1201:137-146. doi: 10.1111/j.1749-6632.2010.05621.x.

[13] Kim HS, Patel K, Muldoon-Jacobs K, Bisht KS, Aykin-Burns N, Pennington JD, van der Meer R, Nguyen P, Savage J, Owens KM, Vassilopoulos A, Ozden O, Park SH, Singh KK, Abdulkadir SA, Spitz DR, Deng CX, Gius D. SIRT3 is a mitochondria-localized tumor suppressor required for maintenance of mitochondrial integrity and metabolism during stress. Cancer Cell 2010;17(1) 41-52.

[14] Mullen AR, Wheaton WW, Jin ES, Chen PH, Sullivan LB, Cheng T, Yang Y, Linehan WM, Chandel NS, DeBerardinis RJ. Reductive carboxylation supports growth in tumour cells with defective mitochondria. Nature 2011;481(7381) 385-388.

[15] Owens KM, Kulawiec M, Desouki MM, Vanniarajan A, Singh KK. Impaired OXPHOS complex III in breast cancer. PLoS One 2011;6(8) e23846.

[16] Cook CC, Kim A, Terao S, Gotoh A, Higuchi M. Consumption of oxygen: a mitochondrial-generated progression signal of advanced cancer. Cell Death and Disease 2012; 3:e258. doi: 10.1038/cddis.2011.141.

[17] Chen PL, Chen CF, Chen Y, Guo XE, Huang CK, Shew JY, Reddick RL, Wallace DC, Lee WH. Mitochondrial genome instability resulting from SUV3 haploinsufficiency leads to tumorigenesis and shortened lifespan. Oncogene 2013;32(9) 1193-1201.

[18] Baysal BE, Ferrell RE, Willett-Brozick JE, Lawrence EC, Myssiorek D, Bosch A, van der Mey A, Taschner PE, Rubinstein WS, Myers EN, Richard CW 3rd, Cornelisse CJ, Devilee P, Devlin B. Mutations in SDHD, a mitochondrial complex II gene, in hereditary paraganglioma. Science 2000;287(5454) 848-851.

[19] Kirches E, Krause G, Warich-Kirches M, Weis S, Schneider T, Meyer-Puttlitz B, Mawrin C, Dietzmann K. High frequency of mitochondrial DNA mutations in glioblastoma multiforme identified by direct sequence comparison to blood samples. International Journal of Cancer 2001;93(4) 534-538.

[20] Wong LJ, Lueth M, Li XN, Lau CC, Vogel H. Detection of mitochondrial DNA mutations in the tumor and cerebrospinal fluid of medulloblastoma patients. Cancer Research 2003;63(14) 3866-3871.

[21] Dai JG, Xiao YB, Min JX, Zhang GQ, Yao K, Zhou RJ. Mitochondrial DNA 4977 BP deletion mutations in lung carcinoma. Indian Journal of Cancer 2006;43(1) 20-25.

[22] Lueth M, Wronski L, Giese A, Kirschner-Schwabe R, Pietsch T, von Deimling A, Henze G, Kurtz A, Driever PH. Somatic mitochondrial mutations in pilocytic astrocytoma. Cancer Genetics and Cytogenetics 2009;192(1) 30-35.

[23] Lueth M, von Deimling A, Pietsch T, Wong LJ, Kurtz A, Henze G, Driever PH. Medulloblastoma harbor somatic mitochondrial DNA mutations in the D-loop region. Journal of Pediatric Hematology/Oncology 2010; 32(2) 156-159.

[24] Li LH, Kang T, Chen L, Zhang W, Liao Y, Chen J, Shi Y. Detection of mitochondrial DNA mutations by high-throughput sequencing in the blood of breast cancer patients. International Journal of Molecular Medicine 2014;33(1) 77-82.

[25] Larman TC, DePalma SR, Hadjipanayis AG; Cancer Genome Atlas Research Network, Protopopov A, Zhang J, Gabriel SB, Chin L, Seidman CE, Kucherlapati R, Seidman JG. Spectrum of somatic mitochondrial mutations in five cancers. Proceedings of the National Academy of Sciences USA 2012;109(35) 14087-14091.

[26] Yin PH, Wu CC, Lin JC, Chi CW, Wei YH, Lee HC. Somatic mutations of mitochondrial genome in hepatocellular carcinoma. Mitochondrion 2010;10(2) 174-182.

[27] Frey TG, Mannella CA. The internal structure of mitochondria. Trends in Biochemical Sciences 2000;25(7) 319-324.

[28] Palade G. The fine structure of mitochondria. Anatomical Record. 1952;114(3) 427-451.

[29] Sjöstrand FS. The ultrastructure of cells as revealed by the electron microscope. International Review of Cytology 1956; 5: 455-533.

[30] Perkins G, Renken C, Martone ME, Young SJ, Ellisman M, Frey T. Electron tomography of neuronal mitochondria: three dimensional structure and organization of cristae and membrane contacts. Journal of Structural Biology 1997;119(3) 260-272.

[31] Perkins GA, Frey TG. Recent structural insight into mitochondria gained by microscopy. Micron 2000;31(1) 97-111.

[32] Frey TG, Renken CW, Perkins GA. Insight into mitochondrial structure and function from electron tomography. Biochimica et Biophysica Acta 2002;1555(1-3) 196-203.

[33] Mitchell P. Coupling of phosphorylation to electron and hydrogen transfer by chemiosmotic type mechanism. Nature 1961;191: 144-148.

[34] Mitchell P, Moyle J. Chemiosmotic hypothesis of oxidative phosphorylation. Nature 1967;213(5072) 137-139.

[35] Voet D, Voet JG, Pratt CW. 2002. Fundamentals of Biochemistry. John Wiley & Sons,Inc., New York

[36] Nass S, Nass MMK. Intramitochondrial fibres with DNA characteristics. Journal of Cell Biology 1963;19: 593-629.

[37] Anderson S, Bankier AT, Barrell BG, de-Bruijn MH, Coulson AR, Drouin J, Eperon IC, Nierlich DP, Roe BA, Sanger F, Schreier PH, Smith AJ, Staden R, Young IG. Sequence and organization of the human mitochondrial genome. Nature 1981;290(5806) 427-465.

[38] Andrews RM, Kubacka I, Chinnery PF, Lightowlers RN, Turnbull DM, Howell N. Reanalysis and revision of the Cambridge reference sequence for human mitochondrial DNA. Nature Genetics 1999;23(2) 147.

[39] Kasamatsu H, Vinograd J. Replication of circular DNA in eukaryotic cells. Annual Review of Biochemistry 1974;43(0) 695-719.

[40] Lutz S, Weisser HJ, Heizmann J, Pollak S. A third hypervariable region in the human mitochondrial D-loop. Human Genetics 1997;101(3) 384.

[41] Taanman JW. The mitochondrial genome: transcription, translation and replication. Biochimica et Biophysica Acta 1999;1410(2) 103-123.

[42] Monnat RJ, Reay DT. Nucleotide sequence identity of mitochondrial DNA from different human tissues. Gene 1986;43(3) 205-211.

[43] Tzagoloff A, Myers AM. Biogenesis of mitochondrial genetics. Annual Review of Biochemistry 1986; 55: 249-285.

[44] Gadaleta G, Pepe G, DeCandia G, Quagliariello C, Sbissá E, Saccone C. The complete nucleotide sequence of the Rattus norvegicus mitochondrial genome: cryptic signals revealed by comparative analysis between vertebrates. Journal of Molecular Evolution 1989;28(6) 497-516.

[45] Lightowlers RN, Chinnery PF, Turnbull DM, Howell N. Mammalian mitochondrial genetics: heredity, heteroplasmy and disease. Trends in Genetics 1997;13(11) 450-455.

[46] Warburg O. On the origin of cancer cells. Science 1956;123(3191) 309-314.

[47] Pedersen PL. Tumor mitochondria and the bioenergetics of cancer cells. Progress in Experimental Tumor Research 1978; 22 190-274.

[48] Cuezva JM, Krajewska M, de Heredia ML, Krajewski S, Santamaría G, Kim H, Zapata JM, Marusawa H, Chamorro M, Reed JC. The bioenergetic signature of cancer: a marker of tumor progression. Cancer Research 2002;62(22) 6674-6681.

[49] Arnould T, Vankoningsloo S, Renard P, Houbion A, Ninane N, Demazy C, Remacle J, Raes M. CREB activation induced by mitochondrial dysfunction is a new signaling pathway that impairs cell proliferation. The EMBO Journal 2002;21(1-2) 53-63.

[50] Rustin P. Mitochondria from cell death to proliferation. Nature Genetics 2002;30(4) 352-353.

[51] Pelicano H, Xu RH, Du M, Feng L, Sasaki R, Carew JS, Hu Y, Ramdas L, Hu L, Keating MJ, Zhang W, Plunkett W, Huang P. Mitochondrial respiration defects in cancer cells cause activation of Akt survival pathway through a redox-mediated mechanism. Journal of Cell Biology 2006;175(6) 913-923.

[52] Elstrom RL, Bauer DE, Buzzai M, Karnauskas R, Harris MH, Plas DR, Zhuang H, Cinalli RM, Alavi A, Rudin CM, Thompson CB. Akt stimulates aerobic glycolysis in cancer cells. Cancer Research 2004;64(11) 3892-3899.

[53] Plas DR, Thompson CB. Akt-dependent transformation: there is more to growth than just surviving. Oncogene 2005; 24(50) 7435-7442.

[54] López-Ríos F, Sánchez-Aragó M, García-García E, Ortega AD, Berrendero JR, Pozo-Rodríguez F, López-Encuentra A, Ballestín C, Cuezva JM. Loss of the mitochondrial bioenergetic capacity underlies the glucose avidity of carcinomas. Cancer Research 2007;67(19) 9013-9017.

[55] Wu M, Neilson A, Swift AL, Moran R, Tamagnine J, Parslow D, Armistead S, Lemire K, Orrell J, Teich J, Chomicz S, Ferrick DA. Multiparameter metabolic analysis reveals a close link between attenuated mitochondrial bioenergetic function and enhanced glycolysis dependency in human tumor cells. American Journal of Physiology-Cell Physiology 2007;292(1) C125-136.

[56] Chance B, Sies H, Boveris A. Hydroperoxide metabolism in mammalian organs. Physiological Reviews 1979;59(3) 527-605.

[57] Burdon RH. Superoxide and hydrogen peroxide in relation to mammalian cell proliferation. Free Radical Biology and Medicine 1995;18(4) 775-794.

[58] Nose K, Shibanuma M, Kikuchi K, Kageyama H, Sakiyama S, Kuroki T. Transcriptional activation of early-response genes by hydrogen peroxide in a mouse osteoblastic cell line. European Journal of Biochemistry 1991;201(1) 99-106.

[59] Amstad PA, Krupitza G, Cerutti PA. Mechanism of c-fos induction by active oxygen. Cancer Research 1992;52(14) 3952-3960.

[60] Nose K, Ohba M. Functional activation of the Egr-1 (early growth response-1) gene by hydrogen peroxide. Biochemical Journal 1996;316 (Pt 2) 381-383.

[61] Sundaresan M, Yu ZX, Ferrans VJ, Sulciner DJ, Gutkind JS, Irani K, Goldschmidt-Clermont PJ, Finkel T. Regulation of reactive-oxygen-species generation in fibroblasts by Rac1. Biochemical Journal 1996;318 (Pt 2) 379-382.

[62] Ha HC, Thiagalingam A, Nelkin BD, Casero RA Jr. Reactive oxygen species are critical for the growth and differentiation of medullary thyroid carcinoma cells. Clinical Cancer Research 2000;6(9) 3783-3787.

[63] Harman D. Free radicals in aging. Molecular and Cellular Biochemistry 1988;84(2) 155-161.

[64] Ames BN, Shigenaga MK. Oxidants are a major contributor to aging. Annals of the New York Academy of Sciences 1992;663 85-96.

[65] Poulsen HE, Prieme H, Loft S. Role of oxidative DNA damage in cancer initiation and promotion. European Journal of Cancer Prevention 1998;7(1) 9-16.

[66] Zanssen S, Schon EA. Mitochondrial DNA mutations in cancer. PLoS Medicine 2005;2(11) e401.

[67] Grzybowska-Szatkowska L, Slaska B. Mitochondrial DNA and carcinogenesis (review). Molecular Medicine Reports 2012;6(5) 923-930.

[68] Kang D, Hamasaki N. Mitochondrial transcription factor A in the maintenance of mitochondrial DNA: overview of its multiple roles. Annals of the New York Academy of Sciences 2005;1042: 101-108.

[69] Chandra D, Singh KK. Genetic insights into OXPHOS defect and its role in cancer. Biochimica et Biophysica Acta 2011;1807(6) 620-625.

[70] Richter C. Pro-oxidants and mitochondrial $Ca^{2+}$: their relationship to apoptosis and oncogenesis. FEBS Letters 1993;325(1-2) 104-107.

[71] Orrenius S. Mitochondrial regulation of apoptotic cell death. Toxicology Letters 2004;149(1-3) 19-23.

[72] Nelson DA, Tan TT, Rabson AB, Anderson D, Degenhardt K, White E. Hypoxia and defective apoptosis drive genomic instability and tumorigenesis. Genes & Development 2004;18(17) 2095-2107.

[73] Kwong JQ, Henning MS, Starkov AA, Manfredi G. The mitochondrial respiratory chain is a modulator of apoptosis. Journal of Cell Biology 2007;179(6) 1163-1177.

[74] Raha S, Robinson BH. Mitochondria, oxygen free radicals, and apoptosis. American Journal of Medical Genetics 2001;106(1) 62-70.

[75] Kang BH, Plescia J, Dohi T, Rosa J, Doxsey SJ, Altieri DC. Regulation of tumor cell mitochondrial homeostasis by an organelle-specific Hsp90 chaperone network. Cell 2007;131(2) 257-270.

[76] Ghosh JC, Dohi T, Kang BH, Altieri DC. Hsp60 regulation of tumor cell apoptosis. Journal of Biological Chemistry 2008;283(8) 5188-5194.

[77] Holt IJ, Harding AE, Morgan-Hughes JA. Deletions of muscle mitochondrial DNA in patients with mitochondrial myopathies. Nature 1988;331(6158) 717-719.

[78] Wallace DC, Singh G, Lott MT, Hodge JA, Schurr TG, Lezza AM, Elsas LJ 2nd, Nikoskelainen EK. Mitochondrial DNA mutation associated with Leber's hereditary optic neuropathy. Science 1988;242(4884) 1427-1430.

[79] Zeviani M, Moraes CT, DiMauro S, Nakase H, Bonilla E, Schon EA, Rowland LP. Deletions of mitochondrial DNA in Kearns-Sayre syndrome. Neurology 1988;38(9) 1339-1346.

[80] Penta JS, Johnson FM, Wachsman JT, Copeland WC. Mitochondrial DNA in human malignancy. Mutation Research 2001;488(2) 119-133.

[81] Chinnery PF, Schon EA. Mitochondria. Journal of Neurology, Neurosurgery, and Psychiatry 2003;74(9) 1188-1199.

[82] DiMauro S, Davidzon G. Mitochondrial DNA and disease. Annals of Medicine 2005;37(3) 222-232.

[83] Schapira AH. Mitochondrial diseases. Lancet. 2012;379(9828) 1825-1834. doi: 10.1016/S0140-6736(11)61305-6.

[84] DiMauro S, Schon EA. Mitochondrial respiratory-chain diseases. New England Journal of Medicine 2003;348(26) 2656-2668.

[85] Chatterjee A, Dasgupta S, Sidransky D. Mitochondrial subversion in cancer. Cancer Prevention Research 2011;4(5) 638-654.

[86] Salas A, Yao YG, Macaulay V, Vega A, Carracedo A, Bandelt HJ. A critical reassessment of the role of mitochondria in tumorigenesis. PLOS Medicine 2005;2(11) e296.

[87] Nie H, Shu H, Vartak R, Milstein AC, Mo Y, Hu X, Fang H, Shen L, Ding Z, Lu J, Bai Y. Mitochondrial common deletion, a potential biomarker for cancer occurrence, is

selected against in cancer background: a meta-analysis of 38 studies. PLoS One 2013;8(7) e67953.

[88] Brandon M, Baldi P, Wallace DC. Mitochondrial mutations in cancer. Oncogene 2006;25(34) 4647-4662.

[89] Chatterjee A, Mambo E, Sidransky D. Mitochondrial DNA mutations in human cancer. Oncogene 2006;25(34) 4663-4674.

[90] Yu M. Somatic mitochondrial DNA mutations in human cancers. Advances in Clinical Chemistry 2012;57 99-138.

[91] Polyak K, Li Y, Zhu H, Lengauer C, Willson JK, Markowitz SD, Trush MA, Kinzler KW, Vogelstein B. Somatic mutations of the mitochondrial genome in human colorectal tumours. Nature Genetics 1998;20(3) 291-293.

[92] Fliss MS, Usadel H, Caballero OL, Wu L, Buta MR, Eleff SM, Jen J, Sidransky D. Facile detection of mitochondrial DNA mutations in tumors and bodily fluids. Science 2000;287(5460) 2017-2019.

[93] Tan DJ, Bai RK, Wong LJC. Comprehensive scanning of somatic mitochondrial DNA mutations in breast cancer. Cancer Research 2002;62(4) 972-976.

[94] Zhu W, Qin W, Bradley P, Wessel A, Puckett CL, Sauter ER. Mitochondrial DNA mutations in breast cancer tissue and in matched nipple aspirate fluid. Carcinogenesis 2005;26(1) 145-152.

[95] Tseng LM, Yin PH, Yang CW, Tsai YF, Hsu CY, Chi CW, Lee HC. Somatic mutations of the mitochondrial genome in human breast cancers. Genes Chromosomes Cancer 2011;50(10) 800-811.

[96] Xu C, Tran-Thanh D, Ma C, May K, Jung J, Vecchiarelli J, Done SJ. Mitochondrial D310 mutations in the early development of breast cancer. British Journal of Cancer 2012;106(9) 1506-1511.

[97] Kumimoto H, Yamane Y, Nishimoto Y, Fukami H, Shinoda M, Hatooka S, Ishizaki K. Frequent somatic mutations of mitochondrial DNA in esophageal squamous cell carcinoma. International Journal of Cancer 2004;108(2) 228-231.

[98] Tan DJ, Chang J, Liu LL, Bai RK, Wang YF, Yeh KT, Wong LJ. Significance of somatic mutations and content alteration of mitochondrial DNA in esophageal cancer. BMC Cancer 2006;6:93.

[99] Lin CS, Chang SC, Wang LS, Chou TY, Hsu WH, Wu YC, Wei YH. The role of mitochondrial DNA alterations in esophageal squamous cell carcinomas. Journal of Thoracic and Cardiovascular Surgery 2010;139(1) 189-197.

[100] Lievre A, Blons H, Houllier AM, Laccourreye O, Brasnu D, Beaune P, Laurent-Puig P. Clinicopathological significance of mitochondrial D-Loop mutations in head and neck carcinoma. British Journal of Cancer 2006;94(5) 692-697.

[101] Lee HC, Li SH, Lin JC, Wu CC, Yeh DC, Wei YH. Somatic mutations in the D-loop and decrease in the copy number of mitochondrial DNA in human hepatocellular carcinoma. Mutation Research 2004;547(1-2) 71-78.

[102] Tamori A, Nishiguchi S, Nishikawa M, Kubo S, Koh N, Hirohashi K, Shiomi S, Inoue M. Correlation between clinical characteristics and mitochondrial D-loop DNA mutations in hepatocellular carcinoma. Journal of Gastroenterology 2004;39(11) 1063-1068.

[103] Yin PH, Wu CC, Lin JC, Chi CW, Wei YH, Lee HC. Somatic mutations of mitochondrial genome in hepatocellular carcinoma. Mitochondrion 2010;10(2) 174-182.

[104] Suzuki M, Toyooka S, Miyajima K, Iizasa T, Fujisawa T, Bekele NB, Gazdar AF. Alterations in the mitochondrial displacement loop in lung cancers. Clinical Cancer Research 2003;9(15) 5636-5641.

[105] Jin X, Zhang J, Gao Y, Ding K, Wang N, Zhou D, Jen J, Cheng S. Relationship between mitochondrial DNA mutations and clinical characteristics in human lung cancer. Mitochondrion 2007;7(5) 347-353.

[106] Choi SJ, Kim SH, Kang HY, Lee J, Bhak JH, Sohn I, Jung SH, Choi YS, Kim HK, Han J, Huh N, Lee G, Kim BC, Kim J. Mutational hotspots in the mitochondrial genome of lung cancer. Biochemical and Biophysical Research Communications 2011;407(1) 23-27.

[107] Liu VW, Shi HH, Cheung AN, Chiu PM, Leung TW, Nagley P, Wong LC, Ngan HY (2001) High incidence of somatic mitochondrial DNA mutations in human ovarian carcinomas. Cancer Research 2001; 61(16) 5998-6001.

[108] Van Trappen PO, Cullup T, Troke R, Swann D, Shepherd JH, Jacobs IJ, Gayther SA, Mein CA. Somatic mitochondrial DNA mutations in primary and metastatic ovarian cancer. Gynecologic Oncology 2007;104(1) 129-133.

[109] Jerónimo C, Nomoto S, Caballero OL, Usadel H, Henrique R, Varzim G, Oliveira J, Lopes C, Fliss MS, Sidransky D. Mitochondrial mutations in early stage prostate cancer and bodily fluids. Oncogene 2001;20(37) 5195-5198.

[110] Gomez-Zaera M, Abril J, Gonzalez L, Aguilo F, Condom E, Nadal M, Nunes V (2006) Identification of somatic and germline mitochondrial DNA sequence variants in prostate cancer patients. Mutation Research 2006;595(1-2) 42-51.

[111] Kloss-Brandstätter A, Schäfer G, Erhart G, Hüttenhofer A, Coassin S, Seifarth C, Summerer M, Bektic J, Klocker H, Kronenberg F. Somatic mutations throughout the entire mitochondrial genome are associated with elevated PSA levels in prostate cancer patients. American Journal of Human Genetics 2010;87(6) 802-812.

[112] Nagy A, Wilhelm M, Sukosd F, Ljungberg B, Kovacs G. Somatic mitochondrial DNA mutations in human chromophobe renal cell carcinomas. Genes Chromosomes Cancer 2002;35(3) 256-260.

[113] Tong BC, Ha PK, Dhir K, Xing M, Westra WH, Sidransky D, Califano JA. Mitochondrial DNA alterations in thyroid cancer. Journal Surgical Oncology 2003;82(3) 170-173.

[114] Carew JS, Zhou Y, Albitar M, Carew JD, Keating MJ, Huang P. Mitochondrial DNA mutations in primary leukemia cells after chemotherapy: clinical significance and therapeutic implications. Leukemia 2003;17(8) 1437-1447.

[115] Grist SA, Lu XJ, Morley AA. Mitochondrial mutations in acute leukemia. Leukemia 2004;18(7) 1313-1316.

[116] Schon EA, DiMauro S, Hirano M. Human mitochondrial DNA: roles of inherited and somatic mutations. Nature Review Genetics 2012;13(12) 878-890.

[117] Kirches E, Michael M, Woy C, Schneider T, Warich M-Kirches, Schneider-Stock R, Winkler K, Wittig H, Dietzmann K. Loss of heteroplasmy in the displacement loop of brain mitochondrial DNA in astrocytic tumors. Genes Chromosomes Cancer 1999;26(1) 80-83.

[118] Kirches E, Mawrin C, Schneider-Stock R, Krause G, Scherlach C, Dietzmann K. Mitochondrial DNA as a clonal tumor cell marker: gliomatosis cerebri. Journal of Neuro-Oncology 2003;61(1) 1-5.

[119] Kurtz A, Lueth M, Kluwe L, Zhang T, Foster R, Mautner VF, Hartmann M, Tan DJ, Martuza RL, Friedrich RE, Driever PH, Wong LJ. Somatic mitochondrial DNA mutations in neurofibromatosis type 1-associated tumors. Molecular Cancer Research 2004;2(8) 433-441.

[120] Vega A, Salas A, Gamborino E, Sobrido MJ, Macaulay V, Carracedo A. mtDNA mutations in tumors of the central nervous system reflect the neutral evolution of mtDNA in populations. Oncogene 2004;23(6) 1314-1320.

[121] Montanini L, Regna-Gladin C, Eoli M, Albarosa R, Carrara F, Zeviani M, Bruzzone MG, Broggi G, Boiardi A, Finocchiaro G. Instability of mitochondrial DNA and MRI and clinical correlations in malignant gliomas. Journal of Neuro-Oncology 2005;74(1) 87-89.

[122] Barthelemy C, de Baulny HO, Lombes A. D-loop mutations in mitochondrial DNA: link with mitochondrial DNA depletion? Human Genetics 2002;110(5) 479-487.

[123] Wong L, Tan D, Bai R, Yeh K, and Chang J. Molecular alterations in mitochondrial DNA of hepatocellular carcinomas: is there a correlation with clinicopathological profile? Journal of Medical Genetics 2004;41(5) e65.

[124] Maximo V, Soares P, Lima J, Cameselle-Teijeiro J, Sobrinho-Simoes M. Mitochondrial DNA somatic mutations (point mutations and large deletions) and mitochondrial DNA variants in human thyroid pathology: A study with emphasis on Hurthle cell tumors. American Journal of Pathology 2002;160(5) 1857-1865.

[125] Abnet CC, Huppi K, Carrera A, Armistead D, McKenney K, Hu N, Tang ZZ, Taylor PR, Dawsey SM. Control region mutations and the 'common deletion' are frequent in the mitochondrial DNA of patients with esophageal squamous cell carcinoma. BMC Cancer 2004;4: 30.

[126] Yin PH, Lee HC, Chau GY, Wu YT, Li SH, Lui WY, Wei YH, Liu TY, Chi CW. Alteration of the copy number and deletion of mitochondrial DNA in human hepatocellular carcinoma. British Journal of Cancer 2004;90(12) 2390-2396.

[127] Wu CW, Yin PH, Hung WY, Li AF, Li SH, Chi CW, Wei YH, Lee HC. Mitochondrial DNA mutations and mitochondrial DNA depletion in gastric cancer. Genes Chromosomes Cancer 2005;44(1) 19-28.

[128] Ye C, Shu XO, Wen W, Pierce L, Courtney R, Gao YT, Zheng W, Cai Q. Quantitative analysis of mitochondrial DNA 4977-bp deletion in sporadic breast cancer and benign breast diseases. Breast Cancer Research and Treatment 2008;108(3) 427-434.

[129] Peng TI, Yu PR, Chen JY, Wang HL, Wu HY, Wei YH, Jou MJ. Visualizing common deletion of mitochondrial DNA-augmented mitochondrial reactive oxygen species generation and apoptosis upon oxidative stress. Biochimica et Biophysica Acta 2006;1762(2) 241-255.

[130] Corral-Debrinski M, Horton T, Lott MT, Shoffner JM, Beal MF, Wallace DC. Mitochondrial DNA deletions in human brain: regional variability and increase with advanced age. Nature Genetics 1992;2(4) 324-329.

[131] Kato T, Stine OC, McMahon FJ, Crowe RR. Increased levels of a mitochondrial DNA deletion in the brain of patients with bipolar disorder. Biological Psychiatry 1997;42(10) 871-875.

[132] Yeung KY, Dickinson A, Donoghue JF, Polekhina G, White SJ, Grammatopoulos DK, McKenzie M, Johns TG, John JC. The identification of mitochondrial DNA variants in glioblastoma multiforme. Acta Neuropathologica Communications 2014;2(1): 1. doi: 10.1186/2051-5960-2-1.

[133] Liang BC. Evidence for association of mitochondrial DNA sequence amplification and nuclear localization in human low-grade gliomas. Mutation Research 1996;354(1) 27-33.

[134] Liang BC, Hays L. Mitochondrial DNA copy number changes in human gliomas. Cancer Letters 1996;105(2)167-173.

[135] Dmitrenko V, Shostak K, Boyko O, Khomenko O, Rozumenko V, Malisheva T, Shamayev M, Zozulya Y, Kavsan V. Reduction of the transcription level of the mitochondrial genome in human glioblastoma. Cancer Letters 2005;218(1) 99-107.

[136] Salas A, Yao YG, Macaulay V, Vega A, Carracedo A, Bandelt HJ. A critical reassessment of the role of mitochondria in tumorigenesis. PLoS Medicine 2005;2:e296.

http://dx.doi.org/10.5772/58965

[137] Fang H, Lu J, Wei J, Shen LJ, Ding Z, Li H, Bai Y. Mitochondrial DNA mutations in the D-loop region may not be frequent in cervical cancer: a discussion on pitfalls in mitochondrial DNA studies. Journal of Cancer Research and Clinical Oncology 2009;135(4) 649-651.

Chapter 2

# Systems Biology of Glioblastoma Multiforme

Caroline Agha, Hannah C. Machemehl and
Hassan M. Fathallah-Shaykh

Additional information is available at the end of the chapter

http://dx.doi.org/10.5772/59642

## 1. Introduction

Gliomas encompass approximately 80% of primary brain malignancies [1]. The five-year survival rate is dependent on the subtype of glioma. According to the Central Brain Tumor Registry there are about 13,000 deaths and 18,000 new cases per year of primary brain cancer in the United States and the overall average annual age-adjusted incidence rate for 2006-2010 for primary brain and CNS tumors was 21.03 per 100,000 [2]. In this chapter, our main focus is glioblastoma (GBM), which is by far the most common and the most malignant of all primary brain tumor [2]. Often described as the most lethal or the most devastating brain tumors, gliomas continue to carry a very poor prognosis at all levels, quantity and quality of life. GBM almost exclusively recurs despite meticulous conventional therapies, including surgical resection, radiation, and chemotherapy and bevacizumab. Despite all advances, the survival rates continue to be low, with a median survival of approximately 15 months in patients with malignant gliomas [3].

The multiple hit theory of cancer speculates that the origin and progression of GBM is the product of complex series of molecular processes like activation of oncogenes and alterations in tumor suppression genes. However, the complexity of the molecular interactions in malignant gliomas imposes a great challenge that indeed has crucial implications on treatment. This cannot be achieved without a meticulous understanding of this multifaceted process and its molecular mechanism, and therefore dictates dissection at systems level. The Cancer Genome Atlas Research Network has sequenced the genome of GBM and deduced that the apparatus of tumor growth and recurrence is the result of complex epigenetic mechanisms and gene interactions [4]. The twenty first century has been referred to as the genomic millennium, thus in an era where genes dictate remedy a comprehensive understanding of the systems biology of gliomas may be a key to the cure. Our goal in this chapter is to touch on the complexity of the molecular networks of GBM by presenting on an overview without delving into details. We will focus on how molecules and pathways are dysregulated in GBM rather than presenting detailed graphs of networks as the latter are readily easily found. To illustrate the clinical relevance of a systems approach to molecular networks, we dissect the case of the use of rapamycin in a GBM clinical trial and discuss the pathogenesis of its adverse effect in causing activation of AKT, an oncogene.

## 2. Classes of GBM

Malignant gliomas develop as part of a multistep process comprising chronological and collective genetic modifications resulting from core and environmental dynamics. Cowden, Turcot, Li-Fraumeni, neurofibromatosis type 1 and type 2, tuberous sclerosis, and familial schwannomatosis are among the predisposing syndromes for glioblastoma occurrence [15]. From a molecular perspective, malignant gliomas are greatly heterogeneous tumors [14]. In a nutshell, 4 transcriptional subclasses of GBM have been proposed: *classical, mesenchymal, proneural,* and *neural* [1]. The classical type glioblastoma typically exhibits chromosome 7 amplifications, chromosome 10 deletions, *EGFR* amplification, *EGFR* mutations (point and vIII mutations), and *Ink4a/ARF* locus deletion. The mesenchymal subclass shows a high frequency of *NF1* mutation/deletion and high expression of *CHI3L1, MET,* and genes involved in tumor necrosis factor and nuclear factor–κB pathways. Proneural type glioblastoma is characterized by changes of *PDGFRA* and mutations in *IDH1* and *TP53;* these are features common to lower-grade gliomas and secondary GBM. A characteristic feature of the neural subclass of GBM is the expression of neuronal markers.

## 3. Gliomagenesis

The multiple hit theory of cancer stipulates sequential molecular events leading to GBM. The following is a summary of current ideas. One of the first steps in tumoregenesis is loss of cell cycle control. The cell cycle checkpoint that has been of most interest is the G1-S phase. This important checkpoint is mainly controlled by p16INK4a/cyclin-dependent kinase (CDK)-4/RB (retinoblastoma) 1 pathway, which involves p16, CDK-4, cyclin D1, and RB1[16]. The CDK/cyclin D1 complex phosphorylates RB1 therefore releasing the E2F transcription factor, which in turn activates the genes, involved in the G1/S transition [17]. Subsequent steps in glioma-genesis include the overexpression of growth factors and their receptors. A diverse array of growth factors such as epidermal growth factor receptor (EGFR), platelet-derived growth factor (PDGF), basic fibroblast growth factor (bFGF, FGF-2), transforming growth factor (TGF)-alpha, and insulin-like growth factor (IGF)-1 are overly expressed in glioblastoma [18, 19]. Malignant gliomas are highly vascular tumors; the angiogenic molecule that has been most widely implicated in GBM is vascular endothelial growth factor (VEGF), an endothelial cell mitogenic [20].

Another key event contributing to gliomagenesis is the abolishment of apoptosis, or programmed cell death. Malignant glioma cells, not only divide uncontrollably, but also intentionally lose the ability to undergo apoptosis. *p53,* a key molecule involved in apoptosis, is often mutated during gliomagenesis [21]. An important process contributing to gliomagenesis is genetic instability, which refers to the property that random mutations are introduced in dividing cancer cells because of the loss of check points and the molecular machinery that ensures that the genome is copied faithfully during mitosis [22]. A clinical correlation to genetic instability is the Turcot syndrome [23].

## 4. Signaling pathways

A large number of signaling pathways exchange information to generate a large molecular network that controls the phenotypes of GBM. A detailed discussion is beyond the scope of this chapter. In this section, we will discuss how the RTK/PI3K/Akt, mTOR, Ras/MEK/MAPK, p53, ATM/Chk2, Rb, and stat3 pathways are affected to GBM. Additional pathways will be briefly discussed in the section on crosstalk.

### 4.1. RTK/PI3K/Akt pathway

This pathway regulates a range of cellular processes such as proliferation, growth, apoptosis, and cytoskeletal rearrangement. It involves receptor tyrosine kinases (RTKs), like EGFR, PDGFR, and VEGFR, as well as tumor suppressor protein phosphatase (PTEN), and protein kinases PI3K, AKT. Irregular activation of RTK/PI3K/AKT is commonly seen in malignant gliomas [24].

#### *4.1.1. Receptor tyrosine kinases*

RTKs relay extracellular signals to activation of intracellular networks through PI3K and AKT. *EGFR* gene amplification is the most widespread alteration present in GBM [25]. The most common is EGFR vIII, which relays ligand independent accumulative growth signals [26, 27]. Some studies have previously shown a correlation between aberrance of EGFR and aggressiveness of tumor and therefore shorter survival [28, 29]. Unfortunately, EGFR inhibitors such as Gefinitib and Erlotinib have not produced promising results in clinical trials of patients with GBM [30, 31]. Overexpression of PDGFR (especially PDGFR-$\alpha$) and PDGF have been documented in astrocytic tumors irrespective of the grade [32], [33]. *PDGFRA* amplification and *IDH1* mutation are a characteristic of the proneural subtype of GBM implying a possible association of the proneural subtype and secondary GBM [4]. Anti-PDGFR therapy such as imatinib has not been promising either [34].

#### *4.1.2. PI3K–PTEN-AKT signaling*

AKT, a serine/threonine kinase that acts to regulate cell growth, proliferation, and apoptosis, is activated in about 80% of human GBMs [35]. PI3K belongs to the family of lipid kinases.

PI3K enzymes produce phosphatidylinositol-3,4,5-trisphosphate (PIP3), a lipid secondary messenger, which is found to be at high levels in cancer cells [36, 37]. Binding of PI3Ks to RTKs results in activation of AKT through PiP3 and PDK1 [38]. Dissecting the PI3K complex, it is composed of a catalytically active protein, p110$\alpha$, encoded by *PIK3CA*, and a regulatory protein, p85$\alpha$, encoded by *PIK3R1*. In primary GBM, *PIK3CA* mutations and amplification are seen in about 5% to 13% of cases [39]. Furthermore, *PIK3R1* mutations have been reported in about 10 % in GBM patients [4].

PTEN (phosphatase and tensin homologue, located on chromosome 10) is a tumor suppressor gene. PTEN mutations are associated with several types of cancer including GBM. Loss of heterozygosity of chromosome 10, which causes deletions or mutations of PTEN, is a common event in GBMs. PTEN negatively regulates the PI3K/AKT/PKB pathway by blocking AKT signaling via the reduction of intracellular levels of PIP3. Furthermore, lower PTEN activity induces activation of the RTKs/PI3K/AKT pathway. This is due to the negative inhibition accomplished by PTEN antagonizing PIK3 [40]. GBMs typically harbor diminished expression of PTEN through homozygous deletion or mutations of PTEN, which contributes the activation of the RTKs/PI3K/Akt pathway [4, 41, 42]. Mesenchymal and classical types of GBM exhibit loss of PTEN (www.cbtrus.org). It is noteworthy that GBM cells expressing EGFRvIII with an intact PTEN appear to have a higher response rate to EGFR inhibitors [35, 43].

### 4.2. mTOR

Signaling through mTOR is mediated by two independent complexes, mTORC1 and mTORC2. mTORC2 is activated by growth factors and ribosomes and in turn activates AKT among other kinases via phosphorylation [44]. mTORC1 controls cellular metabolism, biosynthesis, stress, and by several growth factors such as EGF and its receptor, EGFR [45]. In settings promoting cell growth, mTORC1 phosphorylates substrates to stimulate anabolic processes such as ribosome biogenesis, translation, and synthesis of lipids and nucleotides and to abolish catabolic processes such as autophagy [45]. Likewise, mTORC2 promotes cancer growth by stimulating glucose uptake via activation of AKT and activating serum/glucocorticoid regulated kinase (SGK), which contributes to proliferation and survival [46]. Inhibitors of mTOR, like rapamycin, sirolimus, temsirolimus, everolimus have not shown efficacy in GBM [47, 48]. In fact, inhibitors of mTOR lead to elevated expression and activity of growth factor receptors, which increases PI3K activity and RAS signaling. Below we discuss the effects of rapamycin on the mTOR pathway in detail.

### 4.3. Ras/MAPK pathway

The 3 components of the human Ras genes (Rat Sarcoma) are transmuting oncogenes and include: H-Ras, N-Ras, and K-Ras. Ras is a member of the G protein family, which basically means that it is activated by binding to guanosine triphosphate (GTP), and deactivated by binding to guanosine diphosphate (GDP) [49]. Ras serves to activate serine tyrosine kinases (STK) including Raf, MAPK (ERK1 and ERK2), PI3K, among other proteins that influence cell proliferation, differentiation, and survival [50]. Although the mutual activation of Ras and AKT in neural progenitors contributes to gliomagenesis in mouse models [51], Ras mutations are uncommon in human GBM [4]. Activated Raf phosphorylates and activates MAPK kinase (MAPKK), also called MEK, which in turn phosphorylates and activates MAPK [52, 53][54], which then moves to the nucleus to induce other transcription factors including Elk1, c-myc, Ets, STAT (signal transducers and activators of transcription), and PPARγ (peroxisome proliferator-activated receptor γ), which induce cell cycle progression and anti-apoptosis genes [50, 55].

NF-1, a tumor suppressor gene encoding neurofibromin, negatively regulates Ras and influences adenylate cyclase- and AKT-mTOR-mediated pathways [56]. NF-1 mutation and homozygous deletions are detected in 18% of GBM [4]. Mesenchymal type GBM appears to respond to concomitant chemo-radiation therapy and happens to commonly have inactivation of the NF-1 (37%), p53 (32%), and PTEN genes [57].

### 4.4. The p53 pathway

The *p53* gene, labeled as the "guardian of the genome", is located at chromosome 17q13.1 and encodes a protein that takes action against miscellaneous cellular stresses to regulate the corresponding genes that provoke programmed cell death or apoptosis, cell differentiation, senescence, DNA repair, and neovascularization [58]. The p53 pathway is the most frequently mutated pathway in human cancer and is essentially disrupted in roughly 80% of high-grade gliomas. p53, activated in response to DNA damage, induces transcription of genes such as p21Waf1/Cip1 that arrest the cell cycle progression at the G1 phase [59].

An important regulator of the p53 pathway is MDM2, an E3 ubiquitin ligase that negatively modulates p53 through transcriptional inhibition by direct binding as well as by degradation through its E3 ligase activity [60] [61]. On the other hand, the transcription of the MDM2 gene is induced by wild-type p53 [62]. This creates an autoregulatory feedback loop which controls the function of both the expression of MDM2 and the activity of p53. Another regulator of the p53 pathway is the tumor suppressor protein ARF (p14ARF), which controls p53 transcriptional activities by binding to MDM2 and consequently hindering its E3 ubiquitin ligase activity [63, 64]; conversely p14ARF expression is negatively regulated by p53 [59]. Both low grade and high grade gliomas exhibit inactivation or mutation of p14ARF [65]; homozygous deletion of p16INK4a/p14ARF/p15INK4b locus is one of the common mutations in GBMs [66]. Remarkably, mouse models revealed that co-deletion of ARF and INK4a increased accordingly with tumor progression from low- to high-grade gliomas [67]. This suggests that ARF and INK4a mutations are important steps in gliomagenesis.

### 4.5. ATM/Chk2 pathway

Disruption of the ATM/Chk2 pathway increases the speed of growth and development of glioma [68]; it also contributes to resistance to radiation therapy by helping the malignant cell activate a group of sensor kinases including ATM, ATR, and DNA-dependent protein kinase [69]. The latter phosphorylates multiple downstream mediators such as checkpoint kinases Chk1 and Chk2 that lead to cell-cycle checkpoint initiation and/or apoptosis [70]. Chk2, encoded at chromosome 22q12.1, acts as a tumor suppressor as it regulates p53-dependent apoptosis [71]. Chk2 mutations have in general been rarely reported; however single copy loss of the chromosomal region containing Chk2 has been reported in gliomas [4].

### 4.6. Rb pathway

The retinoblastoma gene, Rb, is implicated in progression from low grade to higher grade astrocytoma [72], and it is inactivated in GBM [73]. The Rb pathway suppresses cell cycle entry and progression and curbs the p53 pathway by binding and inhibiting transcription factors of the E2F family. Of note, Rb controls progression from G1 to S-phase of the cell cycle [16]. Rb is regulated by the complex of cyclin-dependent kinases (CDKs); in the G1 phase, Rb is normally inactivated by Cyclin D/CDK4/CDK6- induced phosphorylation, causing its release from E2F and consequent cell cycle progression into the S phase. CDKN2B, a CDK inhibitor, which is commonly inactivated in GBM, forms a complex with CDK4 or CDK6, thus preventing the activation of CDKs. The outcome of this inhibition is prevention of cell growth. In addition to the inactivation of CDKN2B, amplification of CDK4 and CDK6 is also common in GBM, demonstrating that both CDK4 and CDK6 have a fundamental function in gliomagenesis and progression [74]. The CDKN2A (p16INK4a) protein binds to CDK4 and inhibits the CDK4/ cyclin D1 complex, consequently inhibiting cell cycle transition from G1 to S phase [73]. This implies that any alteration of Rb, CDK4, or CDKN2A causes aberrant dysregulation of the G1-S phase transition. Complete loss of Rb, homozygous deletion or mutation of CDKN2A, CDK4 amplification, CDKN2B (p15INK4b) homozygous deletion, CDKN2C (p18INK4c) homozygous deletion, CCND2 (cyclin D2) amplification, and CDK6 amplification are observed in almost 80% of GBM [75-77].

### 4.7. STAT3

STAT (Signal transducers and activators of transcription) complexes are a family of cytoplasmic proteins that have SH2 (Src Homology-2) domains functioning as transcription factors that control cellular responses to cytokines and growth factors by signal transduction from the plasma membrane to the nucleus [78]. Target genes are then transcribed and contribute to proliferation, invasion, and apoptosis. STAT3 is an example of the STAT family proteins; it is rendered active by EGF and is overexpressed in GBM [79]. STAT3 also plays a role in the development of neural stem cells and astrocytes [80]. Targeting STAT3 may influence glioma cell motility, resistance to temozolomide, as well as clinical outcome [81-83].

## 5. Crosstalk

A distinguished characteristic of signaling networks in GBM is the presence of crosstalk, or communication between subnetworks, which interact to promote gliomagenesis and all the phenotypes of GBM. For example, there is evidence of mutual cross talk between cells inactivation of either Ras/Raf/MAPK or PI3K/AKT/mTOR triggering activation of the other [39]. Other examples are the interactions between Ras and stem cell factor (SCF)/c-kit signaling, mTOR, and MAP kinase pathways and the interactions between PI3Kand STAT3 pathways and NF-κB, nuclear factor kappa-light-chain-enhancer of activated B cells, in gliomas [84] [85]. In this section, we examine selected networks that play a role in glioma stem cells (GSC) and cell motility.

### 5.1. GSC

GSC have the particular ability to auto-renew and initiate gliomagenesis, express neural stem cell markers, and differentiate into multiple phenotypes such as neuronal, astrocytic, and oligodendroglial. Sonic hedgehog homolog (SHH) and Notch are overly expressed in GSC and therefore aberrantly regulate neural progenitor cells [86]. SHH is an important mitogen for medulloblastoma precursor cells. The SHH pathway also contributes to glioma formation as it is activated in GSCs. The SHH pathway is also closely related to the cell cycle as it inactivates Rb and causes over-expression of cell cycle regulators such as N-myc. PDGF signaling in neural stem cells is required for oligodendrogenesis, and amplification of this signal causes an abnormal proliferation of neural stem cells and the formation of large glioma-like lesions [87].

Notch (Notch1-4 in mammals) is a family of transmembrane receptors that control intercellular signaling [88]. They are transmembrane proteins that bind to notch and reveal the receptor to proteolytic activation. Notch is cleaved by presenilin 1 which generates a Notch1 intracellular domain (NICD), a nuclear transcriptional activator. Notch activation induces expression of downstream target genes, such as p53, and promotes neural stem cell growth [89]. BMPs are growth factors that act through binding to cell-surface receptor kinases (BMPRs); the effectors of BMPRs are the Smad proteins, which play a major role in bone and cartilage formation. The overall activity of BMPs is regulation of transcription. BMP ligands exhaust the GSC population by inducing the differentiation of GSCs into astroglial and neuron-like cells. Treating GSCs with BMPs *in vivo* delays tumor growth and diminishes tumor invasion [90].

miRNA is a small non-coding RNA that post-transcriptionally downregulates gene expression. Several studies have identified aberrant miRNA (microRNA-21, miR-326, microRNA-34a) expression in gliomas, and linked some of them to GSC maintenance and growth [91, 92]. Finally, Tumor Necrosis Factor alpha-Induced Protein (TNFAIP) 3 regulates both the NF-κB pathway as well as GSC self-renewal, growth, and apoptotic resistance [93].

### 5.2. Brain invasion and motility

Brain invasion is a hallmark of gliomas. Tumor cell migration requires highly coordinated steps of dissociation of existing cellular adhesions, remodeling of the actin cytoskeleton to project lamellipodium extensions, formation of new adhesions, and tail detachment along with proteolytic processing and secretion of extracellular matrix proteins along the trajectory. This complex phenotype requires crosstalk between networks that control the extracellular matrix, growth factors, cdc42, GTPases, actin polymerization, PAK, src, cadherins, PIP3, integrins, and myosin (see [96] for details).

Furthermore, some GBM exhibit enhanced motility at 5% ambient oxygen, which is higher than the typical 0.3-1% concentrations observed in cancer hypoxia. This result supports an increased propensity for invasion. The phenotype of increased motility in low ambient oxygen conditions is mediated by phosphorylation of src, which in turn phosphorylates NWASP, Neural Wiskott-Aldrich Syndrome Protein (see [97] for details).

## 6. Effects of rapamycin on AKT

In the preceding section we have highlighted the complexity of the molecular interactions in GBM and the large number of subnetworks that communicate to generate the phenotypes. Because rapamycin inhibits the mTOR complex, it was considered a hopeful prospect for pharmaceutical therapy. However, in a clinical trial using rapamycin in the treatment of PTEN-deficient GBM, researchers encountered a paradoxical increase in AKT signaling, which was unexpected and undesirable as the latter promotes oncogenic processes [98]. The exact mechanisms for this finding are not yet known. Although many scientists postulate about a simple loss of negative feedback, there may be more than what meets the eye. To illustrate this point, we will delineate a well-characterized pathway in GBM molecular biology and discuss how intersecting activation and inhibitory pathways can lead to paradoxical downstream effects.

As reviewed in Howell et al. and Huang and Manning, mTORC1 acts ultimately as a negative regulator of AKT through various mechanisms [99-101]. First, mTORC1 directly phosphorylates IRS (insulin receptor substrate), which is thought to hinder the scaffolding ability of PI3K to activate AKT. Additionally, mTORC1 acts through its downstream effector S6K1 (S6 kinase 1), which also phosphorylates IRS at specific serine residues and reduces downstream AKT activation [102-105]. Zhang et al. in 2003 and 2007 showed that mTORC1 activation leads to repression of PDGFR A and B transcription, which inhibits PDGF signaling to AKT and blocks proper transmission of signals from other growth factors [106, 107]. AKT also acts as an activator of mTORC1; but this interaction is irrelevant to our discussion of mTORC1 inhibitors because direct inhibitors of mTORC1 are not influenced by AKT.

Since mTORC1 inhibits AKT (Figure 1, t = 0), bringing down mTORC1 via rapamycin (Figure 1, t = 1) would subsequently lead to an increase in AKT (Figure 1, t = 2).

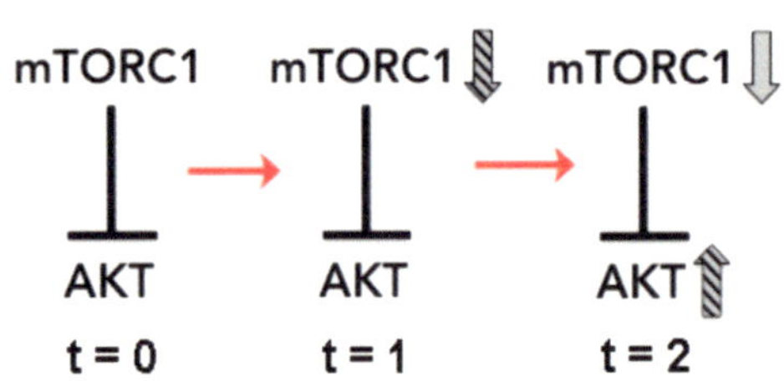


**Figure 1. Cartoon depicting the negative effects of mTORC1 on AKT activation and its response to perturbations.** Blocked arrows indicate repression/deactivation. The arrow pointing down indicates repression of mTORC1 activity at time = 1. The arrow pointing up indicates the response of the network by increasing the activity of AKT at time = 2.

At first sight this explanation is logical, but when we look deeper into the networks we discover additional factors to this relationship that can provide alternate explanations for the clinical trial's findings. The simple diagram of Figure 1a does not appear to be the appropriate explanation.

Subsequent studies have found that at low concentrations, rapamycin treatment leads to an increase in AKT activity; however, at high, super-physiological concentrations rapamycin causes a decrease in AKT activity [108]. Interestingly, at high concentrations of rapamycin, both mTORC1 and mTORC2 are inhibited. Hence, we need to consider the effects of mTORC2 on AKT. In fact, mTORC2 phosphorylates AKT on S473 (serine 473), which activates AKT at the plasma membrane [112]. The observation, that inhibiting both mTORC1 and mTORC2 caused a decrease in AKT activity, indicates that mTORC1 is a weak inhibitor of AKT as compared to mTORC2 as an activator (see Figure 2 for details).

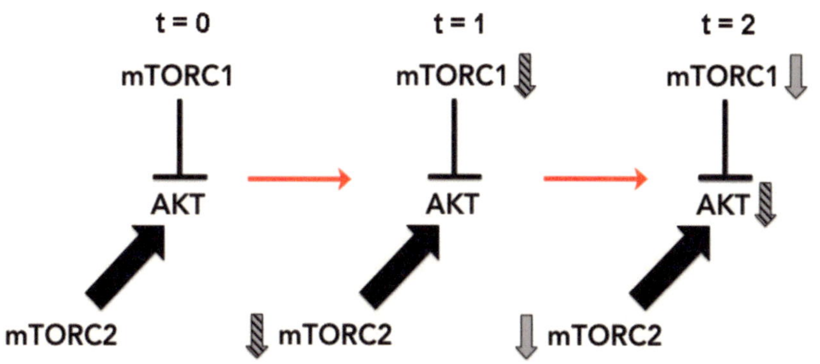


**Figure 2. Cartoon depicting relative effects of mTORC1 and mTORC2 on AKT and the response of the network to high concentrations of rapamycin.** Blocked and regular arrows indicate repression/deactivation and activation, respectively. The thickness of the arrows reflects the level of repression or activation. If mTORC2 is a stronger activator of AKT than mTORC1 is a repressor (time = 0), treating the cells with high concentrations of rapamycin, which inhibits both mTORC1 and mTORC2 (time = 1), causes a decrease in AKT activity (time = 2).

If we delve deeper into these pathways, we learn of a negative loop between AKT, TSC2 (tuberous sclerosis complex 2), and mTORC2 (See Figure 3) [101]. AKT directly inhibits the activity of the TSC2 complex by phosphorylating TSC2 [109-111]. Furthermore, Huang and Manning provide evidence for the subsequent arm of the loop where the TSC2 complex activates mTORC2 in a manner independent of mTORC1 [100]. These relationships together comprise the negative loop illustrated in Figure 3.

We assume that the physiological levels of rapamycin used in the clinical trial inhibit the activity of mTORC1 without any effects on mTORC2; let us now study the reaction of the network in the presence of the AKT/TSC2/mTORC2 negative loop (see Figure 4). Theoretically, if mTORC1 levels go down (Figure 4a), AKT activity should initially increase (Figure 4b). However, higher AKT activity would lead to augmented inhibition of the TSC2 complex (Figure 4c). The lower levels of TSC2 complex would then reduce the activation of mTORC2 (Figure 4c), which in turn feeds back to influence AKT. The ultimate result on AKT depends on the dynamics and the strengths of the connections the negative loop. At this stage, two possibilities arise as follows.

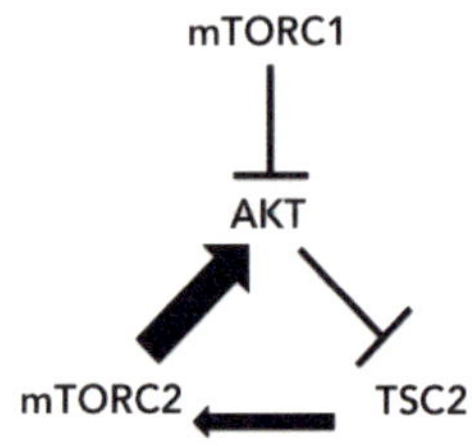


**Figure 3. Cartoon depicting negative loop between AKT, mTORC2 and the TSC2 complex.** Blocked and regular arrows indicate repression/deactivation and activation, respectively.

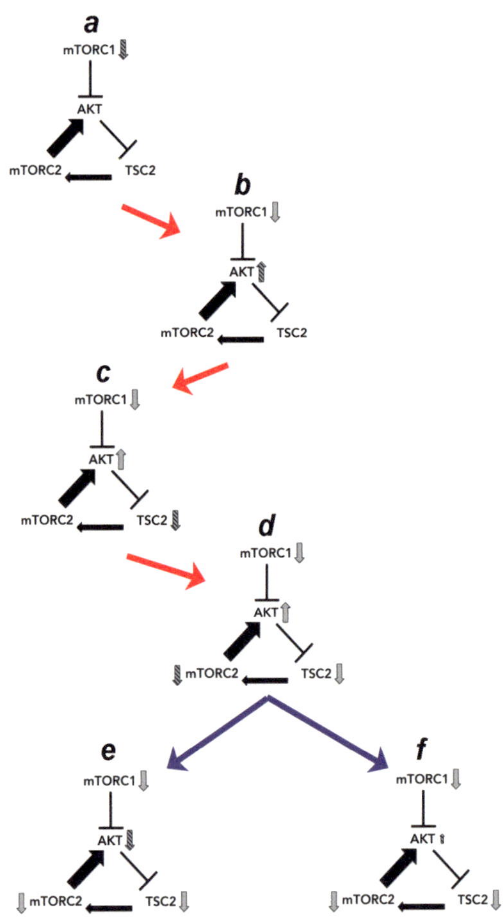


**Figure 4. Cartoon depicting the reaction of the network to rapamycin in the presence of the negative loop.** Blocked and regular arrows indicate repression/deactivation and activation, respectively. Arrows pointing up or down indicate perturbations causing increased or decreased activity, respectively.

*Possibility A*: If both AKT's inhibitory effect on TSC2 and TSC2's activation effect on mTORC2 are strong, then an increase in AKT will lead to a significant decrease in mTORC2. Because the latter is a stronger activator than mTORC1 is a repressor (Figure 3), this causes an ultimate *decrease* in AKT activity (Figure 4e).

*Possibility B*: The negative loop would cause a decrease in mTORC2 activity in any case. This could attenuate but may not reverse the increase in AKT (Figure 4f).

This exercise highlights the profound effects of the presence of a negative loop in the simple network. The results of the clinical trial where rapamycin leads to an increase in AKT activity would be consistent with the explanation of possibility B. However, possibility A cannot be excluded, since other regulatory loops likely influence this pathway as well. In creating treatments and therapeutic strategies in GBM, it is imperative to gain a complete picture of the complexity of intersecting pathways since inhibition can lead to paradoxical, sometimes detrimental results.

## 7. Conclusion

The molecular networks of GBM include a large number of molecules and interactions, as well as multiple subnetworks and crosstalk. These large networks appear to have the ability to not only bypass therapeutic blockade, but to react to therapeutic modalities by activation of oncogenic subnetworks. We are not surprised that little progress has been made against these deadly and intelligent tumors. Success requires a clear understanding of these large networks as well as predictions of their dynamical (time-dependent) behavior in response to perturbations (*ie.* therapeutic interventions). Fortunately, recent advancements in genomics and mathematical biology bring us closer to attaining these goals.

## Author details

Caroline Agha, Hannah C. Machemehl and Hassan M. Fathallah-Shaykh*

*Address all correspondence to: hfathall@uab.edu

The University of Alabama at Birmingham, Department of Neurology, USA

## References

[1] Phillips, H.S., et al., *Molecular subclasses of high-grade glioma predict prognosis, delineate a pattern of disease progression, and resemble stages in neurogenesis.* Cancer Cell, 2006. 9(3): p. 157-73.

[2] Ostrom, Q.T., et al., *CBTRUS statistical report: Primary brain and central nervous system tumors diagnosed in the United States in 2006-2010.* Neuro Oncol, 2013. 15 Suppl 2: p. ii1-56.

[3] Stupp, R., et al., *Radiotherapy plus concomitant and adjuvant temozolomide for glioblastoma.* N Engl J Med, 2005. 352(10): p. 987-96.

[4] Cancer Genome Atlas Research, N., *Comprehensive genomic characterization defines human glioblastoma genes and core pathways.* Nature, 2008. 455(7216): p. 1061-8.

[5] Temple, S., *The development of neural stem cells.* Nature, 2001. 414(6859): p. 112-7.

[6] Kriegstein, A. and A. Alvarez-Buylla, *The glial nature of embryonic and adult neural stem cells.* Annu Rev Neurosci, 2009. 32: p. 149-84.

[7] Richardson, P.M., *Ciliary neurotrophic factor: a review.* Pharmacol Ther, 1994. 63(2): p. 187-98.

[8] Kornblum, H.I., et al., *Multiple trophic actions of heparin-binding epidermal growth factor (HB-EGF) in the central nervous system.* Eur J Neurosci, 1999. 11(9): p. 3236-46.

[9] Powell, E.M., et al., *Mechanisms of astrocyte-directed neurite guidance.* Cell Tissue Res, 1997. 290(2): p. 385-93.

[10] van den Pol, A.N. and D.D. Spencer, *Differential neurite growth on astrocyte substrates: interspecies facilitation in green fluorescent protein-transfected rat and human neurons.* Neuroscience, 2000. 95(2): p. 603-16.

[11] Komuro, H. and P. Rakic, *Distinct modes of neuronal migration in different domains of developing cerebellar cortex.* J Neurosci, 1998. 18(4): p. 1478-90.

[12] Bacci, A., et al., *The role of glial cells in synaptic function.* Philos Trans R Soc Lond B Biol Sci, 1999. 354(1381): p. 403-9.

[13] Rasheed, B.K., et al., *Molecular pathogenesis of malignant gliomas.* Curr Opin Oncol, 1999. 11(3): p. 162-7.

[14] Theeler, B.J., et al., *Moving toward molecular classification of diffuse gliomas in adults.* Neurology, 2012. 79(18): p. 1917-26.

[15] Hottinger, A.F. and Y. Khakoo, *Update on the management of familial central nervous system tumor syndromes.* Curr Neurol Neurosci Rep, 2007. 7(3): p. 200-7.

[16] Serrano, M., G.J. Hannon, and D. Beach, *A new regulatory motif in cell-cycle control causing specific inhibition of cyclin D/CDK4.* Nature, 1993. 366(6456): p. 704-7.

[17] Sherr, C.J. and J.M. Roberts, *CDK inhibitors: positive and negative regulators of G1-phase progression.* Genes Dev, 1999. 13(12): p. 1501-12.

[18] Wong, A.J., et al., *Increased expression of the epidermal growth factor receptor gene in malignant gliomas is invariably associated with gene amplification.* Proc Natl Acad Sci U S A, 1987. 84(19): p. 6899-903.

[19] Westermark, B., C.H. Heldin, and M. Nister, *Platelet-derived growth factor in human glioma.* Glia, 1995. 15(3): p. 257-63.

[20] Louis, D.N., *Molecular pathology of malignant gliomas.* Annu Rev Pathol, 2006. 1: p. 97-117.

[21] Gomez-Manzano, C., et al., *Characterization of p53 and p21 functional interactions in glioma cells en route to apoptosis.* J Natl Cancer Inst, 1997. 89(14): p. 1036-44.

[22] Leung, S.Y., et al., *Chromosomal instability and p53 inactivation are required for genesis of glioblastoma but not for colorectal cancer in patients with germline mismatch repair gene mutation.* Oncogene, 2000. 19(35): p. 4079-83.

[23] Hamilton, S.R., et al., *The molecular basis of Turcot's syndrome.* N Engl J Med, 1995. 332(13): p. 839-47.

[24] Ekstrand, A.J., et al., *Amplified and rearranged epidermal growth factor receptor genes in human glioblastomas reveal deletions of sequences encoding portions of the N- and/or C-terminal tails.* Proc Natl Acad Sci U S A, 1992. 89(10): p. 4309-13.

[25] Ohgaki, H., et al., *Genetic pathways to glioblastoma: a population-based study.* Cancer Res, 2004. 64(19): p. 6892-9.

[26] Yamazaki, H., et al., *Amplification of the structurally and functionally altered epidermal growth factor receptor gene (c-erbB) in human brain tumors.* Mol Cell Biol, 1988. 8(4): p. 1816-20.

[27] Biernat, W., et al., *Predominant expression of mutant EGFR (EGFRvIII) is rare in primary glioblastomas.* Brain Pathol, 2004. 14(2): p. 131-6.

[28] Barker, F.G., 2nd, et al., *EGFR overexpression and radiation response in glioblastoma multiforme.* Int J Radiat Oncol Biol Phys, 2001. 51(2): p. 410-8.

[29] Shinojima, N., et al., *Prognostic value of epidermal growth factor receptor in patients with glioblastoma multiforme.* Cancer Res, 2003. 63(20): p. 6962-70.

[30] Haas-Kogan, D.A., et al., *Epidermal growth factor receptor, protein kinase B/Akt, and glioma response to erlotinib.* J Natl Cancer Inst, 2005. 97(12): p. 880-7.

[31] van den Bent, M.J., et al., *Randomized phase II trial of erlotinib versus temozolomide or carmustine in recurrent glioblastoma: EORTC brain tumor group study 26034.* J Clin Oncol, 2009. 27(8): p. 1268-74.

[32] Guha, A., et al., *Expression of PDGF and PDGF receptors in human astrocytoma operation specimens supports the existence of an autocrine loop.* Int J Cancer, 1995. 60(2): p. 168-73.

[33] Lokker, N.A., et al., *Platelet-derived growth factor (PDGF) autocrine signaling regulates survival and mitogenic pathways in glioblastoma cells: evidence that the novel PDGF-C and*

*PDGF-D ligands may play a role in the development of brain tumors.* Cancer Res, 2002. 62(13): p. 3729-35.

[34] Reardon, D.A., et al., *Multicentre phase II studies evaluating imatinib plus hydroxyurea in patients with progressive glioblastoma.* Br J Cancer, 2009. 101(12): p. 1995-2004.

[35] Haas-Kogan, D., et al., *Protein kinase B (PKB/Akt) activity is elevated in glioblastoma cells due to mutation of the tumor suppressor PTEN/MMAC.* Curr Biol, 1998. 8(21): p. 1195-8.

[36] Zhao, J., et al., *Signal transduction and metabolic flux of beta-thujaplicin and monoterpene biosynthesis in elicited Cupressus lusitanica cell cultures.* Metab Eng, 2006. 8(1): p. 14-29.

[37] Lemmon, M.A., *Membrane recognition by phospholipid-binding domains.* Nat Rev Mol Cell Biol, 2008. 9(2): p. 99-111.

[38] Vivanco, I. and C.L. Sawyers, *The phosphatidylinositol 3-Kinase AKT pathway in human cancer.* Nat Rev Cancer, 2002. 2(7): p. 489-501.

[39] Kita, D., et al., *PIK3CA alterations in primary (de novo) and secondary glioblastomas.* Acta Neuropathol, 2007. 113(3): p. 295-302.

[40] Furnari, F.B., et al., *Malignant astrocytic glioma: genetics, biology, and paths to treatment.* Genes Dev, 2007. 21(21): p. 2683-710.

[41] Li, J., et al., *PTEN, a putative protein tyrosine phosphatase gene mutated in human brain, breast, and prostate cancer.* Science, 1997. 275(5308): p. 1943-7.

[42] Tohma, Y., et al., *PTEN (MMAC1) mutations are frequent in primary glioblastomas (de novo) but not in secondary glioblastomas.* J Neuropathol Exp Neurol, 1998. 57(7): p. 684-9.

[43] Mellinghoff, I.K., et al., *Molecular determinants of the response of glioblastomas to EGFR kinase inhibitors.* N Engl J Med, 2005. 353(19): p. 2012-24.

[44] Zinzalla, V., et al., *Activation of mTORC2 by association with the ribosome.* Cell, 2011. 144(5): p. 757-68.

[45] Laplante, M. and D.M. Sabatini, *mTOR signaling in growth control and disease.* Cell, 2012. 149(2): p. 274-93.

[46] Zoncu, R., A. Efeyan, and D.M. Sabatini, *mTOR: from growth signal integration to cancer, diabetes and ageing.* Nat Rev Mol Cell Biol, 2011. 12(1): p. 21-35.

[47] Chang, S.M., et al., *Phase II study of CCI-779 in patients with recurrent glioblastoma multiforme.* Invest New Drugs, 2005. 23(4): p. 357-61.

[48] Galanis, E., et al., *Phase II trial of temsirolimus (CCI-779) in recurrent glioblastoma multiforme: a North Central Cancer Treatment Group Study.* J Clin Oncol, 2005. 23(23): p. 5294-304.

[49] Hurley, J.B., et al., *Homologies between signal transducing G proteins and ras gene products.* Science, 1984. 226(4676): p. 860-2.

[50] Nakada, M., et al., *Aberrant signaling pathways in glioma.* Cancers (Basel), 2011. 3(3): p. 3242-78.

[51] Holland, E.C., et al., *Combined activation of Ras and Akt in neural progenitors induces glioblastoma formation in mice.* Nat Genet, 2000. 25(1): p. 55-7.

[52] Moodie, S.A., et al., *Complexes of Ras.GTP with Raf-1 and mitogen-activated protein kinase kinase.* Science, 1993. 260(5114): p. 1658-61.

[53] Thomas, S.M., et al., *Ras is essential for nerve growth factor- and phorbol ester-induced tyrosine phosphorylation of MAP kinases.* Cell, 1992. 68(6): p. 1031-40.

[54] Krakstad, C. and M. Chekenya, *Survival signalling and apoptosis resistance in glioblastomas: opportunities for targeted therapeutics.* Mol Cancer, 2010. 9: p. 135.

[55] Kapoor, G.S. and D.M. O'Rourke, *Receptor tyrosine kinase signaling in gliomagenesis: pathobiology and therapeutic approaches.* Cancer Biol Ther, 2003. 2(4): p. 330-42.

[56] Gottfried, O.N., D.H. Viskochil, and W.T. Couldwell, *Neurofibromatosis Type 1 and tumorigenesis: molecular mechanisms and therapeutic implications.* Neurosurg Focus, 2010. 28(1): p. E8.

[57] Verhaak, R.G., et al., *Integrated genomic analysis identifies clinically relevant subtypes of glioblastoma characterized by abnormalities in PDGFRA, IDH1, EGFR, and NF1.* Cancer Cell, 2010. 17(1): p. 98-110.

[58] Bogler, O., et al., *The p53 gene and its role in human brain tumors.* Glia, 1995. 15(3): p. 308-27.

[59] Stott, F.J., et al., *The alternative product from the human CDKN2A locus, p14(ARF), participates in a regulatory feedback loop with p53 and MDM2.* EMBO J, 1998. 17(17): p. 5001-14.

[60] Haupt, Y., et al., *Mdm2 promotes the rapid degradation of p53.* Nature, 1997. 387(6630): p. 296-9.

[61] Kubbutat, M.H., S.N. Jones, and K.H. Vousden, *Regulation of p53 stability by Mdm2.* Nature, 1997. 387(6630): p. 299-303.

[62] Zauberman, A., et al., *A functional p53-responsive intronic promoter is contained within the human mdm2 gene.* Nucleic Acids Res, 1995. 23(14): p. 2584-92.

[63] Kamijo, T., et al., *Functional and physical interactions of the ARF tumor suppressor with p53 and Mdm2.* Proc Natl Acad Sci U S A, 1998. 95(14): p. 8292-7.

[64] Zhang, Y., Y. Xiong, and W.G. Yarbrough, *ARF promotes MDM2 degradation and stabilizes p53: ARF-INK4a locus deletion impairs both the Rb and p53 tumor suppression pathways.* Cell, 1998. 92(6): p. 725-34.

[65] Nakamura, M., et al., *p14ARF deletion and methylation in genetic pathways to glioblastomas.* Brain Pathol, 2001. 11(2): p. 159-68.

[66] Solomon, D.A., et al., *Conspirators in a capital crime: co-deletion of p18INK4c and p16INK4a/p14ARF/p15INK4b in glioblastoma multiforme.* Cancer Res, 2008. 68(21): p. 8657-60.

[67] Labuhn, M., et al., *Quantitative real-time PCR does not show selective targeting of p14(ARF) but concomitant inactivation of both p16(INK4A) and p14(ARF) in 105 human primary gliomas.* Oncogene, 2001. 20(9): p. 1103-9.

[68] Squatrito, M., et al., *Loss of ATM/Chk2/p53 pathway components accelerates tumor development and contributes to radiation resistance in gliomas.* Cancer Cell, 2010. 18(6): p. 619-29.

[69] Durocher, D. and S.P. Jackson, *DNA-PK, ATM and ATR as sensors of DNA damage: variations on a theme?* Curr Opin Cell Biol, 2001. 13(2): p. 225-31.

[70] Stracker, T.H., T. Usui, and J.H. Petrini, *Taking the time to make important decisions: the checkpoint effector kinases Chk1 and Chk2 and the DNA damage response.* DNA Repair (Amst), 2009. 8(9): p. 1047-54.

[71] Hirao, A., et al., *Chk2 is a tumor suppressor that regulates apoptosis in both an ataxia telangiectasia mutated (ATM)-dependent and an ATM-independent manner.* Mol Cell Biol, 2002. 22(18): p. 6521-32.

[72] Henson, J.W., et al., *The retinoblastoma gene is involved in malignant progression of astrocytomas.* Ann Neurol, 1994. 36(5): p. 714-21.

[73] Biernat, W., et al., *Alterations of cell cycle regulatory genes in primary (de novo) and secondary glioblastomas.* Acta Neuropathol, 1997. 94(4): p. 303-9.

[74] Lam, P.Y., et al., *Expression of p19INK4d, CDK4, CDK6 in glioblastoma multiforme.* Br J Neurosurg, 2000. 14(1): p. 28-32.

[75] Schmidt, E.E., et al., *CDKN2 (p16/MTS1) gene deletion or CDK4 amplification occurs in the majority of glioblastomas.* Cancer Res, 1994. 54(24): p. 6321-4.

[76] Hayashi, Y., et al., *Association of EGFR gene amplification and CDKN2 (p16/MTS1) gene deletion in glioblastoma multiforme.* Brain Pathol, 1997. 7(3): p. 871-5.

[77] Hegi, M.E., et al., *Hemizygous or homozygous deletion of the chromosomal region containing the p16INK4a gene is associated with amplification of the EGF receptor gene in glioblastomas.* Int J Cancer, 1997. 73(1): p. 57-63.

[78] Abal, M., et al., *Molecular pathology of endometrial carcinoma: transcriptional signature in endometrioid tumors.* Histol Histopathol, 2006. 21(2): p. 197-204.

[79] Rahaman, S.O., et al., *Inhibition of constitutively active Stat3 suppresses proliferation and induces apoptosis in glioblastoma multiforme cells.* Oncogene, 2002. 21(55): p. 8404-13.

[80] Rajan, P. and R.D. McKay, *Multiple routes to astrocytic differentiation in the CNS.* J Neurosci, 1998. 18(10): p. 3620-9.

[81] Lin, G.S., et al., *STAT3 serine 727 phosphorylation influences clinical outcome in glioblastoma.* Int J Clin Exp Pathol, 2014. 7(6): p. 3141-9.

[82] Ashizawa, T., et al., *Effect of the STAT3 inhibitor STX-0119 on the proliferation of a temozolomide-resistant glioblastoma cell line.* Int J Oncol, 2014. 45(1): p. 411-8.

[83] Liang, Q., et al., *Inhibition of STAT3 reduces astrocytoma cell invasion and constitutive activation of STAT3 predicts poor prognosis in human astrocytoma.* PLoS ONE, 2013. 8(12): p. e84723.

[84] Smith, D., et al., *NF-kappaB controls growth of glioblastomas/astrocytomas.* Mol Cell Biochem, 2008. 307(1-2): p. 141-7.

[85] Romashkova, J.A. and S.S. Makarov, *NF-kappaB is a target of AKT in anti-apoptotic PDGF signalling.* Nature, 1999. 401(6748): p. 86-90.

[86] Sanai, N., A. Alvarez-Buylla, and M.S. Berger, *Neural stem cells and the origin of gliomas.* N Engl J Med, 2005. 353(8): p. 811-22.

[87] Jackson, E.L., et al., *PDGFR alpha-positive B cells are neural stem cells in the adult SVZ that form glioma-like growths in response to increased PDGF signaling.* Neuron, 2006. 51(2): p. 187-99.

[88] Artavanis-Tsakonas, S., M.D. Rand, and R.J. Lake, *Notch signaling: cell fate control and signal integration in development.* Science, 1999. 284(5415): p. 770-6.

[89] Androutsellis-Theotokis, A., et al., *Notch signalling regulates stem cell numbers in vitro and in vivo.* Nature, 2006. 442(7104): p. 823-6.

[90] Lee, J., et al., *Epigenetic-mediated dysfunction of the bone morphogenetic protein pathway inhibits differentiation of glioblastoma-initiating cells.* Cancer Cell, 2008. 13(1): p. 69-80.

[91] Kefas, B., et al., *The neuronal microRNA miR-326 acts in a feedback loop with notch and has therapeutic potential against brain tumors.* J Neurosci, 2009. 29(48): p. 15161-8.

[92] Guessous, F., et al., *microRNA-34a is tumor suppressive in brain tumors and glioma stem cells.* Cell Cycle, 2010. 9(6): p. 1031-6.

[93] Hjelmeland, A.B., et al., *Targeting A20 decreases glioma stem cell survival and tumor growth.* PLoS Biol, 2010. 8(2): p. e1000319.

[94] Chuang, Y.Y., et al., *Role of synaptojanin 2 in glioma cell migration and invasion.* Cancer Res, 2004. 64(22): p. 8271-5.

[95] Salhia, B., et al., *Inhibition of Rho-kinase affects astrocytoma morphology, motility, and invasion through activation of Rac1.* Cancer Res, 2005. 65(19): p. 8792-800.

[96] Tang, Z., L.M. Araysi, and H.M. Fathallah-Shaykh, *c-Src and neural Wiskott-Aldrich syndrome protein (N-WASP) promote low oxygen-induced accelerated brain invasion by gliomas.* PLoS ONE, 2013. 8(9): p. e75436.

[97] Fathallah-Shaykh, H.M., *Logical networks inferred from highly specific discovery of transcriptionally regulated genes predict protein states in cultured gliomas.* Biochem Biophys Res Comm, 2005. 336: p. 1278-1284.

[98] Carracedo, A., et al., *Inhibition of mTORC1 leads to MAPK pathway activation through a PI3K-dependent feedback loop in human cancer.* J Clin Invest, 2008. 118(9): p. 3065-74.

[99] Howell, J.J. and B.D. Manning, *mTOR couples cellular nutrient sensing to organismal metabolic homeostasis.* Trends Endocrinol Metab, 2011. 22(3): p. 94-102.

[100] Huang, J. and B.D. Manning, *A complex interplay between Akt, TSC2 and the two mTOR complexes.* Biochem Soc Trans, 2009. 37(Pt 1): p. 217-22.

[101] Carracedo, A. and P.P. Pandolfi, *The PTEN-PI3K pathway: of feedbacks and cross-talks.* Oncogene, 2008. 27(41): p. 5527-41.

[102] Shah, O.J. and T. Hunter, *Turnover of the active fraction of IRS1 involves raptor-mTOR- and S6K1-dependent serine phosphorylation in cell culture models of tuberous sclerosis.* Mol Cell Biol, 2006. 26(17): p. 6425-34.

[103] Harrington, L.S., G.M. Findlay, and R.F. Lamb, *Restraining PI3K: mTOR signalling goes back to the membrane.* Trends Biochem Sci, 2005. 30(1): p. 35-42.

[104] Tremblay, F., et al., *Identification of IRS-1 Ser-1101 as a target of S6K1 in nutrient- and obesity-induced insulin resistance.* Proc Natl Acad Sci U S A, 2007. 104(35): p. 14056-61.

[105] Manning, B.D., *Balancing Akt with S6K: implications for both metabolic diseases and tumorigenesis.* J Cell Biol, 2004. 167(3): p. 399-403.

[106] Zhang, H., et al., *PDGFRs are critical for PI3K/Akt activation and negatively regulated by mTOR.* J Clin Invest, 2007. 117(3): p. 730-8.

[107] Zhang, H., et al., *Loss of Tsc1/Tsc2 activates mTOR and disrupts PI3K-Akt signaling through downregulation of PDGFR.* J Clin Invest, 2003. 112(8): p. 1223-33.

[108] Costanzo, M., et al., *The genetic landscape of a cell.* Science, 2010. 327: p. 425-431.

[109] Potter, C.J., L.G. Pedraza, and T. Xu, *Akt regulates growth by directly phosphorylating Tsc2.* Nat Cell Biol, 2002. 4(9): p. 658-65.

[110] Inoki, K., et al., *TSC2 is phosphorylated and inhibited by Akt and suppresses mTOR signalling.* Nat Cell Biol, 2002. 4(9): p. 648-57.

[111] Dan, H.C., et al., *Phosphatidylinositol 3-kinase/Akt pathway regulates tuberous sclerosis tumor suppressor* complex by phosphorylation of tuberin. J Biol Chem, 2002. 277(38): p. 35364-70.

[112] Sarbassov, D.D., et al., Phosphorylation and regulation of Akt/PKB by the rictor-mTOR complex. Science, 2005. 307(5712): p. 1098-101.

Chapter 3

# Tumor Microenvironment — Perivascular and Perinecrotic Niches

Davide Schiffer, Marta Mellai, Laura Annovazzi,
Cristina Casalone and Paola Cassoni

Additional information is available at the end of the chapter

http://dx.doi.org/10.5772/58962

## 1. Introduction

Tumor microenvironment is a dynamic concept that includes, beside tumor cells, everything is not tumor cells. It consists of cells, soluble factors, signaling molecules, extracellular matrix (ECM), and mechanical cues that can promote neoplastic transformation, support tumor growth and invasion, protect the tumor from host immunity and foster therapeutic resistance [1]. It is organ-specific and in the brain it is not yet fully understood. In addition to cancer cells, it contains different stromal cells mainly represented by endothelial cells, microglia/macrophages, and reactive astrocytes [2], but other cell types should be considered such as fibroblasts, pericytes, immune cells, *etc.* (Figure 1). These cells are heterogeneously distributed in the tumor, according to its different phenotypes and relevant biological significances.

## 2. Microenvironment cell components

### 2.1. Microglia/macrophages

Malignant gliomas are rich in microglia/macrophages that are classified as ramified or resident microglia, ameboid or activated microglia, macrophages and perivascular microglia [3]. They are called tumor-associated macrophages (TAM) and lack apparent phagocytic activity [4].They are considered as both intrinsic to the central nervous system (CNS) and blood-borne arrived, subjected to the local production of chemoattractant factors [5]; they share surface markers [6], but it has been demonstrated that microglia are chemokine (C-X3-C motif) receptor 1 (CX3CR1)+/chemokine (C-C motif) receptor 2 (CCR2)– and monocytes are CCR2+/

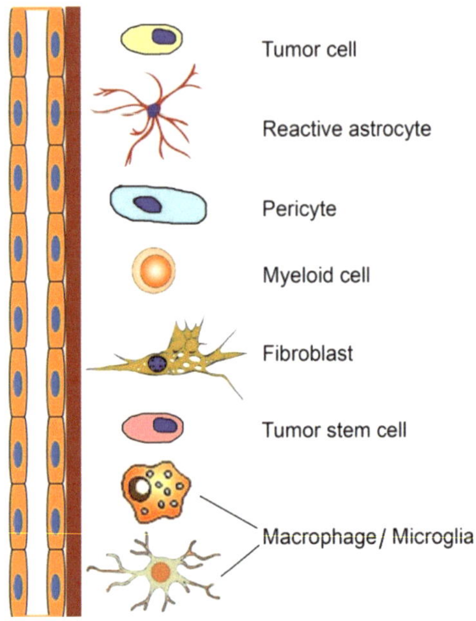


**Figure 1.** Scheme of the relationship between vessels/endothelium and microenvironment cells.

CX3CR1– [7]. In acute conditions microglia is blood-derived, from adult haematopoietic stem cells (HSCs), even though macrophages in adult renew independently from HSCs. Their majority derives from Tie2+ pathway generating eritro-myeloid progenitors, distinct from HSCs, from the yolk sac they migrate in the various organs [8].

It is still debated whether they are included in or they are distinct from pro-inflammatory cells. They increase both in the center and at the periphery of the tumors [9] and it has been calculated that up to one third of the cells in glioma biopsies are represented by macrophages [9,10] (Figure 2A,B). In the tissue, microglia/macrophages are found as small or large clusters around vessels or necroses, whereas at the periphery or around the tumor they are more regularly distributed. Undoubtedly, they proliferate in response to tumor growth and they have a cytotoxic defense function [11], as well as the capacity for antigen presentation [12], but they can also promote tumor infiltration and proliferation [13,14]. An inverse correlation between TAM infiltration and glioblastoma multiforme (GBM) prognosis [15] and promotion of tumor progression have been found [16].

Together with fibroblasts, pericytes, neutrophils, mast cells, lymphocytes, dendritic and endothelial cells, macrophages belong to the category of stromal cells that interact with the tumor, as discussed before, *via* cell-cell or by cytokine or chemokine-mediated signaling. Tumor cells may influence stromal cells to produce growth factors such as vascular endothelial growth factor (VEGF), tumor necrosis factor alpha (TNF-$\alpha$), transforming growth factor beta (TGF-$\beta$), interleukin 1 (IL-1) or CXC ligand 2 (CXCL2), CXCL8, CXCL12 that promote angiogenesis and tumor growth. Conversely, tumor cells are stimulated to produce chemokines that influence angiogenesis [16] and growth. There is both an autocrine and a paracrine tumor growth stimulation [17]. The enrichment in stromal cells, especially microglia/macrophages, in the brain adjacent to tumor (BAT) strongly influences immunoregulation and tumor growth on the one side, and it represents a defense from the tumor on the other side.

The existence of a positive relationship between microglia/macrophages and tumor-initiating cells (TICs) in the two opposite directions is relevant to the problem [18]. The vessels can be associated or not with macrophages (Figure 2C,D) even with only one (Figure 2E). They occur obviously in circumscribed necroses (Figure 2F). Basically, any glioma-associated monocytic cell with macrophage characteristics has been called "tumor associated microglia". It shows a functional phenotype different from the inflammatory one and promotes glioma cell migration and tumor growth [19]. Migration promotion is accomplished through matrix metalloproteinases (MMPs) released by microglia [20,21] and CX3CL1 with its receptor (CX3CR1) [22]. The demonstration that microglia/macrophages promote glioma progression means that their inhibition can be a useful therapeutic tool [23]. Macrophages have long been recognized as critical components of immunity against tumors, because, when appropriately stimulated, they can attack tumor cells by contact interaction or by secreting cytotoxic and cytostatic factors [24]. However, they can also contribute to tumor development, by secretion of growth factors such as angiogenic factors, proteinases, which degrade the matrix, and immunosuppressor factors [25]. Their dual function is mainly exerted through TNF that demonstrates both an anticancer [26] and a tumorigenic activity [27]. However, it has also been shown that TNF can reduce glioma growth and prolong patient survival [28].

One specific question is the role of immune cells in the tumor microenvironment. These cells through cytokines, growth factors, chemokines and cerebrospinal fluid (CSF) interfere with tumor initiation, angiogenesis, proliferation and invasion [29]. IL-1β is the primary factor of microglia that enhances TGF-β, that, in turn, inhibits lymphocyte proliferation by suppressing antiglioma responses [30]. IL-1β also stimulates VEGF, epidermal growth factor receptor (EGFR) and MMP9 for angiogenesis, proliferation and invasion [31].

Macrophages can be subdivided into M1 and M2 subtypes, according their polarization status, supporting tumor suppression or progression, respectively [32]. As shown by the marker MHCII [33], they are strongly M2 in GBM [34]. In summary, it can be stated that macrophages support tumor progression and that tumor recruit macrophages [35]. There is an interrelationship between glioma stem cells (GSCs) and TAMs in GBM and it was shown that the former express Periostin, a member of the Fasciclin family (POSTN) [36] that has a supportive role in various tumors. TAM density correlates with POSTN in GBM and disrupting it TAM density is reduced so that GSCs secrete POSTN to recruit M2 that support tumor growth [37]. It was then showed that POSTN is highly expressed in high grade in comparison with low grade tumors [38]. How POSTN acts in potentiating tumor progression in niches has been widely discussed [39].

### 2.2. Reactive astrocytes

Reactive astrocytes can be sometimes confused with tumor cells, mainly because their phenotype changes over time until their complete maturation. There are analogies between glial reaction and physiological maturation of astrocytes during embryogenesis. In the initial phases, the fine processes originate directly from the cell soma and then from the thick and long processes [40]. Nestin and Vimentin would be the main markers of immature astrocytes whereas glial fibrillary acidic protein (GFAP) is the main marker of mature astrocytes [41,42].

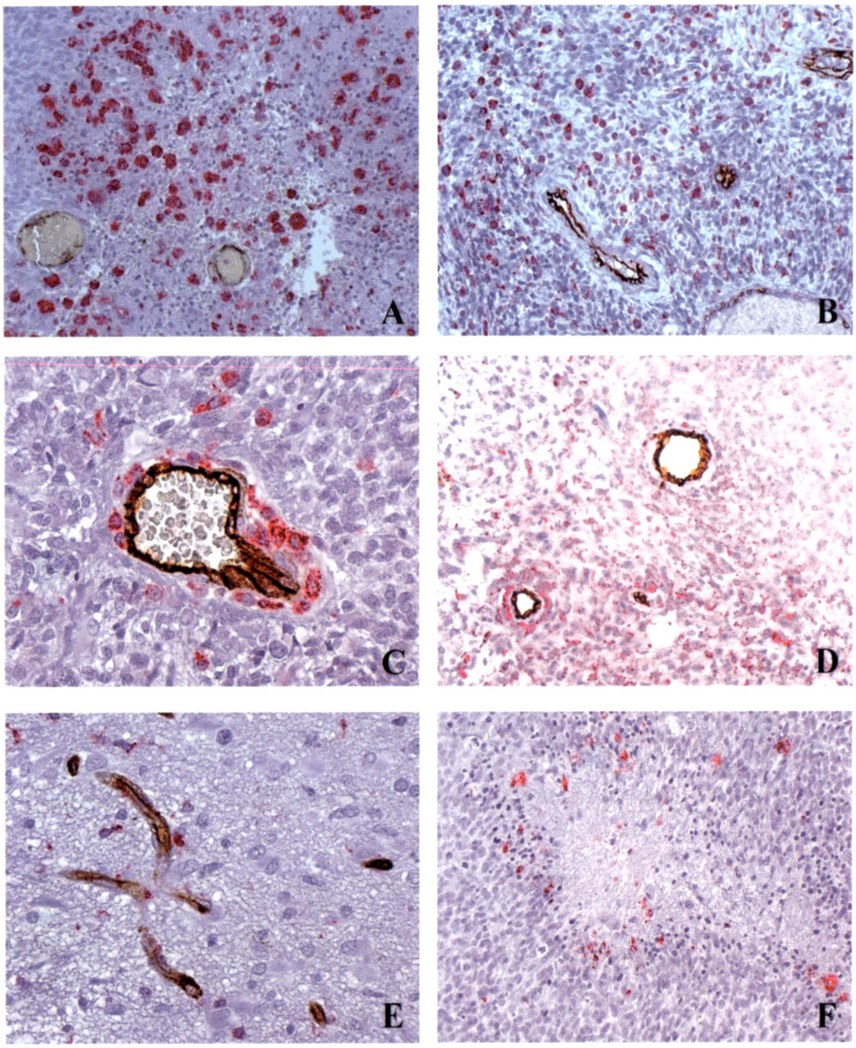


**Figure 2.** Glioblastoma. Macrophages/microglia. A – Cluster of macrophages in a proliferating area, not in relation with vessels; x200. B – Regular distribution of macrophages/microglia in a proliferating area not in relation with vessels; x200. C – Cluster of macrophages around a middle size vessel; x400. D – One vessel is surrounded by a crowd of macrophages, the other has none; x200. E – Capillaries with a macrophage adherent to the wall; x200. F – Macrophages in a perinecrotic palisade; x400. All double staining CD68-CD34, Alkaline Phosphatase Red and DAB, respectively.

It is still a debated question whether tumor infiltration can be recognized by magnetic resonance imaging (MRI), not only when adjacent to tumor, but also at distance. It has been observed, for example, that low grade gliomas, which preferentially locate in the *insula* and in

http://dx.doi.org/10.5772/58962

the supplementary motor area, spread along distinct subcortical *fasciculi* [43]. By analyzing different peritumor areas with different MRI methods, it has been shown that fractional anisotropy and not apparent diffusion coefficient can be used to evaluate glioma cell invasion. An attempt to classify different peritumoral tissues by a voxel-wise analytical solution using serial diffusion MRI has been made [44].

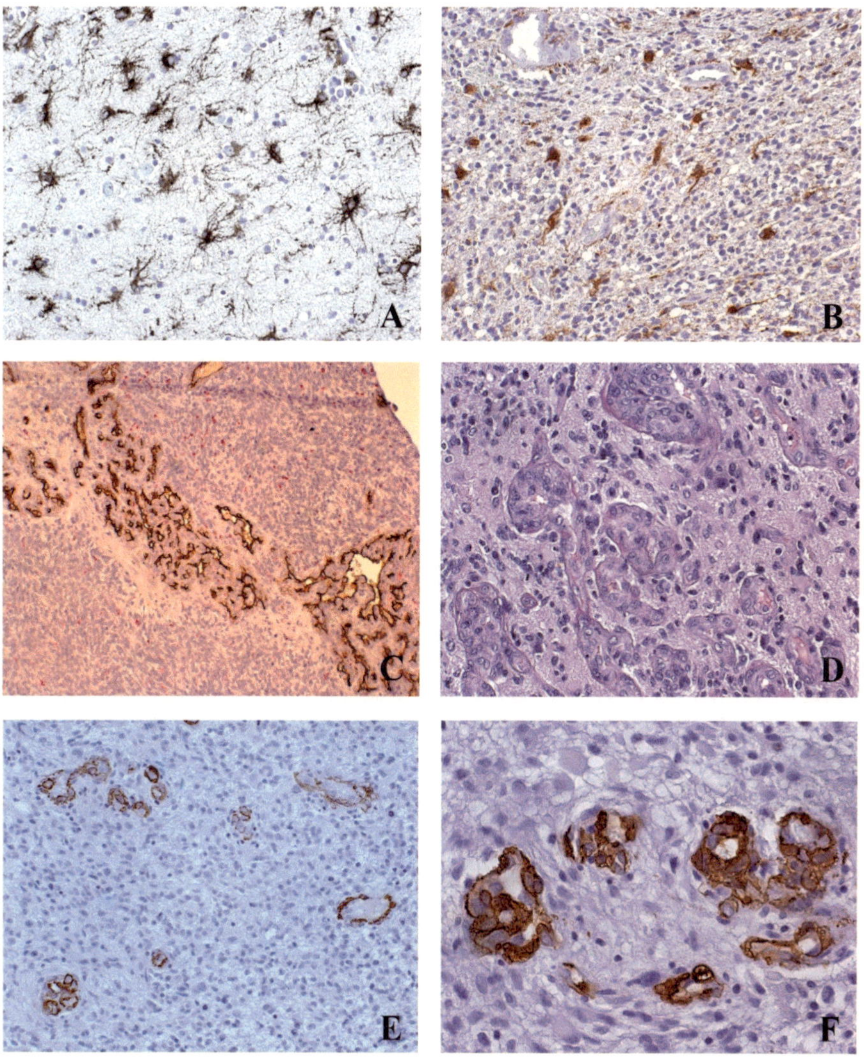


**Figure 3.** Glioblastoma. Reactive astrocytes. A – Regular distribution of reactive astrocytes in a cortex with mild infiltration. Some adhere to small vessels; GFAP, x200, DAB. B – Proliferating area with reactive astrocytes entrapped; almost only the large cytoplasm is visible; GFAP, x200, DAB. C – *Glomeruli*: multi-channel formations; double staining CD68-CD34, x100, DAB and Alkaline Phosphatase Red, respectively; D – Microvascular proliferations; x200, H&E. E – Pericytes; $\alpha$-SMA, x200, DAB. F – *Id.* x400.

Peritumoral reactive gliosis (Figure 3A) has a particular importance because of three main characteristics: reactive astrocytes divide by mitosis as tumor cells do, they progressively lose Nestin and increase GFAP expression, as during development, and they may regionally exert a series of metabolic and molecular influences [45]. The most important point is that reactive astrocytes may be included in the advancing tumor (Figure 3B), in which they progressively become no more recognizable from tumor cells. The question is whether they disappear suffocated by the high tumor cell density, or if they remain, unrecognizable from tumor cells, to contribute to the pleomorphic aspect of gliomas, or if they even can be transformed into tumor cells [46]. There are evidences that reactive astrocytes support tumor progression [2].

## 3. The glioma origin and the stem cell theory

The existence of a similarity between cancer cells and embryonic stem cells is known since Virchow [47]. Glioma cells may derive through tumor transformation from immature glia cells [48,49], or primitive neuroepithelial cells or neural stem cells (NSCs) and many experimental demonstrations are available on this matter [50,51]. Glioma-initiating cells (GICs) and GSCs [52,53] share with NSCs some properties, *i.e.* proliferation and self-renewal, and GSCs share with malignant gliomas similar genetic alterations. In contrast to the hypothesis of the transformation of NSCs or neural progenitor cells (NPCs) into GSCs [54], either occurring *in situ* during embryogenesis or during migration and their relationship with GICs, the origin of GSCs has also been referred to dedifferentiation.

Dedifferentiation may refer to two distinct biological processes. The first one is represented by a multi-step process accompanied by genetic alterations that lead to the progressive transformation of normal cells into highly malignant cells. They require self-sufficiency growth signal, insensitivity to anti-growth signals, escape from apoptosis, proliferation potential, angiogenesis and invasion [55]. By combining activation of specific oncogenes and loss of tumor suppressor genes, it is possible to induce GBM from cortical astrocytes [56]. Examples are the combination of p16(INK4a)-p19(ARF) loss with K-Ras and Akt activation [57], p16(INK4a) and p19(ARF) loss with EGFR activation [58] and p53 loss with myr-Akt and c-Myc overexpression in mature astrocytes [59]. Basically, the capacity of transformation inversely correlates with differentiation. It is easier to get transformation from Nestin+ progenitors than from mature astrocytes by Ras and Akt activation [60].

A second meaning of dedifferentiation refers to tumor cells that would acquire stemness properties instead of reflecting the nature of the primitive cells [50,61].

Today, the existence of cell subpopulations, called cancer stem cells (CSCs) or GSCs, with stem cell-like properties such as multipotency, ability to self-renewal or to form neurospheres *in vitro*, is generally accepted, also for gliomas [62].

The origin of gliomas from NSCs has been repeatedly demonstrated by the experimental induction of brain tumors by nitrosourea derivatives [63]. Moreover, NSCs have been accepted as the source of gliomas, also because the signaling that regulates their self-renewal, proliferation and differentiation occurs, altered, in gliomas. Several studies demonstrated that GBM may arise from the subventricular zone (SVZ) [64,65] that is the source of stem cells and progenitors in adults [66,67]. The latter are represented by neuroblasts (type A cells) and oligodendrocyte precursor cells (OPCs), by quiescent type B cells that give origin to highly proliferative cells, and by transit-amplifying progenitor cells (type C cells), that differentiate into two lineage-restricted progenitor cells [68,69]. These cells accumulate mutations up to give rise to gliomas [70], not excluding the intervention of human Cytomegalovirus (HCMV) [71].

GBM is a heterogeneous tumor and its heterogeneity might be explained by either the hierarchical model mechanism [72] or the stochastic mechanism of development [73]. Progenitor cells are at risk of malignant transformation since they show the activation of the adequate cell machinery, represented by telomerase activity, promitotic and antiapoptotic genes [54]. Abnormal developmental patterns are Sonic hedgehog (Shh) pathway, EGFR and phosphatase and tensin homologue (PTEN) signaling. Although their clonal origin is from a small fraction of transformed NSCs, gliomas are heterogeneous as a consequence of an anomalous tumor cell differentiation [74]. The diversity within gliomas is due to changes of the subclones, being all of them generated by multipotent tumor cells, but also through an arrest of the differentiation process.

Recently, other cells have been supposed to give origin to GBM.

## 4. Origin of GSCs and glioma heterogeneity

The hypothesis of GSCs is based on the concept that a rare subset of cells within GBM may have significant expansion capacity and the ability to generate new tumors [72]. The remainder of tumor cells, which predominantly resemble GBM, may represent partially differentiated cells with limited progenitor capacity or terminally differentiated non-tumorigenic cells. A possible origin of gliomas is also from mature astrocytes by acquiring stemness properties through a dedifferentiation process, as above mentioned [54,75] or from NG2 cells that fit better with tumors arising far from the ventricles or with secondary GBMs [76]. Also reactive astrocytes can be candidate for gliomas [77,78], since they can acquire a stem-like phenotype [79].

In spite of the great similarity between SVZ NSCs or progenitors and GICs, the relationship with GSCs remains unresolved. Are they equivalent, or the latter have nothing to share with the former, if not the stemness properties? An answer can be that over time GICs can acquire sufficient alterations to engender GSCs. GICs are the first genetically aberrant cells that can initiate tumor development and that are responsible for the bulk of tumor cells. OPCs, the major dividing cell population in the adult brain that gives origin to oligodendrocytes, distributed in the SVZ and in the gray and white matter, remain a further unresolved problem. The EGFR and prostaglandin-endoperoxide synthase 2 (PTGS2) inhibition prevents the tumorigenesis of transformed OPCs and GICs for anaplastic oligodendroglioma but not the tumorigenesis of transformed NSCs or GICs for GBM, suggesting that the latter can arise from OPCs or NSCs [80].

In mice models, by using the retrovirus replication-competent avian sarcoma-leukosis virus long terminal repeat with splice acceptor (RCAS) [81], OPCs expressing 2′, 3′-cyclic-nucleotide 3′-phosphodiesterase (CNP) could be targeted later in their development or in the adult. Low grade oligodendrogliomas were obtained by RCAS-platelet-derived growth factor subunit beta (PDGF-β) expressing OPC markers such as sex-determining region Y (SRY)-box2 (SOX2), oligodendrocyte transcription factor 2 (OLIG2), NG2 and PDGF receptor (PDGFR), interpreted as indicating a slight dedifferentiation of tumor cells [82]. OPCs could serve as cells of origin of gliomas [83]. According to the already mentioned experiments by mosaic analysis with double markers (MADM), aberrant growth of precancerous lesions could only be found in cells differentiated along the oligodendrocyte lineage to become OPCs but not in any other lineage or in NSCs [84]. These demonstrations, however, do not exclude that aberrant growth can occur in NSCs, responsible for a direct origin of malignant tumors.

Heterogeneity in gliomas is not due to the occurrence in the same tumor of different non-tumor cells of various species, but to the cellular complexity formed by tumor cells that differ among themselves for a series of phenotypic and molecular characteristics affecting cell proliferation, invasion, *etc.* [85,86]. Cells are at risk of transformation only when demanded to proliferate, such as progenitors, opposite, for example, to B cells of SVZ that are protected [87]. The passage from B cells to amplifying cells implies a chromatin rearrangement from a quiescent to a proliferating status where genetic lesions, if not repaired, pass to the following dividing cells. There are interactions among DNA repair, epigenetics and stem cells. In the niche a homeostatic regulation of stem cells occurs, with a balance between self-renewal and differentiation, and with proliferation starting in response to a stimulating signal. Uncontrolled proliferation would take place when stem cells become independent of growth signal, because of mutations, or they resist anti-growth signals [88]. The homeostatic balance would be regulated by the interaction between Wnt/β-catenin pathway, that promotes cell growth, and bone morphogenetic protein (BMP) signaling that inhibits it. This can be the starting point of heterogeneity, largely dependent on the microenvironment. Gliomas with different genetic signatures may as well originate from different cell subtypes [89].

The same molecular mechanisms of NSCs regulate gliomas [90] that can undergo epigenetic changes and genetic mutations favoring evolution toward malignancy. During their lifespan, they can be exposed to genotoxic stress, to which they respond through repair mechanisms [76]. GBM has many molecular signatures depending on its polyclonality, and the events themselves may have an effect on the clonality. The greater is the potency of stem cells, the more anaplastic is the tumor.

The molecular profile of malignant gliomas has led to the distinction of proneural, proliferative and mesenchymal types associated to NSC profiles [91] or to the distinction of proneural, classic and mesenchymal types, the former expressing genes associated to progenitors and the latter two to stem cells [92]. The stemness would reflect the cell of origin, but it could also be acquired in the niche in adult gliomas [93]. On this basis, the contrasting results obtained on GBM can be explained by the finding of different series of TICs characterized by different phenotypic and molecular profiles [86,94].

## 5. Migration of NSCs or NPCs toward tumors

NPCs can migrate from the SVZ toward a tumor and target it [95]. Today, this migration may represent a new goal for therapeutic purposes. NSCs exhibit tumor-homing capability. In mice experiments, immortalized murine NSCs, implanted into glioma-bearing rodents, distributed within and around tumors, even migrating to the contralateral hemisphere [96]. Genetically engineered NSCs show a tropism for gliomas, on which may have an adverse effect [97-100], especially if they are also transduced with herpes simplex virus-thymidine kinase (HSVtk) gene and followed by the administration of systemic Ganciclovir [101-103]. Human NSCs implanted in rat brains containing a C6 glioma, migrated in the direction of the expanding tumor [104]. The same properties are shown by mesenchymal stem cells (MSCs) injected either into carotid arteries or intracerebrally [105,106] and by hematopoietic progenitor cells [107]. Endogeneous progenitor cells have been observed to migrate from the SVZ toward a murine experimental GBM [108]. The migrated Nestin+ cells were also actively cycling, as shown by Ki-67/MIB.1 positivity, and 35% of them expressed Musashi-1 [109]. In transgenic mice, virally labeled proliferating cells of the SVZ demonstrated that NPCs accumulate around gliomas, diverted from their physiological migratory pathway to the olfactory bulb [110].

Chemokines, angiogenic cytokines and glioma-produced ECM can play a role in the NSC tropism [111]. It is possible to take advantage of the natural capacity of chemokines to initiate migratory responses and to use this ability to enhance the tumor inhibitory capacity by NPCs to target an intracranially growing glioma [112]. The therapeutic possibilities offered by NSCs are continuously increasing. For example, they can be engineered as sources of secreted therapeutics, exploiting their mobility toward CNS lesions. They could function as minipumps [113].

Rat embryonic progenitor cells, transplanted at distance from a glioma grown in the *striatum*, migrate and co-localize with it. They modify their phenotype, express Vimentin and reduce the tumor volume, demonstrating that a cross-talk exists between them and the tumor [114]. It has been shown that hypoxia is a key factor in determining NSC tropism to glioma by stromal-derived factor 1 (SDF-1) and its receptor (CXCR4), urokinase-type plasminogen activator (uPA) and its receptor (uPAR) and VEGF and its receptor (VEGFR) [115]. It could be interesting to try to enhance motility of adult NSCs toward CNS injury or disease and to take into account that EGFR could play a role, because of its participation to malignant transformation [116]. It has also been recognized that a limitation exists to the possibility of migration of neural precursors from SVZ to an induced cortical GBM in mice. The limitation is caused by the age and the proliferation potential of the SVZ. Adult mice supply fewer cells than younger mice, depending on the expression of D-type Cyclins, because with aging Cyclin D1 is lost and only Cyclin D2 is expressed [110]. Recently, novel treatment strategies using NSCs have been proposed, for example the suicide gene therapy using converting enzymes [117]. New strategies will emerge from further NSC and brain tumor stem cell (BTSC) studies [118]. Is it possible that tumors grow from transplanted NSCs [119]?

## 6. Perivascular niches (PVN). Relationship between NPCs/GSCs and endothelial cells

GBM is composed of three concentric zones: a central necrotic area, surrounded by an intermediate zone containing large vessels with thrombosis or altered walls; a surrounding proliferation zone that abruptly or progressively flows into the normal tissue and invades it [63]. Neo-angiogenesis takes place in the proliferating zone or in normal surrounding tissue after tumor cell invasion. In the latter, new capillaries are formed from the pre-existing venules. Basically, new capillary formation is due to the endothelial proliferation that mimics angiogenesis in normal embryonic conditions, with buds and new tubule formation. In comparison with normal angiogenesis, tumor angiogenesis is often dysregulated until the formation of *glomeruli* (Figure 3C). In the invasion zone, tumor cells wrap around vessels (co-option). In invaded cortex, the vascular tree coming down from the meningeal vessels is assailed by advancing and invading tumor cells and it progressively deforms through endothelial cell hypertrophy and hyperplasia. It becomes less adequate to perfuse the increased mass of tumor cells coming up from the white matter, because transformed into a lumpy tree with irregular lumina. The generated microvascular proliferations (MVPs) (Figure 3D) are mainly found at the transition from central necrosis to the proliferation zone, where circumscribed necroses with pseudopalisading develop [120]. As a consequence, areas very rich in capillaries and small vessels, produced by an intense angiogenesis, coexist in tumors beside areas poorly vascularized where necroses develop.

Vasculogenesis is a mechanism of tumor neovascularization that has been also attributed to circulating bone marrow (BM)-derived cells known as endothelial progenitor cells (EPCs). Its importance is debated [121,122], but it was shown that mesenchymal progenitors from bone marrow can differentiate into proliferating endothelial cells [123,124]. Also BM-derived TAMs, including TIE-2 expressing monocytes/macrophages (TEMs), circulate in the blood, home at sites of pathological neovascularization and differentiate into endothelial cells or macrophages [125,126].

Another type of vascularization is represented by the "vascular mimicry" due to the capacity of tumor cells to form a functional net of channels coated by themeselves. Two types of vascular mimicry have been described. The patterned matrix type is composed of a basement membrane, lined by tumor cells, forming channels with flowing blood [127]. Vasculogenic mimicry of the tubular type may be morphologically confused with endothelial cell-lined blood vessels. In both types, cells express endothelium-associated genes, as in embryonic vasculogenesis [128,129]. These properties are associated with CSCs [130]. By fluorescent *in situ* hybridization (FISH) and immunophenotyping, these non-endothelial cell-lined vessels have been demonstrated to be primary tumor cells. *In vitro* CD133+ GSCs are vasculogenetic even with vascular smooth muscle-like cell differentiation. The cells do not express CD34 and show EGFR gene amplification [131]. It must be remarked, however, that usually cells of tumor vessels and MVPs never show either isocitrate dehydrogenase 1 and 2 (IDH1/2) mutations or EGFR gene amplification, never exceeding 1 or 2 copies [132]. They do not share with tumor cells genetic alterations and this is in line with the lack of TP53 mutations in MVPs [133].

In tumors transplanted into mice and irradiated, recruitment through hypoxia of BM-derived cells occurs, able to restore circulation through SDF1 and CXCR4 [134]; among these cells, EPCs prevail [121,135-137]. Vasculogenesis can be blocked by pharmacological inhibition or antibodies toward SDF1 and CXCR4 [134].

Interestingly, also a GBM-endothelial cell transdifferentiation is considered to contribute to tumor vascularization, favored by hypoxia [138], independently of VEGF [139]. It has been observed that a quota of GBM CD31+ endothelial cells shares with tumors cells chromosomal aberrations [140] and that a quota of GBM CD105+ endothelial cells harbours the same somatic mutations identified within tumor cells, such as amplification of EGFR and chromosome 7 [141]. In a GBM model, it was demonstrated that the tumor-derived endothelial cells originated from TICs [138]. This finding is of paramount importance because of the possibility to use an anti-VEGF antibody (Bevacizumab) for therapy [142]. Unfortunately, the effects of the drug are only transient [143] and the reason of the failure is the activation of other pro-angiogenic pathways, the recruitment of BM-derived cells and the increase of pericyte protection and tumor invasion [144,145]. The possibility that the tumor becomes more aggressive after therapy has been contemplated [146].

The problem of transdifferentiation and the role that CSCs play in this process are still under discussion [139]. All the observations have been made in animals or from animal models, and *in vivo* experiments of transdifferentiation have been challenged [85]. In human pathology, the contribution of tumor cells to the GBM vasculature has never been demonstrated and vessel cells with typical genetic changes of tumor cells, such as those of EGFR, PDGFR, PTEN, TP53, IDH1/2 have never been found in GBM [132].

By intussusception, pre-existing brain capillaries can be multiplied by transluminal endothelial bridges and by lumen partitioning; it is an early phenomenon [147].

As NPCs or NSCs reside in the normal SVZ niche at close contact with endothelial cells, in GBM, GSCs and/or NPCs are located in PVN. In the latter, a strict similarity exists with what happens in the normal SVZ niche, where the intimate association between normal NSCs and endothelial cells regulates self-renewal and differentiation of the former. In PVN, angiogenesis is activated by VEGF produced by NSCs/GSCs [88,148], whereas their stemness is maintained by Notch produced by endothelial cells through nitric oxide [19,149,150]. Notch is constitutively active in high grade gliomas and conditions their progression [104]. PVNs are strictly correlated with tumor progression. There would be a bidirectional communication between endothelial cells and TICs or GSCs [151].

The PVN composition has been carefully described in GBM, with the inclusion, beside cells of the environment, of ECM, integrins, cell adhesion signaling, cadherin family, *etc.* [152]. In GBMs, strong evidence for the existence of an endothelial mesenchymal transition (EMT) process is still lacking, but this process is increasingly reported as instrumental to tumor growth and diffusion [153,154]. It is defined by the possibility that differentiated epithelial cells establish stable contacts with neighbor cells, assume a mesenchymal cell phenotype with loss of cell-cell interactions, reduce cellular adhesion, active production of ECM proteases, increase cytoskeletal dynamics and changes in transcription factor expression, and acquire a stem cell program, all of them leading to increased migration and invasion ability [155]. The three major groups of transcription factors, the SNAI, Twist-related protein 1 (TWIST1) and Zinc-finger enhancer binding (ZEB) family members, have been reported to be altered in GBM. Their over-expression follows the activation of Wnt/β-catenin pathway and results *in vitro* in an increased cell migration and invasion [156,157]. It is likely that the high expression of mesenchymal genes in the mesenchymal subset of human GBMs [91] can be considered to be reminiscent of the EMT program [92] or that the aberrant activation of EMT factors during gliomagenesis can trigger the mesenchymal shift in GBM [158].

The influence that GSCs can exert on BM-derived endothelial cells has been summarized as follows [159]: to elicit angiogenesis, to home at the tumor the BM-derived EPCs and to promote their differentiation into blood vessels that incorporate into the existing vasculature. Trans-differentiation into endothelial-like cells contributes to the formation of blood vessels [140,160].

The PVN concept was substantiated by the demonstration of Nestin+ and CD133+ cells on capillaries, forming a microvasculature in which the microenvironment that maintains CSCs and their renewal is given by endothelial cells that, in turn, are stimulated by CSCs [149]. A positive correlation was found between the CD133+ niches and CD133+ blood vessels, similar to the correlation between the Nestin+ niches and Nestin+ blood vessels [161]. A good PVN demonstration has been given [2] and beautiful and useful schemes have been provided [159, 162]. It can be added that angiogenesis and self-renewal would represent a resistance to chemo- and radio-therapy.

The location of GSCs in PVN was confirmed by several studies using either CD133 positivity [163] or side population signature genes, such as aspartate beta-hydroxylase domain-containing protein 2 (ASPHD2) or nuclear factor erythroid 2-related factor 2 (NFE2L2) or hypoxia-inducible factor 2 (HIF-2) [164]; they increase with malignancy [161]. By comparing xenografts of C6 glioma with a high or low fraction of GSCs, it was observed that the former exhibit an increased microvessel density and an increased recruitment of BM-derived endothelial progenitors [123]. The relevance of the hypoxia will be discussed later.

### 6.1. Pericytes

Pericytes, the last PVN component, are perivascular cells that support blood vessels [165], control blood vessel stability, function through paracrine factors and direct cell-cell contacts, and promote vascular maturation (Figure 3E,F). They express different markers including PDGFR-β, α-smooth muscle Actin (α-SMA), Desmin, and NG2. They originate from mesoderm-derived MSCs or from neuroectoderm-derived neural crest cells, depending on their location within the brain. Pericytes are an essential element of the neurovascular unit and contribute to the function of blood-brain-barrier (BBB) [166]. Gliomas can induce the differentiation of MSCs into pericytes [167]. MSCs injected into brain tumors in mouse models have been shown to closely associate with the tumor vasculature and also with up-regulation of the expression of pericyte markers [168].

Pathology observations show that pericytes increase in number in GBM and wrap around vessels with endothelial hyperplasia.

## 7. PVN neuropathology

The description of the niches must be obviously a survey of the different vascular structures in GBM with their surrounding cell components. The first question to give an answer is: does each vascular structure represent a niche, or are they distributed in the tumor and how? The second question is: is the cell composition of the niches a constant one or does it vary from one another? In the literature, GSCs have been demonstrated in perivascular position [149], as well in perinecrotic niches [164,169] as discussed later. Good schemes of PVN are provided including all the cells that can be encountered in such position [62,159,162]. Such schemes, obviously, are not encounted as real occurrences in the histological examination of GBMs.

By examining the vascular structures in the different tumor zones, in infiltration areas capillaries, arterioles, venules or penetrating vessels from the meninges occur. Around them, there are tumor stem cells/progenitors, often forming cuffings (co-option), or Nestin+ cells adherent to the walls, or reactive GFAP+ astrocytes (Figure 4A–D). Scattered in the tissue, microglia/macrophages occur rather regularly, occasionally distributed in perivascular position (Figure 2). Reactive astrocytes continue to be present also in more intense infiltration, recognizable for their GFAP positivity and for what remains of their long and thick processes; however, they are regularly distributed in the tumor tissue and occasionally they can be found in perivascular position.

In areas of intense tumor cell proliferation, many small vessels can be found either with or without endothelial hyperplasia, sometimes forming a dense net. Around them, tumor cells, mostly Nestin+ and SOX2+, crowded, that can easily be considered as undifferentiated and containing sometimes cells with stemness properties, associated with occasional CD68+ cells. In proliferating areas, larger vessels can be found, with walls thicker than in capillaries, surrounded by a dense cuffing of cells that are Nestin+ in the inner part and GFAP+ outside (Figure 4E,F). In most vessels, pericytes appear wrapping the channel outside the endothelial cell layer; they are well evident in MVPs or in *glomeruli* that, on the other hand, do not appear to be surrounded by other cell types, if not tumor cells.

In intermediate areas or near the central necrosis, many vessels of different size and nature are associated with edema or tissue dissociation and they do not show to be surrounded by any special cell kind. Scattered in the tumor, myeloid cells can be found in variable quantity, associated or not with other types of cells among which macrophages seem to be the most frequent. Microglia/macrophages are distributed in small or large clusters around necroses or around vessels where they can be associated or not with some of the other cell types. The association with myeloid cells is the most striking.

The neuropathological study provides the information that PVN represents a theoretical picture where the different cell types can be represented and where cross-talks occur among the different signalings that support some tumor activities such as invasion, growth, *etc.* Of course, the most important dialogue in these structures occurs between GSCs and endothelial cells, and this is feasible around capillaries and small vessels, even though the thickness of the vessel walls could not in absolute be an insuperable obstacle.

## 8. Hypoxia and necroses – Perinecrotic niches

In GBM, there are two main types of necrosis: large necroses, usually at the tumor center, of thrombotic origin, and circumscribed necroses, occurring in the proliferative areas and representing a hallmark of the tumor. Hypoxia is, therefore, a tumor characteristic [170], mediated by HIF-1/2 composed of two subunits, an oxygen insensitive HIF-$\beta$ subunit and an oxygen regulated HIF-$\alpha$ subunit [171]. Under normoxic conditions, HIF-$\alpha$ is rapidly degraded following hydroxylation by the oxygen-dependent prolyl-hydroxylase domain proteins (PHDs), that mark it for ubiquitination and proteasomal degradation [172]. Hypoxia stabilizes HIF-1$\alpha$ by preventing its hydroxylation and degradation; together with HIF-2$\alpha$, it is critically involved in the regulation of GSCs [164]. Hypoxia directly promotes the GSCs expansion. In human GBM biopsies, GSCs are enriched in perinecrotic regions, where the oxygen tension is reduced and HIF-1$\alpha$ and HIF-2$\alpha$ are activated [164,173]. HIF-2$\alpha$ remains elevated under chronic hypoxia, while HIF-1$\alpha$ is only transiently upregulated [174].

Hypoxia through HIF-1$\alpha$ promotes the expansion of GSCs through the phosphatidylinositol 3-kinase (PI3K)/Akt and ERK1/2 pathways, the inhibition of which reduces the fraction of CD133+ GSCs [175]. In perinecrotic regions hypoxia regulates many properties [159]. In GSCs under hypoxic conditions, it activates Notch by inducing its ligands and the activation of target genes Hes1 and Hey2 [164,176]. Blockade of Notch signaling with $\gamma$-secretase inhibitors depletes the GSC population, reduces the expression of GSC markers such as CD133, Nestin, Bmi1 and OLIG2 and inhibits the growth of tumor neurospheres and xenografts [177].

GSCs can be demonstrated to lie around circumscribed necroses or scattered in the tissue by CD133 positivity [169] or other specific antigens [164].

Hypoxia is generally realized when tumor growth exceeds neovascularization, and it would not only regulate tumor cell proliferation, metabolism, differentiation, but also induce key stem cell genes such as Nanog, Oct4 and c-Myc [178].

Necroses are the place where hypoxia occurs, but it must be taken into account that usually its occurrence is histologically deduced from its pathologic effects, *i.e.*, necrosis in the tissue. Hypoxia at its very beginning could not yet be visible as necrosis, but already efficient for other signs. It is possible that tissue features in an area not suspected to be hypoxic, are indeed due to hypoxia. An example is given by apoptosis. Apoptotic nuclei are found in proliferating tumor areas due to an intrinsic or transcriptional pathway *via* mitochondria and focused on TP53 [179], or in hypoxic areas through an extrinsic pathway or TNF [180].

It is, however, possible that isolated apoptotic nuclei in a proliferating area are not due to the first type of apoptosis, *i.e.* the intrinsic one, but to the extrinsic type, consequence of a not yet morphologically evident hypoxia [181]. As a matter of fact, HIF-1$\alpha$ expression can be mainly demonstrated around circumscribed necroses, but also in scattered cells in proliferating areas (Figure 5A,B) [45].

Circumscribed necroses in GBM are the hallmark of the tumor, but their origin and development are still discussed. They have been carefully described and codified [139,182,183] as due to an ischemic process following a vascular occlusion or to a pathology of the endothelium.

http://dx.doi.org/10.5772/58962

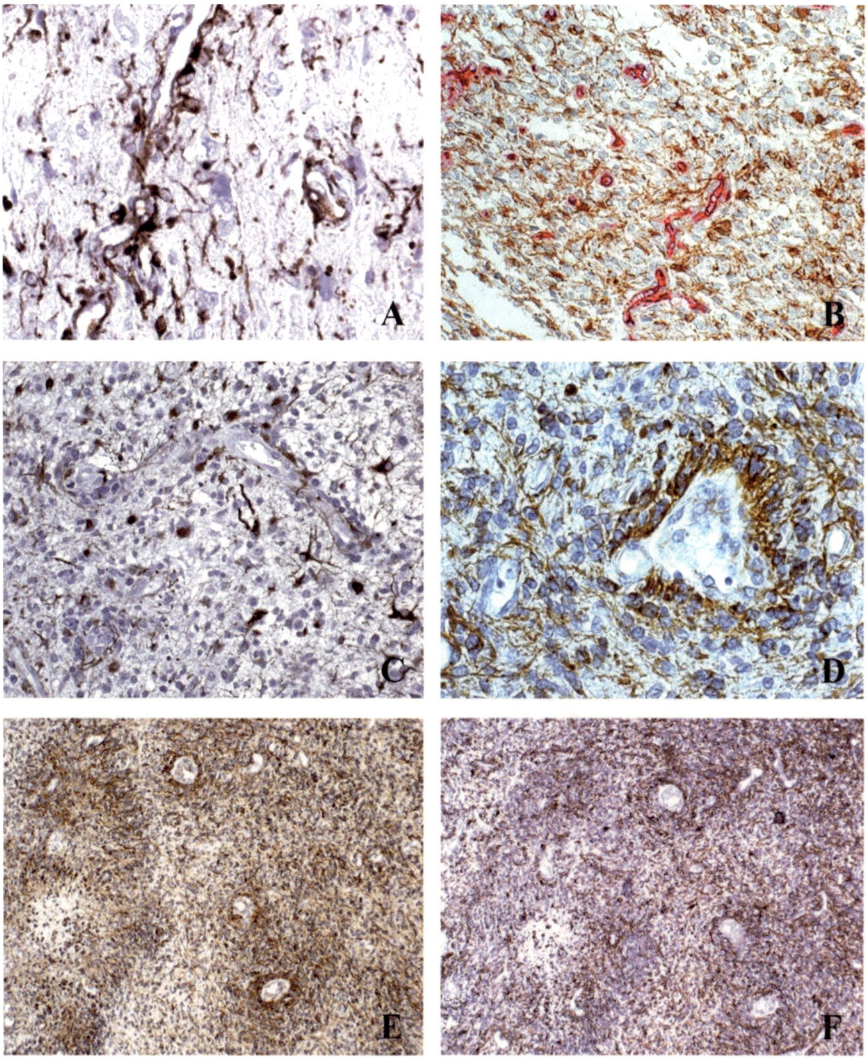


**Figure 4.** Glioblastoma. D – Nestin+ tumor cells adhere to small vessels; Nestin, x200, DAB. B – GFAP+ cells scattered in the tissue or in relation with vessels directly or by vascular feet: tumor cells or reactive astrocytes; double staining GFAP-CD34, x200, DAB and Alkaline Phosphatase Red, respectively. C – *Id.* with a cuffing of GAFP+ cells in the outer layer; GFAP, x200, DAB. D – Cuffing of Nestin+ cells on a medium size vessel; Nestin, DAB, x200. E – Infiltrative area with Nestin+ cells on small vessels; Nestin, x200, DAB. F – *Id.* Some GFAP+ tumor cells adhere to vessels; GFAP, x200, DAB.

The consequent hypoxia would stimulate angiogenesis, through HIF-1 and VEGF. Another interpretation can be given: necroses develop in hyperproliferating areas, with a high Ki-67/ MIB.1 labeling index (LI) and a high Nestin expression in comparison with GFAP, due to the focal insufficiency of angiogenesis to feed a very large number of tumor cells, because of the imbalance between the high tumor cell proliferation capacity and the low one of endothelial cells (Figure 6A–F and Figure 7) [184-186].

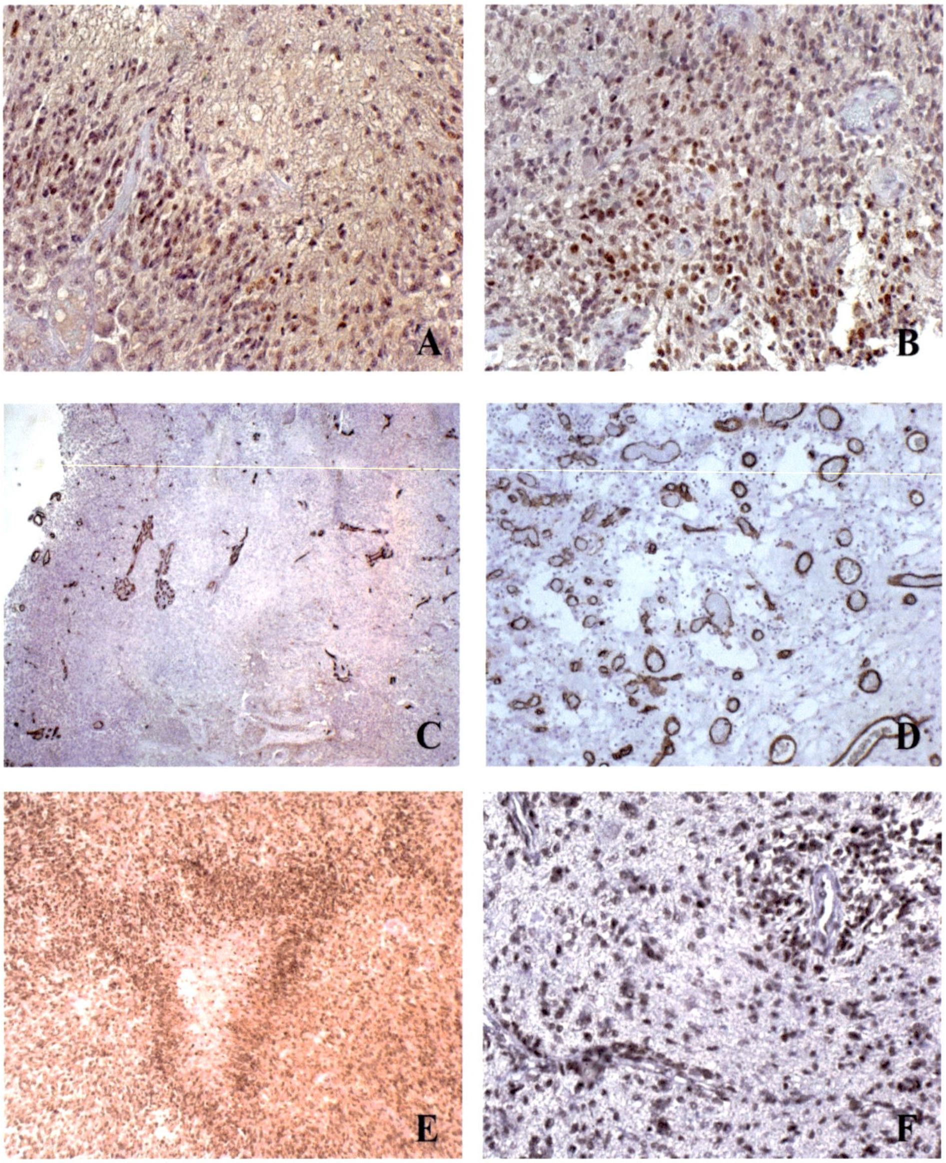


**Figure 5.** Glioblastoma. A – HIF-1+ cells in perinecrotic position; HIF-1, x200, DAB. B – HIF-1+ cells scattered in a proliferative area; HIF-1, x200, DAB. C – A large avascular area; CD34, x25, DAB. D – High vessel density; CD34, x100, DAB. E – Perinecrotic palisade with high density of SOX2+ cells; SOX2, x200, DAB. F – Cuffing of SOX2+ cells around vessels; SOX2, x200, DAB.

This observation does not exclude that inside necroses regressive pathological vessels occur [183]. In GBMs, beside areas with a high vessel density due to an active neoangiogenesis, large avascular areas occur where necroses develop (Figure 5C,D).

http://dx.doi.org/10.5772/58962

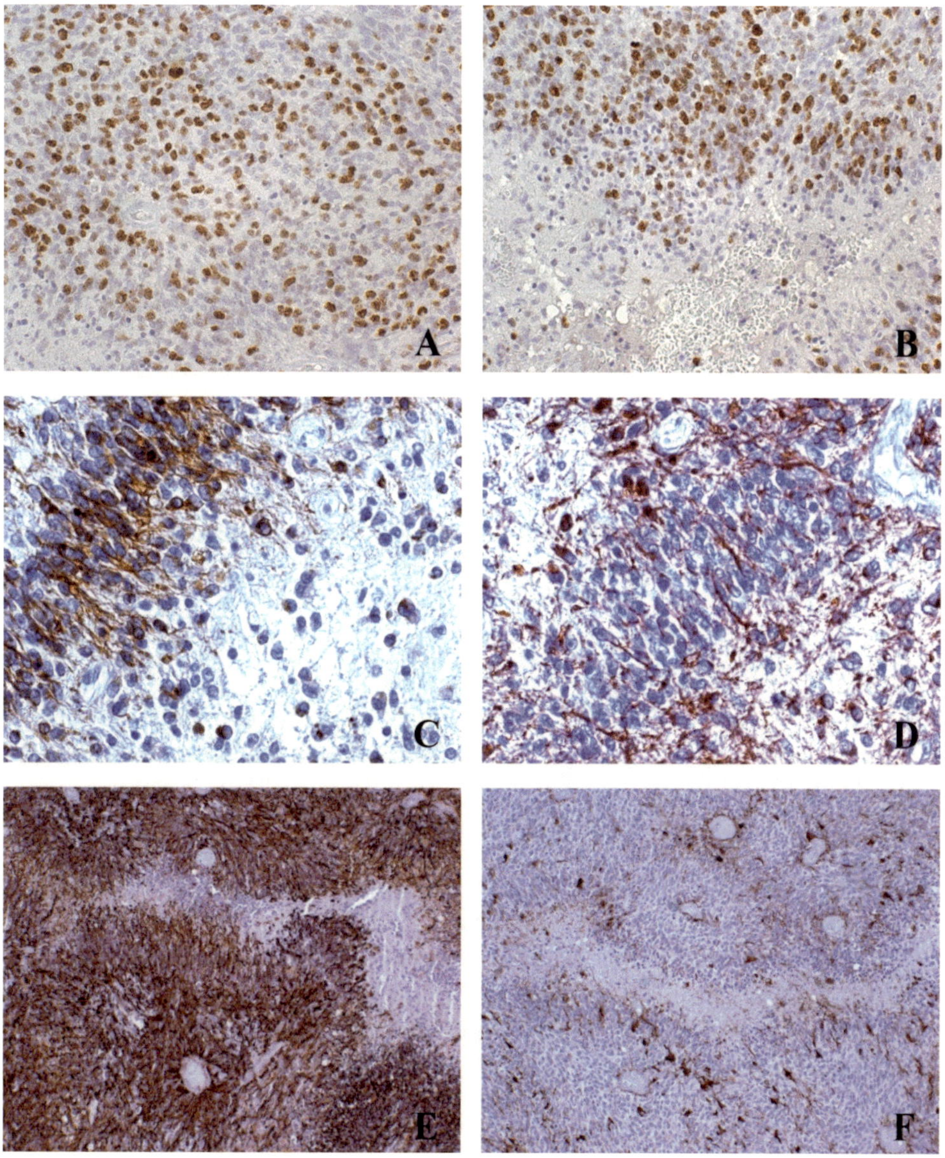


**Figure 6.** Glioblastoma. A – High Ki-67/MIB.1 labeling index (LI) in a hyperproliferating area; Ki-67/MIB.1, x200, DAB. B – High Ki67/MIB.1 LI in the perinecrotic palisade; Ki-67/MIB.1, x200, DAB. C – Perinecrotic palisade with high density of Nestin+ cells; Nestin, x400, DAB. D – *Id.* with only rare GFAP+ cells; GFAP, x400, DAB. E – A circumscribed necrosis in hyperproliferating Nestin+ area; Nestin, x200, DAB. F – *Id.* only rare GFAP+ tumor cells; GFAP, x200, DAB.

The palisades would be the remnants of the hyperproliferating area after necrosis development. Both are composed of a high number of cells positive for stemness markers such as CD133, Nestin, SOX2, and RE-1-silencing transcription factor (REST), and have a high proliferation index (Figure 5E,F) [163,187,188]. GSCs can be conceived as deriving from dedifferentiated tumor cells that acquired stemness properties [189]; they would be concentrated in the above mentioned malignant tumor areas where circumscribed necroses develop because of the vascular insufficiency. It is likely that GSCs around necroses represent the quota of GSCs that populated the hyperproliferating areas and remained unaffected by necrosis development. The palisadings themselves would be the remnants of hyperproliferating areas, spared by necrosis [45,189].

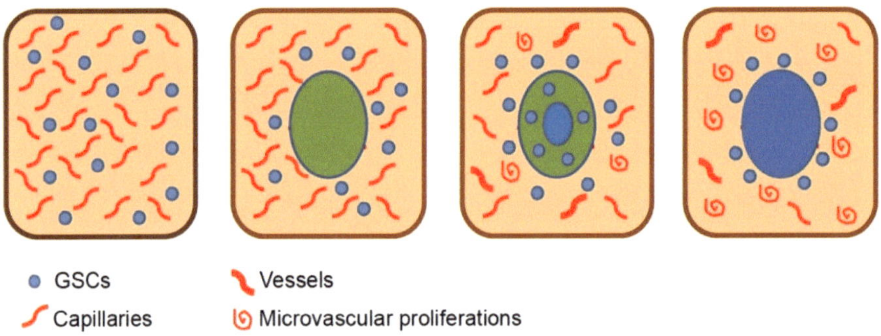


**Figure 7.** Progression from hyperproliferating areas with GSCs/progenitors → development of avascular area → appearance of necrosis → necrosis surrounded by GSCs/progenitors.

## 9. Functions of the niches in the tumor and their interdependence

The GSC maintenance is provided by the signalings that occur in the niches; they can expand and form new ones that, in turn, drive the tumor growth [190]. Signalings involved in the GSC regulation are Oct4, c-Myc, Notch, TGF-β, Wnt/β-catenin pathways. Genes associated with shorter patient survival, as already observed [91], are overexpressed in the side population found by Seidel *et al* [164] and, *viceversa,* downregulated in those associated with longer survival. The overexpression concerns more primary than secondary glioblastomas that show a reduced CSC component [191] that, however, may still support tumor growth.

Perivascular and perinecrotic niches are not separated entities, first of all for temporal reasons. Hypoxia is the main cause of angiogenesis, but this is realized through factors, such as VEGF, Angiopoietin 1 and 2, SDF1 produced by GSCs and, at the same time, the imbalance between the high proliferation rate of tumor cells and the low one of endothelial cells makes angiogenesis insufficient and causes necrosis development. Moreover, besides tumor areas rich in small neo-formed vessels and capillaries, MVPs due to a dysregulated angiogenesis do not show sufficient exchanges with tumor cells and are responsible for hypoxia [63]. Another important question, widely discussed [172], is how hypoxia and the vasculature regulate macrophages and immune cells through HIFs and nuclear factor kappa-light-chain-enhancer of activated B cells (NF-kB) [192,193] and CXCR4 [194].

It cannot be established whether GSCs of perivascular and perinecrotic niches belong to the same population, because, although showing the same stemness antigens, they still represent progenitors that can be in different state of differentiation. The significance conferred to GSCs in perinecrotic position as dedifferentiated tumor cells which reached stemness beyond a certain point of dedifferentiation, cannot be recognized to GSCs in perivascular niches [45,189]. Letting aside the transdifferentiation of tumor cells into endothelial cells, which did not received sufficient support, another point of link between the two microenvironments is represented by cell migration through EMT that is promoted by hypoxia and bound to GSCs [155]. GSCs can migrate along newly formed vessels and favor tumor diffusion.

The most important question in this topic is the occurrence of circumscribed necroses in the tumor areas with the highest malignant phenotype including both avascular districts and districts with a high vessel density, so that perinecrotic niches appear to be associated with perivascular niches to characterize these malignant areas [45,189,195].

## 10. Conclusions

The origin of gliomas has been outlined as traceable back to the transformation of primitive neuroepithelial cells or NSCs, capable of self-renewal and proliferation, *i.e.* endowed with stemness properties, or to the dedifferentiation of adult glia to reach stemness properties. The CSC responsibility for tumor proliferation, recurrence and resistance to therapies falls today into the most credited hypothesis. Many experiments have shown that GSCs derive by transformation of NSCs or they represent a simple functional stemness status. Some aspects of the problem remain unresolved, for example, the relationship between TICs and CSCs or the CSCs location in the tumor, as well as the existence in the tumor of NSCs that continuously renew the CSCs quota.

Recently, a new concept arose to indicate everything in the tumor, outside cancer cells, that regulates tumor proliferation, invasion, differentiation, resistance to therapies as the microenvironment, with its innumerable molecular pathways and numberless signalings and cross-talks. Major expressions of the microenvironment are in GBM the perivascular and the perinecrotic niches. The former are important for the endothelial cell/CSC relationship that, on one side, maintains the stemness status of CSCs and, on the other side, gives origin to angiogenesis. The latter are important for the occurrence of hypoxia through HIF-1/2 that can induce CSC formation.

The neuropathological study of GBMs with the final goal to find a concrete expression to the perinecrotic niche concept, provides an alternative interpretation to that considering perinecrotic CSCs as induced by hypoxia. They can be the remnants of CSCs that crowded the hyperproliferating and malignant areas of the tumor in which necrosis developed for insufficient vascularization. Perivascular niches are usually very well depicted as schemes that contemplate all the cells that can be in contact with vessels/endothelial cells. This event, however, is not observed to be realized with all the identified cells in all the vessels, going from capillaries or small vessels to larger vessels, MVPs or *glomeruli* in the different tumor areas. The cells described in the schemes never occur concurrently in one or all the vessels, so that the schemes themselves remain as a theoretical indication of possible relationships that can be established between tumor cells and vessels as a consequence of a general molecular regulation that is realized in the microenvironment.

## Acknowledgements

This work was supported by Grant n. 4011 SD/cv 2011-0438 from Compagnia di San Paolo, Turin, Italy.

## Author details

Davide Schiffer[1*], Marta Mellai[1], Laura Annovazzi[1], Cristina Casalone[2] and Paola Cassoni[3]

*Address all correspondence to: davide.schiffer@unito.it

1 Neuro-Bio-Oncology Research Center / Policlinico di Monza Foundation, Consorzio di Neuroscienze, University of Pavia, Vercelli, Italy

2 Istituto Zooprofilattico, Turin, Italy

3 Dpt. Medical Sciences, University of Turin, Turin, Italy

## References

[1] Swartz MA, Iida N, Roberts EW, Sangaletti S, Wong MH, et al. Tumor microenvironment complexity: emerging roles in cancer therapy. Cancer Res. 2012; 72(10): 2473–2480.

[2] Lorger M. Tumor microenvironment in the brain. Cancers (Basel). 2012; 4(1): 218–243.

[3] Graeber MB, Streit WJ. Microglia: immune network in the CNS. Brain Pathol. 1990; 1(1): 2–5.

[4] Hao C, Parney IF, Roa WH, Turner J, Petruk KC, et al. Cytokine and cytokine receptor mRNA expression in human glioblastomas: evidence of Th1, Th2 and Th3 cytokine dysregulation. Acta Neuropathol. 2002; 103(2): 171–178.

[5] Frei K, Nohava K, Malipiero UV, Schwerdel C, Fontana A. Production of macrophage colony-stimulating factor by astrocytes and brain macrophages. J Neuroimmunol. 1992; 40(2-3): 189–195.

[6] Deininger MH, Seid K, Engel S, Meyermann R, Schluesener HJ. Allograft inflammatory factor–1 defines a distinct subset of infiltrating macrophages/microglialcells in rat and human gliomas. Acta Neuropathol. 2000; 100(6): 673–680.

[7] Mizutani M, Pino PA, Saederup N, Charo IF, Ransohoff RM, et al. The fractalkine receptor but not CCR2 is present on microglia from embryonic development throughout adulthood. J Immunol. 2012; 188(1): 29–36.

[8] Gomez Perdiguero E, Schulz C, Geissmann F. Development and homeostasis of "resident" myeloid cells: the case of the microglia. Glia. 2013; 61(1): 112–120.

[9] Roggendorf W, Strupp S, Paulus W. Distribution and characterization of microglia/macrophages in human brain tumors. Acta Neuropathol. 1996; 92(3): 288–293.

[10] Morimura T, Neuchrist C, Kitz K, Budka H, Scheiner O, et al. Monocyte subpopulations in human gliomas: expression of Fc and complement receptors and correlation with tumor proliferation. Acta Neuropathol. 1990; 80(3): 287–294.

[11] Sutter A, Hekmat A, Luckenbach GA. Antibody-mediated tumor cytotoxicity of microglia. Pathobiology. 1991; 59(4): 254–258.

[12] Flügel A, Bradl M, Kreutzberg GW, Graeber MB. Transformation of donor-derived bone marrow precursors into host microglia during autoimmune CNS inflammation and during the retrograde response to axotomy. J Neurosci Res. 2001; 66(1): 74–82.

[13] Huettner C, Czub S, Kerkau S, Roggendorf W, Tonn JC. Interleukin 10 is expressed in human gliomas in vivo and increases glioma cell proliferation and motility in vitro. Anticancer Res. 1997; 17(5A): 3217–3224.

[14] Graeber MB, Streit WJ. Microglia: biology and pathology. Acta Neuropathol. 2010; 119(1): 89–105.

[15] Abou-Ghazal M, Yang DS, Qiao W, Reina–Ortiz C, Wei J, et al. The incidence, correlation with tumor–infiltrating inflammation, and prognosis of phosphorylated STAT3 expression in human gliomas. Clin Cancer Res. 2008; 14(24): 8228–8235.

[16] Kanamori M, Kawaguchi T, Berger MS, Pieper RO. Intracranial microenvironment reveals independent opposing functions of host alphaVbeta3expression on glioma growth and angiogenesis. J Biol Chem. 2006; 281(48): 37256–37264.

[17] Somasundaram R, Herlyn D. Chemokines and the microenvironment in neuroectodermal tumor-host interaction. Semin Cancer Biol. 2009; 19(2): 92–96.

[18] Yi L, Xiao H, Xu M, Ye X, Hu J, et al. Glioma-initiating cells: a predominant role in microglia/macrophages tropism to glioma. J Neuroimmunol. 2011; 232(1-2): 75–82.

[19] Charles N, Ozawa T, Squatrito M, Bleau AM, Brennan CW, et al. Perivascular nitric oxide activates notch signaling and promotes stem-like character in PDGF-induced glioma cells. Cell Stem Cell. 2010; 6(2): 141–152.

[20] Markovic DS, Glass R, Synowitz M, Rooijen Nv, Kettenmann H. Microglia stimulate the invasiveness of glioma cells by increasing the activity of metalloprotease-2. Neuropathol Exp Neurol. 2005; 64(9): 754–762.

[21] Markovic DS, Vinnakota K, Chirasani S, Synowitz M, Raguet H, et al. Gliomas induce and exploit microglial MT1-MMP expression for tumor expansion. Proc Natl Acad Sci U S A. 2009; 106(30): 1230–1235.

[22] Held-Feindt J, Hattermann K, Müerköster SS, Wedderkopp H, Knerlich-Lukoschus F, et al. CX3CR1 promotes recruitment of human glioma-infiltrating microglia/macrophages (GIMs). Exp Cell Res. 2010; 316(9): 1553–1566.

[23] Zhai H, Heppner FL, Tsirka SE. Microglia/macrophages promote glioma progression. Glia. 2011; 59(3): 472–485.

[24] Burke B, Sumner S, Maitland N, Lewis CE. Macrophages in gene therapy: cellular delivery vehicles and in vivo targets. J Leukoc Biol. 2002; 72(3): 417–428.

[25] Bingle L, Brown NJ, Lewis CE. The role of tumor-associated macrophages in tumor progression: implications for new anticancer therapies. J Pathol. 2002; 196(3): 254–265.

[26] Lejeune F, Liénard D, Eggermont A. Regional administration of recombinant tumor necrosis factor-alpha in cancer, with special reference to melanoma. BioDrugs. 1998; 9(3): 211–218.

[27] Orosz P, Echtenacher B, Falk W, Rüschoff J, Weber D, et al. Enhancement of experimental metastasis by tumor necrosis factor. J Exp Med. 1993; 177(5): 1391–1398.

[28] Villeneuve J, Tremblay P, Vallières L. Tumor necrosis factor reduces brain tumor growth by enhancing macrophage recruitment and microcyst formation. Cancer Res. 2005; 65(9): 3928–3936.

[29] Pollard JW. Tumor-educated macrophages promote tumor progression and metastasis. Nat Rev Cancer. 2004; 4(1): 71–78.

[30] Naganuma H, Sasaki A, Satoh E, Nagasaka M, Nakano S, et al. Transforming growth factor-beta inhibits interferon-gamma secretion by lymphokine-activated killer cells stimulated with tumor cells. Neurol Med Chir (Tokyo). 1996; 36(11): 789–795.

[31] Watters JJ, Schartner JM, Badie B. Microglia function in brain tumors. Neurosci Res. 2005; 81(3): 447–455.

[32] Sielska M, Przanowski P, Wylot B, Gabrusiewicz K, Maleszewska M, et al. Distinct roles of CSF family cytokines in macrophage infiltration and activation in glioma progression and injury response. J Pathol. 2013; 230(3): 310–321.

[33] Tran CT, Wolz P, Egensperger R, Kösel S, Imai Y, et al. Differential expression of MHC class II molecules by microglia and neoplastic astroglia: relevance for the escape of astrocytoma cells from immune surveillance. Neuropathol Appl Neurobiol. 1998; 24(4): 293–301.

[34] Komohara Y, Ohnishi K, Kuratsu J, Takeya M. Possible involvement of the M2 anti–inflammatory macrophage phenotype in growth of humangliomas. J Pathol. 2008; 216(1): 15–24.

[35] Zhou W, Bao S. Reciprocal Supportive Interplay between Glioblastoma and Tumor-Associated Macrophages. Cancers (Basel). 2014; 6(2): 723–740.

[36] Bao S, Ouyang G, Bai X, Huang Z, Ma C, et al. Periostin potently promotes metastatic growth of colon cancer by augmenting cell survival viathe Akt/PKB pathway. Cancer Cell. 2004; 5(4): 329–339.

[37] Zhou W, Ke SQ, Huang Z, Flavahan W, Fang X, et al. Periostin secreted by glioblastoma stem cells recruits M2 tumour–associated macrophages and promotes malignant growth. Nat Cell Biol. 2015; 17(2): 170–182.

[38] Mikheev AM, Mikheeva SA, Trister AD, Tokita MJ, Emerson SN, et al. Periostin is a novel therapeutic target that predicts and regulates glioma malignancy. Neuro Oncol. 2014. pii: nou161.

[39] Squadrito ML, De Palma M. A niche role for periostin and macrophages in glioblastoma. Nat Cell Biol. 2015; 17(2): 107–109.

[40] Bushong EA, Martone ME, Ellisman MH. Maturation of astrocyte morphology and the establishment of astrocyte domains during postnatal hippocampal development. Int J Dev Neurosci. 2004; 22(2): 73–86.

[41] Clarke SR, Shetty AK, Bradley JL, Turner DA. Reactive astrocytes express the embryonic intermediate neurofilament nestin. Neuroreport. 1994; 5(15): 1885–1888.

[42] Eliasson C, Sahlgren C, Berthold CH, Stakeberg J, Celis JE, et al. Intermediate filament protein partnership in astrocytes. J Biol Chem. 1999; 274(34): 23996–24006.

[43] Mandonnet E, Capelle L, Duffau H. Extension of paralimbic low grade gliomas: toward an anatomical classification based on white matter invasion patterns. J Neurooncol. 2006; 78(2): 179–185.

[44] Ellingson BM, LaViolette PS, Rand SD, Malkin MG, Connelly JM, et al. Spatially quantifying microscopic tumor invasion and proliferation using a voxel-wise solution to a glioma growth model and serial diffusion MRI. Magn Reson Med. 2011; 65(4): 1131–1143.

[45] Schiffer D, Mellai M, Annovazzi L, Caldera V, Piazzi A, et al. Stem cell niches in glioblastoma: a neuropathological view. Biomed Res Int. 2014; 2014: 725921.

[46] Tamagno I, Schiffer D. Nestin expression in reactive astrocytes of human pathology. J Neurooncol. 2006; 80(3): 227–233.

[47] Virchow R. Die krankhaften Geschwülste. Berlin: Hirschwald; 1863-1865.

[48] Reynolds BA, Weiss S. Generation of neurons and astrocytes from isolated cells of the adult mammalian central nervous system. Science. 1992; 255(5052): 1707–1710.

[49] Doetsch F, Caillé I, Lim DA, García-Verdugo JM, Alvarez-Buylla A. Subventricular zone astrocytes are neural stem cells in the adult mammalian brain. Cell. 1999; 97(6): 703–716.

[50] Visvader JE, Lindeman GJ. Cancer stem cells in solid tumors: accumulating evidence and unresolved questions. Nat Rev Cancer. 2008; 8(10): 755–768.

[51] De Filippis L, Binda E. Concise review: self-renewal in the central nervous system: neural stem cells from embryo to adult. Stem Cells Transl Med. 2012; 1(4): 298–308.

[52] Singh SK, Clarke ID, Terasaki M, Bonn VE, Hawkins C, et al. Identification of a cancer stem cell in human brain tumors. Cancer Res. 2003; 63(18): 5821–5828.

[53] Singh SK, Clarke ID, Hide T, Dirks PB. Cancer stem cells in nervous system tumors. Oncogene. 2004; 23(43): 7267–7273.

[54] Sanai N, Alvarez-Buylla A, Berger MS. Neural stem cells and the origin of gliomas. N Engl J Med. 2005; 353(8): 811–822.

[55] Hanahan D, Weinberg RA. The hallmarks of cancer. Cell. 2000; 100(1): 57–70.

[56] Stiles CD, Rowitch DH. Glioma stem cells: a midterm exam. Neuron. 2008; 58(6): 832–846.

[57] Uhrbom L, Dai C, Celestino JC, Rosenblum MK, Fuller GN, et al. Ink4a-Arf loss cooperates with KRas activation in astrocytes and neural progenitors to generate glioblastomas of various morphologies depending on activated Akt. Cancer Res. 2002; 62(19): 5551–5558.

[58] Bachoo RM, Maher EA, Ligon KL, Sharpless NE, Chan SS, et al. Epidermal growth factor receptor and Ink4a/Arf: convergent mechanisms governing terminal differentiation and transformation along the neural stem cell to astrocyte axis. Cancer Cell. 2002; 1(3): 269–277.

[59] Radke J, Bortolussi G, Pagenstecher A. Akt and c-Myc induce stem-cell markers in mature primary $p53^{-}/^{-}$ astrocytes and render these cells gliomagenic in the brain of immunocompetent mice. PLoS One. 2013; 8(2): e56691.

[60] Holland EC, Celestino J, Dai C, Schaefer L, Sawaya RE, et al. Combined activation of Ras and Akt in neural progenitors induces glioblastoma formation in mice. Nat Genet. 2000; 25(1): 55–57.

[61] Schiffer D, Mellai M, Annovazzi L, Piazzi A, Monzeglio O, et al. Glioblastoma cancer stem cells: basis for a functional hypothesis. Stem Cell Discovery 2012; 2(3): 122–131.

[62] Goffart N, Kroonen J, Rogister B. Glioblastoma-initiating cells: relationship with neural stem cells and the micro-environment. Cancers (Basel). 2013; 5(3): 1049-1071.

[63] Schiffer D. Brain tumors: biology, pathology and clinical references. Berlin, Heidelberg, New York: Springer; 1997.

[64] Lim DA, Cha S, Mayo MC, Chen MH, Keles E, et al. Relationship of glioblastoma multiforme to neural stem cell regions predicts invasive and multifocal tumor phenotype. Neuro Oncol. 2007; 9(4): 424–429.

[65] Alcantara Llaguno S, Chen J, Kwon CH, Jackson EL, Li Y, et al. Malignant astrocytomas originate from neural stem/progenitor cells in a somatic tumor suppressor mouse model. Cancer Cell. 2009; 15(1): 45–56.

[66] Luskin MB. Restricted proliferation and migration of postnatally generated neurons derived from the forebrain subventricular zone. Neuron. 1993; 11(1): 173–189.

[67] Lois C, Alvarez-Buylla A. Long-distance neuronal migration in the adult mammalian brain. Science. 1994; 264(5162): 1145–1148.

[68] Hack MA, Saghatelyan A, de Chevigny A, Pfeifer A, Ashery-Padan R, et al. Neuronal fate determinants of adult olfactory bulb neurogenesis. Nat Neurosci. 2005; 8(7): 865–872.

[69] Menn B, Garcia-Verdugo JM, Yaschine C, Gonzalez-Perez O, Rowitch D, et al. Origin of oligodendrocytes in the subventricular zone of the adult brain. J Neurosci. 2006; 26(30): 7907–7918.

[70] Jackson EL, Garcia-Verdugo JM, Gil-Perotin S, Roy M, Quinones-Hinojosa A, et al. PDGFR alpha-positive B cells are neural stem cells in the adult SVZ that form glioma-like growths in response to increased PDGF signaling. Neuron. 2006; 51(2): 187–199.

[71] Price RL, Song J, Bingmer K, Kim TH, Yi JY, et al. Cytomegalovirus contributes to glioblastoma in the context of tumor suppressor mutations. Cancer Res. 2013; 73(11): 3441–3450.

[72] Holland EC. Progenitor cells and glioma formation. Curr Opin Neurol. 2001; 14(6): 683–688.

[73] Adams JM, Strasser A. Is tumor growth sustained by rare cancer stem cells or dominant clones? Cancer Res. 2008; 68(11): 4018–4021.

[74] Reya T, Morrison SJ, Clarke MF, Weissman IL. Stem cells, cancer, and cancer stem cells. Nature. 2001; 414(6859): 105–111.

[75] Assanah M, Lochhead R, Ogden A, Bruce J, Goldman J, et al. Glial progenitors in adult white matter are driven to form malignant gliomas by platelet-derived growth factor-expressing retroviruses. J Neurosci. 2006; 26(25): 6781–6790.

[76] Siebzehnrubl FA, Reynolds BA, Vescovi A, Steindler DA, Deleyrolle LP. The origins of glioma: E Pluribus Unum? Glia. 2011; 59(8): 1135–1147.

[77] Dufour C, Cadusseau J, Varlet P, Surena AL, de Faria GP, et al. Astrocytes reverted to a neural progenitor-like state with transforming growth factor alpha are sensitized to cancerous transformation. Stem Cells. 2009; 27(10): 2373–2382.

[78] Silver DJ, Steindler DA. Common astrocytic programs during brain development, injury and cancer. Trends Neurosci. 2009; 32(6): 303–311.

[79] Buffo A, Rite I, Tripathi P, Lepier A, Colak D, et al. Origin and progeny of reactive gliosis: A source of multipotent cells in the injured brain. Proc Natl Acad Sci U S A. 2008; 105(9): 3581–3586.

[80] Hide T, Takezaki T, Nakatani Y, Nakamura H, Kuratsu J, et al. Combination of a ptgs2 inhibitor and an epidermal growth factor receptor-signaling inhibitor prevents tumorigenesis of oligodendrocyte lineage-derived glioma-initiating cells. Stem Cells. 2011; 29(4): 590–599.

[81] Moore LM, Holmes KM, Fuller GN, Zhang W. Oncogene interactions are required for glioma development and progression as revealed by a tissue specific transgenic mouse model. Chin J Cancer. 2011; 30(3): 163–172.

[82] Persson AI, Petritsch C, Swartling FJ, Itsara M, Sim FJ, et al. Non-stem cell origin for oligodendroglioma. Cancer Cell. 2010; 18(6): 669–682.

[83] Lindberg N, Kastemar M, Olofsson T, Smits A, Uhrbom L. Oligodendrocyte progenitor cells can act as cell of origin for experimental glioma. Oncogene. 2009; 28(23): 2266–2275.

[84] Jiang Y, Uhrbom L. On the origin of glioma. Ups J Med Sci. 2012; 117(2): 113–121.

[85] Lathia JD, Gallagher J, Myers JT, Li M, Vasanji A, et al. Direct in vivo evidence for tumor propagation by glioblastoma cancer stem cells. PLoS One. 2011; 6(9): e24807.

[86] Mazzoleni S, Galli R. Gliomagenesis: a game played by few players or a team effort? Front Biosci (Elite Ed). 2012; 4: 205–213.

[87] Foroni C, Galli R, Cipelletti B, Caumo A, Alberti S, et al. Resilience to transformation and inherent genetic and functional stability of adult neural stem cells ex vivo. Cancer Res. 2007; 67(8): 3725–3733.

[88] Li L, Neaves WB. Normal stem cells and cancer stem cells: the niche matters. Cancer Res. 2006; 66(9): 4553–4557.

[89] Furnari FB, Fenton T, Bachoo RM, Mukasa A, Stommel JM, et al. Malignant astrocytic glioma: genetics, biology, and paths to treatment. Genes Dev. 2007; 21(21): 2683–2710.

[90] Zheng H, Ying H, Yan H, Kimmelman AC, Hiller DJ, et al. p53 and Pten control neural and glioma stem/progenitor cell renewal and differentiation. Nature. 2008; 455(7216): 1129–1133.

[91] Phillips HS, Kharbanda S, Chen R, Forrest WF, Soriano RH, et al. Molecular subclasses of high-grade glioma predict prognosis, delineate a pattern of disease progression, and resemble stages in neurogenesis. Cancer Cell. 2006; 9(3): 157–173.

[92] Verhaak RG, Hoadley KA, Purdom E, Wang V, Qi Y, et al. Integrated genomic analysis identifies clinically relevant subtypes of glioblastoma characterized by abnormalities in PDGFRA, IDH1, EGFR, and NF1. Cancer Cell. 2010; 17(1): 98–110.

[93] Swartling FJ, Hede SM, Weiss WA. What underlies the diversity of brain tumors? Cancer Metastasis Rev. 2013; 32(1-2): 5–24.

[94] Chen R, Nishimura MC, Bumbaca SM, Kharbanda S, Forrest WF, et al. A hierarchy of self-renewing tumor-initiating cell types in glioblastoma. Cancer Cell. 2010; 17(4): 362–375.

[95] Shah K, Bureau E, Kim DE, Yang K, Tang Y, et al. Glioma therapy and real-time imaging of neural precursor cell migration and tumor regression. Ann Neurol. 2005; 57(1): 34–41.

[96] Aboody KS, Brown A, Rainov NG, Bower KA, Liu S, et al. Neural stem cells display extensive tropism for pathology in adult brain: evidence from intracranial gliomas. Proc Natl Acad Sci U S A. 2000; 97(23): 12846–12851.

[97] Ehtesham M, Kabos P, Kabosova A, Neuman T, Black KL, et al. The use of interleukin 12-secreting neural stem cells for the treatment of intracranial glioma. Cancer Res. 2002; 62(20): 5657–5663.

[98] Shah AC, Benos D, Gillespie GY, Markert JM. Oncolytic viruses: clinical applications as vectors for the treatment of malignant gliomas. J Neurooncol. 2003; 65(3): 203–226.

[99] Kim SK, Cargioli TG, Machluf M, Yang W, Sun Y, et al. PEX-producing human neural stem cells inhibit tumor growth in a mouse glioma model. Clin Cancer Res. 2005; 11(16): 5965–5970.

[100] Uhl M, Weiler M, Wick W, Jacobs AH, Weller M, et al. Migratory neural stem cells for improved thymidine kinase-based gene therapy of malignant gliomas. Biochem Biophys Res Commun. 2005; 328(1): 125–129.

[101] Li ZB, Zeng ZJ, Chen Q, Luo SQ, Hu WX. Recombinant AAV-mediated HSVtk gene transfer with direct intratumoral injections and Tet-On regulation for implanted human breast cancer. BMC Cancer. 2006; 6: 66.

[102] Rath P, Shi H, Maruniak JA, Litofsky NS, Maria BL, et al. Stem cells as vectors to deliver HSV/tk gene therapy for malignant gliomas. Curr Stem Cell Res Ther. 2009; 4(1): 44–49.

[103] Tyler MA, Ulasov IV, Sonabend AM, Nandi S, Han Y, et al. Neural stem cells target intracranial glioma to deliver an oncolytic adenovirus in vivo. Gene Ther. 2009; 16(2): 262–278.

[104] Jeon JY, An JH, Kim SU, Park HG, Lee MA. Migration of human neural stem cells toward an intracranial glioma. Exp Mol Med. 2008; 40(1): 84–91.

[105] Nakamura K, Ito Y, Kawano Y, Kurozumi K, Kobune M, et al. Antitumor effect of genetically engineered mesenchymal stem cells in a rat glioma model. Gene Ther. 2004; 11(14): 1155–1164.

[106] Nakamizo A, Marini F, Amano T, Khan A, Studeny M, et al. Human bone marrow-derived mesenchymal stem cells in the treatment of gliomas. Cancer Res. 2005; 65(8): 3307–3318.

[107] Tabatabai G, Bähr O, Möhle R, Eyüpoglu IY, Boehmler AM, et al. Lessons from the bone marrow: how malignant glioma cells attract adult haematopoietic progenitor cells. Brain. 2005; 128(Pt 9): 2200–2211.

[108] Glass R, Synowitz M, Kronenberg G, Walzlein JH, Markovic DS, et al. Glioblastoma-induced attraction of endogenous neural precursor cells is associated with improved survival. J Neurosci. 2005; 25(10): 2637–2646.

[109] Pirzkall A, Nelson SJ, McKnight TR, Takahashi MM, Li X, et al. Metabolic imaging of low-grade gliomas with three-dimensional magnetic resonance spectroscopy. Int J Radiat Oncol Biol Phys. 2002; 53(5): 1254–1264.

[110] Walzlein JH, Synowitz M, Engels B, Markovic DS, Gabrusiewicz K, et al. The antitumorigenic response of neural precursors depends on subventricular proliferation and age. Stem Cells. 2008; 26(11): 2945–2954.

[111] Xu F, Zhu JH. Stem cells tropism for malignant gliomas.Neurosci Bull. 2007; 23(6): 363–369.

[112] Honeth G, Staflin K, Kalliomäki S, Lindvall M, Kjellman C. Chemokine-directed migration of tumor-inhibitory neural progenitor cells towards an intracranially growing glioma. Exp Cell Res. 2006; 312(8): 1265–1276.

[113] Chen HI, Bakshi A, Royo NC, Magge SN, Watson DJ. Neural stem cells as biological minipumps: a faster route to cell therapy for the CNS? Curr Stem Cell Res Ther. 2007; 2(1): 13–22.

[114] Staflin K, Lindvall M, Zuchner T, Lundberg C. Instructive cross-talk between neural progenitor cells and gliomas. J Neurosci Res. 2007; 85(10): 2147–2159.

[115] Zhao D, Najbauer J, Garcia E, Metz MZ, Gutova M, et al. Neural stem cell tropism to glioma: critical role of tumor hypoxia. Mol Cancer Res. 2008; 6(12): 1819–1829.

[116] Ayuso-Sacido A, Graham C, Greenfield JP, Boockvar JA. The duality of epidermal growth factor receptor (EGFR) signaling and neural stem cell phenotype: cell enhancer or cell transformer? Curr Stem Cell Res Ther. 2006; 1(3): 387–394.

[117] Barresi V, Belluardo N, Sipione S, Mudò G, Cattaneo E, et al. Transplantation of prodrug-converting neural progenitor cells for brain tumor therapy. Cancer Gene Ther. 2003; 10(5): 396–402.

[118] Oh MC, Lim DA. Novel treatment strategies for malignant gliomas using neural stem cells. Neurotherapeutics. 2009; 6(3): 458–464.

[119] Amariglio N, Hirshberg A, Scheithauer BW, Cohen Y, Loewenthal R, et al. Donor-derived brain tumor following neural stem cell transplantation in an ataxia telangiectasia patient. PLoS Med. 2009; 6(2): e1000029.

[120] Schiffer D, Chiò A, Giordana MT, Mauro A, Migheli A, et al. Vascular response to irradiation in malignant gliomas. J Neurooncol. 1990; 8(1): 73–84.

[121] Lyden D, Hattori K, Dias S, Costa C, Blaikie P, et al. Impaired recruitment of bone-marrow-derived endothelial and hematopoietic precursor cells blocks tumor angiogenesis and growth. Nat Med. 2001; 7(11): 1194–1201.

[122] Machein MR, Renninger S, de Lima-Hahn E, Plate KH. Minor contribution of bone marrow-derived endothelial progenitors to the vascularization of murine gliomas. Brain Pathol. 2003; 13(4): 582–597.

[123] Folkins C, Shaked Y, Man S, Tang T, Lee CR, et al. Glioma tumor stem-like cells promote tumor angiogenesis and vasculogenesis via vascular endothelial growth factor and stromal-derived factor 1. Cancer Res. 2009; 69(18): 7243–7251.

[124] Burrel K, Zadeh G. Molecular mechanism of Tumor angiogenesis. In: Lichtor T. (ed.) Tumor angiogenesis. Rijeka: InTech; 2012. p275–296.

[125] Lewis CE, De Palma M, Naldini L. Tie2-expressing monocytes and tumor angiogenesis: regulation by hypoxia and angiopoietin-2. Cancer Res. 2007; 67(18): 8429–8432.

[126] Venneri MA, De Palma M, Ponzoni M, Pucci F, Scielzo C, et al. Identification of proangiogenic TIE2-expressing monocytes (TEMs) in human peripheral blood and cancer. Blood. 2007; 109(12): 5276–5285.

[127] Maniotis AJ, Folberg R, Hess A, Seftor EA, Gardner LM, et al. Vascular channel formation by human melanoma cells in vivo and in vitro: vasculogenic mimicry. Am J Pathol. 1999; 155(3): 739–752.

[128] Seftor EA, Meltzer PS, Schatteman GC, Gruman LM, Hess AR, et al. Expression of multiple molecular phenotypes by aggressive melanoma tumor cells: role in vasculogenic mimicry. Crit Rev Oncol Hematol. 2002; 44(1): 17–27.

[129] Liu C, Huang H, Doñate F, Dickinson C, Santucci R, et al. Prostate-specific membrane antigen directed selective thrombotic infarction of tumors. Cancer Res. 2002; 62(19): 5470–5475.

[130] Bonnet D, Dick JE. Human acute myeloid leukemia is organized as a hierarchy that originates from a primitive hematopoietic cell. Nat Med. 1997; 3(7): 730–737.

[131] El Hallani S, Boisselier B, Peglion F, Rousseau A, Colin C, et al. A new alternative mechanism in glioblastoma vascularization: tubular vasculogenic mimicry. Brain. 2010; 133(Pt 4): 973–982.

[132] Rodriguez FJ, Orr BA, Ligon KL, Eberhart CG. Neoplastic cells are a rare component in human glioblastoma microvasculature. Oncotarget. 2012; 3(1): 98–106.

[133] Kulla A, Burkhardt K, Meyer-Puttlitz B, Teesalu T, Asser T, et al. Analysis of the TP53 gene in laser-microdissected glioblastoma vasculature. Acta Neuropathol. 2003; 105(4): 328–332.

[134] Kioi M, Vogel H, Schultz G, Hoffman RM, Harsh GR, et al. Inhibition of vasculogenesis, but not angiogenesis, prevents the recurrence of glioblastoma after irradiation in mice. J Clin Invest. 2010; 120(3): 694–705.

[135] Takahashi T, Kalka C, Masuda H, Chen D, Silver M, et al. Ischemia- and cytokine-induced mobilization of bone marrow-derived endothelial progenitor cells for neovascularization. Nat Med. 1999; 5(4): 434–438.

[136] Orlic D, Kajstura J, Chimenti S, Bodine DM, Leri A, et al. Bone marrow stem cells regenerate infarcted myocardium. Pediatr Transplant. 2003; 7 (S3): 86–88.

[137] Greenfield JP, Cobb WS, Lyden D. Resisting arrest: a switch from angiogenesis to vasculogenesis in recurrent malignant gliomas. J Clin Invest. 2010; 120(3): 663–667.

[138] Soda Y, Marumoto T, Friedmann-Morvinski D, Soda M, Liu F, et al. Transdifferentiation of glioblastoma cells into vascular endothelial cells. Proc Natl Acad Sci U S A. 2011; 108(11): 4274–4280.

[139] Hardee ME, Zagzag D. Mechanisms of glioma-associated neovascularization. Am J Pathol. 2012; 181(4): 1126–1141.

[140] Ricci-Vitiani L, Pallini R, Biffoni M, Todaro M, Invernici G, et al. Tumor vascularization via endothelial differentiation of glioblastoma stem-like cells. Nature. 2010; 468(7325): 824–828.

[141] Wang Y, Zhu M, Zhang R, Yang H, Wang Y, et al. Whole genome amplification of the rust Puccinia striiformis f. sp. tritici from single spores. J Microbiol Methods. 2009; 77(2): 229–234.

[142] Jain RK, di Tomaso E, Duda DG, Loeffler JS, Sorensen AG, et al. Angiogenesis in brain tumors. Nat Rev Neurosci. 2007; 8(8): 610–622.

[143] Vredenburgh JJ, Desjardins A, Herndon JE 2nd, Dowell JM, Reardon DA, et al. Phase II trial of bevacizumab and irinotecan in recurrent malignant glioma. Clin Cancer Res. 2007; 13(4): 1253–1259.

[144] Bergers G, Hanahan D. Modes of resistance to anti-angiogenic therapy. Nat Rev Cancer. 2008; 8(8): 592–603.

[145] Shojaei F, Ferrara N. Refractoriness to antivascular endothelial growth factor treatment: role of myeloid cells. Cancer Res. 2008; 68(14): 5501–5504.

[146] Pàez-Ribes M, Allen E, Hudock J, Takeda T, Okuyama H, et al. Antiangiogenic therapy elicits malignant progression of tumors to increased local invasion and distant metastasis. Cancer Cell. 2009; 15(3): 220–231.

[147] Winkler F, Kienast Y, Fuhrmann M, Von Baumgarten L, Burgold S, et al. Imaging glioma cell invasion in vivo reveals mechanisms of dissemination and peritumoral angiogenesis. Glia. 2009; 57(12): 1306–1315.

[148] Bao S, Wu Q, Sathornsumetee S, Hao Y, Li Z, et al. Stem cell-like glioma cells promote tumor angiogenesis through vascular endothelial growth factor. Cancer Res. 2006; 66(16): 7843–7848.

[149] Calabrese C, Poppleton H, Kocak M, Hogg TL, Fuller C, et al. A perivascular niche for brain tumor stem cells. Cancer Cell. 2007; 11(1): 69–82.

[150] Hambardzumyan D, Becher OJ, Rosenblum MK, Pandolfi PP, Manova-Todorova K, et al. PI3K pathway regulates survival of cancer stem cells residing in the perivascular niche following radiation in medulloblastoma in vivo. Genes Dev. 2008; 22(4): 436–348.

[151] Gilbertson RJ, Rich JN. Making a tumor's bed: glioblastoma stem cells and the vascular niche. Nat Rev Cancer. 2007; 7(10): 733–736.

[152] Brooks MD, Sengupta R, Snyder SC, Rubin JB. Hitting them where they live: targeting the glioblastoma perivascular stem cell niche. Curr Pathobiol Rep. 2013; 1(2): 101–110.

[153] Pala A, Karpel-Massler G, Wirtz CR, Halatsch ME. Epithelial to mesenchymal transition and progression of Glioblastoma. In: Lichtor T. (ed.) Clinical menagment and evolving novel therapeutic strategies for patients with brain Tumors. Rijeka: InTech; 2013. p277–289.

[154] Ortensi B, Setti M, Osti D, Pelicci G. Cancer stem cell contribution to glioblastoma invasiveness. Stem Cell Res Ther. 2013; 4(1): 18.

[155] Mani SA, Guo W, Liao MJ, Eaton EN, Ayyanan A, et al. The epithelial-mesenchymal transition generates cells with properties of stem cells. Cell. 2008; 133(4): 704–715.

[156] Jin X, Jeon HY, Joo KM, Kim JK, Jin J, et al. Frizzled 4 regulates stemness and invasiveness of migrating glioma cells established by serial intracranial transplantation. Cancer Res. 2011; 71(8): 3066–3075.

[157] Kahlert UD, Maciaczyk D, Doostkam S, Orr BA, Simons B, et al. Activation of canonical WNT/β-catenin signaling enhances in vitro motility of glioblastoma cells by activation of ZEB1 and other activators of epithelial-to-mesenchymal transition. Cancer Lett. 2012; 325(1): 42–53.

[158] Bhat KP, Salazar KL, Balasubramaniyan V, Wani K, Heathcock L, et al. The transcriptional coactivator TAZ regulates mesenchymal differentiation in malignant glioma. Genes Dev. 2011; 25(24): 2594–2609.

[159] Filatova A, Acker T, Garvalov BK. The cancer stem cell niche(s): the crosstalk between glioma stem cells and their microenvironment. Biochim Biophys Acta. 2013; 1830(2): 2496–2508.

[160] Wang R, Chadalavada K, Wilshire J, Kowalik U, Hovinga KE, et al. Glioblastoma stem-like cells give rise to tumor endothelium. Nature. 2010; 468(7325): 829–833.

[161] He H, Li MW, Niu CS. The pathological characteristics of glioma stem cell niches. J Clin Neurosci. 2012; 19(1): 121–127.

[162] Charles NA, Holland EC, Gilbertson R, Glass R, Kettenmann H. The brain tumor microenvironment. Glia. 2012; 60(3): 502–514.

[163] Christensen K, Schrøder HD, Kristensen BW. CD133 identifies perivascular niches in grade II-IV astrocytomas. J Neurooncol. 2008; 90(2): 157–170.

[164] Seidel S, Garvalov BK, Wirta V, von Stechow L, Schänzer A, et al. A hypoxic niche regulates glioblastoma stem cells through hypoxia inducible factor 2 alpha. Brain. 2010; 133(Pt 4): 983–995.

[165] Bergers G, Song S. The role of pericytes in blood-vessel formation and maintenance. Neuro Oncol. 2005; 7(4): 452–464.

[166] Armulik A, Genové G, Mäe M, Nisancioglu MH, Wallgard E, et al. Pericytes regulate the blood-brain barrier. Nature. 2010; 468(7323): 557–561.

[167] Birnbaum T, Hildebrandt J, Nuebling G, Sostak P, Straube A. Glioblastoma-dependent differentiation and angiogenic potential of human mesenchymal stem cells in vitro. J Neurooncol. 2011; 105(1): 57–65.

[168] Bexell D, Gunnarsson S, Tormin A, Darabi A, Gisselsson D, et al. Bone marrow multipotent mesenchymal stroma cells act as pericyte-like migratory vehicles in experimental gliomas. Mol Ther. 2009; 17(1): 183–190.

[169] Christensen K, Schrøder HD, Kristensen BW. CD133+ niches and single cells in glioblastoma have different phenotypes. J Neurooncol. 2011; 104(1): 129–143.

[170] Evans SM, Judy KD, Dunphy I, Jenkins WT, Hwang WT, et al. Hypoxia is important in the biology and aggression of human glial brain tumors. Clin Cancer Res. 2004; 10(24): 8177–8184.

[171] Keith B, Johnson RS, Simon MC. HIF1$\alpha$ and HIF2$\alpha$: sibling rivalry in hypoxic tumor growth and progression. Nat Rev Cancer. 2011; 12(1): 9–22.

[172] Wang GL, Jiang BH, Rue EA, Semenza GL. Hypoxia-inducible factor 1 is a basic-helix-loop-helix-PAS heterodimer regulated by cellular O2 tension. Proc Natl Acad Sci U S A. 1995; 92(12): 5510–5514.

[173] Rankin EB, Giaccia AJ. The role of hypoxia-inducible factors in tumorigenesis. Cell Death Differ. 2008; 15(4): 678–685.

[174] Holmquist-Mengelbier L, Fredlund E, Löfstedt T, Noguera R, Navarro S, et al. Recruitment of HIF-1alpha and HIF-2alpha to common target genes is differentially regulated in neuroblastoma: HIF-2alpha promotes an aggressive phenotype. Cancer Cell. 2006; 10(5): 413–423.

[175] Soeda A, Park M, Lee D, Mintz A, Androutsellis-Theotokis A, et al. Hypoxia promotes expansion of the CD133-positive glioma stem cells through activation of HIF-1alpha. Oncogene. 2009; 28(45): 3949–3959.

[176] Bar EE, Lin A, Mahairaki V, Matsui W, Eberhart CG. Hypoxia increases the expression of stem-cell markers and promotes clonogenicity in glioblastoma neurospheres. Am J Pathol. 2010; 177(3): 1491–1502.

[177] Fan X, Khaki L, Zhu TS, Soules ME, Talsma CE, et al. NOTCH pathway blockade depletes CD133-positive glioblastoma cells and inhibits growth of tumor neurospheres and xenografts. Stem Cells. 2010; 28(1): 5–16.

[178] Heddleston JM, Li Z, McLendon RE, Hjelmeland AB, Rich JN. The hypoxic microenvironment maintains glioblastoma stem cells and promotes reprogramming towards a cancer stem cell phenotype. Cell Cycle. 2009; 8(20): 3274–3284.

[179] Green DR, Reed JC. Mitochondria and apoptosis. Science. 1998; 281(5381): 1309–1312.

[180] Ashkenazi A, Dixit VM. Apoptosis control by death and decoy receptors. Curr Opin Cell Biol. 1999; 11(2): 255–260.

[181] Mellai M, Schiffer D. Apoptosis in brain tumors: prognostic and therapeutic considerations. Anticancer Res. 2007 Jan; 27(1A): 437–448.

[182] Fischer I, Gagner JP, Law M, Newcomb EW, Zagzag D. Angiogenesis in gliomas: biology and molecular pathophysiology. Brain Pathol. 2005; 15(4): 297–310.

[183] Rong Y, Durden DL, Van Meir EG, Brat DJ. 'Pseudopalisading' necrosis in glioblastoma: a familiar morphologic feature that links vascular pathology, hypoxia, and angiogenesis. J Neuropathol Exp Neurol. 2006; 65(6): 529–539.

[184] Schiffer D, Chiò A, Giordana MT, Mauro A, Migheli A, Vigliani MC. The vascular response to tumor infiltration in malignant gliomas. Morphometric and reconstruction study. Acta Neuropathol. 1989; 77(4): 369–378.

[185] Kargiotis O, Rao JS, Kyritsis AP. Mechanisms of angiogenesis in gliomas. J Neurooncol. 2006; 78(3): 281–293.

[186] Schiffer D, Manazza A, Tamagno I. Nestin expression in neuroepithelial tumors. Neurosci Lett. 2006; 400(1-2): 80–85.

[187] Annovazzi L, Mellai M, Caldera V, Valente G, Schiffer D. SOX2 expression and amplification in gliomas and glioma cell lines. Cancer Genomics Proteomics. 2011; 8(3): 139–147.

[188] Conti L, Crisafulli L, Caldera V, Tortoreto M, Brilli E, et al. REST controls self-renewal and tumorigenic competence of human glioblastoma cells. PLoS One. 2012; 7(6): e38486.

[189] Caldera V, Mellai M, Annovazzi L, Piazzi A, Lanotte M, et al. Antigenic and genotypic similarity between primary glioblastomas and their derived neurospheres. J Oncol. 2011; 2011: 314962.

[190] Clarke MF, Fuller M. Stem cells and cancer: two faces of eve. Cell. 2006; 124(6): 1111–1115.

[191] Beier D, Hau P, Proescholdt M, Lohmeier A, Wischhusen J, et al. CD133(+) and CD133(-) glioblastoma-derived cancer stem cells show differential growth characteristics and molecular profiles. Cancer Res. 2007; 67(9): 4010–4015.

[192] Cummins EP, Berra E, Comerford KM, Ginouves A, Fitzgerald KT. Prolyl hydroxylase-1 negatively regulates IkappaB kinase-beta, giving insight into hypoxia-induced NFkappaB activity. Proc Natl Acad Sci U S A. 2006; 103(48): 18154–18159.

[193] Taylor CT, Cummins EP. The role of NF-kappaB in hypoxia-induced gene expression. Ann N Y Acad Sci. 2009; 1177: 178–184.

[194] Tafani M, Di Vito M, Frati A, Pellegrini L, De Santis E, et al. Pro-inflammatory gene expression in solid glioblastoma microenvironment and in hypoxic stem cells from human glioblastoma. J Neuroinflammation. 2011; 8: 32.

[195] Bar EE. Glioblastoma, cancer stem cells and hypoxia. Brain Pathol. 2011; 21(2): 119–129.

Chapter 4

# Brain Tumor Metabolism — Unraveling Its Role in Finding New Therapeutic Targets

Vera Miranda Gonçalves, Fátima Baltazar and
Rui Manuel Reis

Additional information is available at the end of the chapter

http://dx.doi.org/10.5772/59606

## 1. Introduction

Primary tumors of brain account for approximately 2-3% of all cancers, with annual incidence approximately 15 patients per 100,000 people and the prevalence has been estimated in 69 patients per 100,000 people. Several brain tumor types evolve from glial or neuronal precursors, being the tumors of glial cells the most common and denominated gliomas [1, 2]. Gliomas are histologically classified according to the World Health Organization (WHO) classification into four malignancy grades[3, 4]. Pilocytic astrocytomas (WHO grade I) are benign tumors that can usually be cured after surgical resection. Diffuse astrocytomas (WHO grade II) exhibit a slow growth, but have an inevitable tendency to progress to higher grade lesions, such as anaplastic gliomas (WHO grade III) and glioblastomas (WHO grade IV). Anaplastic gliomas are rapidly growing malignant tumors that, in addition to surgery, require aggressive adjuvant therapy. Glioblastomas (GBMs) are the most malignant and frequent type of gliomas, which are preferentially manifested in aged adults with a peak of incidence between 50-60 years old [4]. Glioblastomas may evolve from lower grade tumors as described and are mentioned secondary glioblastomas, although most of GBMs arise rapidly without the evidence of less malignant lesion, and are denominated *de novo* or primary glioblastomas [2, 4].

The current standard therapy for GBM includes tumor resection followed by radiation and concomitant chemotherapy, with temozolomide being the only approved drug that shows some efficacy in this disease [5]. In the last decade, specific inhibitors of oncogenic signaling pathways such as EGFR, PI3K/Akt, and VEGF have made progress with some of them currently tested in clinical trials. Nowadays, bevacizumab (avastin®), a humanized monoclonal antibody against VEGF is approved as a second line of treatment for recurrent GBMs and is currently in phase III clinical trials for the treatment of initial GBMs [6]. Antiangiogenic therapy with avastin improved radiographic response and 6 month of progression free survival, however with modest or little effect on overall survival, when in combination with TMZ during and after radiotherapy [7, 8]. Besides, its role in promoting vascular normalization, the effect on tumor cell invasion is still controversial. Avastin treatment induces infiltration in U87 xenograft model and also was associated with diffusing invasive recurrence in some GBM patients [9, 10]. Additionally, it was observed that vasculature normalization with bevacizumab treatment leads to increased hypoxia and consequently acquisition of resistance [11]. Despite progress in new molecular-based therapies, the prognosis of glioblastomas patients is still very dismal [12, 13]. Thus, exploitation of new molecular targets becomes crucial in neuro-oncology.

In recent years, understanding the regulation of tumor metabolism has significantly improved. Accumulating evidence showed that tumor cells reprogram their metabolism to meet high energy demands, coordinate markedly elevated biosynthetic processes and energy production, which in turn promote rapid growth and division of tumor cells [14-17]. Thus, targeting metabolism has become a novel promising strategy for treating cancers, particularly glioblastomas.

## 2. Tumor metabolism

During cancer progression, molecular changes are associated to metabolic reprogramming [18, 19], which is nowadays defined as a new hallmark of cancer [20]. In mammalian cells, namely quiescent cells or differentiated tissues, glycolysis is reduced in the presence of oxygen and energy production arises from mitochondrial oxidative phosphorylation which oxidizes pyruvate to $CO_2$ and $H_2O$, known as "Pasteur effect" (Figure 1) [21]. However, in tumor cells, like proliferating tissues, there is high glycolytic activity even in the presence of oxygen, being glycolysis the major source of energy. This phenomenon is known as "Warburg effect". As a result, tumor cells convert most of the incoming glucose into lactate (around 85 %) rather than metabolizing pyruvate in the mitochondria through oxidative phosphorylation (around 5%) (Figure 1) [16, 21, 22].

### 2.1. Glycolytic metabolism in brain tumors

As above mentioned, in tumor cells, even in the presence of oxygen, glucose is converted into lactate instead of being oxidized in mitochondria, being glycolysis the major source of energy [16]. It has been described that glioblastomas present metabolic remodeling, increasing glycolytic activity about 3-fold when compared to normal brain tissue [23, 24]. Thus, an increase in several glycolytic enzymes was observed, such as hexokinase II (HKII), pyruvate kinase (PKM), as well as the glucose transporters (GLUTs). Importantly, several studies reported these molecules as important mediators in glycolytic metabolism, constituting attractive molecular targets (Figure 2).

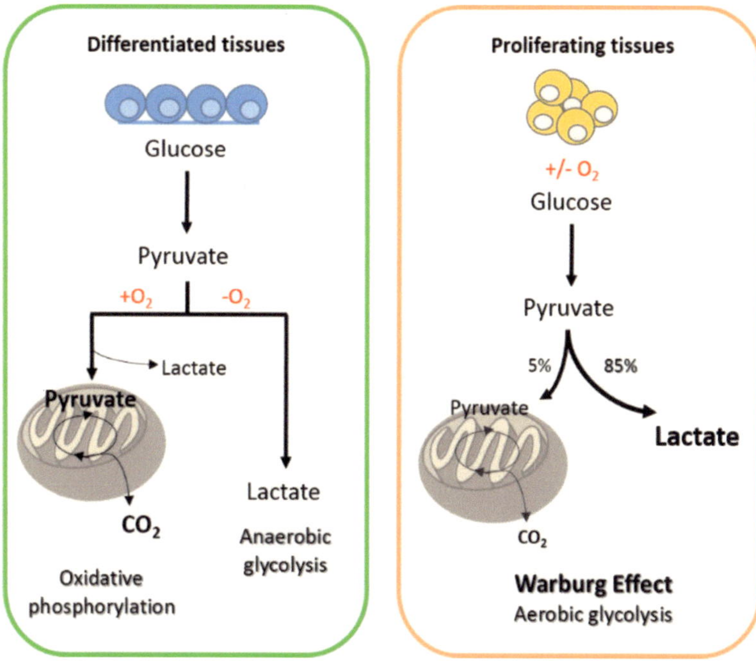


**Figure 1. Schematic representation of the metabolic differences between differentiated tissues and proliferating tissues.** In the presence of oxygen, non-proliferating tissues metabolize glucose to pyruvate and oxidize it in mitochondria through oxidative phosphorylation. On the other hand, glucose is metabolized to lactate when in the absence of oxygen. In proliferative tissues, like tumor cells, glucose is metabolized to pyruvate and even in the presence of oxygen pryruvate is converted into lactate,a phenomenon denominated aerobic glycolysis or Warburg effect.

#### *2.1.1. Glucose Transporters (GLUTs)*

Glucose is the main source of energy in most tissues, including brain. GLUTs are transmembrane transporters that perform the uptake of glucose into the cell. The GLUT family is composed by 12 isoforms, however only GLUT1, GLUT3, and GLUT12 have been described as transporters of glucose [25]. GLUT1 is ubiquitously expressed and it is responsible for providing basal glucose to different tissues and cells. In brain, GLUT1 is expressed in astrocytes, whereas GLUT3 is observed in neurons [26].

In the tumoral context, overexpression of specific isoforms of GLUTs has been reported [27, 28]. Most frequently, an increase in GLUT1 expression has been observed in several solid tumors compared with the corresponding normal tissue [27, 28]. However, it has been verified that their expression is tissue specific and some tumors overexpressed other isoforms, such as GLUT12 in prostate cancer [29]. Concerning brain tumors, few studies have evaluated GLUT expression, where it is described that glioblastomas have an increased expression of GLUT1 and GLUT3 when compared with low grade gliomas and normal brain [30, 31]. In fact, both the isoforms are downstream targets of hypoxia-inducible factor 1$\alpha$ (HIF-1$\alpha$), a transcription factor that is frequently present in glioblastomas. GLUT1 expression is observed in vessels of the normal brain tissues and presents a focal expression in the perinecrotic regions of GBMs, suggesting that their expression is associated with hypoxic regions in glioblastomas (Miranda-

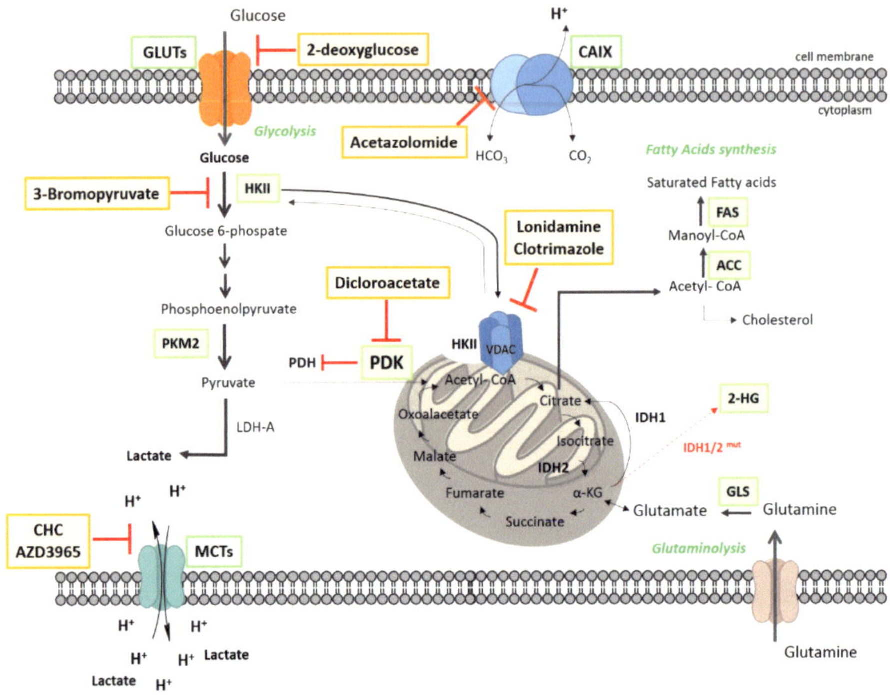


**Figure 2. Potential molecular targets in metabolic remodeling of glioblastomas.** The green boxes represent the potential metabolic molecular targets in glioblastomas: enzymes involved in glycolytic metabolism, glutamine metabolism, lipid metabolism; different transporters and also the oncometabolite 2-hydroxyglutarate. Yellow boxes represent the different inhibitors of the specific molecular targets described. Abbreviations: GLUTs, glucose transporters; MCTs, monocarboxylate transporters; CAIX, carbonic anhydrase IX; HKII, hexokinase II, PKM2, pyruvate kinase M2; LDH-A, lactate dehydrogenase A; PDH, pyruvate dehydrogenase; PDK, pyruvate dehydrogenase kinase; IDH1/2, isocitrate dehydrogenase 1/2; IDH1/2 $^{mut}$, isocitrate dehydrogenase ½ mutation; 2-HG, 2-hydroxyglutarate; GLS, glutaminase; ACC, acetyl-CoA carboxylase; FAS, fatty acid synthase; α-KG, α-ketoglutarate; VDAC, voltage-dependent anion channel; CHC, α-cyanohydroxycinnamic acid.

Gonçalves V. *et al*, submitted). Several *in vitro* studies also reported overexpression of GLUT1 expression in GBMs cells when compared with normal astrocytes [32].

These findings raise the importance of GLUT inhibition in tumor therapy, however, at the moment, a glucose transporter inhibitor is not available at the clinical level. Nevertheless, *in vitro* studies have been using 2-deoxy-D-glucose has an inhibitor of glucose uptake promoting a decrease on tumor cell proliferation [33] (Figure 2). These studies reported the high dependence of brain tumors on glucose as source of energy and also for catabolic processes.

### 2.1.2. Hexokinase II

HK is one of the most important enzymes of the glycolytic pathway, which is responsible for the phosphorylation of glucose to glucose-6-phosphate (G6P), thereby preventing the efflux of glucose from the cell [34]. This enzyme has four isoforms (I-IV) identified in different mammalian tissues [35].

In most solid tumors, hexokinases type I and II are the most frequently upregulated [36]. In glioblastomas, HKII is highly expressed, whereas HKI is predominantly expressed in normal brain and low grade gliomas [37]. Additionally, HKII is expressed at low levels in neuronal tissue, but is highly expressed in mesenchymal subtype of glioblastomas [37]. As the first enzyme involved in the glycolytic pathway, HK controls glucose flux in glycolysis or the pentose phosphate pathway (PPP) [38]. HKII is a highly regulated form of hexokinase, being regulated by HIF-1$\alpha$, glucose, p53, insulin, glucagon, cAMP, among others [36]. The four hexokinase types are normally expressed in the cytoplasm, however type I and II can bind to the outer membrane of the mitochondria *via* voltage-dependent anion channel (VDAC) (Figure 2) [39]. The translocation of HKII to mitochondria is regulated by growth factors and signaling pathways, such as EGFR and PI3K/AKT activation, which are known to be upregulated in glioblastomas [40]. Moreover, the association of HKII with mitochondria in gliomas, besides maintaining high glucose influx, also renders cells resistant to apoptosis, due to the prevention of cytochrome c release [41].

Several studies have described that the expression of HKII in gliomas promotes proliferation and increase in lactate production, being dependent on both mitochondrial localization and kinase activity [42]. Additionally, HKII overexpression in glioblastomas confers resistance to treatment with both temozolomide and radiation, being associated with poor overall survival [43]. Furthermore, silencing of HKII in glioma cells leads to decrease in glycolytic metabolism, observed by a decrease in lactate production and increase expression of OXPHOS proteins and oxygen consumption [43]. Finally, it was also demonstrated that reduction of HKII expression impaired tumor growth *in vivo* both on subcutaneous and intracranial xenograft models [37, 43].

Some drugs have been proposed for chemical inhibition of HKII (Figure 2). 3-bromopyruvate (3-BrPA), a pyruvate analogue, is an alkylating agent and also an inhibitor of glycolysis that decreases tumor growth, without apparent toxicity in subcutaneous hepatocellular carcinoma [44]. However, it is effective only at high concentrations (mM) and to the best our knowledge is not under clinical trials. Other known inhibitor is lonidamine, an inhibitor of HKII binding to the mitochondria, which is currently in clinical trials. *In vitro* studies showed a decrease in lactate production in high grade gliomas but not in low grade [33]. Despite that lonidamine treatment leads to a decrease in tumor growth in different solid tumors without adverse effects, the results of a phase I/II efficacy trial was disappointing in gliomas [45, 46]. Clotrimazole is another inhibitor of HKII localization that demonstrated promising results *in vivo*. In gliomas, clotrimazole increased the sensitivity to radiotherapy and also leads to decrease in tumor growth [47, 48].

#### *2.1.3. Pyruvate Kinase (PK)*

PK is an enzyme involved in the last irreversible step of the glycolytic pathway, converting phosphoenolpyruvate (PEP) to pyruvate [49, 50]. It is also regulated allosterically by the phosphotyrosine binding or phosphorylation and its expression is regulated by isoform selection [50]. Thus, PKM1 is mostly present in adult tissues, such as adult brain and muscle, whereas PKM2 is more frequent in proliferating tissues and embryonic tissues, namely in fetal brain and tumor cancer cells [49]. PKM1 and PKM2 presented different properties, which results in different activities. PKM1 is constitutively active, but PKM2 is regulated by fructose-1,6-biphosphate, presenting reduced activity, which allows the accumulation of glycolytic intermediates and promotes the entry of G6P into the oxidative metabolism of PPP for the production of energy and biosynthesis of proteins, lipids and nucleotides (macromolecules) [50-53]. In cancer cells, like glioblastomas, there is upregulation of PKM2 that favors aerobic glycolysis, increasing lactate production [51, 54, 55]. On the other hand, PKM2 favors the biosynthetic pathway, leading to increased biomass. This dual function potentiates tumor proliferation and aggressiveness. The dimeric form of PKM2 delays pyruvate formation and allows the accumulation of upstream glycolytic intermediates for biosynthetic pathways, whereas the tetrameric form favors aerobic glycolysis, increasing lactate production [56].

In lung cancer cell lines, replacing PKM2 by PKM1 decreases lactate production and increases oxygen consumption (reverse Warburg effect) and also decreases the proliferative capacity of cancer cells in nude mice [54]. It was demonstrated in glioblastomas that knockdown of PKM2 decreased cell proliferation and survival but this did not favor the switch from aerobic glycolysis to oxidative phosphorylation, unlike HKII knockdown [43]. Interestingly, PKM2 was identified as essential for survival of glioma stem cells [57].

Another important function of PKM2 has been associated to epigenetic regulation, being a regulator of histone phosphorylation and acetylation of EGFR-driven glioblastomas [58, 59]. Additionally, in glioblastomas, it was demonstrated that PKM2 is involved in the EGFR signaling pathway that induces its phosphorylation and translocation into the nucleus, which in turn promotes activation of the transcription factor *c-Myc* with consequent activation of downstream targets, namely genes involved in glycolytic metabolism [60]. Taken together, inhibition of PKM2, in order to deplete the dimer and tetramer formation, can be a new therapeutic strategy, since it can lead to inhibition of glycolysis, decreasing energy production and at the same time blocking the anabolic process in tumor cells (Figure 2).

### 2.2. Mitochondrial metabolism in brain tumors

In addition to glycolytic dependence, most tumors present abnormalities in the number and function of mitochondria, as the case of glioblastomas [61]. Otto Warburg hypothesized that the increase on glycolytic metabolism in cancer was due to mitochondrial dysfunction, however nowadays we know that most tumors maintain functional mitochondria [22, 62-64]. Moreover, increased glycolytic metabolism can be a consequence of mitochondrial metabolism impairment, due to abnormalities in components of the tricarboxylic acid (TCA) cycle, alterations in electron transport chain or deficiencies in oxidative phosphorylation [65, 66]. Concerning the selection theory in cancer cells, the dependence on glycolysis occurs gradually in order to compensate the respiratory failure. In contrast to normal brain cells, in which glycolysis and respiration are tightly coupled, tumor cells are defective in their ability to connect glycolysis and respiration [66].

Two mitochondrial enzymes are important in glioblastomas, such as pyruvate dehydrogenase kinase (PDK) and isocitrate dehydrogenases 1 and 2 (IDH1 and IDH2). The presence of mutations in IDH1 and IDH2 has been recently associated with gliomagenesis.

### 2.2.1. *Pyruvate Dehydrogenase Kinase (PDK)*

Pyruvate dehydrogenase (PDH) is a mitochondrial enzyme that controls the entry of pyruvate into mitochondria, promoting its oxidative decarboxylation into acetyl-CoA [67, 68]. The activity of PDH is inhibited by phosphorylation through PDK, resulting in its accumulation in the cytosol and consequent conversion into lactate [67, 68]. PDK is an important mitochondrial matrix protein comprising four isoforms (PDK1 to PDK4), being PDK2 highly expressed in glioblastomas compared to normal adjacent brain tissue [69].

Tumor cells present high levels of glycolysis as a consequence of increased hypoxic microenvironment, which leads to activation of HIF-1$\alpha$ and consequent upregulation of downstream target genes involved in glycolytic metabolism, such as PDK [67]. This enzyme is responsible for the uncoupling between glycolysis and mitochondrial oxidation of glucose, preventing the entry of pyruvate into the mitochondria with consequent increase in glycolytic rates, which confers resistance to apoptosis [67, 68]. Thus, PDK became an important target for glycolytic tumors (Figure 2). Dichloroacetate (DCA), a chemical PDK inhibitor, has been studied in several *in vitro* and *in vivo* models [68]. DCA promotes dephosphorylation of PDH, leading to entry of pyruvate into the mitochondria, decreasing glycolytic rates and lactate production [68, 70]. This leads to activation of oxidative phosphorylation, depolarization of mitochondria and consequent increase in production of reactive oxygen species (ROS), which promotes apoptosis of cancer cells, decreasing tumor cell proliferation [68, 70]. DCA treatment has demonstrated promising results in some tumors, particularly in non-small cell lung, breast and endometrial cancer, either experimentally using *in vitro* and *in vivo* models, as well as in clinical trials [70-73]. In glioblastomas, inhibition of PDK with DCA was evaluated pre-clinically. In C6 glioma cells, it was observed a decrease in lactate production, increase in ROS production, as well as depolarization of mitochondria, which results in a decrease on cell proliferation and induction of apoptosis [74]. *In vivo* it was verified that DCA decreased not only tumor growth but also the angiogenic capacity of glioma cells [74]. The effect of DCA was also tested in a series of glioblastoma patients with congenital acidosis, with a reduction in lactate levels, decrease in HKII localization in the mitochondria, as well as a decrease in mitochondrial polarization, which rendered tumor cells more sensitive to apoptosis [69]. Despite these encouraging results, no exact conclusions can yet be made regarding the efficacy and toxicity of DCA in glioblastoma patients. Thus, a large and randomized clinical study would be important to define the efficacy and toxicity of DCA. Additionally, whether DCA can sensitize GBM cells to temozolomide and radiotherapy remains undetermined.

### 2.2.2. *Isocitrate Dehydrogenase (IDH)*

IDH is an enzyme that catalyzes the oxidative decarboxylation of isocitrate to $\alpha$-ketoglutarate, generating NADH in the mitochondria or NADPH in the cytoplasm [75]. It is composed by 5 genes, being the *IDH1* and *IDH2* the most explored and important in gliomas. IDH1 is presented in the cytoplasm and peroxisome, whereas IDH2 is presented in the mitochondria [76].

In 2008, recurrent somatic hotspot mutations of *IDH1* and *IDH2* were found in low grade gliomas and secondary glioblastomas [77, 78]. These mutations cause amino acid single change in one of the two alleles of the gene (arginine 132 for *IDH1* and arginine 172 for *IDH2*), being classified has a dominant mutation [79]. It is described that the arginine mutation occurs in the binding site of the substrate isocitrate [42]. *IDH1* mutations are reported in more than 80% secondary glioblastomas, but only 5% in primary glioblastomas [76, 80, 81]. Additionally, it occurs in 80% of diffuse astrocytomas (WHO grade II). These mutations are more frequent in younger patient secondary glioblastomas, associated with a proneural subtype and also with increased survival [82]. It was reported that the presence of IDH mutations leads to a decrease in $\alpha$-ketoglutarate that is required for prolyl hydroxylase (PHD) activity that promote degradation of HIF-1$\alpha$ (ref). Thus, downregulation of intracellular $\alpha$-ketoglutarate contributes to stabilization of HIF-1$\alpha$, leading to pseudohypoxia [83]. Nevertheless, subsequent studies did not verify an alteration in $\alpha$-ketoglutarate on mutant IDH1/2, instead, a gain of function activity it was found, which converts $\alpha$-ketoglutarate to 2-hydroxyglutarate (Figure 2) [84, 85]. The latter has been recognized as an oncometabolite, which inhibits enzymes involved in the $\alpha$-ketoglutarate pathway. Additionally, it was described that 2-hydroxyglutarate is involved in epigenetic regulation, promoting a hypermethylator phenotype in gliomas [86] and also keep cells in an undifferentiated *status*, or stem cell-like, which can be more permissive to transformation [17]. The presence of pseudohypoxia, due to the constitutive stabilization of HIF-1$\alpha$, indicates that *IDH1/2* mutations are involved in HIF-1$\alpha$ signaling pathway, which promotes glucose metabolism, angiogenesis and invasion [83]. These results suggest the paramount role of IDH mutations on the metabolic remodeling of glioblastomas, contributing to the "Warburg effect". Therefore, study the involvement of *IDH1/2* mutations in metabolic remodelling and in aerobic glycolysis opens a new window for investigation. Overall, IDH1 is an attractive target for therapy (Figure 2) since they are early events in the progression from low grade to high grade gliomas.

### 2.3. Glutamine metabolism and lipid synthesis in brain tumors

Like glucose, glutamine is a source of energy for tumor cells, functioning as a nitrogen donor [87, 88]. Glutamine metabolism has been reported to be upregulated in some tumors, being crucial for the biosynthetic processes, namely synthesis of cholesterol and fatty acids [14, 89, 90]. The shift to glutamine metabolism to produce the precursor acetyl-CoA for lipid biosynthesis is a mechanism of adaptation to glycolytic metabolism that prevents the entry of pyruvate into mitochondria, due to upregulation of PDK [91]. In fact, it has been observed an increased expression of glutaminase (GLS) enzyme in tumor cells. GLS is located in the mitochondria and catalyzes the conversion of glutamine to glutamate being transcriptionally regulated by the oncogenes *c-Myc* and *NF$\kappa$B*. [92-94], An increased concentration of glutamine in glioblastomas compared to normal brain tissue was demonstrated by nuclear magnetic resonance (NMR) [95]. Additionally, there is a low expression of glutamine synthase that correlates with a better prognosis in glioblastomas [96].

Beyond the altered glycolytic and glutamine metabolism in tumor cells, the alteration in lipid metabolism is also recognized as a component of the metabolic reprogramming. It has been observed that tumor cells present reactivation of *de novo* fatty acid synthesis, important for the biogenesis of cellular membranes [97, 98]. Glioblastomas contain higher levels of unsaturated fatty acids compared to normal brain, indicating the presence of exacerbated lipogenesis, which is regulated by several key genes, such as SREBP-1 and its downstream-targeted genes acetyl-CoA carboxylase (ACC), fatty acid synthase (FAS) and low-density lipoprotein receptor (LDLR), which are upregulated in these tumors [99]. Importantly, the EGFR/PI3K/AkT signaling pathway regulates the metabolic reprogramming in glioblastomas [100]. Cholesterol is also an important component of cell membranes and cholesterol esters have been found to be abundantly present in high grade gliomas, but undetectable in normal tissues by NMR techniques [101, 102]. Recently, low density lipoprotein receptor (LDLR) has been described to be upregulated in GBM patients, xenografts and cell lines, and this upregulation was correlated with high levels of cholesterol esters in GBM cells [103]. Interestingly, LDLR is also be upregulated by EGFR/PI3K/Akt signaling, which was been shown to be mediated by SREBP-1 in GBMs [100]. However, little is known about the altered lipid metabolism in cancer cells, namely glioblastomas, and their role in the tumor context, being possible that lipogenesis in cancer cells could support the cell growth located within nutrient-limited areas, thereby contributing to symbiotic relationships within tumors. Once more, lipid metabolism, as well as glutamine metabolism, and their key enzymes are interesting targets in glioblastomas (Figure 2)

## 3. Lactate transport and pH regulation in brain tumors

A constitutive increase in the glycolytic phenotype of cancer cells leads to acute and chronic acidification of tumor microenvironment. Important proteins involved in acidification of the extracellular space are monocarboxylate transporters (MCTs) that co-transport H+and lactate, and carbonic anhydrases (CAIXs), which are activated by growth factors, oncogenic transformation, hypoxia, and low intracellular pH [21]. As it is known, tumor acidity is associated with cancer cell invasion behavior, i.e. increased migration, invasion and metastasis [104]. Further, tumor acidosis and lactate contributes to several features of tumor progression and malignancy, like immune escape, angiogenesis, and radioresistance, making lactate a key player in cancer aggressiveness. [105]. Still in line with a potential involvement of lactate in the invasion behavior, it has been shown that lactate up-regulates the expression of transforming growth factor (TGF-β2), which is associated with increased migration in glioblastomas [106].

### 3.1. Monocarboxylate transporters

The MCT family comprises 14 members with similar topology; however, only 4 isoforms (MCT1–MCT4) are proton-linked monocarboxylate transporters, performing the transmembrane transport of monocarboxylates, such as lactate, coupled with a proton, in an equimolar manner [107, 108].

In the last years, several studies reported up-regulation of MCTs in different human solid tumors, showing the importance of MCTs in cancer biology [109]. In brain tumors, the scare studies point to the importance of MCT expression, especially MCT1. Strong expression of MCT1 in the plasma membrane was found in high grade gliomas compared with low-grade lesions and normal adjacent tissues, which exhibited negative or weak MCT1 staining [110, 111],. A study in neuroblastomas showed, by mRNA quantification, that MCT1 was differently expressed and that its activity was highly associated with MYCN amplification, leading to the hypothesis that expression of MCT1 could be associated with higher malignancy [112]. Further, expression analysis revealed that SLC16A1 transcript, encoding MCT1, was elevated in 90% of the medulloblastomas analyzed [113]. It was also reported that inhibition of MCT activity, particularly MCT1, decreased the glycolytic phenotype (low glucose consumption and lactate production), cell proliferation and invasion, promoting increase in cell death [111, 114, 115]. This elucidates the importance of MCT1 activity in intracellular pH homeostasis and tumor aggressiveness of glioblastomas.

Although MCTs are not the major $H^+$ transporters, the data available in the literature support the hypothesis of a major contribution of MCTs to the hyper-glycolytic and acid-resistant phenotype, as major adaptation to the hypoxic microenvironment [116]. Thus, MCT inhibition may be a useful therapeutic approach in brain tumors (Figure 2). Actually, it was demonstrated that *in vitro* MCT1 inhibition decreases intracellular pH, leads to cell death and, importantly, enhances cancer cell radiosensivity in gliomas [114, 115]. Importantly, promising results using *in vivo* models have also been reported, where treatment with the chemical inhibitor CHC retarded tumor growth, rendered tumor cells sensitive to radiation and decreased invasion [114, 117]. However, CHC is not a specific MCT inhibitor, having also other targets. Recently, novel MCT1 inhibitors have been designed and may constitute an effective strategy to block MCT1 activity in cancer [118]. A orally administered related compound, AZD3965 (AstraZeneca), is currently in Phase I/II clinical trials for advanced solid tumors [119].

### 3.2. Carbonic anhydrases

Carbonic anhydrase catalyzes the conversion of extracellular bicarbonate to $CO_2$ and protons ($H^+$), thereby contributing to extracellular acidification [120]. This family is composed by 15 isoforms described in mammals, which differ in cellular localization, catalytic activity and susceptibility to different class of inhibitors. Two carbonic anhydrases are overexpressed in many solid tumors, namely CAIX and CAXII, being associated with tumor progression and response to therapy [121]. It is verified that CAIX is mostly negative in normal tissues but increase in the corresponding tumor tissues, whereas CAXII present a diffuse distribution in healthy tissues [122, 123]. Glioblastomas present high levels of intratumoral hypoxia, with consequent HIF-1$\alpha$ activation which contributes to increased expression of glycolysis-related genes [124], including CAIX [125]. CAIX is overexpressed in these tumors with focal plasma membrane expression close to peri-necrotic regions (hypoxic) [126], being negative in normal adjacent tissues, making it a feasible treatment target [127]. Furthermore, it has been described that CAIX is associated to poor overall survival, because it confers resistance to chemotherapy, radiotherapy and anti-angiogenic therapy [128]. Increased expression of CAIX in advanced stages/grades of many tumor types also suggests its association with dedifferentiation [129].

*In vitro* and *in vivo* approaches have demonstrated the potential of CAIX inhibition (Figure 2). Knockdown of CAIX decreased tumor cell ATP levels under hypoxic and glycolytic conditions [126]. In addition, the susceptibility of U251 glioblastoma cells to chemotherapy and radiation treatment was strongly enhanced after CAIX downregulation, which is supported by a recent *in vivo* study [126]. Similarly, CAIX inhibition enhanced the effect of anti-angiogenic therapy with the anti-VEGF antibody bevacizumab [130]. Some inhibitors have been developed to inhibit CA activity, particularly CAIX and CAXII. Acetazolomide, enhances the apoptotic response of glioma cells to temozolomide [131] and an *in vivo* study using derivatives of acetazolamide showed retardation of mice carcinoma xenograft growth after 1 month of treatment [131]. Other studies have identified coumarins as CA inhibitors, however they were not tested yet in the cancer context [132, 133]. Furthermore, specific monoclonal antibodies for the mostly expressed isoforms in tumors, namely CAIX, have been developed, *i.e,* the M75 and WX-G250 for colorectal cancer and renal cell carcinoma, respectively [134, 135].

## 4. Future perspectives and conclusions

Metabolic transformation plays a major role in gliomas development, tumor progression and adaptation to tumor microenvironment. The interplay between tumor angiogenesis, hypoxia, pH regulation and energy metabolism, glycolysis related enzymes and transporters, as well as pH regulator transporters, may provide promising molecular targets for drug development. In addition to glycolysis, glutaminolysis and fatty acid synthesis represent key metabolic events with potentially interesting drug targets. Furthermore, mutations in *IDH1/2*, detected in a genome wide screen on GBMs, point to new specific transforming events in gliomas. These metabolic pathways are tightly linked and also controlled by signaling events often deregulated in gliomas, underlying the flexibility of glioma cells to develop adaptive mechanisms when exposed to oxygen or nutrient deprivation. This highlights the need of targeting several pathways simultaneously and linking the metabolic targets to the genetic makeup of GBM tumors.

## Author details

Vera Miranda Gonçalves[1,2], Fátima Baltazar[1,2] and Rui Manuel Reis[1,2,3*]

*Address all correspondence to: ruireis.hcb@gmail.com

1 Life and Health Sciences Research Institute (ICVS), School of Health Sciences, University of Minho, Braga, Portugal

2 ICVS/3B's-PT Government Associate Laboratory, Braga/Guimarães, Portugal

3 Molecular Oncology Research Center, Barretos Cancer Hospital, Barretos, São Paulo, Brazil

## References


[1] Ohgaki, H. and P. Kleihues, *Epidemiology and etiology of gliomas.* Acta Neuropathol, 2005. 109(1): p. 93-108.

[2] Huse, J.T. and E.C. Holland, *Targeting brain cancer: advances in the molecular pathology of malignant glioma and medulloblastoma.* Nat Rev Cancer, 2010. 10(5): p. 319-31.

[3] Louis, D.N., et al., *The 2007 WHO classification of tumours of the central nervous system.* Acta Neuropathol, 2007. 114(2): p. 97-109.

[4] Riemenschneider, M.J. and G. Reifenberger, *Molecular neuropathology of gliomas.* Int J Mol Sci, 2009. 10(1): p. 184-212.

[5] Stupp, R., et al., *Radiotherapy plus concomitant and adjuvant temozolomide for glioblastoma.* N Engl J Med, 2005. 352(10): p. 987-96.

[6] Lai, A., et al., *Phase II study of bevacizumab plus temozolomide during and after radiation therapy for patients with newly diagnosed glioblastoma multiforme.* J Clin Oncol, 2011. 29(2): p. 142-8.

[7] Chinot, O.L., et al., *Bevacizumab plus radiotherapy-temozolomide for newly diagnosed glioblastoma.* N Engl J Med, 2014. 370(8): p. 709-22.

[8] Weathers, S.P. and M.R. Gilbert, *Advances in treating glioblastoma.* F1000Prime Rep, 2014. 6: p. 46.

[9] de Groot, J.F., et al., *Tumor invasion after treatment of glioblastoma with bevacizumab: radiographic and pathologic correlation in humans and mice.* Neuro Oncol, 2010. 12(3): p. 233-42.

[10] Narayana, A., et al., *Bevacizumab in recurrent high-grade pediatric gliomas.* Neuro Oncol, 2010. 12(9): p. 985-90.

[11] Mesti, T., et al., *Metabolic impact of anti-angiogenic agents on U87 glioma cells.* PLoS One, 2014. 9(6): p. e99198.

[12] Gaspar, N., et al., *MGMT-independent temozolomide resistance in pediatric glioblastoma cells associated with a PI3-kinase-mediated HOX/stem cell gene signature.* Cancer Res, 2010. 70(22): p. 9243-52.

[13] Costa, B.M., et al., *Prognostic value of MGMT promoter methylation in glioblastoma patients treated with temozolomide-based chemoradiation: a Portuguese multicentre study.* Oncol Rep, 2010. 23(6): p. 1655-62.

[14] DeBerardinis, R.J., et al., *The biology of cancer: metabolic reprogramming fuels cell growth and proliferation.* Cell Metab, 2008. 7(1): p. 11-20.

[15] DeBerardinis, R.J. and C.B. Thompson, *Cellular metabolism and disease: what do metabolic outliers teach us?* Cell, 2012. 148(6): p. 1132-44.

[16] Vander Heiden, M.G., L.C. Cantley, and C.B. Thompson, *Understanding the Warburg effect: the metabolic requirements of cell proliferation.* Science, 2009. 324(5930): p. 1029-33.

[17] Schulze, A. and A.L. Harris, *How cancer metabolism is tuned for proliferation and vulnerable to disruption.* Nature, 2012. 491(7424): p. 364-73.

[18] Dang, C.V. and G.L. Semenza, *Oncogenic alterations of metabolism.* Trends Biochem Sci, 1999. 24(2): p. 68-72.

[19] Gatenby, R.A. and R.J. Gillies, *A microenvironmental model of carcinogenesis.* Nat Rev Cancer, 2008. 8(1): p. 56-61.

[20] Hanahan, D. and R.A. Weinberg, *Hallmarks of cancer: the next generation.* Cell, 2011. 144(5): p. 646-74.

[21] Gatenby, R.A. and R.J. Gillies, *Why do cancers have high aerobic glycolysis?* Nat Rev Cancer, 2004. 4(11): p. 891-9.

[22] Warburg, O., *On respiratory impairment in cancer cells.* Science, 1956. 124(3215): p. 269-70.

[23] Oudard, S., et al., *High glycolysis in gliomas despite low hexokinase transcription and activity correlated to chromosome 10 loss.* Br J Cancer, 1996. 74(6): p. 839-45.

[24] Tabatabaei, P., et al., *Glucose metabolites, glutamate and glycerol in malignant glioma tumours during radiotherapy.* J Neurooncol, 2008. 90(1): p. 35-9.

[25] Zhao, F.Q. and A.F. Keating, *Functional properties and genomics of glucose transporters.* Curr Genomics, 2007. 8(2): p. 113-28.

[26] Leybaert, L., *Neurobarrier coupling in the brain: a partner of neurovascular and neurometabolic coupling?* J Cereb Blood Flow Metab, 2005. 25(1): p. 2-16.

[27] Medina, R.A. and G.I. Owen, *Glucose transporters: expression, regulation and cancer.* Biol Res, 2002. 35(1): p. 9-26.

[28] Macheda, M.L., S. Rogers, and J.D. Best, *Molecular and cellular regulation of glucose transporter (GLUT) proteins in cancer.* J Cell Physiol, 2005. 202(3): p. 654-62.

[29] Chandler, J.D., et al., *Expression and localization of GLUT1 and GLUT12 in prostate carcinoma.* Cancer, 2003. 97(8): p. 2035-42.

[30] Boado, R.J., K.L. Black, and W.M. Pardridge, *Gene expression of GLUT3 and GLUT1 glucose transporters in human brain tumors.* Brain Res Mol Brain Res, 1994. 27(1): p. 51-7.

[31] Flynn, J.R., et al., *Hypoxia-regulated protein expression, patient characteristics, and preoperative imaging as predictors of survival in adults with glioblastoma multiforme.* Cancer, 2008. 113(5): p. 1032-42.

[32] Jensen, R.L., *Brain tumor hypoxia: tumorigenesis, angiogenesis, imaging, pseudoprogression, and as a therapeutic target.* J Neurooncol, 2009. 92(3): p. 317-35.

[33] Stieber, D., S.A. Abdul Rahim, and S.P. Niclou, *Novel ways to target brain tumour metabolism.* Expert Opin Ther Targets, 2011. 15(10): p. 1227-39.

[34] Smith, T.A., *Mammalian hexokinases and their abnormal expression in cancer.* Br J Biomed Sci, 2000. 57(2): p. 170-8.

[35] Wilson, J.E., *Isozymes of mammalian hexokinase: structure, subcellular localization and metabolic function.* J Exp Biol, 2003. 206(Pt 12): p. 2049-57.

[36] Pedersen, P.L., et al., *Mitochondrial bound type II hexokinase: a key player in the growth and survival of many cancers and an ideal prospect for therapeutic intervention.* Biochim Biophys Acta, 2002. 1555(1-3): p. 14-20.

[37] Wolf, A., et al., *Hexokinase 2 is a key mediator of aerobic glycolysis and promotes tumor growth in human glioblastoma multiforme.* J Exp Med, 2011. 208(2): p. 313-26.

[38] Agnihotri, S., et al., *A GATA4-regulated tumor suppressor network represses formation of malignant human astrocytomas.* J Exp Med, 2011. 208(4): p. 689-702.

[39] Mathupala, S.P., Y.H. Ko, and P.L. Pedersen, *Hexokinase-2 bound to mitochondria: cancer's stygian link to the "Warburg Effect" and a pivotal target for effective therapy.* Semin Cancer Biol, 2009. 19(1): p. 17-24.

[40] Mellinghoff, I.K., et al., *Molecular determinants of the response of glioblastomas to EGFR kinase inhibitors.* N Engl J Med, 2005. 353(19): p. 2012-24.

[41] Pastorino, J.G., N. Shulga, and J.B. Hoek, *Mitochondrial binding of hexokinase II inhibits Bax-induced cytochrome c release and apoptosis.* J Biol Chem, 2002. 277(9): p. 7610-8.

[42] Wolf, A., S. Agnihotri, and A. Guha, *Targeting metabolic remodeling in glioblastoma multiforme.* Oncotarget, 2010. 1(7): p. 552-62.

[43] Wolf, A., et al., *Developmental profile and regulation of the glycolytic enzyme hexokinase 2 in normal brain and glioblastoma multiforme.* Neurobiol Dis, 2011. 44(1): p. 84-91.

[44] Ko, Y.H., et al., *Advanced cancers: eradication in all cases using 3-bromopyruvate therapy to deplete ATP.* Biochem Biophys Res Commun, 2004. 324(1): p. 269-75.

[45] Oudard, S., et al., *Phase II study of lonidamine and diazepam in the treatment of recurrent glioblastoma multiforme.* J Neurooncol, 2003. 63(1): p. 81-6.

[46] Carapella, C.M., et al., *The potential role of lonidamine (LND) in the treatment of malignant glioma. Phase II study.* J Neurooncol, 1989. 7(1): p. 103-8.

[47] Liu, H., Y. Li, and K.P. Raisch, *Clotrimazole induces a late G1 cell cycle arrest and sensitizes glioblastoma cells to radiation in vitro.* Anticancer Drugs, 2010. 21(9): p. 841-9.

[48] Khalid, M.H., et al., *Inhibition of tumor growth and prolonged survival of rats with intracranial gliomas following administration of clotrimazole.* J Neurosurg, 2005. 103(1): p. 79-86.

[49] Altenberg, B. and K.O. Greulich, *Genes of glycolysis are ubiquitously overexpressed in 24 cancer classes.* Genomics, 2004. 84(6): p. 1014-20.

[50] Mazurek, S., et al., *Pyruvate kinase type M2 and its role in tumor growth and spreading.* Semin Cancer Biol, 2005. 15(4): p. 300-8.

[51] Mazurek, S., et al., *Pyruvate kinase type M2: a crossroad in the tumor metabolome.* Br J Nutr, 2002. 87 Suppl 1: p. S23-9.

[52] Christofk, H.R., et al., *Pyruvate kinase M2 is a phosphotyrosine-binding protein.* Nature, 2008. 452(7184): p. 181-6.

[53] Eigenbrodt, E., et al., *Double role for pyruvate kinase type M2 in the expansion of phosphometabolite pools found in tumor cells.* Crit Rev Oncog, 1992. 3(1-2): p. 91-115.

[54] Christofk, H.R., et al., *The M2 splice isoform of pyruvate kinase is important for cancer metabolism and tumour growth.* Nature, 2008. 452(7184): p. 230-3.

[55] Kefas, B., et al., *Pyruvate kinase M2 is a target of the tumor-suppressive microRNA-326 and regulates the survival of glioma cells.* Neuro Oncol, 2010. 12(11): p. 1102-12.

[56] Soga, T., *Cancer metabolism: key players in metabolic reprogramming.* Cancer Sci, 2013. 104(3): p. 275-81.

[57] Goidts, V., et al., *RNAi screening in glioma stem-like cells identifies PFKFB4 as a key molecule important for cancer cell survival.* Oncogene, 2012. 31(27): p. 3235-43.

[58] Yang, W., et al., *PKM2 phosphorylates histone H3 and promotes gene transcription and tumorigenesis.* Cell, 2012. 150(4): p. 685-96.

[59] Yang, W., et al., *EGFR-induced and PKCepsilon monoubiquitylation-dependent NF-kappaB activation upregulates PKM2 expression and promotes tumorigenesis.* Mol Cell, 2012. 48(5): p. 771-84.

[60] Yang, W., et al., *ERK1/2-dependent phosphorylation and nuclear translocation of PKM2 promotes the Warburg effect.* Nat Cell Biol, 2012. 14(12): p. 1295-304.

[61] Katsetos, C.D., H. Anni, and P. Draber, *Mitochondrial dysfunction in gliomas.* Semin Pediatr Neurol, 2013. 20(3): p. 216-27.

[62] Warburg, O., *On the origin of cancer cells.* Science, 1956. 123(3191): p. 309-14.

[63] Pedersen, P.L., *Tumor mitochondria and the bioenergetics of cancer cells.* Prog Exp Tumor Res, 1978. 22: p. 190-274.

[64] Meixensberger, J., et al., *Metabolic patterns in malignant gliomas.* J Neurooncol, 1995. 24(2): p. 153-61.

[65] Seyfried, T.N. and P. Mukherjee, *Targeting energy metabolism in brain cancer: review and hypothesis.* Nutr Metab (Lond), 2005. 2: p. 30.

[66] Seyfried, T.N., et al., *Metabolic management of brain cancer.* Biochim Biophys Acta, 2011. 1807(6): p. 577-94.

[67] Kim, J.W., et al., *HIF-1-mediated expression of pyruvate dehydrogenase kinase: a metabolic switch required for cellular adaptation to hypoxia.* Cell Metab, 2006. 3(3): p. 177-85.

[68] Michelakis, E.D., L. Webster, and J.R. Mackey, *Dichloroacetate (DCA) as a potential metabolic-targeting therapy for cancer.* Br J Cancer, 2008. 99(7): p. 989-94.

[69] Michelakis, E.D., et al., *Metabolic modulation of glioblastoma with dichloroacetate.* Sci Transl Med, 2010. 2(31): p. 31ra34.

[70] Bonnet, S., et al., *A mitochondria-K+channel axis is suppressed in cancer and its normalization promotes apoptosis and inhibits cancer growth.* Cancer Cell, 2007. 11(1): p. 37-51.

[71] Cairns, R.A., et al., *Metabolic targeting of hypoxia and HIF1 in solid tumors can enhance cytotoxic chemotherapy.* Proc Natl Acad Sci U S A, 2007. 104(22): p. 9445-50.

[72] Cao, W., et al., *Dichloroacetate (DCA) sensitizes both wild-type and over expressing Bcl-2 prostate cancer cells in vitro to radiation.* Prostate, 2008. 68(11): p. 1223-31.

[73] Wong, J.Y., et al., *Dichloroacetate induces apoptosis in endometrial cancer cells.* Gynecol Oncol, 2008. 109(3): p. 394-402.

[74] Duan, Y., et al., *Antitumor activity of dichloroacetate on C6 glioma cell: in vitro and in vivo evaluation.* Onco Targets Ther, 2013. 6: p. 189-98.

[75] Reitman, Z.J. and H. Yan, *Isocitrate dehydrogenase 1 and 2 mutations in cancer: alterations at a crossroads of cellular metabolism.* J Natl Cancer Inst, 2010. 102(13): p. 932-41.

[76] Kim, W. and L.M. Liau, *IDH mutations in human glioma.* Neurosurg Clin N Am, 2012. 23(3): p. 471-80.

[77] Parsons, D.W., et al., *An integrated genomic analysis of human glioblastoma multiforme.* Science, 2008. 321(5897): p. 1807-12.

[78] Yan, H., et al., *IDH1 and IDH2 mutations in gliomas.* N Engl J Med, 2009. 360(8): p. 765-73.

[79] Fu, Y., et al., *Glioma-derived mutations in IDH: from mechanism to potential therapy.* Biochem Biophys Res Commun, 2010. 397(2): p. 127-30.

[80] DeAngelis, L.M. and I.K. Mellinghoff, *Virchow 2011 or how to ID(H) human glioblastoma.* J Clin Oncol, 2011. 29(34): p. 4473-4.

[81] Watanabe, T., et al., *IDH1 mutations are early events in the development of astrocytomas and oligodendrogliomas.* Am J Pathol, 2009. 174(4): p. 1149-53.

[82] Verhaak, R.G., et al., *Integrated genomic analysis identifies clinically relevant subtypes of glioblastoma characterized by abnormalities in PDGFRA, IDH1, EGFR, and NF1.* Cancer Cell, 2010. 17(1): p. 98-110.

[83] Zhao, S., et al., *Glioma-derived mutations in IDH1 dominantly inhibit IDH1 catalytic activity and induce HIF-1alpha.* Science, 2009. 324(5924): p. 261-5.

[84] Ward, P.S., et al., *The common feature of leukemia-associated IDH1 and IDH2 mutations is a neomorphic enzyme activity converting alpha-ketoglutarate to 2-hydroxyglutarate.* Cancer Cell, 2010. 17(3): p. 225-34.

[85] Dang, L., et al., *Cancer-associated IDH1 mutations produce 2-hydroxyglutarate.* Nature, 2009. 462(7274): p. 739-44.

[86] Lu, C. and C.B. Thompson, *Metabolic regulation of epigenetics.* Cell Metab, 2012. 16(1): p. 9-17.

[87] Zielke, H.R., C.L. Zielke, and P.T. Ozand, *Glutamine: a major energy source for cultured mammalian cells.* Fed Proc, 1984. 43(1): p. 121-5.

[88] Reitzer, L.J., B.M. Wice, and D. Kennell, *Evidence that glutamine, not sugar, is the major energy source for cultured HeLa cells.* J Biol Chem, 1979. 254(8): p. 2669-76.

[89] DeBerardinis, R.J., et al., *Beyond aerobic glycolysis: transformed cells can engage in glutamine metabolism that exceeds the requirement for protein and nucleotide synthesis.* Proc Natl Acad Sci U S A, 2007. 104(49): p. 19345-50.

[90] Rajagopalan, K.N. and R.J. DeBerardinis, *Role of glutamine in cancer: therapeutic and imaging implications.* J Nucl Med, 2011. 52(7): p. 1005-8.

[91] Daye, D. and K.E. Wellen, *Metabolic reprogramming in cancer: unraveling the role of glutamine in tumorigenesis.* Semin Cell Dev Biol, 2012. 23(4): p. 362-9.

[92] Dang, C.V., A. Le, and P. Gao, *MYC-induced cancer cell energy metabolism and therapeutic opportunities.* Clin Cancer Res, 2009. 15(21): p. 6479-83.

[93] Rathore, M.G., et al., *The NF-kappaB member p65 controls glutamine metabolism through miR-23a.* Int J Biochem Cell Biol, 2012. 44(9): p. 1448-56.

[94] Wang, J.B., et al., *Targeting mitochondrial glutaminase activity inhibits oncogenic transformation.* Cancer Cell, 2010. 18(3): p. 207-19.

[95] Kallenberg, K., et al., *Untreated glioblastoma multiforme: increased myo-inositol and glutamine levels in the contralateral cerebral hemisphere at proton MR spectroscopy.* Radiology, 2009. 253(3): p. 805-12.

[96] Rosati, A., et al., *Epilepsy in glioblastoma multiforme: correlation with glutamine synthetase levels.* J Neurooncol, 2009. 93(3): p. 319-24.

[97] Menendez, J.A. and R. Lupu, *Fatty acid synthase and the lipogenic phenotype in cancer pathogenesis.* Nat Rev Cancer, 2007. 7(10): p. 763-77.

[98] Abramson, H.N., *The lipogenesis pathway as a cancer target.* J Med Chem, 2011. 54(16): p. 5615-38.

[99] Gopal, K., et al., *Lipid Composition of Human Intracranial Tumors: A Biochemical Study.* Acta Neurochir (Wien), 1963. 11: p. 333-47.

[100] Guo, D., et al., *EGFR signaling through an Akt-SREBP-1-dependent, rapamycin-resistant pathway sensitizes glioblastomas to antilipogenic therapy.* Sci Signal, 2009. 2(101): p. ra82.

[101] Tugnoli, V., et al., *Characterization of lipids from human brain tissues by multinuclear magnetic resonance spectroscopy.* Biopolymers, 2001. 62(6): p. 297-306.

[102] Yates, A.J., et al., *Lipid composition of human neural tumors.* J Lipid Res, 1979. 20(4): p. 428-36.

[103] Rudling, M.J., et al., *Low density lipoprotein receptor activity in human intracranial tumors and its relation to the cholesterol requirement.* Cancer Res, 1990. 50(3): p. 483-7.

[104] Dhup, S., et al., *Multiple biological activities of lactic acid in cancer: influences on tumor growth, angiogenesis and metastasis.* Curr Pharm Des, 2012. 18(10): p. 1319-30.

[105] Hirschhaeuser, F., U.G. Sattler, and W. Mueller-Klieser, *Lactate: a metabolic key player in cancer.* Cancer Res, 2011. 71(22): p. 6921-5.

[106] Baumann, F., et al., *Lactate promotes glioma migration by TGF-beta2-dependent regulation of matrix metalloproteinase-2.* Neuro Oncol, 2009. 11(4): p. 368-80.

[107] Halestrap, A.P. and N.T. Price, *The proton-linked monocarboxylate transporter (MCT) family: structure, function and regulation.* Biochem J, 1999. 343 Pt 2: p. 281-99.

[108] Enerson, B.E. and L.R. Drewes, *Molecular features, regulation, and function of monocarboxylate transporters: implications for drug delivery.* J Pharm Sci, 2003. 92(8): p. 1531-44.

[109] Pinheiro, C., et al., *Role of monocarboxylate transporters in human cancers: state of the art.* J Bioenerg Biomembr, 2012. 44(1): p. 127-39.

[110] Froberg, M.K., et al., *Expression of monocarboxylate transporter MCT1 in normal and neoplastic human CNS tissues.* Neuroreport, 2001. 12(4): p. 761-5.

[111] Miranda-Goncalves, V., et al., *Monocarboxylate transporters (MCTs) in gliomas: expression and exploitation as therapeutic targets.* Neuro Oncol, 2013. 15(2): p. 172-88.

[112] Fang, J., et al., *The H+-linked monocarboxylate transporter (MCT1/SLC16A1): a potential therapeutic target for high-risk neuroblastoma.* Mol Pharmacol, 2006. 70(6): p. 2108-15.

[113] Li, K.K., et al., *miR-124 is frequently down-regulated in medulloblastoma and is a negative regulator of SLC16A1.* Hum Pathol, 2009. 40(9): p. 1234-43.

[114] Colen, C.B., et al., *Metabolic targeting of lactate efflux by malignant glioma inhibits invasiveness and induces necrosis: an in vivo study.* Neoplasia, 2011. 13(7): p. 620-32.

[115] Colen, C.B., et al., *Metabolic remodeling of malignant gliomas for enhanced sensitization during radiotherapy: an in vitro study.* Neurosurgery, 2006. 59(6): p. 1313-23; discussion 1323-4.

[116] Pouyssegur, J., F. Dayan, and N.M. Mazure, *Hypoxia signalling in cancer and approaches to enforce tumour regression.* Nature, 2006. 441(7092): p. 437-43.

[117] Sonveaux, P., et al., *Targeting lactate-fueled respiration selectively kills hypoxic tumor cells in mice.* J Clin Invest, 2008. 118(12): p. 3930-42.

[118] Bueno, V., et al., *The specific monocarboxylate transporter (MCT1) inhibitor, AR-C117977, a novel immunosuppressant, prolongs allograft survival in the mouse.* Transplantation, 2007. 84(9): p. 1204-7.

[119] Porporato, P.E., et al., *Anticancer targets in the glycolytic metabolism of tumors: a comprehensive review.* Front Pharmacol, 2011. 2: p. 49.

[120] Damaghi, M., J.W. Wojtkowiak, and R.J. Gillies, *pH sensing and regulation in cancer.* Front Physiol, 2013. 4: p. 370.

[121] Supuran, C.T., *Carbonic anhydrases: novel therapeutic applications for inhibitors and activators.* Nat Rev Drug Discov, 2008. 7(2): p. 168-81.

[122] Tureci, O., et al., *Human carbonic anhydrase XII: cDNA cloning, expression, and chromosomal localization of a carbonic anhydrase gene that is overexpressed in some renal cell cancers.* Proc Natl Acad Sci U S A, 1998. 95(13): p. 7608-13.

[123] Hilvo, M., et al., *Biochemical characterization of CA IX, one of the most active carbonic anhydrase isozymes.* J Biol Chem, 2008. 283(41): p. 27799-809.

[124] Brahimi-Horn, M.C., G. Bellot, and J. Pouyssegur, *Hypoxia and energetic tumour metabolism.* Curr Opin Genet Dev, 2011. 21(1): p. 67-72.

[125] Chiche, J., M.C. Brahimi-Horn, and J. Pouyssegur, *Tumour hypoxia induces a metabolic shift causing acidosis: a common feature in cancer.* J Cell Mol Med, 2010. 14(4): p. 771-94.

[126] Proescholdt, M.A., et al., *Function of carbonic anhydrase IX in glioblastoma multiforme.* Neuro Oncol, 2012. 14(11): p. 1357-66.

[127] Zatovicova, M., et al., *Carbonic anhydrase IX as an anticancer therapy target: preclinical evaluation of internalizing monoclonal antibody directed to catalytic domain.* Curr Pharm Des, 2010. 16(29): p. 3255-63.

[128] Sedlakova, O., et al., *Carbonic anhydrase IX, a hypoxia-induced catalytic component of the pH regulating machinery in tumors.* Front Physiol, 2014. 4: p. 400.

[129] Currie, M.J., et al., *Immunohistochemical analysis of cancer stem cell markers in invasive breast carcinoma and associated ductal carcinoma in situ: relationships with markers of tumor hypoxia and microvascularity.* Hum Pathol, 2013. 44(3): p. 402-11.

[130] McIntyre, A., et al., *Carbonic anhydrase IX promotes tumor growth and necrosis in vivo and inhibition enhances anti-VEGF therapy.* Clin Cancer Res, 2012. 18(11): p. 3100-11.

[131] De Simone, G., et al., *Carbonic anhydrase inhibitors: Hypoxia-activatable sulfonamides incorporating disulfide bonds that target the tumor-associated isoform IX.* J Med Chem, 2006. 49(18): p. 5544-51.

[132] Maresca, A., et al., *Non-zinc mediated inhibition of carbonic anhydrases: coumarins are a new class of suicide inhibitors.* J Am Chem Soc, 2009. 131(8): p. 3057-62.

[133] Maresca, A., et al., *Deciphering the mechanism of carbonic anhydrase inhibition with coumarins and thiocoumarins.* J Med Chem, 2010. 53(1): p. 335-44.

[134] Chrastina, A., S. Pastorekova, and J. Pastorek, *Immunotargeting of human cervical carcinoma xenograft expressing CA IX tumor-associated antigen by 125I-labeled M75 monoclonal antibody.* Neoplasma, 2003. 50(1): p. 13-21.

[135] Siebels, M., et al., A clinical phase I/II trial with the monoclonal antibody cG250 (RENCAREX(R)) and interferon-alpha-2a in metastatic renal cell carcinoma patients. World J Urol, 2011. 29(1): p. 121-6.

Chapter 5

# BMI Transcription Factor as a Novel Target for the Treatment of Brain Tumors

Mohammad M. Hossain, Bárbara Meléndez,
Juan A. Rey, Javier S. Castresana and Mehdi H. Shahi

Additional information is available at the end of the chapter

http://dx.doi.org/10.5772/59194

## 1. Introduction

Recent studies have hypothesized that brain tumor stem cells (BTSCs) are responsible for the poor survival outcome of brain tumor patients. Sonic hedgehog (Shh) is one of the crucial signaling pathways to regulate stem cell self-renewable capacity. Disruption of this pathway activate Gli transcription factors, which further activate other downstream target genes including BMI1 to promote brain tumor development (medulloblastoma and glioblastoma among other tumors) (Leung *et al.,* 2004; Bruggeman *et al.,* 2007; Godlewski *et al.,* 2008). BMI1 is a polycomb complex protein also known as polycomb group RING finger protein 4 (PCGF4) or RING finger protein 51 (RNF51). BMI1 gene (B cell-specific Moloney Murin leukemia virus integration site 1) is located on human chromosome 10 (10p13). Interestingly, BMI1 showed high expression in medulloblastoma and glioblastoma (Leung *et al.,* 2004; Natsume *et al.,* 2011). Shh treatment induced both BMI1 and Gli1 expression. Gli1 overexpression also promoted high expression of BMI1. High expression of BMI1 in tumor cells indicates high capacity of self-renewing characteristics (Hemmati *et al.,* 2003). Most of the BTSCs showed high expression of BMI1. Inhibition of Gli with specific inhibitor GANT61 and Gli siRNAs mediated knock-down inhibited brain tumor cell proliferation and also decreased the expression of BMI1 in medulloblastoma and glioblastoma (Shahi *et al.,* unpublished). Therefore, all these studies suggest that BMI1 would be a novel therapeutic transcription factor to target BTSCs and enhance the survival of brain tumor patients.

INTECH
open science | open minds

## 2. BMI1: An oncogene and stem cell marker

BMI1 is one of the crucial genes for the development of various tissues including the nervous system. This gene is located at chromosome 10p13 in humans. BMI1 was initially identified as a murin leukemia viral oncogene [1]. BMI1 was the first gene reported to belong to the Polycomb-group of genes [2]. These genes express the proteins which form a large multimeric structure to silence other genes via modification in chromatin organization [3]. Polycomb repressive complexes are divided into two groups.

Polycomb repressive complex 1 (PRC1)

Polycomb repressive complex 2 (PRC2)

PRC1 includes BMI1, and PRC2 includes enhancer of zeste homolog 2 (EZHZ) to facilitate stable silencing of gene expression [4]

## 3. Role of BMI1 in normal development

BMI1 polycomb protein is essential for the self-renewal of stem cells of different tissues of the body besides the central nervous system (CNS) [5]. One study showed that Nestin-BMI1-GFP transgenic mice cells increased the development of neural stem cell colonies and the self-renewal capability of fetal and adult CNS cells *(He et al., 2009).* Ink4a and Arf genes encode tumor suppressor proteins p16Ink4a and p19Arf respectively, which are involved in the inhibition of cell cycle progression [6]. Interestingly, BMI1 promotes the maintenance of CNS stem cells from the embryonic stage to adulthood by suppressing Ink4a and Arf genes [5]. BMI1 is also involved in Shh signaling mediated postnatal cerebellar neurogenesis by binding to the promoter of p21waf1/cip1 [7]. Moreover, BMI1 is a crucial gene for the development of embryonic and adult stem cells and brain tumors. Interestingly, selective conditional knockout of BMI1 based on Cre/LoXP in transgenic mouse showed that BMI1 has potential to induce neural stem cells proliferation and self-renewal both *in vitro* and *in vivo* [8]. In this process BMI1 down-regulates both Ink4a/ARF and p21/FoxG1. Moreover, increased ectopic expression of BMI1 in progenitors committed to a neuronal lineage during embryonic cortical development, triggered apoptosis via a survivin-mediated mechanism, and caused a reduction in brain size [8]. However, the self-renewable capability of adult neural stem progenitor cells is independent of FoxG1, while apoptosis resistance of neural progenitor cells depends on high expression of BMI1 [8].

## 4. Role of BMI1 in glioblastoma development

Gliomas are the most common brain tumors of the central nervous system comprising astrocytic gliomas, oligodendrogliomas, or a mixture of both. The most malignant glioma is glioblastoma multiforme (GBM) (WHO grade IV) comprising about 50% of glioma. Post-therapy survival rate of GBM patients is 24% for 1 year and 12% for 2 years only [9]. There are ample amount of evidence suggesting that gliomas have stem-like cells called glioma initiating cells (GICs). These cells have self-renewal capability and cause gliomagenesis. The GICs are under the regulation of several signaling pathways including Shh, Notch, Wnt and BMI1. Effective targeting of GICs could become a novel strategy to target glioma [10]. The 10p13 region is highly significant in brain tumorigenesis especially glioblastoma. BMI1 is part of the polycomb repressive complex 1, which epigenetically regulates gene expression by acetylation, methylation, and mono-ubiquitination of histones [11]. These modifications cause transcriptional repression of differentiation and pluripotency of embryonic stem cells [12]. BMI1 is essential for the proliferation and transformation of primary glial cells. BMI1 deficient glial cells have less proliferating and tumorigenic capacities. BMI1 is also involved in pathways including proliferation, adhesion, and differentiation. All these pathways play a significant contribution to stem cell renewal and glioblastoma development [13]. One report demonstrates a high copy number of BMI1 in glioma samples [11]. Even, a murine tumor model showed a role for BMI1 in the genesis of glioma and high fold expression of BMI1 in high-grade gliomas [13]. BMI1 shows functional diversity in different cell types including embryonic stem cells and mature neurons [12]. Moreover, BMI1 sometimes behaves as a tumor suppressor gene or oncogene in different tumors. According to one study most of the glioma samples showed BMI1 gene allelic imbalance. BMI1 negatively regulates p16 in astrocytoma. However, they also suggest that BMI1 is not very significant for prognosis of astrocytic tumors [2]. Interestingly, BMI1 is considered as a transgene, which helps MYC to promote hematopoietic malignancies [14-16]. High expression of BMI1 has been noted in brain tumors irrespective of tumor grades [5]. BMI1 has a role in glioma and glioma stem cell growth which is both dependent and independent of InK4a-Arf [13]. GBM showed an association of BMI1 overexpression and enrichment in CD133+ cells [Xia *et al.*, 2012]. Stable knockdown of BMI1 in GBM reveals that BMI1 prevented the clonogenic nature of GBM cells and also these cells were not able to develop brain tumors *in vivo*. Accordingly, BMI1 is a potent inhibitor of apoptosis in CD133+ cells and of differentiation into neurons and astrocytes [17]. BMI1 is also capable to inhibit alternate tumor suppressor pathways that attempt to compensate for INK4A-ARF/p53 deletion and hyperactivity of the PI3K/AKT pathway [17]. Interestingly, one study suggests that BMI1 causes apoptotic resistance to glioma cells through the activation of IKK-Nuclear factor-kB pathway and could therefore be a good prognostic factor for glioma [20]. IKK-Nuclear factor-kB pathway is very active in high grade GBM and glioma cell lines [18, 19]. High expression of BMI1 protects brain tumor cells from cytotoxic reagents-induced apoptosis, while attenuated BMI1 expression promotes apoptosis inducer factors. BMI1 also controls apoptosis in glioma cell lines by activation of the IKK-NF-kB pathway and promoting anti-apoptotic genes [20]. Co-expression of BMI1 and p65 protein, a subunit of NF-kB in glioma is in favour of BMI1 and NF-kB pathways involvement in glioma chemoresistance. GBM is resistant to all types of therapies. It has been postulated that most CD133+ cells are resistant to gamma radiation via activation of DNA double-strand break (DSB) response mechanism, including the participation of the ataxia-telangiectasia-mutated kinase gene (ATM). After purification of BMI1 with DNA DSB responsive factors and nonhomologous end joining (NHEJ) repair proteins in GBM cells [21], a BMI1 enrichment was observed after irradiation, being colocalized and co-purified with ATM and histone gammaH2AX. Deficient BMI1 glioma cells showed inactive DNA DSB response, which promoted sensitivity of radiation in glioma cells. Overexpressed BMI1 modulated the neural stem cells radiation resistance by enhancing the ATM activity. Therefore, a combined effect of BMI1 inhibition together with radiation therapy might efficiently target GBM stem cells [21]. Interestingly, a recent report suggested that expression of BMI1 and c-Myc correlated in glioma. This finding further reveals that c-Myc, either directly or indirectly, activates several epigenetic modulators including acetylase GCN5 and polycomb-group (PcG) gene BMI1 [22, 23]. It is interesting to know that BMI1 promoter contains functional E-box and c-Myc binding regions [24, 25]. Moreover, c-Myc was able to activate BMI1; and BMI1 further facilitated the oncogenic expression of c-Myc in glioblastoma development [17]. It has been speculated that c-Myc and BMI1 might be good biomarkers of glioblastoma due to their high expression and involvement in gliomagenesis. Inhibition of both genes could give glioblastoma a greater sensitivity to combined anticancer therapy. A recent study revealed that Tamoxifen (TAM) has the ability to reduce the expression of neural stem cell markers, like Nestin, Bmi1 and Vimentin, in glioma cell lines. Moreover, the action of TAM in glioma cells apoptosis is assisted by prostate apoptosis response-4(par-4) [26]. It has been published that AR-A 014418 inhibits GSK3 beta kinase activation which further regulates the cancer escape pathway via downregulation of anti-apoptotic gene BMI1 [27].

## 5. BMI1 and miRNAs

Low expression of miRNA-128 was reported in GBM samples. High expression of miRNA-128 in GBM down-regulates ARP5 (ANGPTL 6), BMI1 and E2F-3a, factors which are key regulator for brain cell proliferation [28]. miRNA-128 also targets BMI1 and down-regulates its expression. Most of the glioma samples show less expression of miRNA-128. Overexpression of miRNA-128 shows inhibition of GICs proliferation and self-renewable capacity [10]. Normal brain has abundant expression of miRNA-124, however, miRNA-124 expression is diminished during the development of glioma. Interestingly, overexpression of miRNA-124 reduced the formation of neurospheres, the CD133+ cell subpopulation, and the expression of stem cells markers like BMI1, Nanog and Nestin [29]. Smoothened inhibitor NPV-LDE-225 (Erismodegib) inhibits BMI1 in GICs via upregulation of miRNA-128, miRNA-21 and miRNA-200 [30]. Interestingly, NPV-LDE-225 was used in topical cream for basal cell carcinoma treatment and it inhibited the Shh pathway [31]. A recent study suggested that NPV-LDE-225 mediated inhibition of Shh signaling downregulates Bmi1 via upregulation of miRNA-128 [30]. Another study also suggested that polycomb repressor complex BMI1 is targeted by miRNA-128 in glioma stem cells [32]. Another miRNA-218 also inhibited the expression of BMI1 which further retarded glioma invasion, migration, and glioma stem cell renewal capability. Most gliomas showed less expression of miRNA-218 and overexpression of miRNA-128, which further inhibited glioma tumor characteristics. It was assumed that BMI1 is the downstream target gene of miRNA-218. miRNA-218 regulates many genes which are involved in glioma tumorigenesis [33]. Interestingly, we illustrate a model diagram for the role of BMI1 in gliomagenesis (Figure 1).

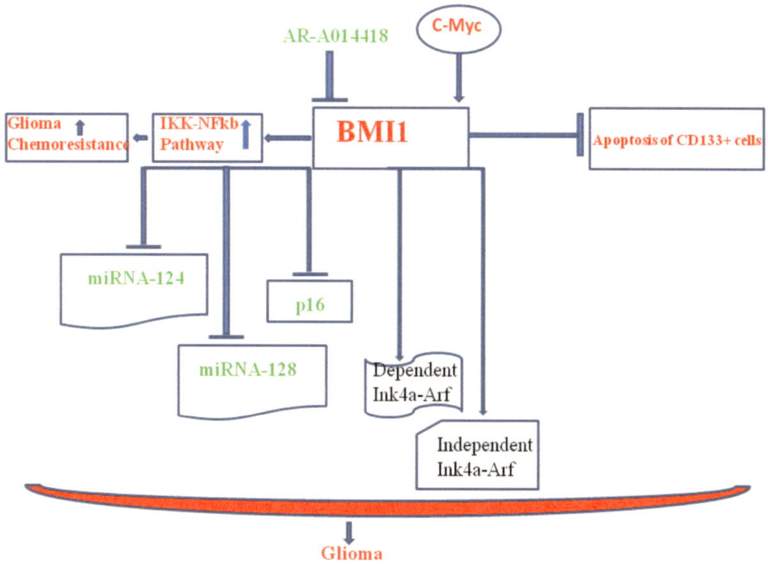


**Figure 1.** BMI1 networking in gliomagenesis

## 6. Role of BMI1 in medulloblastoma

Medulloblastoma is a primitive neuroectodermal tumor of the cerebellum. Medulloblastoma is the most common pediatric malignant brain tumor, representing 20% of newly identified CNS tumors in children [34]. Medulloblastoma is driven by several signaling pathways, among which, Shh plays a critical role for the majority of these tumors [35, 36]. Mutations of the Shh pathway regulators are present in about 20-25% of medulloblastomas [37]. Shh-driven medulloblastoma showed high expression of BMI1. A recent study reveals the role of BMI1 in Shh-driven medulloblastoma. Transgenic mice showed the expression of Shh signaling activator SmoA1 with the help of glial fibrillary acidic protein (GFAP) promoter. They found that SmoA1/BMI1+/+; SmoA1/BMI1+/-postnatal mice (p=26) between days P14 to P26 showed prominent potential to develop medulloblastoma compared to SmoA1/BMI1-/-post natal mice (n=6) [38]. Interestingly, cells with BMI1 deficiency BMI1-/- even in the presence of SmoA1 were non-proliferative compared to BMI1+/+ cells [38]. Two down-stream genes which are inversely regulated by BMI1 in Shh-driven medulloblastoma development were reported. Cyclin D1 expression was downregulated and cyclin-dependent kinase inhibitor p19Arf was upregulated. Moreover, it was concluded that BMI1 is crucial for the Shh-driven medulloblastoma development and that BMI1 facilitates medulloblastoma development de novo [38]. During embryonic development Shh signaling pathway regulates proliferation of granular neuron precursors (GNPs). GNPs are progenitors for medulloblastoma development, comprising the transient external granular layer of cerebellum [39]. BMI1 seems to promote the expression of downstream target genes during cerebellum development [40]. BMI1-null mice developed reduced cerebellum and impaired production of granular neurons. Altered expression of BMI1 in medulloblastoma as well as correlation of BMI1 expression and Shh activation was reported in medulloblastoma [38, 41]. It was suggested that polycomb gene expression could be used as a predictor of poor clinical outcome in medulloblastoma [42]. BMI1 overexpression caused cell proliferation and assisted Shh signaling driven tumorigenesis [43]. BMI1 expression and Shh ligand concentration were positively correlated during development. Chromatin immunoprecipitation experiments revealed that Shh signaling pathway main transcriptional activator Gli1 preferentially binds to the promoter regions of BMI1. Moreover, overexpression and downregulation of Gli1 controls high and low expression of BMI1 respectively. Interestingly, BMI1 is not only a Shh-Gli1 downstream target gene but also promotes a feedback mechanism which further activates Shh-Gli1 signaling. This finding suggested that both BMI1 and Shh signaling pathways are mutually indispensable pathways in brain tumor initiating cells (BTICs) of medulloblastoma [43]. One study reported that overexpressed BMI1 was unable to induce tumors in mice from granule cell progenitors (GCPs). Therefore, it was concluded that overexpression of BMI1 in GCP-derived human medulloblastoma, could promote later stages of tumorigenesis and further sustain tumor cell survival [44]. Apart from cell proliferation other characteristic of tumors include anti-apoptotic nature and sustaining of high metabolic rate, both supported by high BMI1 and low TP53 levels of expression which are characteristic of group 4 human medulloblastoma [44]. BMI1 overexpression alone was not sufficient to induce medulloblastoma; however BMI1 overexpression and loss of p53 induced medulloblastoma in mice, producing similar tumors to group 4 human medulloblastomas [44]. Recently, medulloblastomas have been categorized in 4 subgroups on the basis of prognosis and predicted therapeutics (Kool et al., 2012, Ramaswamy et al., 2013 and Gottardo et al., 2014). Group 1 and group 2 are under the good clinical outcome and regulated by Shh and Wnt signaling, respectively [45]. Groups 3 and 4 medulloblastoma are not Shh/Wnt signaling mediated tumors, have metastatic potencial, and poor patient outcome and lack of known molecular pathways. Current gene expression analysis is unable to detect self-renewal gene and brain tumor-initiating cells (BTIC) in group 3 and group 4 medulloblastoma. BTICs constitute a minority of the tumor mass, and their detection can be difficult in medulloblastoma. High BTIC promoted tumors to increase tumor aggressiveness and poor patient outcome. They investigated the potential stem cells candidate genes among the different subgroups of 251 human medulloblastoma samples from the 4 overlapping MB transcriptional data bases (Amsterdam, Memphis, Toronto and Boston) and 74 nano-string sub-grouped medulloblastoma (Vancouver) [45]. This analysis showed two crucial genes BMI1 and FoxG1, which presented abundant expression in non-Shh/wnt medulloblastoma groups. These genes are responsible to promote MB stem cells and tumor initiation in mice [45]. We also depicted a model for the different group of medulloblastoma development on the basis of cell signaling pathways and gene expression profile (Figure 3). This study also identified a reciprocal promoter in CD15+ medulloblastoma stem cells. The finding could be used as a novel target therapy against BTIC self-renewal. They also found BMI1 is a downstream target of FoxG1 and further promotes tumorigenicity. BMI1 also exerts feedback to FoxG1 expression and facilitates *in vivo* tumor malignancy and enhances in vitro stem cell self-renewal capability. Moreover, high expression of BMI1 can be considered as a strong molecular prognostic marker in pediatric brain tumors. We attempted to show a model for the role of BMI1 in medulloblastoma development (Figure 2).

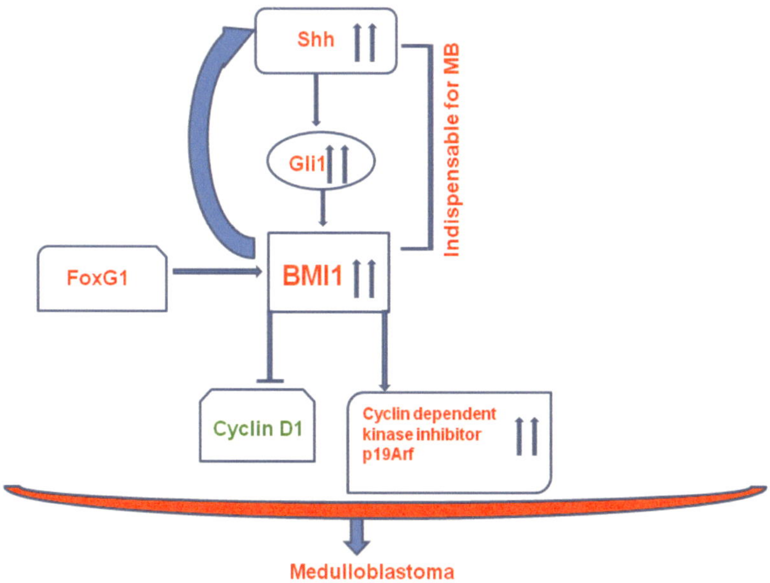


**Figure 2.** BMI1 networking in medulloblastoma development

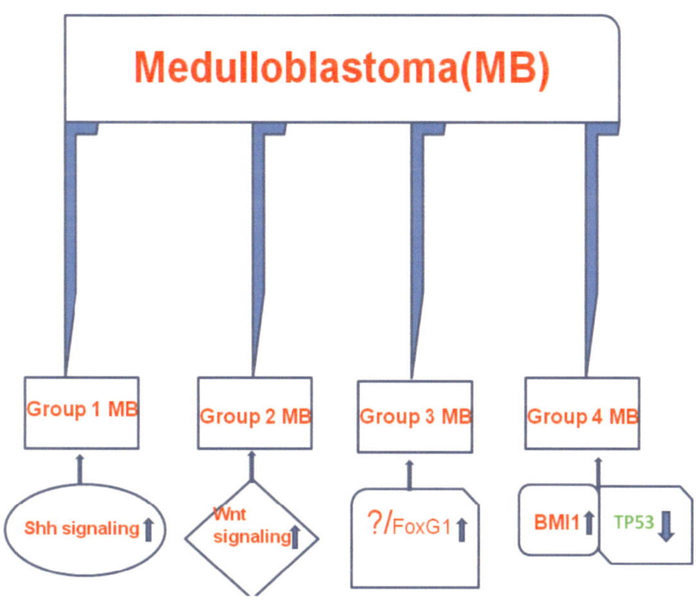


**Figure 3.** Division of medulloblastoma on the basis of gene and cell signaling expression

## 7. Conclusion

BMI1 is a very significant stem cell marker gene which contributes to the development of glioblastoma and medulloblastoma. Therefore, the treatment of glioblastoma and medulloblastoma would improve with the addition of BMI1 inhibitors. Moreover, high expression of BMI1 could be used as one of the earliest markers to diagnose brain tumors.

## Acknowledgements

Authors are thankful to all members of Interdisciplinary Brain Research Centre, Aligarh Muslim University, Aligarh, India for their constant supports.

## Author details

Mohammad M. Hossain[1], Bárbara Meléndez[2], Juan A. Rey[3], Javier S. Castresana[4] and Mehdi H. Shahi[1*]

*Address all correspondence to: mehdihayat@gmail.com

1 Interdisciplinary Brain Research Centre, Faculty of Medicine, Aligarh Muslim University,Aligarh, , India

2 Molecular Pathology Research Unit, Virgen de la Salud Hospital, Toledo, Spain

3 IdiPaz Research Unit, La Paz University Hospital, Madrid, Spain

4 Department of Biochemistry and Genetics, University of Navarra School of Sciences, Pamplona, Spain

## References

[1] Jacobs, J.J., et al., *The oncogene and Polycomb-group gene bmi-1 regulates cell proliferation and senescence through the ink4a locus.* Nature, 1999. 397(6715): p. 164-8.

[2] Tirabosco, R., et al., *Expression of the Polycomb-Group protein BMI1 and correlation with p16 in astrocytomas an immunohistochemical study on 80 cases.* Pathol Res Pract, 2008. 204(9): p. 625-31.

[3] Sparmann, A. and M. van Lohuizen, *Polycomb silencers control cell fate, development and cancer.* Nat Rev Cancer, 2006. 6(11): p. 846-56.

[4] Dellino, G.I., et al., *Polycomb silencing blocks transcription initiation*. Mol Cell, 2004. 13(6): p. 887-93.

[5] He, S., et al., *Bmi-1 over-expression in neural stem/progenitor cells increases proliferation and neurogenesis in culture but has little effect on these functions in vivo*. Dev Biol, 2009. 328(2): p. 257-72.

[6] Lowe, S.W. and C.J. Sherr, *Tumor suppression by Ink4a-Arf: progress and puzzles*. Curr Opin Genet Dev, 2003. 13(1): p. 77-83.

[7] Subkhankulova, T., et al., *Bmi1 directly represses p21Waf1/Cip1 in Shh-induced proliferation of cerebellar granule cell progenitors*. Mol Cell Neurosci, 2010. 45(2): p. 151-62.

[8] Yadirgi, G., et al., *Conditional activation of Bmi1 expression regulates self-renewal, apoptosis, and differentiation of neural stem/progenitor cells in vitro and in vivo*. Stem Cells, 2011. 29(4): p. 700-12.

[9] Zhou, Y.H., et al., *Establishment of prognostic models for astrocytic and oligodendroglial brain tumors with standardized quantification of marker gene expression and clinical variables*. Biomark Insights, 2010. 5: p. 153-68.

[10] Natsume, A., et al., *Glioma-initiating cells and molecular pathology: implications for therapy*. Brain Tumor Pathol, 2011. 28(1): p. 1-12.

[11] Hayry, V., et al., *Copy number alterations of the polycomb gene BMI1 in gliomas*. Acta Neuropathol, 2008. 116(1): p. 97-102.

[12] Spivakov, M. and A.G. Fisher, *Epigenetic signatures of stem-cell identity*. Nat Rev Genet, 2007. 8(4): p. 263-71.

[13] Bruggeman, S.W., et al., *Bmi1 controls tumor development in an Ink4a/Arf-independent manner in a mouse model for glioma*. Cancer Cell, 2007. 12(4): p. 328-41.

[14] Haupt, Y., et al., *bmi-1 transgene induces lymphomas and collaborates with myc in tumorigenesis*. Oncogene, 1993. 8(11): p. 3161-4.

[15] Jacobs, J.J., et al., *Bmi-1 collaborates with c-Myc in tumorigenesis by inhibiting c-Myc-induced apoptosis via INK4a/ARF*. Genes Dev, 1999. 13(20): p. 2678-90.

[16] van Lohuizen, M., et al., *Sequence similarity between the mammalian bmi-1 proto-oncogene and the Drosophila regulatory genes Psc and Su(z)2*. Nature, 1991. 353(6342): p. 353-5.

[17] Abdouh, M., et al., *BMI1 sustains human glioblastoma multiforme stem cell renewal*. J Neurosci, 2009. 29(28): p. 8884-96.

[18] Lefranc, F., J. Brotchi, and R. Kiss, *Possible future issues in the treatment of glioblastomas: special emphasis on cell migration and the resistance of migrating glioblastoma cells to apoptosis*. J Clin Oncol, 2005. 23(10): p. 2411-22.

[19] Nagai, S., et al., *Aberrant nuclear factor-kappaB activity and its participation in the growth of human malignant astrocytoma.* J Neurosurg, 2002. 96(5): p. 909-17.

[20] Li, J., et al., *Oncoprotein Bmi-1 renders apoptotic resistance to glioma cells through activation of the IKK-nuclear factor-kappaB Pathway.* Am J Pathol, 2010. 176(2): p. 699-709.

[21] Facchino, S., et al., *BMI1 confers radioresistance to normal and cancerous neural stem cells through recruitment of the DNA damage response machinery.* J Neurosci, 2010. 30(30): p. 10096-111.

[22] Cole, M.D. and V.H. Cowling, *Transcription-independent functions of MYC: regulation of translation and DNA replication.* Nat Rev Mol Cell Biol, 2008. 9(10): p. 810-5.

[23] Martinato, F., et al., *Analysis of Myc-induced histone modifications on target chromatin.* PLoS One, 2008. 3(11): p. e3650.

[24] Guney, I., S. Wu, and J.M. Sedivy, *Reduced c-Myc signaling triggers telomere-independent senescence by regulating Bmi-1 and p16(INK4a).* Proc Natl Acad Sci U S A, 2006. 103(10): p. 3645-50.

[25] Guo, W.J., et al., *Mel-18, a polycomb group protein, regulates cell proliferation and senescence via transcriptional repression of Bmi-1 and c-Myc oncoproteins.* Mol Biol Cell, 2007. 18(2): p. 536-46.

[26] Jagtap, J.C., et al., *Expression and regulation of prostate apoptosis response-4 (Par-4) in human glioma stem cells in drug-induced apoptosis.* PLoS One, 2014. 9(2): p. e88505.

[27] Yadav, A.K., et al., *AR-A 014418 Used against GSK3beta Downregulates Expression of hnRNPA1 and SF2/ASF Splicing Factors.* J Oncol, 2014. 2014: p. 695325.

[28] Cui, J.G., et al., *Micro-RNA-128 (miRNA-128) down-regulation in glioblastoma targets ARP5 (ANGPTL6), Bmi-1 and E2F-3a, key regulators of brain cell proliferation.* J Neurooncol, 2010. 98(3): p. 297-304.

[29] Xia, H., et al., *Loss of brain-enriched miR-124 microRNA enhances stem-like traits and invasiveness of glioma cells.* J Biol Chem, 2012. 287(13): p. 9962-71.

[30] Fu, J. and W. Hsu, *Epidermal Wnt controls hair follicle induction by orchestrating dynamic signaling crosstalk between the epidermis and dermis.* J Invest Dermatol, 2013. 133(4): p. 890-8.

[31] Skvara, H., et al., *Topical treatment of Basal cell carcinomas in nevoid Basal cell carcinoma syndrome with a smoothened inhibitor.* J Invest Dermatol, 2011. 131(8): p. 1735-44.

[32] Peruzzi, P., et al., *MicroRNA-128 coordinately targets Polycomb Repressor Complexes in glioma stem cells.* Neuro Oncol, 2013. 15(9): p. 1212-24.

[33] Tu, Y., et al., *MicroRNA-218 inhibits glioma invasion, migration, proliferation, and cancer stem-like cell self-renewal by targeting the polycomb group gene Bmi1.* Cancer Res, 2013. 73(19): p. 6046-55.

[34] Packer, R.J., et al., *Medulloblastoma: clinical and biologic aspects*. Neuro Oncol, 1999. 1(3): p. 232-50.

[35] Goodrich, L.V., et al., *Altered neural cell fates and medulloblastoma in mouse patched mutants*. Science, 1997. 277(5329): p. 1109-13.

[36] Wetmore, C., D.E. Eberhart, and T. Curran, *The normal patched allele is expressed in medulloblastomas from mice with heterozygous germ-line mutation of patched*. Cancer Res, 2000. 60(8): p. 2239-46.

[37] Ellison, D.W., et al., *What's new in neuro-oncology? Recent advances in medulloblastoma*. Eur J Paediatr Neurol, 2003. 7(2): p. 53-66.

[38] Michael, L.E., et al., *Bmi1 is required for Hedgehog pathway-driven medulloblastoma expansion*. Neoplasia, 2008. 10(12): p. 1343-9, 5p following 1349.

[39] Marino, S., *Medulloblastoma: developmental mechanisms out of control*. Trends Mol Med, 2005. 11(1): p. 17-22.

[40] Leung, C., et al., *Bmi1 is essential for cerebellar development and is overexpressed in human medulloblastomas*. Nature, 2004. 428(6980): p. 337-41.

[41] Glinsky, G.V., O. Berezovska, and A.B. Glinskii, *Microarray analysis identifies a death-from-cancer signature predicting therapy failure in patients with multiple types of cancer*. J Clin Invest, 2005. 115(6): p. 1503-21.

[42] Zakrzewska, M., et al., *Polycomb genes expression as a predictor of poor clinical outcome in children with medulloblastoma*. Childs Nerv Syst, 2011. 27(1): p. 79-86.

[43] Wang, X., et al., *Sonic hedgehog regulates Bmi1 in human medulloblastoma brain tumor-initiating cells*. Oncogene, 2012. 31(2): p. 187-99.

[44] Behesti, H., et al., *Bmi1 overexpression in the cerebellar granule cell lineage of mice affects cell proliferation and survival without initiating medulloblastoma formation*. Dis Model Mech, 2013. 6(1): p. 49-63.

[45] Manoranjan, B., et al., *FoxG1 interacts with Bmi1 to regulate self-renewal and tumorigenicity of medulloblastoma stem cells*. Stem Cells, 2013. 31(7): p. 1266-77.

Chapter 6

# Metalloproteinases in Brain Tumors

Krzysztof Siemianowicz, Wirginia Likus and
Jarosław Markowski

Additional information is available at the end of the chapter

http://dx.doi.org/10.5772/58964

## 1. Introduction

Metalloproteinases (MMPs) were first described by Gross more than fifty years ago. They are a family of zinc-dependent endopeptidases. They comprise a group of 25 enzymes. MMPs were first described as proteases degrading extracellular matrix (ECM) proteins such as collagens, elastin, proteoglycans and laminins, hence they were named matrix metalloproteinases. MMPs were divided according to their substrate specificity into collagenases, gelatinases, stromolysins and matrilysins. This classification was later replaced by numbering the enzymes according to the chronology of their identification.

Four metalloproteinases (MMP-14, MMP-15, MMP-16 and MMP-24) have a transmembrane and cytosolic domains. They constitute a subgroup of membrane-type metalloproteinases (MT-MMPs). Recently an intracellular, nuclear localization and functions of metalloproteinases have been discovered [1-4].

## 2. Physiological role of metalloproteinases

MMP-1 (collagenase 1) hydrolyzes collagen types I, II, III, VII, VIII, X and XI, as well as gelatin, fibronectin, vitronectin, laminin, tenascin, aggrecan, links protein, myelin basic protein and versican. MMP-2 (gellatinase) degrades collagen types I, II, III, IV, V, VII, X and XI, gelatin, elastin, fibronectin, vitronectin, laminin, entactin, tenascin, SPARC and aggrecan, links protein, galectin-3, versican, decanin and myelin basic protein. One of the most important differences between these two metalloproteinases is the possibility of the hydrolysis of elastin and collagen type IV by MMP-2, but not by MMP-1. Researchers have also focused their interest on MMP-9 which can degrade collagen types IV, V, VII, X and XIV, fibronectin, laminin, nidogen, proteoglycan link protein and versican.

For a long time metalloproteinases have been viewed solely as enzymes of matrix proteins breakdown. Results of researches performed in recent years indicate that there is a group of non-matrix proteins which can be substrates for various MMPs. Metalloproteinases are involved in the activation of latent forms of effective proteins. For example, MMP-2, MMP-3 and MMP-9 can activate interleukin 1β (IL-1β). They can also act on active cytokines, IL-1β undergoes subsequent degradation catalyzed by MMP-3. Metalloproteinases can alter cell surface proteins such as receptors and act on microbial peptides.

Metalloproteinases are not indiscriminately released by cells. They are secreted to or anchored to cell membrane. MT-MMPs have a specific transmembrane domain placing them in a certain position. Other metalloproteinases can be bound by specific cell-MMP interactions. This phenomenon allows an exact localization of their proteolytic activity [1-3].

## 3. Activation of metalloproteinases

Metalloproteinases are encoded as inactive proenzymes, zymogens. They undergo proteolytic activation. This process can take place either intracellulary or extracellulary. One third of MMPs are activated by intracellular serine protease, furin. This process takes place in trans-Golgi network. A number of MMPs has a cleavage site for other metalloproteinases. MMP-3 activates proMMP-1 and pro-MMP-7. Some metalloproteinases have been described to be activated by kallikrein or plasmin.

*In vivo* studies indicate that reactive oxygen species (ROS) generated by neutrophils can both activate and subsequently inactivate MMPs. Hypochlorus acid (HClO) generated by neutrophil myeloperoxidase and hydroxyl radicals can activate proMMP-1, proMMP-7 and proMMP-9, whereas peroxynitrate can activate proenzymes of MMP-1, MMP-2 and MMP-9. This process enables a control of burst of proteolytic activity within an inflammatory setting.

Like some other proteases, activity of MMPs is controlled also by two other mechanisms, regulation of gene expression and specific inhibitors. MMP-2 is constitutively expressed and regulation of its activity occurs by either activation or inhibition. Expression of a number of metalloproteinases is up-regulated during various pathological conditions. Among them inflammation is the most studied setting. MMPs are inhibited by $\alpha$-2 macroglobulin and tissue inhibitors of metalloproteinases (TIMPs). There are four TIMPs. Their secretion is also regulated and represents another point in a network of control of the activity of metalloproteinases. TIMP-3 is primarily bond to ECM and allows a regulation of MMPs' activity in the very site of their action. The network of the control of the activity of metalloproteinases is complex and very precise. Sometimes TIMP interacts with proMMP and inactivate other MMP, e.g. a complex of TIMP-1 and proMMP-9 inactivates MMP-3.

Protection from MMP degradation represents the next step in this sophisticated network of diverse interactions. Neutrophil gelatinase-associated lipocalin (NGAL) bounds to MMP-9 protecting this metalloproteinase from its degradation [1-3].

http://dx.doi.org/10.5772/58964

## 4. Metalloproteinases in central nervous system

Metalloproteinases in central nervous system can be produced by cells constituting it, by cells of blood vessels' wall or by blood cells. The production of MMPs in central nervous system under normal conditions is low, however it can be augmented in several neoplastic and non-neoplastic conditions. The expression of MMP-14 (MT1-MMP) in microglia is very low under physiological conditions. It can be increased in neurodegenerative and neuroinflammatory pathologies, e.g. Alzheimer's disease, multiple sclerosis, amyotrophic lateral sclerosis (ALS) or even in a stroke. Astrocytes were reported to secrete MMP-2 and MMP-9 [5,6].

For a long time MMPs were thought to be enzymes acting exclusively in extracellular compartment. Studies carried in last few years have revealed nontraditional roles for MMPs in extracellular space as well as in the cytosol and nucleus. MMP-2 and MMP-9 which were largely studied in central nervous system have been shown to present an increased activity in cortex neuronal nuclei after focal cerebral ischemia. These two MMPs, MMP-2 and MMP-9, are also termed gelatinase A and gelatinase B. The increased gelanolytic activity in nucleus occurs to be linked with MMP-dependent cell death triggering neuroinflammatory reactions. MMP-13, named also collagenase-3, was found to be activated mostly in neurons and oligodendrocytes. Its function in cell nucleus may be linked to the apoptosis cascade following ischemic stimulus. MMPs localized in cell nucleus can have a different set of target proteins than MMPs acting in extracellular space. Poly-ADP-ribose polymerase-1 (PARP-1) and X-ray cross-complementary factor-1 (XRCC-1) can be the substrates for MMP-dependent cleavage [4].

## 5. Metalloproteinases in brain tumors

Gliomas are the most common malignant tumors in the brain, and the overall prognosis for patients suffering from this neoplasm is poor. Glioblastoma multiforme (GBM) is the most aggressive type of glioma. Molecular mechanisms of invasiveness of this neoplasm have been most widely studied. Many factors are involved in the migration and invasiveness of GBM. MMPs have gained a large interest of researchers. The role of MMPs is significant in the degradation of ECM, thereby facilitating tumor cell invasion into surrounding stroma. Neoplastic cell invades in three steps. The first one is the attachment of tumor cell to the basement membrane through binding of neoplastic cell receptors to the basement membrane receptors. The next one is the secretion of hydrolytic enzymes, MMPs, which locally degrade ECM by extracellular proteolysis. The third step comprises the movement of the tumor cell to the free space obtained by degradation of ECM. MMP-13 is involved in the initiation of progression of invasion due to its proteolytic activity. Expression of MMP-13 is higher in glioma than in the surrounding normal brain tissue. High expression of this MMP is more often detected in advanced grades of glioma. Some researchers suggest that MMP-13 can be used as a biomarker of GBM progression. A study of Hsieh *et al.* revealed that GBM cells express higher amount of endothelin-1 receptors $ET_A$ and $ET_B$. The stimulation of one of the most invasive glioma cell lines *in vivo*, U251, with endothelin resulted in an increased expression of MMP-13, MMP-9 and increased cell migration. The addition of MMP-13 and MMP-9 inhibitors attenuated this increased cell migration [7-9].

Other scientists have shown that GBM cells can present an increased expression of other metalloproteinases: MMP-1, MMP-2, MMP-3, MMP-7, MMP-9 and MMP-14. Some researchers tried to reveal the molecular markers of invasiveness in gliomas. In the results of their studies various MMPs can be found. Bakalova *et al.* found that patients in terminal stages of brain tumors had elevated plasma levels of MMP-2 and MMP-9. Mariani *et al.* measured levels of MMP-2 and MMP-9 in cerebrospinal fluid (CSF) of dogs with intracranial tumors. Latent, but not active form of MMP-2 was found in all samples. MMP-9 was found in CSF of a minority of studied animals. Xu *et al.* analyzed brain samples obtained from patients undergoing surgery for GBM and non-malignant condition, epilepsy. Overexpression of both MMP-1 and vascular endothelial growth factor-1 (VEGF-1) was an independent poor prognostic factor in gliomas. Wang and co-workers analyzed frozen glioma samples and found out an increased expression of stromal periostin (POSTN) gene. This protein took part in both cell invasion and migration. In glioma cells POSTN signaling led to increased MMP-9 expression. The expression of POSTN correlated with both grade and progression of glioma being a poor prognostic factor [10-13].

MT1-MMP (MMP-14) activates directly proMMP-2 and indirectly MMP-2 and MMP-9. Expression of MMP-14 was shown to correlate with invasiveness of glioma and to increase with glioma grade. MMP-14 expression was also shown to correlate with brain tumor progression. This metalloproteinase, MMP-14, has been proposed as a biomarker to determine the type and grade of specific tumor. MMP-14 has a very interesting set of digested proteins. Apart from ECM proteins it can hydrolyze the most potent central nervous myelin inhibitory proteins, including BN-220. MMP-14 can also digest some proteins having adhesion functions. MMP-14 can also be involved in some intracellular processes. It can be trafficked along the tubulin cytoskeleton and be involved in intracellular recycling pathway. MMP-14 expression abnormalities were linked to mitotic spindle aberrations and chromosome instability leading to malignant transformation of neoplastic cells. MMP-14 may also be involved in regulation of VEGF-A expression. VEGF-A induces angiogenesis and inhibits apoptosis. MMP-14 seems to promote malignant glioma transformation, invasion and metastasis through intracellular signaling pathways [14].

## 6. Metalloproteinases and intracellular signaling pathways

Increased expression of various MMPs observed in brain tumors is a result of multiple intracellular events which may be termed as dysregulated pathways. These intracellular molecular mechanisms leading to increased invasion of neoplasmatic cells have focused scientists' interest. Understanding these complex mechanisms may be a key to design a molecular targeted therapy for patients with brain tumors. Signaling pathways leading to increased expression of MMPs are of special interest.

Tsai *et al.* observed that inhibition of focal adhesion kinase (FAK) phosporylation by osthole reduced MMP-13 expression in human glioma cells. This inhibition led to a reduction of cells migration even in a subgroup of glioma cells selected for high migratory ability. Lee *et al.* observed GMB U251 cell line presented increased FAK activation which led to an augmented expression of MMP-2. This study also revealed that examined GBM cells had an increased Bcl-w (B-cell lymphoma-w) expression. This protein is a prosurvival member of Bcl-2 family. The augmented expression of this protein is associated with infiltration properties and aggressiveness of various cancers. Bcl-w promotes the mesenchymal traits of glioblastoma cells by inducing vimentin expression of transcription factors, β-catenin, Twist1 and Snail. The increased expression of MMP-2 is accompanied by and results from the FAK activation, i.e. phosphorylation, via the PI3K-p-Akt-p-GSK3β-β-catenin pathway. The role of Bcl-w in promoting invasiveness of GBM by increasing MMP-2 activation was also confirmed in another study of this researchers team which proposed Bcl-w induced activation of β-catenin, also termed specificity protein-1 (Sp1), as a putative marker for aggressiveness of GBM. Nuclear factor of activated T cell (NFAT) family has been identified as a group of regulators of oncogenic transformation in several human malignancies. NFAT1 (NFATc2) is the prevalent family member expressed in peripheral T lymphocytes and many other cells outside the immune system. It is associated with tumor cell survival, apoptosis, migration and invasion. Clustering analysis of microarray data revealed that in glioma cells the expression of invasion related genes, cyclooxygenase-2 (COX-2), MMP-7 and MMP-9, was correlated with the expression of NFAT1. In vitro analysis confirmed the role of NFAT1, as in a specific NFAT1 knock down in U87 glioma cell line led to a marked reduction of COX-2, MMP-7 and MMP-9 expression [7,15-17].

MMP-2 has been discovered to posses intracellular activity and play some role in cell nucleus. A study by Kesanakurti *et al.* put new light on a role of MMP-2 in molecular mechanisms engaged in aggressiveness of glioma cells. p21 activated kinase 4 (PAK4) is one of down stream effectors of small GTPases Rac1 and Cdc42 which have diverse cellular functions by regulating cytoskeletal reorganization, cell survival and angiogenesis. Abberant PAK4 expression was found to be associated with enhanced tumor progression in various carcinomas. MMP-2 directly interacts with PAK-4 and augments the activation of $\alpha v\beta 3$-mediated phospho-epidermal growth factor receptor (phospho-EGFR) in GBM. MMP-2 is supposed to bind to PAK4 and the complex PAK4/MMP-2 is supposed to regulate integrin mediated pathways in gliomas. Earlier study of Kesanakurti study group revealed that MMP-2 knock down glioma cells entered on apoptosis pathway [18-20].

Understanding the molecular pathways enhancing aggressiveness of glioma cells may lead to introducing a complex therapy focused on several targets which may give a better effectiveness.

## 7. Metalloproteinases in other cells supporting tumor and metastasis development

In last few years scientists have paid more attention to interactions between glioma cells and microglia as well as on inreactions between metastatic cancer cells and astrocytes. Ellert-

Miklaszewska *et al.* observed that glioma attracted microglia and polarized them into tumor-supporting cells that participated in matrix-remodeling, invasion, angiogenesis and suppression of adaptative immunity. In her experiment rat microglial cultures exposed to glioma conditioned medium polarized into pro-inflammatory or alternatively activated cells. Glioma derived factors increased cell motility, phagocytosis and sustained proliferation. Glioma induced activation of microglia was associated with induction of expression of several genes. One of them was MT1-MMP. Vinnakota *et al.* also observed that microglia promoted glioma through upregulation of MT1-MMP. This conversion of microglia into glioma supportive phenotype was dependent on activation of Toll-like receptor 2 (TLR 2) along with TLR 1 and or TLR 6 signaling [21, 22].

Brain metastasis is a defining component of tumor pathophysiology and underlying mechanisms urgently need deeper elucidation. The relationship between metastatic cells and astrocytes is crucial for tumor cell sustenance in brain. Some researchers postulate that tumor cell metastasis to the brain are influenced by astrocyte secretome and astrocytes play a direct role in tumor metastasis. Wang *et al.* revealed that astrocyte conditioned tumor cells displayed highly invasive and metastatic behavior both *in vitro* and *in vivo* as well. MMP-2 and MMP-9 were two factors in the astrocyte secretome that were responsible for that response. Blocking these MMPs proteins partially prevented the invasion and metastasis of tumor cells both *in vitro* and *in vivo* as well. A very important question arises. What are the mechanisms by which MMPs secreted by astrocytes trigger invasion of tumor cells? MMP-2 and MMP-9 may increase the permeability of blood-brain barrier and allow the transfer of metastatic cells reaching brain via blood stream. The alternative hypothesis is that latent MMPs substrates on tumor cells or cells of tumor microenvironment may be activated upon cleavage by astrocyte secreted MMP-2 and MMP-9 leading to an invasive phenotype. The precise elucidation of these interactions is urgent as astrocytes may be a novel target for therapy aimed at prevention of brain metastases in patients with various cancers [21-23].

## 8. Blocking MMPs expression and/or activity

Scientists have widely studied the possibilities of attenuating MMPs expression and activity in order to reduce the invasiveness of gliomas. They efforts have combined various directions.

Atorvastatin is a well known statin, an inhibitor of β-hydroxy-β-methylglutaryl-CoA reductase. By inhibiting the key enzyme in a mevalonate synthesis pathway atorvastatin has pleiotropic effects. The main mode of action of this drug is the inhibition of *de novo* cholesterol synthesis. However, this drug has some other advantages resulting in its pleiotropic antiatherogenic properties due to the inhibition of synthesis of other biologically important mevalonate pathway derivates: dolichol, ubichinon, farnesyl and geranyl residues. This inhibition leads to disturbances in some signaling pathways. The possible anticancer properties of statins have been postulated since a long time.

Yongjun and co-workers have observed that atorvastatin reduced pro-tumorigenic effects of microglia on glioma migration and invasion by reducing microglial expression of MT1-MMP

(MMP-14). Mohebbi *et al.* observed that atorvastatin 40 mg administered twice daily seven from days before till three weeks after the neurosurgical procedure led to better outcome after the neurosurgical treatment of brain tumors and raised significantly Karnofsky score. The biochemical analysis showed that two weeks after the surgical treatment patients on atorvastatin therapy had significantly reduced plasma level of MMP-9 compared to patients receiving placebo [24,25].

Locatelli *et al.* evaluated a composition of polymeric nanoparticles containing a composition of two cytotoxic agents, drug alisertib and nanosilver conjugated with chlorotoxin, a peptide binding specifically to MMP-2. Their experimental *in vitro* and *in vivo* studies showed the tumor reduction [26].

Researchers are trying to investigate drugs aimed at inhibiting MT1-MMP (MMP-14). DX-2400, a fully human antibody was shown to reduce MMP-14 activity, retard tumor progression, metastasis, migration and invasion. Two natural isoflavonoid phytoestrogens, genistein and biochain A, were shown to reduce MMP-14 activity in a dose dependent manner in U87MG cell line. The green tea polyphenol, (Q)-epigallocatechin gallate (EGCg), has been found to inhibit MMP-14 mediated cell migration. This compound also disrupted proMMP-2 activation via downregulation of MMP-14 gene expression. Marimastat, an orally administered MMP inhibitor, was tested in two clinical trials in GBM patients after neurosurgery or irradiation. Marimastat alone did not improve survival, but in conjunction with cytotoxic chemotherapy gave promising results [27-30].

The next point of scientists interest are microRNAs (miRNAs). These small, non-coding RNA molecules containing 18-25 nucleotides in length can inhibit gene expression by binding to the 3′ untranslated region of their target genes and suppress translation. Several studies have shown that various miRNAs can inhibit expression of MMP-14, MMP-2 and inhibit tumor cell adhesion, migration, invasion and angiogenesis [31-35].

Lei *et al.* proposed a new strategy combining a cytotoxic drug paclitaxel and RNA interference suppressing MMP-2 expression. This conception was aimed at blocking tumor growth and proliferation by Paclitaxel and blocking tumor angiogenesis and invasion by inhibiting MMP-2 expression [36].

## 9. Conclusions

In last few years MMPs have been shown to exert new biochemical properties. Their extracellular mode of action as well as intracellular, intranuclear activities were shown to be involved in invasiveness of brain tumors, especially gliomas. Inhibiting their expression may be a new therapeutical approach. So far some drugs being MMPs inhibitors have some serious adverse effects. Inhibiting MMPs expression and activity seems to be rather a supplement to chemotherapy, radiotherapy or neurosurgical procedures than a new single method of treatment of brain tumors.

## Author details

Krzysztof Siemianowicz[1*], Wirginia Likus[2] and Jarosław Markowski[3]

*Address all correspondence to: ksiem@mp.pl

1 Department of Biochemistry, School of Medicine in Katowice, Medical University of Silesia, Poland

2 Department of Human Anatomy, School of Medicine in Katowice, Medical University of Silesia, Poland

3 Department of Laryngology, School of Medicine in Katowice, Medical University of Silesia, Poland

Sections 1-3 contain text originally published in [3].

## References

[1] Pearce WH, Shively VP. Abdominal aortic aneurysm as a complex multifactorial disease. Annals of New York Academy of Sciences 2006;1085 117-132.

[2] Ra H-J, Parks WC. Control of matrix metalloproteinase catalytic activity. Matrix Biology 2007;26: 587-596.

[3] Siemianowicz K. The role of metalloproteinases in the development of aneurysm. in: „Aneurysm" (ed.) Yasuo Murai, Rijeka, InTech, 2012, p65-74.

[4] Mannello F, Medda V. Nuclear localization of matrix metalloproteinases. Progress in Histochemistry and Cytochemistry 2012;47 27-58.

[5] Langenfurth A, Rinnenthal JL, Vinnakota K, Prinz V, Carlo AS, Stadelmann C, Siffrin V, Peaschke S, Endres M, Heppner F, Glass R, Wolf SA, Kettenmann H. Membrane-type 1 metalloproteinase is upregulated in microglia/brain macrophages in neurodegenerative and neuroinflammatory diseases. Journal of Neuroscience Research 2014;92(3) 275-286.

[6] Wang L, Cossette SM, Rarick KR, Gershan J, Dwinell MB, Harder DR, Ramchandran R. Astrocytes directly influence tumor cell invasion and metastasis *in vivo*. PLoS ONE 8(12): e80933, doi: 10.1371/journal.pone.0080933.

[7] Tsai CF, Yeh WL, Chen JH, Lin C, Huang SS, Lu DY. Osthole suppresses the migratory ability of human glioblastoma multiforme cells via inhibition of focal adhesion kinase-mediated matrix metalloproteinase-13 expression. International Journal of Molecular Sciences 2014;15 3889-3903.

[8] Wang J, Li Y, Li C, Yu K, Wang Q. Increased expression of metalloproteinase-13 in glioma is associated with poor overall survival of patients. Medical Oncology 2012; 29, 2432-2437.

[9] Hsieh WT, Yeh Wl, Cheng RY, Lin C, Tsai CF, Huang BR, Wu CY, Lin HY, Huang SS, Lu DY. Exogenous endothelin-1 induces cell migration and matrix metalloproteinase expression in U251 glioblastoma multiforme. Journal of Neuro-Oncology 2014;118(2) 257-69.

[10] Bakalova R, Zhelev Z, Aoki I, Saga T. Tissue redox activity as a hallmark of carcinogenesis: from early to terminal stages of cancer. Clinical Cancer Research 2013;19(9) 2503-2517.

[11] Mariani CL, Boozer LB, Braxton AM, Platt SR, Vernau KM, McDonnell JJ, Guevar J. Evaluation of matrix metalloproteinase-2 and -9 in the cerebrospinal fluid of dogs with intracranial tumors. American Journal of Veterinary Research 2013;74(1) 122-129.

[12] Xu Y, Zhong Z, Yuan J, Zhang Z, Wei Q, Song W, Chen H. Collaborative overexpression of matrix metallloproteianse-1 and vascular endothelial growth factor-C predicts adverse prognosis in patients with gliomas. Cancer Epidemiology 2013;37(5) 697-702.

[13] Wang H, Wang Y, Jiang C. Stromal protein periostatin identified as a progression associated and prognostic biomarker in glioma via inducing an invasive and proliferative phenotype. International Journal of Oncology 2013;42(5) 1716-1724.

[14] Ulasof I, Yi R, Guo D, Sarvaiya, Cobbs C. The emerging role of MMP-14 in brain tumorigenesis and future therapeutics. Biochimica et Biophysica Acta 2014;1846 113-120.

[15] Lee WS, Woo EZ, Kwon J, Park MJ, Lee JS, Han YH, Bae IH. Bcl-w enhances mesenchymal changes and invasiveness of glioblastoma cells by inducing nuclear accumulation of β-catenin. PLoS ONE 8(6): e68030. doi: 10.1371/journal.pone.0068030.

[16] Lee SL, Kwon J, Yun DH, Lee YN, Woo EY, Park MJ, Lee JS, Han YH, Bae IH. Specifity protein 1 expression contributes to Bcl-w-induced aggressiveness in glioblastoma multiforme. Molecules and Cells 2014;37(1) 17-23.

[17] Tie X, Han S, Meng L, Wang Y, Wu A. NFAT1 is highly expressed in, and regulates the invasion of, glioblastoma multiforme cells. PLoS ONE 2013;8(6): e66008. doi: 10.1371/journal.pone.0068008.

[18] Kesanakurti D, Chetty C, Maddirela DR, Gujrati M, Rao JS. Functional cooperativity by direct interaction between PAK4 and MMP-2 in the regulation of anoikis resistance, migration and invasion in glioma. Cell Death and Disease 2012;3, e445; doi: 10.1038/cddis.2012.182.

[19] Kesanakurti D, Chetty C, Bhoopathi P, Lakka SS, Gorantla B, Tsung AJ, Rao JS. Suppression of MMP-2 attenuates TNF-alpha induced NF-kappaB activation and leads to JNK mediated cell death in glioma. PLoS One 2011; 6: e19341.

[20] Kesanakurti D, Chetty C, Dinh DH, Gujrati M, Rao JS. Role of MMP-2 in the regulation of IL-6/Stat3 survival signaling via interaction with a5b1 integrin in glioma. Oncogene 2013;32(3) 327-40.

[21] Ellert-Miklaszewska A, Dabrowski M, Lipko M, Sliwa M, Maleszewska M, Kaminska B, Molecular definition of the pro-tumorigenic phenotype of glioma-activated microglia. Glia 2013;61(7) 1178-1190.

[22] Vinnakota K, Hu F, Ku MC, Georgieva PB, Szulzewsky F, Polhmann A, Waiczies S, Waiczies H, Niedorf T, Lehnardt S, Hanisch S, Synowitz M, Markovic D, Wolf SA, Glass R, Kettenmann H. Toll-like receptor-2 mediates microglia/brain macrophage MT1-MMP expression and glioma expansion. Neuro-Oncology 2013;15(11) 1457-1468.

[23] Wang L, Cossette SM, Rarick KR, Gershan J, Dwinell MB, Harder DR, Ramchandran R. Astrocytes directly influence tumor cell invasion and metastasis in vivo. PLos ONE 2013;8(12): e80933. doi:10.1371/journal.pone.0080933.

[24] Yongjun Y, Shuyun H, Lei C, Xiangrong C, Zhilin Y, Yiquan K. Atorvastatin suppresses glioma invasion and migration by reducing microglial MT1-MMP expression. Journal of Neuroimmunology 2013;260(1-2) 1-8.

[25] Mohebbi N, Khoshnevisan A, Naderi S, Abdollahzade S, Salamzadeh J, Javadi M, Mojtahezadeh M, Gholami K. Effects of atorvastatin on plasma matrix metalloproteinase-9 concentration after glial tumor resection; a randomized, double blind, placebo controlled trial. Daru. Journal of Pharmaceutical Sciences 2014;7;22(1): 10. doi: 10.1186/2008-2231-22-10.

[26] Locatelli E, Naddaka M, Uboldi C, Loudos G, Fragogeorgi E, Molinari V, Pucci A, Tsotakos T, Psimadas D, Ponti J, Franchini MC. Targeted delivery of silver nanoparticles and alisertib: in vitro and in vivo synergistic effect against glioblastoma. Nanomedicine (Lond) 2014;9(6) 839-49.

[27] Devy L, Huang L, Naa L, Yanamandra N, Pieters H, Frans N, Chang E, Tao Q, Vanhove M, Lejeune A, van Gool R, Sexton DJ, Kuang G, Rank D, Hogan S, Pazmany C, Ma YL, Schoonbroodt S, Nixon AE, Ladner RC, Hoet R, Henderikx P, Tenhoor C, Rabbani SA, Valentino ML, Wood CR, Dransfield DT. Selective inhibition of matrix metalloproteinase-14 blocks tumor growth, invasion, and angiogenesis. Cancer Research 2009;69 1517-1526.

[28] Puli S, Lai JC, Bhushan A. Inhibition of matrix degrading enzymes and invasion in human glioblastoma (U87MG) cells by isoflavones. Journal of Neuro-Oncology 2006;79 135-142.

[29] Annabi B, Lachambre MP, Bousquet-Gagnon N, Page M, Gingras D, Beliveau R. Green tea polyphenol (−)-epigallocatechin 3-gallate inhibits MMP-2 secretionand MT1-MMP-driven migration in glioblastoma cells, Biochim. Biophys. Acta 2002;1542 209-220.

[30] Groves MD, Puduvalli VK, Hess KR, Jaeckle KA, Peterson P, Yung WK, Levin VA. Phase II trial of temozolomide plus the matrix metalloproteinase inhibitor, marimastat, in recurrent and progressive glioblastoma multiforme. Journal of Clinical Oncology 2002;20(5) 1383-1388.

[31] Zhang H, Qi M, Li S, Qi T, Mei H, Huang K, Zheng I, Tong Q. microRNA-9 targets matrix metalloproteinase 14 to inhibit invasion, metastasis, and angiogenesis of neuroblastoma cells. Molecular Cancer Therapeutics 2012;11 1454-1466.

[32] Hu X, Chen D, Cui Y, Li Z, Huang J. Targeting microRNA-23a to inhibit glioma cell invasion via HOXD10. Scientific Reports 2013; 3 : 3423 DOI: 10.1038/srep03423.

[33] Pratt J, Annabi B. Induction of autophagy biomarker BNIP3 requires a JAK2/STAT3 and MT1-MMP signaling interplay in Concavalin-A-activated U87 glioblastoma cells. Cellular Signalling 2014; 26(5) 917-924.

[34] Dontula R, Dinasarapu A, Chetty C, Pannuru P, Herbert E, Ozer H, Lakka S. MicroRNA 203 modulates glioma cell migration via Robo I/ERK/MMP-9 signaling. Genes & Cancer 2013;4(7-8) 285-296.

[35] Yang TQ, Lu XJ, Wu TF, Ding DD, Zhao ZH, Chen GL, Xie XS, LI B, Wei YX, Guo LC, Zhang Y, Huang YL, Zhou YX, Du ZW. MicroRNA-16 inhibits glioma cell growth and invasion through suppression of BCL2 and the nuclear factor-κB1/MMP-9 signaling pathway. Cancer Science 2014;105(3) 265-71.

[36] Lei C, Cui Y, Zheng L, Chow PK, Wang CH. Development of a gene/drug dual delivery system for brain tumor therapy: potent inhibition via RNA interference and synergistic effects. Biomaterials 2013;34(30) 7483-7494.

Section 2

# Clinical Management of Brain Tumor Patients

Chapter 7

# Radiation-Induced Glioma

Ryuya Yamanaka and Azusa Hayano

Additional information is available at the end of the chapter

http://dx.doi.org/10.5772/59047

## 1. Introduction

Radiation therapy is widely used for patients with intracranial tumors. However, there are many complications, including cerebral atrophy, calcifying microangiopathy, radiation necrosis, leukoencephalopathy and development of radiation-induced tumors [1-5]. Radiation-induced central nervous system (CNS) neoplasms are recognized in patients who have had therapeutic radiotherapy to the head or face [6]. Radiation-induced CNS neoplasms are rare, but the cumulative risk of brain tumor after therapeutic cranial irradiation is reported as 0.5-2.7% at 15 years [7]. Among radiation-induced CNS neoplasms, meningiomas are about 70%, gliomas about 20% and sarcomas less than 10% [4,6,8]. In children, high-grade gliomas are the most common radiation-induced tumor [9]. Type of post-radiation gliomas are glioblastoma (GBM) in 75% and anaplastic astrocytoma in 25% [7]. Brada et al. [6] described a relative risk of secondary glioma of 7.92 times higher than that of the normal non-irradiated population, with an average latency period to glioma diagnosis of 7 years, in 334 patients with pituitary lesions, irradiated to a median dose of 45 Gy for the sellar region. Cahan et al. [10] established criteria to diagnose a radiotherapy induced brain tumor. These criteria were modified in 1972 by Schrantz and Araoz [11] as follows:(1) the tumor must appear within the irradiated field; (2) the tumor was not present prior to the radiotherapy; (3) a sufficient latency period must elapse between irradiation and appearance of the tumor (usually>5 years); (4) the radiation induced tumor must be histologically proven and a different histological type from the original neoplasm treated by the radiation therapy.

## 2. Radiation-induced gliomas in the literature

In a review of the literature, 191 cases of radiation-induced glioma that analyzed in detail were identified in the period 1960-2014 [9,12-120]. The latency period from the irradiation to the onset of the secondary glioma ranged from 6 months to 50 years, with an average of 11.1 years. More than 40 Gy irradiation was delivered in 50% of cases, with an average of 37.2 Gy. As shown in Table 1, 29 grade II, 37 grade III and 97 grade IV gliomas had been reported, and no specific grade had been shown in other 28 cases. Grade II gliomas developed after 10.7 years, and grade IV gliomas developed after 10.6 years from the time of irradiation. The radiation dose of grade II gliomas for primary lesion is 29.7 Gy, grade III 37.4 Gy and grade IV 37.3 Gy, respectively. There was a significant difference of radiation dose between grade II and grade IV glioma ($p<0.05$). In Table 2 and 3, the relation of primary lesion and radiation dose, latency to radiation induced glioma occurrence, glioma grade are shown. The latency in acute lymphoblastic leukemia (ALL) / acute myeloblastic leukemia (AML), Hodgkin/non-Hodgkin lymphoma and cancer patients is short compared to that of intracranial and scalp lesion. And, the irradiated dose in ALL/AML patients is rather small compared to that of intracranial lesion. Patients with ALL/AML and Hodgkin/non-Hodgkin lymphoma are usually intensively treated with anticancer agents with carcinogenic effects, so the patients may suffer from glioma by the synergistic effects of prophylactic irradiation and chemotherapy.

| WHO grade | Number of cases | Irradiated dose (Gy) | Latency (years) |
|---|---|---|---|
| Grade II | 29 | 29.7±18.4 | 10.7±7.7 |
| Grade III | 37 | 37.4±15.9 | 12.6±8.6 |
| Grade IV | 97 | 37.3±17.5 | 10.7±6.6 |

**Table 1.** Radiation induced glioma

| | Number of cases | Irradiated dose (Gy) | Latency (years) | Radiation induced glioma |
|---|---|---|---|---|
| Pituitary adenoma | 20 | 52.2±12.7 | 13.5±7.5 | Grade III/IV 16, II 3 |
| Craniopharyngioma | 15 | 63.9±7.0 | 11.7±7.0 | Grade III/IV 13, II 1 |
| Medulloblastoma | 16 | 44.9±9.5 | 15.8±12.2 | Grade III/IV 12, II 4 |
| Germ cell tumor | 10 | 44.9±8.5 | 15.2±13.4 | Grade III/IV 9, II 1 |
| Optic glioma/ Retinoblastoma | 6 | 46.5±10.9 | 7.2±2.4 | Grade IV 6 |
| Menigioma/Neurinoma | 6 | 38.4±14.2 | 10±5.7 | Grade III/IV 5, II 1 |
| Low grade glioma | 12 | 47.0±7.8 | 13.5±10.1 | Grade III/IV 11, II 1 |

**Table 2.** Radiation induced glioma of intracranial primary lesion

http://dx.doi.org/10.5772/59047

| | Number of cases | Irradiated dose (Gy) | Latency (years) | Radiation induced glioma |
|---|---|---|---|---|
| ALL/AML | 64 | 23.6±7.6 | 8.6±3.9 | Grade III/IV 52, II 10 |
| Hodgkin/non-Hodgkin Lymphoma | 6 | 35.6±10.7 | 8±5.7 | Grade III/IV 6 |
| Cancer | 6 | 60.5±15.4 | 8±3.2 | Grade III/IV 6 |
| Scalp lesion (non-cancer) | 14 | 12.2±12.1 | 15.5±9.2 | Grade III/IV 9, II 5 |

ALL: acute lymphoblastic leukemia, AML: acute myeloblastic leukemia

**Table 3.** Radiation induced glioma of extracranial primary lesion

## 3. Genetic characteristics of radiation-induced glioma

In a patient reported by Gessi [36], the genetic alterations were p53 mutation (C to G transition at codon 176 of Exon 5), loss of heterozygosity (LOH) of 17p and 19q, O(6)-methylguanine DNA methyltransferase (MGMT) promoter methylation, and no amplification of epidermal growth factor receptor (EGFR). In Yang's case [115], p53 mutation (deletion at codon 233 of Exon 7 and a C to G transition at codon 278 of Exon 8) and no amplification of EGFR were reported. In Tada's case [104], 3-bp homozygous deletion in exon 7 of the p53 gene was described. In Kon's case [58], although LOH and amplification of EGFR, phosphatase and tensin analog (PTEN) was not observed, LOH of 1p, K-ras, p16, p53 were observed. In Alexous's two cases, LOH of 1p was found in both cases [15]. Nine radiation-induced high-grade gliomas were studied for possible molecular alterations in p53, PTEN, K-ras, EGFR, and p16 by Brat [121]. Exon 8 of p53 gene mutation (G to A substitution in codon 285) is detected in one case, EGFR amplification in 2 cases and p16/ methylthioadenosine phosphorylase (MTAP) gene deletion in 2 cases [121]. However, genetic alterations similar to those described in spontaneous, sporadic primary GBM, except the absence of PTEN mutations in the radiation-induced group were found. Radiation-induced GBMs have a lower percent of EGFR and p16 alterations than primary GBM [121]. Donson et al. [122] demonstrated by gene expression analysis genetic homogenity relative to de-novo gliomas, suggesting a common precursor cell for radiation-induced gliomas. It is not well known about the molecular alteration of radiation-induced gliomas, due to the limited number of cases and limited genes were analyzed.

## 4. Therapeutic implications

Radiation-induced glioma is difficult to treat; radiotherapy is not always a therapeutic option because the patient has already been exposed to radiation. However there are several patients reported who had a sustained remission following chemotherapy alone or radiochemotherapy. About the reports of treatment of radiation-induced glioma, a dramatic response and prolonged survival by carmustine, nimustine hydrochloride and temozolomide were reported [52, 58, 71, 75]. These tumors have a poor prognosis due to their intrinsic resistance to treatment and the difficulty using aggressive therapies in previously irradiated patients. However, vigorous chemotherapeutic approaches may yield prolonged disease control in some patients with radiation-induced glioma. The relationship of 1p LOH and chemosensitivity in oligodendroglial tumors is well known [123]. 1p LOH may account for the marked response to chemotherapy [52,58], although the reason of the chemosensitivity is not discussed in other case. In Fukui's case [32], 40 Gy of local radiotherapy and chemotherapy with nimustine hydrochloride and Interferone-β yielded dramatic response. The patient received 15 Gy of whole brain radiotherapy 7 years prior to the onset of radiation-induced glioma. Although the tolerable radiation dose is not well known after initial radiation therapy, additional radiotherapeutic approaches may yield prolonged disease control in some patients with radiation-induced glioma. The marked chemo and radiosensitivity should be further investigated for the development of glioma therapy.

## 5. Conclusion

In case that intracranial and extracranial lesions are treated by standard fractionated radiation or stereotatic radiosurgery, radiation-induced gliomas should be considered as possible long-term side effect. And the patients should be followed for a long term, even long after the period of risk for relapse of the primary site has passed.

## Author details

Ryuya Yamanaka* and Azusa Hayano

*Address all correspondence to: ryaman@koto.kpu-m.ac.jp

Graduate School for Health Care Science, Kyoto Prefectural University of Medicine, Kyoto, Japan

## References

[1] Mikhael MA. Radiation necrosis of the brain: correlation between patterns on computed tomography and dose of radiation. J Comput Assist Tomogr 1979;3(2):241-9.

[2] Jacoby CG, Tewfik HH, Blackwelder JT. Cerebellar atrophy developing after cranial irradiation. J Comput Assist Tomogr 1982;6(1):159-62.

[3] Dooms GC, Hecht S, Brant-Zawadzki M, Berthiaume Y, Norman D, Newton TH. Brain radiation lesions. MR imaging. Radiology 1986;158(1):149-55.

[4] Ron E, Modan B, Boice JD Jr, Alfandary E, Stovall M, Chetrit A, Katz L. Tumors of the brain and nervous system after radiotherapy in childhood. N Engl J Med 1988; 319(16):1033-9.

[5] Devivo DC, Malas D, Nelson JS, Land VJ. Leukoencephaly in childhood leukemia. Neurology 1997;27(7):609-13.

[6] Brada M, Ford D, Ashley S, Bliss JM, Crowley S, Mason M, Rajan B, Traish D. Risk of second brain tumour after conservative surgery and radiotherapy for pituitary adenoma. Br Med J 1992;304(6838):1343-6.

[7] Paulino AC, Mai WY, Chintagumpala M, Taher A, Teh BS. Radiation-induced malignant gliomas: is there a role for reirradiation? Int J Radiat Oncol Biol Phys 2008;71:1381-7.

[8] Musa BS, Pople IK, Cummins BH. Intracranial meningiomas following irradiation--a growing problem? Br J Neurosurg 1995;9(5):629-37.

[9] Pettorini BL, Park YS, Caldarelli M, Massimi L, Tamburrini G, Di Rocco C. Radiation-induced brain tumours after central nervous system irradiation in childhood: a review. Childs Nerv Syst 2008; 24: 793–805.

[10] Cahan WG, Woodard HQ, Higinbotham NL, Stewart FW, Coley EL. Sarcoma arising in irradiated bone; report of 11 cases. Cancer1948; 1(1):3-29.

[11] Schrantz JL, Araoz CA. Radiation induced meningeal fibrosarcoma. Arch Pathol 1972;93(1):26-31.

[12] Ahn SJ, Kim IO. Spinal cord glioblastoma induced by radiation therapy of nasopharyngeal rhabdomyosarcoma with MRI findings: case report. Korean J Radiol 2012;13(5):652-7.

[13] Albert RE, Omran AR, Brauer EW, Freed R. Follow-up study of patients treated by X-ray for tinea capitis. Am J Public Health 1966; 56:2114–20.

[14] Alexander MJ, DeSalles AA, Tomiyasu U. Multiple radiation-induced intracranial lesions after treatment for pituitary adenoma. Case report. J Neurosurg 1998;88(1): 111-5.

[15] Alexiou GA, Moschovi M, Georgoulis G, Neroutsou R, Stefanaki K, Sfakianos G, Prodromou N. Anaplastic oligodendrogliomas after treatment of acute lymphoblastic leukemia in children: report of 2 cases. J Neurosurg Pediatr 2010;5(2):179-83.

[16] Anderson JR, Treip CS. Radiation-induced intracranial neoplasms: a report of three possible cases. Cancer 1984; 53:426–9.

[17] Bachman DS, Ostrow PT. Fatal long-term sequela following radiation "cure" for ependymoma. Ann Neurol 1978; 4:319–21.

[18] Balasubramaniam A, Shannon P, Hodaie M, Laperriere N, Michaels H, Guha A. Glioblastoma multiforme after stereotactic radiotherapy for acoustic neuroma: case report and review of the literature. Neuro Oncol 2007;9(4):447-53.

[19] Barnes ARE, Liwnicz BH, Schellhas HE, Altshuller G, Aron BS, Lippert WR. Successful treatment of placental choriocarcinoma metastatic to brain followed by primary brain glioblastoma. Gynecol Oncol 1982;13:108–14.

[20] Bazan C, New PZ, Kaghan-Hallet KS. MRI of radiation-induced spinal cord glioma. Neuroradiology 1990;32:331–3.

[21] Berman EL, Eade TN, Brown D, Weaver M, Glass J, Zorman G, Feigenberg SJ. Radiation-induced tumor after stereotactic radiosurgery for an arteriovenous malformation: case report. Neurosurgery 2007;61(5):E1099.

[22] Beute BJ, Fobben ES, Hubschmann O, Zablow A, Eanelli T, Solitare G. Cerebellar gliosarcoma: report of a probable radiation-induced neoplasm. AJNR 1991;12:554–6.

[23] Bonilha L, Borges G, Fernandes YB, Ramina R, Carelli EF, Alvarenga M. Pilocytic astrocytoma following radiotherapy for craniopharyngioma: case report. Arq Neuropsiquiatr 2000;58(3A):731-5.

[24] Chung CK, Stryker JA, Cruse R, Vanucci R, Towfighi J. Glioblastoma multiforme following prophylactic cranial irradiation and intrathecal methotrexate in a child with acute lymphoblastic leukaemia. Cancer 1980; 47:2563–6.

[25] Clifton MD, Amromin GD, Perry MC, Abadir R, Watts C, Levy N. Spinal cord glioma following irradiation for Hodgkin's disease. Cancer 1980; 45:2051–5.

[26] Cohen MS, Kushner MJ, Dell S. Frontal lobe astrocytoma following radiotherapy for medulloblastoma. Neurology 1988; 31:616–9.

[27] Diersse G, Alvarez G, Figols J. Anaplastic astrocytoma associated with previous radiotherapy: report of three cases. Neurosurgery 1988; 6:1095–7.

[28] Doskaliyev A, Yamasaki F, Kenjo M, Shrestha P, Saito T, Hanaya R, Sugiyama K, Kurisu K. Secondary anaplastic oligodendroglioma after cranial irradiation: a case report. J Neurooncol 2008;88(3):299-303.

[29] Edwards MK, Terry JG, Montebello JF, Hornback NB, Kuharik MA. Gliomas in children following radiation therapy for lymphoblastic leukemia. Acta Radiol Suppl 1986;369:651-3.

[30] Enchev Y, Ferdinandov D, Kounin G, Encheva E, Bussarsky V. Radiation-induced gliomas following radiotherapy for craniopharyngiomas: a case report and review of the literature. Clin Neurol Neurosurg 2009;111(7):591-6.

[31] Fontana M, Stanton C, Pompili A, Amadori S, Mandelli F, Meloni G, Riccio A, Rubinstein LJ. Late multifocal gliomas in adolescents previously treated for lymphoblastic leukaemia. Cancer 1987; 60:1510–8.

[32] Fukui K, Inamura T, Nakamizo A, Ikezaki K, Inoha S, Nakamura K, Matsuzaki A, Fukui M. A case showing effective radiotherapy for a radiation-induced glioblastoma. No Shinkei Geka 2001;29(7):673-7.

[33] Fuller GN, Kaba SE, Ginsberg LE, McCutcheon IE, Langford LA. Late sequelae of treated pleomorphic xanthoastrocytoma: malignant brain stem astrocytoma occurring 15 years after radiation therapy. J Neurooncol 1997;32(1):57-61.

[34] Furuta T, Sugiu K, Tamiya T, Matsumoto K, Ohmoto T. Malignant cerebellar astrocytoma developing 15 years after radiation therapy for a medulloblastoma. Clin Neurol Neurosurg 1998;100(1):56-9.

[35] García-Navarro V, Tena-Suck ML, Celis MA, Vega R, Rembao D, Salinas C. Anaplastic astrocytoma post radiotherapy of pineal germinoma. Arq Neuropsiquiatr 2009;67(3A):707-9.

[36] Gessi M, Maderna E, Guzzetti S, Cefalo G, Massimino M, Solero CL, Finocchiaro G, Pollo B. Radiation-induced glioblastoma in a medulloblastoma patient: a case report with molecular features. Neuropathology 2008;28(6):633-9.

[37] Grabb PA, Kelly DR, Fulmer BB, Palmer C. Radiation-induced glioma of the spinal cord. Pediatr Neurosurg 1996;25:214–9.

[38] Guthjahr P, Dietrich E. Risiko zweiter maligner neoplasien nach erfolgreicher Tumorbehadlung in Kindersalter. Deutch Med Wochenshr 1979; 104:969–72.

[39] Hamasaki K, Nakamura H, Ueda Y, Makino K, Kuratsu J. Radiation-induced glioblastoma occurring 35 years after radiation therapy for medulloblastoma: case report. Brain Tumor Pathol 2010;27(1):39-43.

[40] Haselow RE, Nesbit M, Dehner LP, Knam FM, McHugh R, Lewitt SH. Second neoplasm following megavoltage radiation in a pediatric population. Cancer 1978; 42:1185–91.

[41] Hill MD, Mackenzie I, Mason WP. Radiation-induced glioma presenting as diffuse leptomeningeal gliomatosis: a case report. J Neurooncol 2001;55(2):113-6.

[42] Huang CI, Chiou WH, Ho DM. Oligodendroglioma occurring after radiation therapy for pituitary adenoma. J Neurol Neurosurg Psychiatry 1987;50(12):1619-24.

[43] Hufnagel TJ, Kim JH, Lesser R, Miller JM, Abrahams JJ, Piepmeier J, Manuelidis EE. Malignant glioma of optic chiasm eight years after radiotherapy for prolactinoma. Arch Ophtalmol 1988;106:1701–5.

[44] Jones A. Supervoltage X-ray therapy after of intracranial tumors. Ann R Soc Surg Eng1960;27:310–54.

[45] Judge MR, Eden OB, O'Neill P. Cerebral glioma after cranial prophylaxis for acute lymphoblastic leukaemia. Br Med J (Clin Res Ed) 1984; 289:1038–9.

[46] Kaido T, Hoshida T, Uranishi R, Akita N, Kotani A, Nishi N, Sakaki T. Radiosurgery-induced brain tumor: case report. J Neurosurg 2001;95:710–3.

[47] Kamide T, Nakada M, Hayashi Y, Suzuki T, Hayashi Y, Uchiyama N, Kijima T, Hamada J. Radiation-induced cerebellar high-grade glioma accompanied by meningioma and cavernoma 29 years after the treatment of medulloblastoma: a case report. J Neurooncol 2010;100(2):299-303.

[48] Kaschten B, Flandroy P, Reznik M, Hainaut H, Stevenaert A. Radiation-induced gliosarcoma: case report and review of the literature. J Neurosurg 1995;83:154–62.

[49] Kato N, Kayama T, Sakurada K, Saino M, Kuroki A. Radiation-induced glioblastoma: a case report. No To Shinkei 2000;52:413–8.

[50] Kawaguchi S, Kashiwaba T, Koiwa M, Shimoyama M, Kobayashi N, Fukushi Y, Tokuda K. Two autopsied cases of radiation-induced gliosarcoma. No Shinkei Geka 1991;19(3):285-90.

[51] Kawanabe Y, Sawada M, Yukawa H, Ueda S, Sasaki N, Koizumi T, Kihara S, Hoshimaru M. Radiation-induced spinal cord anaplastic astrocytoma subsequent to radiotherapy for testicular seminoma. Neurol Med Chir (Tokyo) 2012;52(9):675-8.

[52] Khoo HM, Kishima H, Kinoshita M, Goto Y, Kagawa N, Hashimoto N, Maruno M, Yoshimine T. Radiation-induced anaplastic ependymoma with a remarkable clinical response to temozolomide: a case report. Br J Neurosurg 2013;27(2):259-61.

[53] Kikkawa Y, Suzuki SO, Nakamizo A, Tsuchimochi R, Murakami N, Yoshitake T, Aishima S, Okubo F, Hata N, Amano T, Yoshimoto K, Mizoguchi M, Iwaki T, Sasaki T. Radiation-induced spinal cord glioblastoma with cerebrospinal fluid dissemination subsequent to treatment of lymphoblastic lymphoma. Surg Neurol Int. 2013;4:27.

[54] Kitanaka C, Shitara N, Nakagomi T, Nakamura H, Genka S, Nakagawa K, Akanuma A, Aoyama H, Takakura K. Postradiation astrocytoma: report of two cases. J Neurosurg 1989;70:469–74.

[55] Kleriga E, Sher JH, Nallainathan SK, Stein SC, Sacher M. Development of cerebellar malignant astrocytoma at site of medulloblastoma treated 11 years earlier. J Neurosurg 1979;49:445–9.

[56] Komaki S, Komaki R, Chol H, Correa-Paz F. Radiation and drug-induced intracranial neoplasm with angiographic demonstration. Neurol Med Chir (Tokio) 1977;17:55–62.

[57] Komatsu F, Kawaguchi H, Tsugu H, Oshiro S, Komatsu M, Fukushima T, Nabeshima K, Inoue T. Radiation-induced astrocytoma with rapid malignant transformation: case report. Neurol Med Chir (Tokyo) 2011;51(3):243-6.

[58] Kon T, Natsumeda M, Taki T, Takahashi H, Fujii Y, Yamanaka R. Radiation-induced glioblastoma following radiotherapy for pituitary adenomas: marked response to chemotherapy. J Neurol Neurophysiol 2013;4:155.

[59] Lach M, Wallace CJ, Krcek J, Curry B. Radiation-associated gliosarcoma. Can Assoc Radiol J 1996;47(3):209-12.

[60] Leung J, Guiney M. Secondary tumours after prophylactic cranial irradiation. Australas Radiol 1996;40(1):43-4.

[61] Liwnicz BH, Berger TS, Liwnicz RG. Radiation associated gliomas. A report of four cases and analysis of postradiation tumors of the central nervous system. Neurosurgery 1985;17:436–45.

[62] Loeffler JS, Niemierko A, Chapman P. Second tumors after radiosurgery: tip of the iceberg or a bump in the road? Neurosurgery 2003; 52:1436–42.

[63] Maat-Schieman MLC, Bots GTAM, Thomeer RTWM. Malignant astrocytoma following radiotherapy for craniopharyngioma. Br J Radiol 1985; 58:480–2.

[64] Malde R, Jalali R, Muzumdar D, Shet T, Kurkure P. Gliosarcoma occurring 8 years after treatment for a medulloblastoma. Childs Nerv Syst 2004;20(4):243-6.

[65] Malone M, Lumley H, Erdohazi M. Astrocytoma as a second malignancy in patients with acute lymphoblastic leukaemia. Cancer 1986;57:1979–85.

[66] Marus G, Levin V, Rutherford GS. Malignant glioma following radiotherapy for unrelated primary tumors. Cancer 1986; 58:886–94.

[67] Matsumura H, Takimoto H, Shirata M, Hirata M, Ohnishi T, Hayakawa T. Glioblastoma following radiotherapy in a patient with tuberous sclerosis. Neurol Med Chir (Tokio) 1998; 38:287–91.

[68] McWhirter WR, Pearn JH, Smith H, O'Regan P. Cerebral astrocytoma as a complication of acute lymphoblastic leukaemia. Med J Aust 1986;45:96–7.

[69] Menon G, Nair S, Rajesh BJ, Rao BR, Radhakrishnan VV.Malignant astrocytoma following radiotherapy for craniopharyngioma. J Cancer Res Ther 2007;3(1):50-2.

[70] Miyazawa T, Aida S, Shima K. Hemorrhagic cerebellar anaplastic glioma appearing 12 years after prophylactic cranial radiotherapy for acute lymphocytic leukemia. Neurol Med Chir (Tokyo) 2008;48(3):126-30.

[71] Monje ML, Ramakrishna NR, Young G, Drappatz J, Doherty LM, Wen PY, Kesari S. Durable response of a radiation-induced, high-grade cerebellar glioma to temozolomide. J Neurooncol 2007;84(2):179-83.

[72] Myong NH, Park BJ. Malignant glioma arising at the site of an excised cerebellar hemangioblastoma after irradiation in a von Hippel-Lindau disease patient. Yonsei Med J 2009;50(4):576-81.

[73] Muzumdar DP, Desai K, Goel A. Glioblastoma multiforme following prophylactic cranial irradiation and intrathecal methotrexate on a child with acute lymphoblastic leukaemia: a case report. Neurol India 1999; 47:142–4.

[74] Ng C, Fairhall J, Rathmalgoda C, Stening W, Smee R. Spinal cord glioblastoma multiforme induced by radiation after treatment for Hodgkin disease. Case report. J Neurosurg Spine 2007;6(4):364-7.

[75] Nicolardi L, DeAngelis LM. Response to chemotherapy of a radiation-induced glioblastoma multiforme. J Neurooncol 2006;78(1):55-7.

[76] Nishio S, Morioka T, Inamura T, Takeshita I, Fukui M, Sasaki M, Nakamura K, Wakisaka S. Radiation-induced brain tumors: potential late complications of radiation therapy for brain tumors. Acta Neurochir 1998;140:763–70.

[77] Okamoto S, Handa H, Yamashita J. Post-irradiation brain tumors. Neurol Med Chir (Tokyo) 1985;25:528–33.

[78] Osumi AK, Mclendon RE, Tien RD, Friedman HS, Graham M, Hockenberger B, Halperin EC, Oakes WJ. Well differentiated astrocytoma occurring nine years after radiation therapy for medulloblastoma. Clin Neuropathol 1994;13(5):281-5.

[79] Palma L, Vagnozzi R, Annino L, Ciappetta P, Maleci A, Cantore GP. Post-radiation glioma in a child. Case report and review of the literature. Child's Nervous System 1988;4:296–301.

[80] Pearl GS, Mirra SS, Miles ML. Glioblastoma multiforme occurring 13 years after treatment of a medulloblastoma. Neurosurgery 1980;6:546–51.

[81] Platt JH, Blue JM, Schold SC, Burger PC. Glioblastoma multiforme after radiotherapy for acromegaly. Neurosurgery 1983;13:85–9.

[82] Preissig SH, Bohmfalk GL, Reichel GW, Smith M. Anaplastic astrocytoma following radiation for a glomus jugulare tumor. Cancer 1979;43:2243–7.

[83] Raffel C, Edwards MSB, Davis RL, Albin AR. Postirradiation cerebellar glioma: case report. J Neurosurg 1985;63:300–3.

[84] Rappaport ZH, Loren D, Ben-Ahron A. Radiation-induced cerebellar glioblastoma multiforme subsequent to treatment of an astrocytoma of the cervical spinal cord. Neurosurgery 1991;4:606–8.

[85] Riffaud L, Bernard M, Lesimple T, Morandi X. Radiation-induced spinal cord glioma subsequent to treatment of Hodgkin's disease: case report and review. J Neurooncol 2006;76(2):207-11.

[86] Rimm IL, Li FC, Tarbell NJ, Winston KR, Sallan SE. Brain tumors after cranial irradiation for childhood acute lymphoblastic leukaemia: a 13-years experience from Dana-Farber Cancer Institute and The Children's Hospital. Cancer 1987;59:1506–8.

[87] Rittinger O, Kranzinger M, Jones R, Jones N. Malignant astrocytoma arising 10 years after combined treatment of craniopharyngioma. J Pediatr Endocrinol Metab 2003; 16: 97–101.

[88] Robinson RG. A second brain tumor and irradiation. J Neurol Neurosurg Psychiatry 1978;41:1005–12.

[89] Saenger EL, Silverman FN, Sterling FT, Turner ME. Neoplasia following therapeutic irradiation for benign conditions in childhood. Radiology 1960;74:889–904.

[90] Saiki S, Kinouchi T, Usami M, Nakagawa H, Kotake T. Glioblastoma multiforme after radiotherapy for metastatic brain tumor of testicular cancer. Int J Urol 1997;4(5): 527-9.

[91] Salvati M, D'Elia A, Melone GA, Brogna C, Frati A, Raco A, Delfini R. Radio-induced gliomas: 20-year experience and critical review of the pathology. J Neurooncol 2008;89(2):169-77.

[92] Sanders J, Sale GE, Ramberg R, Clift R, Buckner CD, Thomas ED. Glioblastoma multiforme in a patient with acute lymphoblastic leukaemia who received a marrow transplant. Transplant Proc 1982;14:770–4.

[93] Schmidbauer M, Budka H, Bruckner CD, Vorkapic P. Glioblastoma developing at the site of a cerebellar medulloblastoma treated six years earlier. J Neurosurg 1987;71:77–82.

[94] Shamisa A, Bance M, Nag S, Tator C, Wong S, Noren G, Guha A. Glioblastoma multiforme occurring in a patient treated with gamma knife surgery: case report and review of the literature. J Neurosurg 2001;94:816–21.

[95] Shapiro S, Mcaly JJ. Late anaplastic glioma in children previously treated for acute lymphoblastic leukaemia. Pediatr Neurosci 1989;15:176–89.

[96] Shapiro S, Mcaly JJ, Sartorius C. Radiation-induced intracranial malignant gliomas. J Neurosurg 1989;71:77–82.

[97] Shore RE, Albert RE, Pasternack BS. Follow-up study of patients treated by X-ray epilation for tinea capitis. Arch Environ Health 1976;31:21–8.

[98] Simmons NE, Laws ER Jr. Glioma occurrence after sellar irradiation: case report and review. Neurosurgery 1998;42(1):172-8.

[99] Snead OC, Acker JD, Morawetz RW, Benton JW. High resolution computerized tomography with coronal and sagittal reconstruction in the diagnosis of brain tumors in children. Childs Brain 1982; 9:1–9.

[100] Soffer D, Gomori JM, Pomeranz S, Siegal T. Gliomas following low dose irradiation to the head: report of three cases. J Neurooncol 1998;6:67–72.

[101] Sogg RL, Donaldson SS, Yorke CH. Malignant astrocytoma following radiotherapy for craniopharyngioma. J Neurosurg 1978;48:622–7.

[102] Suda Y, Mineura K, Kowada M, Ohishi H. Malignant astrocytoma following radiotherapy in pituitary adenoma: case report. No Shinkei Geka 1989;17(8):783-8.

[103] Tada M, Sawamura Y, Abe H, Iggo R. Homozygous p53 gene mutation in a radiation-induced glioblastoma 10 years after treatment for an intracranial germ cell tumor: a case report. Neurosurgery 1997;40:393–6.

[104] Tamura M, Misumi S, Kurosaki S, Shibasaki T, Ohye C. Anaplastic astrocytoma 14 years after radiotherapy for pituitary adenoma. No Shinkei Geka 1992;20(4):493-7.

[105] Tanriover N, Ulu MO, Sar M, Uzan M. Anaplastic oligoastrocytoma: previous treatment as a possible cause in a child with acute lymphoblastic leukemia. Childs Nerv Syst 2007;23(4):469-73.

[106] Tolnay M, Kaim A, Probst A, Ulrich J. Subependymoma of the third ventricle after partial resection of a craniopharyngioma and repeated postoperative irradiation. Clin Neuropathol 1996;15(2):63-6.

[107] Tomita H, Nogaki H, Shibata Y, Tamaki N. Brain stem glioma induced by radiotherapy: report of a case. No Shinkei Geka 1995;23:151–5.

[108] Tsang RW, Lapierre NJ, Simpson WJ, Brierley MB, Panzarella T, Smyth S. Glioma arising after radiation therapy for pituitary adenoma: a report of four patients and estimation of risk. Cancer 1993;72:2227–33.

[109] Tsutsumi S, Yasumoto Y, Ito M. Pediatric multicentric glioma occurring after cranial irradiation. J Clin Neurosci 2009;16(8):1086-8.

[110] Ushio Y, Anta N, Yoshimine T, Nagatami N, Mogami H. Glioblastoma after radiotherapy for craniopharyngioma: case report. Neurosurgery 1987;21:33–8.

[111] Utsunomiya A, Uenohara H, Suzuki S, Nishimura S, Nishino A, Arai H, Sakurai Y, Suzuki H. A case of anaplastic astrocytoma arising 8 years after initial treatment by partial resection and irradiation for central neurocytoma. No To Shinkei 2001;53(8): 747-51.

[112] Walter AW, Hancock ML, Pui C-H, Hudson MM, Ochs J, Rivera G, Pratt C, Boyett J, Kun L. Secondary brain tumors in children treated for acute lymphoblastic leukaemia at St. Jude Children's Research Hospital. J Clin Oncol 1998;16(12):3761–7.

[113] Walters TR. Childhood acute lymphocytic leukemia with a second neoplasm. Am J Pediatr Hematol Oncol 1979;1:285–7.

[114] Yang SY, Wang KC, Cho BK, Kim YY, Lim SY, Park SH, Kim IH, Kim SK. Radiation-induced cerebellar glioblastoma at the site of a treated medulloblastoma: case report. J Neurosurg 2005;102(4 Suppl):417-22.

[115] Yeung YF, Wong GK, Zhu XL, Ma BB, Hk NG, Poon WS. Radiation-induced spinal glioblastoma multiforme. Acta Oncol 2006;45(1):87-90.

[116] Yu J, Yong WH, Wilson D, Black KL. Glioblastoma induction after radiosurgery for meningioma. Lancet 2000;356:1576–7.

[117] Zagzag D, Miller DC, Cangiarella J, Allen JC, Greco MA. Brainstem glioma after radiation therapy for acute myeloblastic leukemia in a child with Down syndrome. Possible pathogenetic mechanisms. Cancer 1992;70(5):1188-93.

[118] Zampieri P, Zorat PL, Mingrino S, Soattin GB. Radiation-associated cerebral gliomas. Report of two cases and review of the literature. J Neurosurg Sci 1989;3:271–9.

[119] Zochodne DW, Cairncross JG, Arce FP, MacDonald JC, Blume WT, Girvin JP, Kaufmann JC. Astrocytoma following scalp radiotherapy in infancy. Can J Neurol Sci 1984;11:475–8.

[120] Zuccarello M, Sawaya R, DeCourten-Myers G. Glioblastoma after radiation therapy for meningioma: case report and review of the literature. Neurosurgery 1986;19:114–9.

[121] Brat DJ, James CD, Jedlicka AE, Connolly DC, Chang E, Castellani RJ, Schmid M, Schiller M, Carson DA, Burger PC. Molecular genetic alterations in radiation-induced astrocytomas. Am J Pathol1999; 154:1431–8.

[122] Donson AM, Erwin NS, Kleinschmidt-DeMasters BK, Madden JR, Addo-Yobo SO, Foreman NK. Unique molecular characteristics of radiation-induced glioblastoma. J Neuropathol Exp Neurol 2007;66(8):740-9.

[123] Thiessen B, Maguire JA, McNeil K, Huntsman D, Martin MA, Horsman D. Loss of heterozygosity for loci on chromosome arms 1p and 10q in oligodendroglial tumors: relationship to outcome and chemosensitivity. J Neurooncol 2003;64(3):271-8.

Chapter 8

# Radiation-Induced Brain Injury After Radiotherapy for Brain Tumor

Zhihua Yang, Shoumin Bai, Beibei Gu, Shuling Peng,
Wang Liao and Jun Liu

Additional information is available at the end of the chapter

http://dx.doi.org/10.5772/59045

## 1. Introduction

Radiation therapy is used widely for the treatment of diffuse primary and metastatic brain tumors [1]. Especially for nasopharyngeal carcinoma (NPC), the most common type of cancer in southern China, radiation therapy is the first-choice treatment and sometimes the only effective management of the disease. As many as 200,000 patients receive partial large-field or whole-brain irradiation every year, and the population of long-term cancer survivors keeps on growing. During treatment, however, some healthy brain tissues are also exposed to the radiation inevitably, and consequently many patients may experience neurological symptoms associated with damage to these healthy tissues after radiotherapy. Some of these symptoms may even last for months or years. This is known as acute and chronic radiation-induced brain injury (RIBI), also known as radiation encephalopathy (RE). Approximately 100,000 primary and metastatic brain tumor patients each year in the US survive long enough (>6 months) to experience RIBI [2]. For example, the incidence of RIBI for patients with NPC in Guangdong province is up to 3 per 100,000, to our knowledge, 40 times higher than the world average and is the most common one among head and neck tumor. RIBI includes a series of clinical manifestations, such as focal neurological deficits, secondary epilepsy, mental and behavioural disorders, elevated intracranial pressure, and the progressive deterioration of the hippocampal-associated learning and memory functions [3],which can be especially devastating to patients and caregivers.

The American Cancer Society center (ACS) stresses that in order to maximize the quality of life for tumor patients after radiotherapy, the future research should focus on preventing and curing complications of cancer therapy. RIBI, a common and devastating complication of radiotherapy for brain tumor, is now emerging as a major health problem in the treatment of brain tumor.

## 2. Pathogenesis

Based on the time between onset of clinical expression and radiation therapy administration, RIBI has been classified into acute, early delayed, and late delayed injury, which was first reported by Sheline [4]. Acute brain injury occurs during and/or in days to weeks after irradiation. Early delayed brain injury occurs 6–12 weeks post-irradiation [5], while some other researchers consider this time course is 1-6 months [6]. Although both of these early injuries can result in severe reactions, they rarely occur and normally resolve spontaneously or reversible after short-term treatment. In contrast, late delayed brain injury, usually developing 6 months post-irradiation, which is most significantly higher than that of acute and early delayed RIBI, have been viewed as irreversible and progressive continuously due to the pathogenesis [7].

The knowledge of the mechanisms underlying the RIBI following irradiation is the basis for improving the therapies and prophylaxes, but it is not wholly clear.

The most direct affecting risk of RIBI is the radiation doses, fractionation schemes, and adjuvant treatments. [8, 9] Liu Y and Xiao S et al. found that single-dose irradiation at 10Gy failed to induce any significant effects in young male rats whereas an exposure at 20 to 40Gy induced acute brain injury at both cognitive and pathologic levels. [10] Zhou H. and Liu Z. et al. reported that fractionated irradiation of 20 to 40Gy could also induce acute brain injury in young rats which indicated the role of fractionation schemes. [11] Furthermore, Ruben JD et al. not only demonstrated the risk of radiation dose and fraction size, but the subsequent administration of chemotherapy as well. [9]

In general, ionizing radiation can cause RIBI by either direct or indirect way and it is likely that the successful unraveling of this puzzle will not come true without the basic study of subtle molecular, cellular, or microanatomic changes in the brain. Hereon, we will discuss the pathogenesis of RIBI from oxidative stress, nonspecific inflammation, blood brain barrier(BBB) disruption as well as apoptosis and inhibition of neurogenesis which act alone or accompanied.

### 2.1. Oxidative stress

It is reported that in the unilaterally irradiated animals, irradiated hemispheres showed similarly significant changes in oxygenation compared to unirradiated controls. [12]

Due to radiation therapy, the microglia is activated and immune cells begin to infiltrate the brain. These cells then produce reactive oxygen species (ROS) whose production and detoxification are normal physiological processes. Nevertheless, an imbalance between ROS production and ROS removal may lead to oxidative stress [13, 14].Several components of ROS can cause damage to cardinal cellular components, such as lipids, proteins, and DNA, initiating subsequent cell death via necrosis or apoptosis [15]. Thus, ROS can be contributed to neuronal toxicity and implicated in both acute injury and chronic neuropathological conditions [16].

Many related molecules have been reported. Jun showed hydrogen peroxide ($H_2O_2$)-induced oxidative stress and apoptosis in HT22 cells accompany by up-regulated expression of p-ERK 1/2, p-JNK, and p-P38 [13]. What is more, the effectiveness of edaravone(a new agent of ROSscavenger), peroxisome proliferator-activated receptor (PPAR) gamma agonists, and antioxidants/antioxidant enzymes in preventing or mitigating the severity of RIBI also provided an evidence of the oxidative stress. [13, 17]

### 2.2. Nonspecific inflammation

Irradiation can caused an acute endothelial cell apoptosis which lead to BBB breakdown, chronic hypoxia and peritumoral tissue edema. [18] Meanwhile, nonspecific inflammation cascades which further promote the microenvironmental changes, radiation necrosis, and neurogenesis inhibition was activated [19].

Radiation could induce astrocytes proliferation and secrete a great quantity of pro-inflammatory mediators after irradiation, which may aid the infiltration of leukocytes into the brain via blood-brain barrier (BBB) breakdown [20, 21]. Microglias could also be activated by quantity of irradiation through rapid proliferation, as well as increased production of ROS and other cytokines which are involved in mediating neuroinflammation [22].

Plenty of experiments have found up-regulation of pro-inflammatory transcription factors after irradiation which constituted the evidence of nonspecific inflammation cascades in the process of RIBI. Moore, A. H. suggest that radiation-induced changes in vascular permeability are dependent on cyclooxygenase 2 (COX2), one of two isoforms of the obligate enzyme in prostanoid synthesis and the principal target of non-steroid anti-inflammatory drugs activity. [23] Lee et al. found mRNA and protein of pro-inflammatory mediators including tumour necrosis factor-alpha (TNF-alpha), interleukin-1beta (IL-1beta), and monocyte chemoattractant protein-1 (MCP-1) activated significantly in regions isolated from irradiated in rat brain. [24] TNF-alpha is thought to be able to up-regulate other pro-inflammatory cytokines and increase BBB permeability, increase leukocyte adhesion, activate astrocytes, and induce endothelial apoptosis. And the further research demonstrated that anti-inflammation factor (TNF-alpha) successfully inhibited radiation-induced effects in the local as well as abscopal region in the brain. [12] Peroxisome proliferator-activated receptor (PPAR) gamma is ligand-activated transcription factor that belong to the steroid/thyroid hormone nuclear receptor superfamily. And the effectiveness of PPAR-gamma agonists is also a strong demonstration of nonspecific inflammation. [25]

What is more, radiation could induce the loss of oligodendrocyte type-2 astrocyte (O-2A) progenitor cell, the most radiosensitive type of glial cell, which leads to transient demyelination soon after irradiation. Since all the brain gliocytes including oligodendrocyte, astrocytes and microglia would participate in the radioactive damage process in different ways and RIBI is predominated by white matter necrosis and demyelination, the pathological mechanism is well known as Gliocyte Hypothesis. However, there is conflicting conclusion that the targeted anti-inflammatory agent has no effect on gliocytes, but can still ameliorate RIBI [26]. Consequently, pathological mechanism of RIBI cannot be explained so simply by the Gliocyte Hypothesis despite the large amount of evidence supporting this hypothesis.

Due to the synergistic effect of oxidative stress and nonspecific inflammation after irradiation, endothelial cell nuclear, blood vessel density, and blood vessel length are vulnerable to have a reduction. The vascular damage can result in brain ischemia and even white matter necrosis. [7]. All of this elicited the Vascular Hypothesis. Paradoxically, radiation-induced necrosis has also been reported in the absence of vascular changes [27]. In addition, the PPARγ agonist, pioglitazone, and the ACE inhibitor, ramipril, which are believed to prevent RIBI in the rat do not reverse the reduction in vascular density and length that occurs after fWBI [28, 29].

Therefore, RIBI cannot be completely explained by any single cell or tissue despite a host of evidence supporting these hypotheses. It is supposed to occur and develop due to active interactions between the multiple cells. These participating cells are considered to play a synergistic rather than initial role in the radiation brain injury [30].

### 2.3. Blood Brain Barrier(BBB) disruption

A number of data from laboratory animals has demonstrated acute BBB disruption which was initiated by apoptosis of endothelial cells and mediated by the ASMase pathway after irradiation [18]. As a result, change of BBB permeability has been thought to be the most sensitive and reliable index for detection of early RIBI. [31] Breakdown of the BBB may also enhance the effectiveness of chemotherapeutic agents, with the unintended consequence of contributing to injury of the peritumoral tissue. Liu Y. and Xiao S. et al. found that a single-dose exposure at 20 to 40 Gy induced acute brain injury at cognitive is more or less accompanied with increased brain water content and deteriorated BBB function, though mild histopathologic alternations were only noticed in the 40-Gy-irradiated rats at 20 days. [10] Zhou H. and Liu Z. et al. reported disrupted BBB permeability was detected after fractionated irradiation of 20 to 40Gy in young rats and thus proved that the change in BBB permeability could be one of the most sensitive and reliable indices of fractionated-radiation-induced acute RIBI. [11] Besides, increased astrogliosis in the hippocampus could be detected at 4 weeks' postirradiation for 40-Gy group.

### 2.4. Apoptosis and neurogenesis inhibition

The pathogenesis of RIBI may also relate to the process of neuronal apoptosis and inhibition of neurogenesis.

Even gray matter contains neuronal cell bodies which is quite oxygen-dependent, neurons have been considered radioresistant since they could no longer divide. However, it is reported that apoptosis occurs in the young adult rat brain after ionizing irradiation and recent studies also demonstrated that there exists direct radiation-induced damage to hippocampal neurons with associated cognitive decline. The hippocampus consists of the DG, CA3, and CA1 regions. Irradiating the hippocampus resulted in an increase in apoptosis in the subgranular zone of the DG which are capable of both self-renewal and generating neurons, astrocytes, and oligodendrocytes [32, 33]. And blocking neurogenesis which was associated with alterations of microenvironment including disruption of the microvascular angiogenesis and increase in the number and activation status of microglia within the neurogenic zone can contribute to the deleterious side effects of radiation treatment. [14]

Neurogenesis is also related to inflammation for the reason that anti-inflammatory drug was proved to be capable of restoring and augments neurogenesis after cranial irradiation. [19]However, these changes could also be observed in the absence of demyelination, blood vessel density alternation and inflammatory cellular infiltration by a doses of ≤2 Gy that fail to produce these changes [34].

## 3. Clinical characteristics of RIBI

### 3.1. Latency

The latency of RIBI exists a long time span. Chandler reported the time interval between the end of radiotherapy to the onset of RIBI was 1 month to 16 years [35]. JY Qin et al. documented the latency of RIBI was 3 months to 38 months, median time of which was 21.7 months [36]. We collected data of 130 NPC cases who suffered RIBI post radiotherapy, the latency of them underwent a large time span from 0 to 32 years, the mean time was about 6 years [37].

Therefore, being focus on the mechanism research to get early differentiation, diagnosis, explore therapeutic strategies of late delayed RIBI become more and more urgent.

### 3.2. Clinical features and classification

Acute effects occur during and/or shortly after the radiation exposure and are characterized by symptoms of fatigue, dizziness, and signs of increased intracranial pressure. The acute effects are considered to be secondary to edema and disruption of the BBB. Early delayed effects of post-irradiation and usually show reversible symptoms generalized weakness and somnolence, partly resulting from a transient demyelination. It is, however, the late delayed effects that may lead to severe irreversible neurological consequences.

According to the site of involvement and corresponding clinical manifestations, the subtypes of RIBI were divided into cerebellum type, brain stem and cranial type, cerebellum type and mixed type.

#### *3.2.1. Cerebral hemisphere type*

Focal delivery of one large radiation fraction during radiotherapy can lead to focal injury of the brain adjacent to the irradiated lesion [38].Clinically, patients present with focal neurological deficits, which are often accompanied by focal increased intracranial pressure.

The most common and serious delayed complication of cerebral radiotherapy is cognitive dysfunction. Take NPC for example, since inferior temporal lobes inevitably expose to the radiation, the prominent and earliest seen symptom of RIBI is distinctive cognitive impairment. Recently, Hsiao demonstrated that nasopharyngeal cancer patients treated with intensity-modulated radiotherapy (IMRT) had a worse cognitive outcome if >10% of their temporal lobe volume received a total fractionated dose of >60 Gy than patients who received < 60 Gy [39]. The feature of cognitive impairment is different from those with Alzheimer's disease, it is characterized by decreased verbal memory, spatial memory, attention, novel problem-solving ability, and even executive function. Patients usually accompanied with negative emotions including depression, anxiety as well as somatization. Mental disorders such as stupor state, hallucinations and delusions could also be observed as the injury progresses [20].

It should be noted that significant cognitive impairment can be seen in the absence of radiographic or clinical evidence of demyelination or white matter necrosis after irradiation [40]. Therefore, conducting cognitive evaluations shortly post-irradiation at regular intervals is becoming more and more important. Once cognitive decline is detected, no matter whether there is imaging findings of brain lesions, prophylactic treatment should be given to the patients immediately. The mini-mental status examination (MMSE), a test to assess global cognitive function, is relatively insensitive to radiation-induced cognitive impairment [39, 41]. As the cognitive domains that are most affected by brain irradiation is distinct from the common causes of dementia such as Alzheimer's disease and vascular dementia, current Radiation Therapy Oncology Group (RTOG) study has established a series of tests that focuses on the cognitive domains affected by brain irradiation, such as Dutch adult reading test for assessing intelligence, vline bisection test for perception, visual verbal learning test for memory and stroop color word test for executive function [42]. The Montreal cognitive assessment (MoCA) is used to assess different cognitive domains including attention and concentration, executive functions, memory, language, visuoconstructional skills, conceptual thinking, calculations, and orientation. Sensitivity and specificity of MoCA application in radiation-induced cognitive impairment has not been reported.

Another most common injury after radiotherapy is unilateral or/and bilateral temporal lobe edema which might elevate intracranial pressure. If the pathogenesis develops persistently, the area of edema could expand to the parietal lobes and then cause rapidly deteriorating clinical course. Signs of increased intracranial pressure such as headache, nausea and vomiting would get worse progressively. Severe cerebral edema could result in compression of cerebral peduncle and cerebral hernia, which would lead to hemiplegia and even to death. Once that occurs, surgical treatment will be needed. Moreover, cerebral edema could at last get liquefactive necrosis with formation of cystic spaces. Figure.1

*3.2.2. Brain stem and cranial type*

It has been reported that each pair of cranial nerve could get involved in injury after irradiation in NPC patients [43]. Due to the irradiation fields mainly cover the lower part of brain stem, the last four cranial nerves, glossopharyngeal nerve, vagus nerve, accessory nerve and hypoglossal nerve, were commonly affected and leading to corresponding clinical manifestations, such as atrophy of tongue muscle, dysphagia, dysphonia and dysdipsia. Severe bulbar

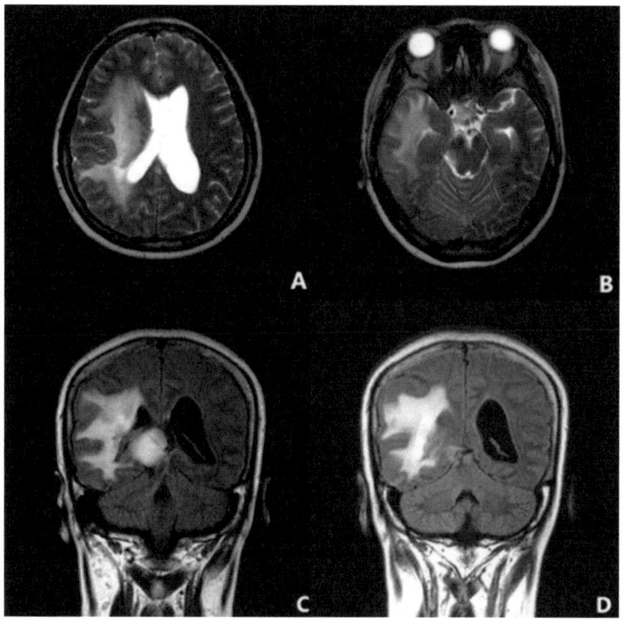


**Figure 1.** Cerebral edema and atrophy of a 39-year-old female cerebral hemangioma patient. 8 years after the treatment of gamma knife. Lumps-like abnormal signal was shown in the right-basolateral region, heterogeneous high signal was shown on T2W, surrounded by low signal, a large fingerlike high signal of the white matter around lesions on T2W. Cerebral gyrus of the frontal and parietal lobe narrow and cerebral sulcus widen which is the sign of cerebral atrophy. A.T2WI B. T2WI C.FLARE D.FLARE

palsy may significantly decrease the life quality of patients and sometime is fatal caused by subsequent lung infection and/or malnutrition [43]. And the frequency of upper cranial nerve injury increased greatly if the patients have to conduct re-radiotherapy.

Some other common involved cranial nerve is cochleovestibular nerve caused by not only direct effect of irradiation to the nerve but also the indirect effect of the inner ear damage after radiotherapy such as secretory otitis media or even intractable suppurative otitis media. The prime symptoms of disorders of the cochleovestibular nerve are vertigo, tinnitus and pain. Irreversible hearing loss caused by nerve deafness, conduction deafness and mixed deafness will happen in the end [43].

Radiation-induced optic neuropathy (RION) is a rare but usually devastating side effect of radiotherapy for NPC. The most frequent clinical symptoms of RION typically present with sudden, painless, irreversible vision loss in one or both eyes after radiotherapy, and occur most commonly from 3 months to more than 9 years after radiotherapy. Liu et al. reported RION in NPC patients [44]. Ophthalmologic examinations showed flake bleeding in the retina, optic nerve atrophy and cotton-wool spots. T1-weighted enhanced MRI images showed enhancement of the optic nerve and optic chiasm in six cases.

One more severe clinical manifestation is syncope. Damage to descending sympathetic nerve fibers, which anatomically run along the brain stem, may result in hazardous syncope as well

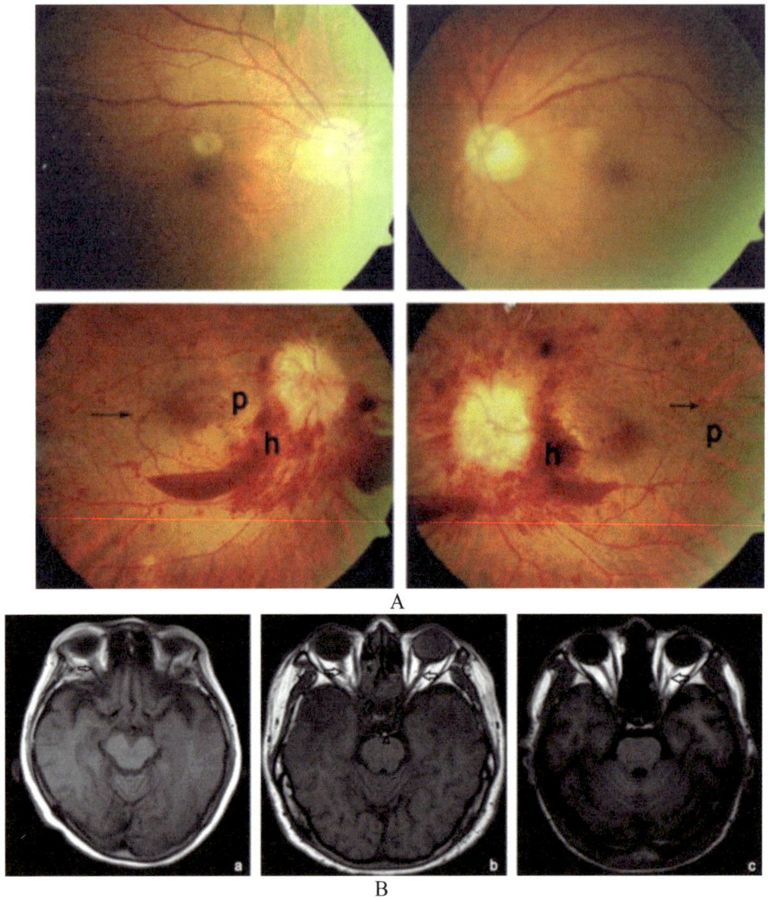


**Figure 2.** A. Fundus examination in radiation-induced optic neuropathy: ocular fundus showing flame-shaped and dot hemorrhage (bottom row, h, arrow) and cotton-wool spots (top row, bottom row, p). B. Axial MRI of three patients showing: (a, b) tortuous optic nerve with blurring of edges, and (b) optic nerve atrophy; (b, c) T1-weighted enhanced MRI showing enhancement of the optic nerves and optic chiasm.

as Horner syndrome. Crossed hemiplegia might also occur when pyramidal tract is involved simultaneously [43].

### 3.2.3. *Cerebellum type*

It is the least common type of RIBI. Damage to cerebellum results in edema of cerebellar hemisphere and leads to symptoms such as vertigo, stumbling, ataxia and other discomfort. The injury to cerebellum has the same prognosis as that in cerebral hemisphere and eventually develop into the tonsillar hernia.

### 3.2.4. *Mixed type*

It is a combination of two or more subtypes mentioned above.

http://dx.doi.org/10.5772/59045

## 4. Value of neuroimaging in RIBI diagnosis

Neuroimaging, including computed tomography (CT), magnetic resonance imaging (MRI) especially neurological functional imaging technology, provide valuable information in early diagnosis and differential diagnosis of RIBI. In this paragraph, we will provide a variety of neuroimaging information to readers. Including not only traditional CT/MRI imaging, but also proton magnetic resonance spectroscopy (MRS) and iffusion tensor imaging (DTI).

### 4.1. Computed Tomography (CT)

CT foundings of focal radiation brain edema and necrosis are generally low density, while the affected white matter is usually symmetric and exhibit no enhancement or irregular peripheral enhancement with contrast material. The brain lesions would range from small foci near the frontal or occipital horns to a confluent band extending from the ventricles to the corticomedullary junction. Figure.3

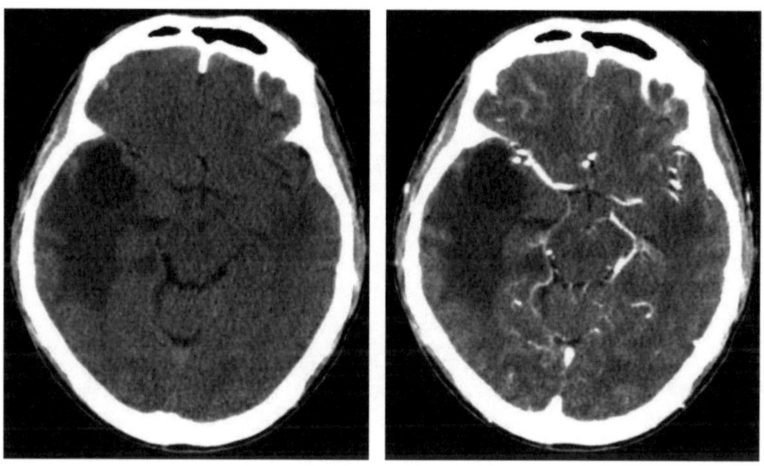

**Figure 3.** CT founding of a 59-year-old male patient with NPC after radiotherapy for over 10 years. A. cystic liquetactive necrosis of the right temporal lobe with edema around lesions. B. no enhancement.

### 4.2. Magnetic resonance Imaging (MRI)

MRI is definitely more valuable for the diagnosis of RIBI than CT. The appearence of finger like edema and focal necrosis which shows low signal intensity on T1WI and high signal on T2WI are typical feature of MR imaging in patients with RIBI. Ringlike or irregular enhancement in the bilateral temporal lobes are also frequently seen on T1WI enhanced MR imaging while haemorrhage with heterogeneous signals is relative rare. (Figure.4)These findings on conventional MRI technology are not specific and insufficient to distinguish RIBI from tumor recurrence or other diseases. Thus various new technologies of MRI are employed to make up for this shortcoming.

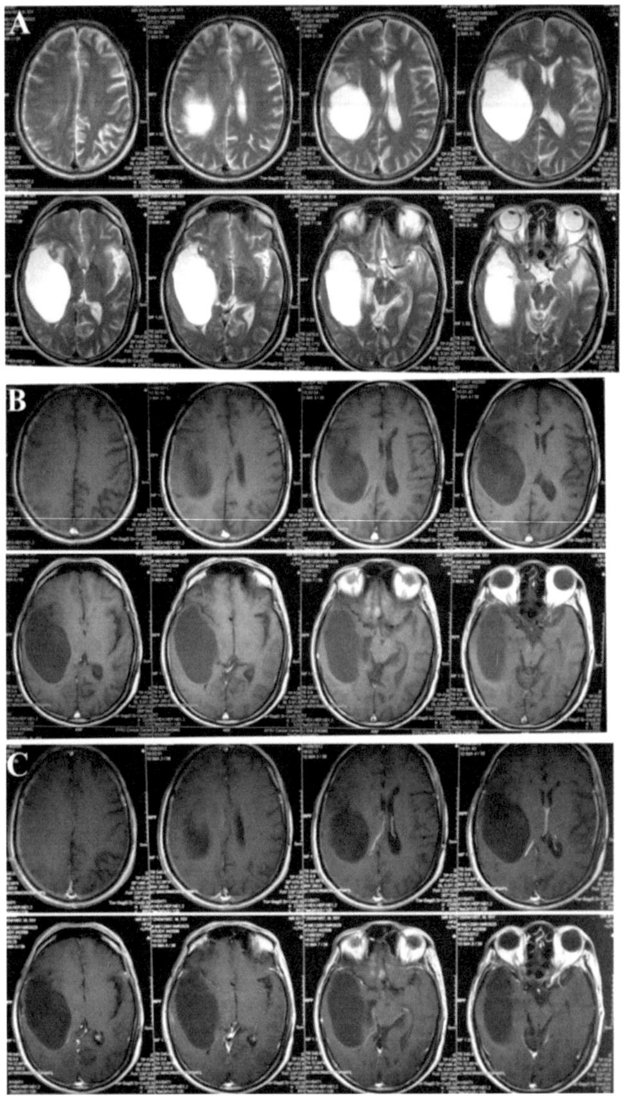

**Figure 4.** Radiation necrosis and edema. MRI performed 8 years after radiotherapy of one 54-years-old male patient with NPC. Necrosis of right-temporal and right-parietal lobe shows low signal intensity on T1WI and high signal on T2WI with enhanced boundary. Edema of the left-temporal lobe shows finger like low signal intensity on T1WI and high signal on T2WI with non-enhanced boundary. A. T2WI; B. T1WI; C.T1WI+C

### 4.3. Proton magnetic Resonance Spectroscopy (MRS)

MRS is used to display metabolite changes in normal appearing white matter after fWBI in the brain. Brain metabolites are quantified including choline(Cho), creatine(Cr), glutamate(Glu), glutamine(Gln), N-acetyl-aspartate (NAA) and lactate. It is reported that NAA, Cr and Cho change regularly from the center of the visible lesions. In the liquefaction and necrosis foci,

NAA, Cr and Cho are nearly absent. In the visible lesions, the levels of NAA increase slightly, while the contents of Cr and Cho decreased obviously. Certain extent away from the visible lesions, the contents of NAA decrease and the levels of Cr and Cho increase. Farther away from the lesions, the levels of the three substances gradually become normal. Consequently the ratios of NAA/Cr and Cho/Cr alter from periphery to the lesion, decrease from a value above 1 to one less than 1. A ratio of NAA/Cr and Cho/Cr less than 1 may be highly indicative of nerve and cell structure damage in the brain tissue [45, 46]. In view of this, MRS is supposed to indentify a larger area of abnormal metabolism in RIBI than visible lesion in MRI, which makes it possible to detect RIBI in early stage.

### 4.4. Diffusion Tensor Imaging (DTI)

DTI is a novel way to assess tissue microstructure by measuring the diffusion of water molecules in three-dimensional (3D) space. It is often applied to distinguish demyelination from axonal injury within white matter bundle. In a DTI study of childhood survivors after fWBI for acute lymphoblastic leukemia, fractional anisotropy (FA) decreases significantly in the frontal and parietal lobes related to declines in intelligence quotient [47]. In another study of adult survivors post fWBI for acute leukemia, FA values reduced obviously in normal appearing cerebral white matter of the temporal lobe, hippocampus, and thalamus [48]. DTI is thought to be a promising technique to detect early changes in white matter integrity before image evidence of radiation-induced demyelination or necrosis. However, the application of DTI to RIBI is just in its infancy. Figure.5

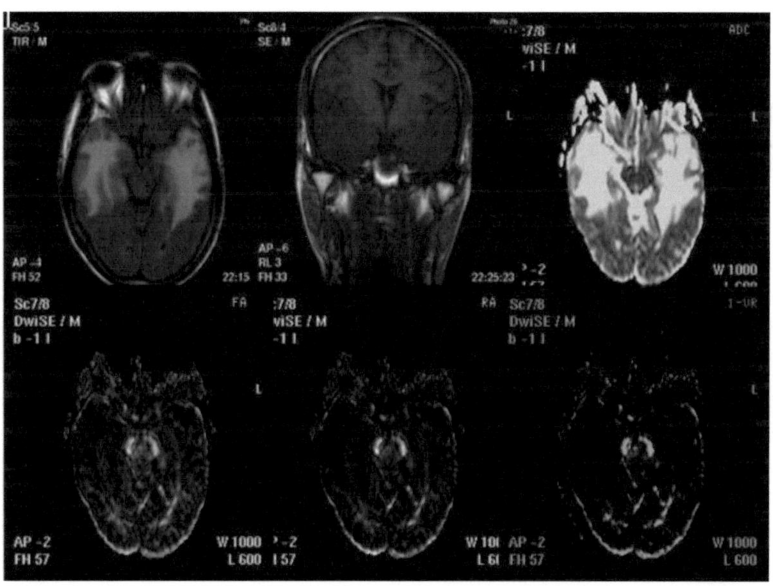

**Figure 5.** Delayed RIBI of bilateral temporal. Edema is obvious. Isotropic map shows high signal in the lesion area which is wider than FLAIR. Anisotropic map shows low signal in the bilateral temporal lobe and white matter fiber of the normal temporal lobe shows high signal and blurred.

## 5. Treatment strategies

Up to now, there has been no proven effective treatment to reverse or terminate the pathogenesis brain irradiation injury, which could be particularly devastating to patients and caregivers since the exact mechanisms of RIBI is unclear. Potential therapeutic strategies to prevent RIBI will be discussed in this part.

### 5.1. Glucocorticoids

Glucocorticoids play a vital role in the comprehensive therapy for RIBI. A large number of experimental and clinical studies have confirmed its polyvalent efficacy of narrowing lesions, relieving symptoms as well as improving their prognosis by counteracting the radiation-induced vascular endothelial damage and inflammatory cascade [49]. Dispute still remains over the opportunity, dose and course of glucocorticoid therapy. Many a researchers recommend maintenance therapy with regular dose for more than 3 months while some others affirm the effect of early large dosage of corticosteroids for shorter periods [49]. Some patients may be weaned off after a period of symptomatic exacerbation while in some cases symptoms can return after steroid cessation and lead to necessitating long-term steroid use. Unfortunately, the prolonged systemic administration will result in immunosupression, psychiatric distrubances, myopathy and sequelae of endocrinologic compromise such as hypertension, diabetes mellitus, osteoporosis, weight changes and thickening of facial subcutis [49].

### 5.2. Antiplatelets and anticoagulation

Radiation induced vascular endothelial injury may lead to subsequent mural thrombosis, thus antiplatelets may play a crucial part in preventing the RIBI. Currently exsisted antiplatelet drugs mainly include cyclooxygenase(COX) inhibitors and adenosine diphosphate (ADP) receptor antagonists. Phosphodiesterase inhibitors, a new type of antiplatelet agents, have been proved to be protective for intravascular thrombosis after radiation [2].

Another kind of drug to control thrombosis is anticoagulation drugs. It's reported that the use of heparin and warfarin lead to partial recovery of function in five of eight patients with cerebral radiation necrosis when they were proved to be unresponsive to steroid therapy [50]. One case concerning a patient experienced a recurrence of symptoms following discontinuation of anticoagulation therapy and was reversed again by resuming anticoagulation treatment [50] demonstrated the limited success of anticoagulation drug. However, this treatment need to be validated in larger trials before clinical application.

### 5.3. Reactive Oxygen Species (ROS) scavengers

Edaravone, a new agent of ROS scavenger, has been verified effective in reducing the vascular endothelial cell injury, inhibiting brain encephaledema and preventing neuronal cell necrosis [51]. Our clinical trails on 42 NPC patients suffered RIBI has demonstrated that efficiency (50.0%) and total efficiency (88.9%) in the edaravone administration group were significantly higher than that in the contrast group (14.3% and 42.9%). After a 4-week treatment, the lesion volume on MRI was smaller than before in edaravone group, and the scores of 6 domains, 19 aspects and the overall quality of life in edaravone group were significantly higher than those in non-edaravone group [52]. However, ROS scavengers have received not so much attention because they are likely to protect brain tumors to the same extent as they protect normal brain [2]. Another antioxidant and radioprotective drug is vitamin E. The administration of Vitamin E significantly reduced the severity of radiation-induced brain damages and increased the activity of superoxide dismutase and catalase enzymes in the brain. [53]

### 5.4. Refactoring microcirculation

The butyl-phthalide, a neotype of drugs reforming the microcirculation, has multiple effects of increasing the perfusion in the ischemia area, protecting the mitochondria from hypoxic injury, and also reducing neuronal apoptosis. Human urinary kallidinogenase for injection, another new agent of this type, may be instrumental in vasodilation of brain blood vessels, increasing haemoglobin in the cerebral blood flow, and also improving glucose metabolism in ischemic brain tissues [54].

### 5.5. Reconstructing the nerve function

Radiation injury could destroy the nerve structure and then lead to loss of neuron function. Therefore neural plasticity is thought to play a vital role in the comprehensive treatment for RIBI. As our data from animals and humans shows that gangliosides is helpful in promoting the recovery of nerve function in lesioned brain, spinal cord and also peripheral nerve. A host of in vivo and in vitro studies also demonstrated that neurotrophic factors are neuroprotective in radiation-induced nouropathy. Curative effect has been proved in patients with temporal lobe injury after two-month injection with mouse nerve growth factor, both MR imaging and cognitive function of them were improved significantly [55].

### 5.6. Renin–Angiotensin System(RAS) inhibitors

The RAS has been viewed as a classical systemic hormonal system. Recently several intra-organ RAS including a brain RAS have been identified. The brain RAS is involved in modulation of the BBB, stress, memory, and cognition. Both angiotensin-converting enzyme inhibitors (ACEI) and angiotensin receptor blockers (ARB) have been proved effective in treating experimental radiation nephropathy and pneumopathy [56, 57]. As for their effect on encephalopathy, studies of Jenrow et al. (2010) show that administration of the ACEI, ramipril has modest protection against WBI-induced decreases in neurogenesis, but did not modulate radiation-induced neuroinflammation while other report has different conclusion with a different timing of chronic administration of theramipril and/or the response after single or fractionated doses on rodent [58, 59]. Whether all of the drug mentioned above can be useful for the patient of RIBI remains to be further elucidated.

### 5.7. Symptomatic treatment

Dehydration medicine such as mannitol and albumin should be given to patients with high cranial pressure. Antiepileptic drugs (AED) should be chosen according to the forms of epilepsy seizures. Serotonin (5-HT) reuptake inhibitors and psychological therapies might be preferred when anxiety and depression are the cardinal symptoms.

It should be mentioned that there has been no known preventive medications for radiation-induced cognitive impairment in humans, although several pharmacologic agents have been assessed for symptomatic management [2]. The Wake Forest Community Clinical Oncology Program Research Base completed a phase II study using 10mg/day of a cholinesterase inhibitor namely donepezil, which showed significant improvement in energy level, mood, and cognitive function in radiation-induced brain injury survivors [60]. Memantine, an NMDA receptor antagonist being able to block ischemia-induced NMDA excitation, was proven to be effective in vascular dementia. Thus it is supposed to be conducive to radiation-induced cognitive impairment if radiation-induced ischemia occurs after fWBI. Other potential pharmacological mediators based on preclinical researches suggesting that anti-inflammatory agents could prevent or ameliorate radiation-induced cognitive function. As for anti-inflammatory peroxisome proliferator-activated PPARγ agonists, researchers have found some evidence that they maight prevent/ameliorate radiation-induced cognitive impairment when given for only a few weeks after fWBI on rodent [61].

### 5.8. Surgical management

Surgical resection can be considered when the patient's necrosis are symptomatic and have no take a turn for the better after medical treatments. For example, when suffering from large area-cerebral edema, and the condition progressively exacerbated active medications although has been given, patients should also be recommended to surgically remove the focal brain lesions in time when the location is in a region that is surgically accessible. During this process, the surgeon should avoid incurring additional significant neurologic morbidity. [85]

### 5.9. Neural Stem Cells(NSCs) therapies

In addition to drug therapeutics, there has been increased interest in the use of various NSCs therapies. Pioneering researchers directly inject NSCs into rodent brains after WBI and found it partially restores cognitive function [62, 63]. Interestingly, these NSCs not only differentiate into neurons, but also oligodendrocytes, astrocytes and endothelial cells that can alter the hippocampal microenvironment [63]. However, the use of exercise or NSCs transplantation to prevent/ameliorate RIBI in humans will require considerably more research before it can be translated to the clinic.

### 5.10. Organ-sparing approach

To date, one of the strategies to prevent RIBI in the clinic involves organ-sparing approach which is based on neuroanatomical target theory. Technology has evolved to potentially allow for selective avoidance of the regions of adult neurogenesis, including the hippocampus and neural stem cell niche in the periventricular regions. With the help of advanced radiation techniques, such as 3D conformal image guidance [64], inverse-planned intensity modulated radiotherapy (IMRT) [65] and proton beam radiotherapy [66], it is expected to reduce the occurrence of RIBI by limiting the dose to critical organs and possibly increasing locoregional tumor control. [67]

### 5.11. Anti-VEGF antibody

As is mentioned above, the necrosis is partly due to increasing capillary permeability which is caused by cytokine release leading to extracellular edema. The edema is the most common pathology of RIBI is just sustained by endothelial dysfunction, tissue hypoxia as well as subsequent necrosis. Consequently, it is a logical option to block the vascular endothelial growth factor (VEGF) at an early stage to reduce the development of radiation necrosis and thus decrease the vascular permeability. After the patient with radiation-induced necrosis was treated with an anti-VEGF antibody (bevacizumab), the improvement neurologic signs and symptoms in accordance with the decrease in T1-weighted fluid-attenuated inversion recovery signals put bevacizumab as a treatment direction for patients with RIBI [68].

### 5.12. Hyperbaric Oxygen Treatment (HBOT)

HBOT is proven to be able to stimulate angiogenesis and restore the regional blood supply by reaching the goal of increasing parenchymal oxygen concentration. HBOT treatment has been demonstrated to be beneficial in pediatric patients with radiation necrosis [69]and in smaller series and case reports [70, 71]. However, Jun L et al. reported that HBOT treatment did not reduce visual loss or blindness in patients with RION [44]. As single institution studies vary widely due to patient selection bias, it would be necessary to conduct more randomized trials to delineate the true benefit of HBOT. [72]

## 6. Problems and prospects

Although a great many treatment strategies have eliminated acute and early delayed brain injury as well as most delayed demyelination and white matter necrosis, radiotherapy is still carries a risk of RIBI which may seriously affect the life quality of survivors. This risk is further exacerbated while the patient need to use chemotherapeutic agents at the same time [2].

To get more knowledge about the mechanism of RIBI is the key to the solution. Although many theories have been proposed, it is likely that the pathogenesis in long term survivors of various tumors like small cell lung cancer, NPC, low-grade glioma, non-parenchymal tumors, primary brain tumors and metastatic brain tumors are different just because they were treated differently. There is not a solely theory that can be used to fully answer this question.

As a result, it is imperative to detect the pathological change non-invasively as early as possible. However, there still a lot of difficulties which need to be solved in clinical practice. It is explicit that the most important issue is to differentiate radiation necrosis and tumor progression. Fortunately, there are multiple radiological and nuclear medicine techniques available to help us even these anatomic and metabolic imaging techniques all have inherent limitations in sensitivity and specificity.

Researchers all over the world have tried hard but have had only modest success in modulating RIBI to date. However, the future looks promising since we have attached importance to RIBI and find some innovative treatments such as the NECs or anti-VEGF therapy which can be the alternative offer [72].

Over the next decade, we will continue paying more attention to the investigation that how radiation-induced brain injury develops and how it can be treated [2].

## Acknowledgements

We are grateful for support from the National Natural Science Foundation of China (no. 81372919) and the Natural Science Foundation of Guangdong Province, China(no. S2013010013964).

## Author details

Zhihua Yang[1], Shoumin Bai[2], Beibei Gu[3], Shuling Peng[3], Wang Liao[4] and Jun Liu[4*]

*Address all correspondence to: docliujun@hotmail.com

1 Department of Neurology, the First Affiliated Hospital, Guangzhou Medical University, Guangdong, China

2 Department of Oncology, Sun Yat-Sen Memorial Hospital, Sun Yat-Sen University, Guangdong, China

3 Department of Anesthesiology, Sun Yat-Sen Memorial Hospital, Sun Yat-Sen University, Guangdong, China

4 Department of Neurology, Sun Yat-Sen Memorial Hospital, Sun Yat-Sen University, Guangdong, China

## References

[1] Tsao, M.N., et al., Radiotherapeutic management of brain metastases: a systematic review and meta-analysis. Cancer Treat Rev, 2005. 31(4): p. 256-73.

[2] Greene-Schloesser, D., et al., Radiation-induced brain injury: A review. Front Oncol, 2012. 2: p. 73.

[3] Roman, D.D. and P.W. Sperduto, Neuropsychological effects of cranial radiation: current knowledge and future directions. Int J Radiat Oncol Biol Phys, 1995. 31(4): p. 983-98.

[4] Sheline, G.E., Radiation therapy of brain tumors. Cancer, 1977. 39(2 Suppl): p. 873-81.

[5] Schultheiss, T.E. and L.C. Stephens, Invited review: permanent radiation myelopathy. Br J Radiol, 1992. 65(777): p. 737-53.

[6] Yan, L., Z. Xi and B. Drettner, Epidemiological studies of nasopharyngeal cancer in the Guangzhou area, China. Preliminary report. Acta Otolaryngol, 1989. 107(5-6): p. 424-7.

[7] Brown, W.R., et al., Capillary loss precedes the cognitive impairment induced by fractionated whole-brain irradiation: a potential rat model of vascular dementia. J Neurol Sci, 2007. 257(1-2): p. 67-71.

[8] Lee, A.W., et al., Factors affecting risk of symptomatic temporal lobe necrosis: significance of fractional dose and treatment time. Int J Radiat Oncol Biol Phys, 2002. 53(1): p. 75-85.

[9] Ruben, J.D., et al., Cerebral radiation necrosis: incidence, outcomes, and risk factors with emphasis on radiation parameters and chemotherapy. Int J Radiat Oncol Biol Phys, 2006. 65(2): p. 499-508.

[10] Liu, Y., et al., An experimental study of acute radiation-induced cognitive dysfunction in a young rat model. AJNR Am J Neuroradiol, 2010. 31(2): p. 383-7.

[11] Zhou, H., et al., Fractionated radiation-induced acute encephalopathy in a young rat model: cognitive dysfunction and histologic findings. AJNR Am J Neuroradiol, 2011. 32(10): p. 1795-800.

[12] Ansari, R., et al., Anti-TNFA (TNF-alpha) treatment abrogates radiation-induced changes in vacular density and tissue oxygenation. Radiat Res, 2007. 167(1): p. 80-6.

[13] Zhao, Z.Y., et al., Edaravone protects HT22 neurons from H2O2-induced apoptosis by inhibiting the MAPK signaling pathway. CNS Neurosci Ther, 2013. 19(3): p. 163-9.

[14] Monje, M.L., et al., Irradiation induces neural precursor-cell dysfunction. Nat Med, 2002. 8(9): p. 955-62.

[15] Gorman, A.M., et al., Oxidative stress and apoptosis in neurodegeneration. J Neurol Sci, 1996. 139 Suppl: p. 45-52.

[16] Pettmann, B. and C.E. Henderson, Neuronal cell death. Neuron, 1998. 20(4): p. 633-47.

[17] Ramanan, S., et al., Role of PPARs in Radiation-Induced Brain Injury. PPAR Res, 2010. 2010: p. 234975.

[18] Li, Y.Q., et al., Endothelial apoptosis initiates acute blood-brain barrier disruption after ionizing radiation. Cancer Res, 2003. 63(18): p. 5950-6.

[19] Monje, M.L., H. Toda and T.D. Palmer, Inflammatory blockade restores adult hippocampal neurogenesis. Science, 2003. 302(5651): p. 1760-5.

[20] Zhou, H., et al., Fractionated radiation-induced acute encephalopathy in a young rat model: cognitive dysfunction and histologic findings. AJNR Am J Neuroradiol, 2011. 32(10): p. 1795-800.

[21] Wilson, C.M., et al., Radiation-induced astrogliosis and blood-brain barrier damage can be abrogated using anti-TNF treatment. Int J Radiat Oncol Biol Phys, 2009. 74(3): p. 934-41.

[22] Conner, K.R., et al., Effects of the AT1 receptor antagonist L-158,809 on microglia and neurogenesis after fractionated whole-brain irradiation. Radiat Res, 2010. 173(1): p. 49-61.

[23] Moore, A.H., et al., Radiation-induced edema is dependent on cyclooxygenase 2 activity in mouse brain. Radiat Res, 2004. 161(2): p. 153-60.

[24] Lee, W.H., et al., Irradiation induces regionally specific alterations in pro-inflammatory environments in rat brain. Int J Radiat Biol, 2010. 86(2): p. 132-44.

[25] Zhao, W. and M.E. Robbins, Inflammation and chronic oxidative stress in radiation-induced late normal tissue injury: therapeutic implications. Curr Med Chem, 2009. 16(2): p. 130-43.

[26] Persson, H.L., et al., Radiation-induced cell death: importance of lysosomal destabilization. Biochem J, 2005. 389(Pt 3): p. 877-84.

[27] Schultheiss, T.E. and L.C. Stephens, Invited review: permanent radiation myelopathy. Br J Radiol, 1992. 65(777): p. 737-53.

[28] Zhao, W., et al., Administration of the peroxisomal proliferator-activated receptor gamma agonist pioglitazone during fractionated brain irradiation prevents radiation-induced cognitive impairment. Int J Radiat Oncol Biol Phys, 2007. 67(1): p. 6-9.

[29] Zhao, W., D.I. Diz and M.E. Robbins, Oxidative damage pathways in relation to normal tissue injury. Br J Radiol, 2007. 80 Spec No 1: p. S23-31.

[30] Tofilon, P.J. and J.R. Fike, The radioresponse of the central nervous system: a dynamic process. Radiat Res, 2000. 153(4): p. 357-70.

[31] Nakata, H., et al., Early blood-brain barrier disruption after high-dose single-fraction irradiation in rats. Acta Neurochir (Wien), 1995. 136(1-2): p. 82-6; discussion 86-7.

[32] Palmer, T.D., J. Takahashi and F.H. Gage, The adult rat hippocampus contains primordial neural stem cells. Mol Cell Neurosci, 1997. 8(6): p. 389-404.

[33] Gage, F.H., et al., Multipotent progenitor cells in the adult dentate gyrus. J Neurobiol, 1998. 36(2): p. 249-66.

[34] Machida, M., G. Lonart and R.A. Britten, Low (60 cGy) doses of (56)Fe HZE-particle radiation lead to a persistent reduction in the glutamatergic readily releasable pool in rat hippocampal synaptosomes. Radiat Res, 2010. 174(5): p. 618-23.

[35] Sundgren, P.C. and Y. Cao, Brain irradiation: effects on normal brain parenchyma and radiation injury. Neuroimaging Clin N Am, 2009. 19(4): p. 657-68.

[36] Ji-yong, Q., Diagnosis, prevention and treatment of radiation brain damage of nasopharyngeal carcinoma patients treated by radiotherapy, L.K.J. Yun-he, L.K.J. Yun-he^Editors. 2006. p. 942-943.

[37] Gu, B., et al., Radiation-induced Brachial Plexus Injury After Radiotherapy for Nasopharyngeal Carcinoma. Jpn J Clin Oncol, 2014. 44(8): p. 736-42.

[38] Flickinger, J.C., et al., Development of a model to predict permanent symptomatic postradiosurgery injury for arteriovenous malformation patients. Arteriovenous Malformation Radiosurgery Study Group. Int J Radiat Oncol Biol Phys, 2000. 46(5): p. 1143-8.

[39] Kondziolka, D., et al., Radiosurgery with or without whole-brain radiotherapy for brain metastases: the patients' perspective regarding complications. Am J Clin Oncol, 2005. 28(2): p. 173-9.

[40] Sundgren, P.C. and Y. Cao, Brain irradiation: effects on normal brain parenchyma and radiation injury. Neuroimaging Clin N Am, 2009. 19(4): p. 657-68.

[41] Herman, M.A., et al., Neurocognitive and functional assessment of patients with brain metastases: a pilot study. Am J Clin Oncol, 2003. 26(3): p. 273-9.

[42] Chang, E.L., et al., Neurocognition in patients with brain metastases treated with radiosurgery or radiosurgery plus whole-brain irradiation: a randomised controlled trial. Lancet Oncol, 2009. 10(11): p. 1037-44.

[43] Rong, X., et al., Radiation-induced cranial neuropathy in patients with nasopharyngeal carcinoma. A follow-up study. Strahlenther Onkol, 2012. 188(3): p. 282-6.

[44] Zhao, Z., et al., Late-onset radiation-induced optic neuropathy after radiotherapy for nasopharyngeal carcinoma. J Clin Neurosci, 2013. 20(5): p. 702-6.

[45] Qiu, S.J., et al., Proton magnetic resonance spectroscopy for radiation encephalopathy induced by radiotherapy for nasopharyngeal carcinoma. Nan Fang Yi Ke Da Xue Xue Bao, 2007. 27(3): p. 241-6.

[46] Rabin, B.M., et al., Radiation-induced changes in the central nervous system and head and neck. Radiographics, 1996. 16(5): p. 1055-72.

[47] Khong, P.L., et al., White matter anisotropy in post-treatment childhood cancer survivors: preliminary evidence of association with neurocognitive function. J Clin Oncol, 2006. 24(6): p. 884-90.

[48] Dellani, P.R., et al., Late structural alterations of cerebral white matter in long-term survivors of childhood leukemia. J Magn Reson Imaging, 2008. 27(6): p. 1250-5.

[49] Shaw, P.J. and D. Bates, Conservative treatment of delayed cerebral radiation necrosis. J Neurol Neurosurg Psychiatry, 1984. 47(12): p. 1338-41.

[50] Glantz, M.J., et al., Treatment of radiation-induced nervous system injury with heparin and warfarin. Neurology, 1994. 44(11): p. 2020-7.

[51] He, F., et al., Effect of edaravone on Abeta1-40 induced enhancement of voltage-gated calcium channel current. CNS Neurosci Ther, 2012. 18(1): p. 89-90.

[52] Tang, Y., et al., Psychological disorders, cognitive dysfunction and quality of life in nasopharyngeal carcinoma patients with radiation-induced brain injury. PLoS One, 2012. 7(6): p. e36529.

[53] Sezen, O., et al., Vitamin E and L-carnitine, separately or in combination, in the prevention of radiation-induced brain and retinal damages. Neurosurg Rev, 2008. 31(2): p. 205-13; discussion 213.

[54] Brown, W.R., et al., Vascular damage after fractionated whole-brain irradiation in rats. Radiat Res, 2005. 164(5): p. 662-8.

[55] Liu, Y., et al., An experimental study of acute radiation-induced cognitive dysfunction in a young rat model. AJNR Am J Neuroradiol, 2010. 31(2): p. 383-7.

[56] Moulder, J.E., B.L. Fish and E.P. Cohen, ACE inhibitors and AII receptor antagonists in the treatment and prevention of bone marrow transplant nephropathy. Curr Pharm Des, 2003. 9(9): p. 737-49.

[57] Molteni, A., et al., Control of radiation-induced pneumopathy and lung fibrosis by angiotensin-converting enzyme inhibitors and an angiotensin II type 1 receptor blocker. Int J Radiat Biol, 2000. 76(4): p. 523-32.

[58] Jenrow, K.A., et al., Ramipril mitigates radiation-induced impairment of neurogenesis in the rat dentate gyrus. Radiat Oncol, 2010. 5: p. 6.

[59] Lee, T.C., et al., Chronic administration of the angiotensin-converting enzyme inhibitor, ramipril, prevents fractionated whole-brain irradiation-induced perirhinal cortex-dependent cognitive impairment. Radiat Res, 2012. 178(1): p. 46-56.

[60] Shaw, E.G., et al., Phase II study of donepezil in irradiated brain tumor patients: effect on cognitive function, mood, and quality of life. J Clin Oncol, 2006. 24(9): p. 1415-20.

[61] Robbins, M.E., et al., The AT1 receptor antagonist, L-158,809, prevents or ameliorates fractionated whole-brain irradiation-induced cognitive impairment. Int J Radiat Oncol Biol Phys, 2009. 73(2): p. 499-505.

[62] Acharya, M.M., et al., Rescue of radiation-induced cognitive impairment through cranial transplantation of human embryonic stem cells. Proc Natl Acad Sci U S A, 2009. 106(45): p. 19150-5.

[63] Joo, K.M., et al., Trans-differentiation of neural stem cells: a therapeutic mechanism against the radiation induced brain damage. PLoS One, 2012. 7(2): p. e25936.

[64] Gutierrez, A.N., et al., Whole brain radiotherapy with hippocampal avoidance and simultaneously integrated brain metastases boost: a planning study. Int J Radiat Oncol Biol Phys, 2007. 69(2): p. 589-97.

[65] Barani, I.J., et al., Neural stem cell-preserving external-beam radiotherapy of central nervous system malignancies. Int J Radiat Oncol Biol Phys, 2007. 68(4): p. 978-85.

[66] Munck, A.R.P., et al., Photon and proton therapy planning comparison for malignant glioma based on CT, FDG-PET, DTI-MRI and fiber tracking. Acta Oncol, 2011. 50(6): p. 777-83.

[67] Wang, X., C. Hu and A. Eisbruch, Organ-sparing radiation therapy for head and neck cancer. Nat Rev Clin Oncol, 2011. 8(11): p. 639-48.

[68] Matuschek, C., et al., Bevacizumab as a treatment option for radiation-induced cerebral necrosis. Strahlenther Onkol, 2011. 187(2): p. 135-9.

[69] Chuba, P.J., et al., Hyperbaric oxygen therapy for radiation-induced brain injury in children. Cancer, 1997. 80(10): p. 2005-12.

[70] Bui, Q.C., et al., The efficacy of hyperbaric oxygen therapy in the treatment of radiation-induced late side effects. Int J Radiat Oncol Biol Phys, 2004. 60(3): p. 871-8.

[71] Kishi, K., et al., Preferential enhancement of tumor radioresponse by a cyclooxygenase-2 inhibitor. Cancer Res, 2000. 60(5): p. 1326-31.

[72] Siu, A., et al., Radiation necrosis following treatment of high grade glioma--a review of the literature and current understanding. Acta Neurochir (Wien), 2012. 154(2): p. 191-201; discussion 201.

Chapter 9

# Minimally Invasive but Maximally Effective Treatment of Anterior Skull Based Tumors — The Combination of Advanced Neuroendoscopy and Intraoperative Imaging with iMRI and O-Arm

Kaveh Asadi-Moghaddam, Joseph C. Taylor and Todd W. Vitaz

Additional information is available at the end of the chapter

http://dx.doi.org/10.5772/59051

## 1. Introduction

The use of endoscopic techniques for the treatment of anterior skull based tumors has seen and exponential rise over the past 15 years. As a result of this rapid growth newer more powerful endoscopic systems with better surgical instruments have been developed which has increased the armamentarium and further broadened the scope of potentially treatable lesions [1,2]. However, even with these newer systems as well as angled surgical telescopes; visual lines of sight and normal anatomical structures can still hinder visualization. In addition, the steep learning curve associated with this type of procedure as well as the loss of the normal surgical feedback such as direct 3d visualization and tactile feedback also increase the challenges associated with such procedures. Therefore, in many cases it may be difficult to determine when the surgical goals of complete resection or safest maximal debulking have been obtained. The addition of advanced intraoperative imaging with intraoperative MRI or O-Arm (Medtronic, Minneapolis, MN) technology to some of these cases enables surgeons to obtain radiographic feedback during the procedure and thus further assess their work and adds another factor into surgical decision making [3].

## 2. Surgical corridors and types of lesion approaches treatable with extended endonasal approach

The treatment of both benign and malignant lesions of the anterior skull base can be performed with this approach. This technique requires a team approach with an ENT and neurosurgeon who both must be experienced in endoscopic principles, skull base anatomy and have a vast understanding of all potential treatment options[1,2,4-6]. An enormous learning curve exists not only for performing the surgical approach but also for dissection and removal of the lesion and subsequent reconstruction of the surgical defect and complication avoidance. Most authors have reported this learning curve with much higher complication rates in the earlier portions of their series[1,6-8]. We like most other teams have modified and fine-tuned our technique as we have continued to gain experience. Most authors recommend starting with straight forward midline lesions (figure 1.) and then broadening their technique to more challenging and invasive para-midline lesions as their comfort level and experience grows. In addition, the inclusion of frameless navigation systems and even more modern advanced imaging techniques such as O-Arm and intraoperative MRI also improve the safety and broaden the scope of lesions that may be amenable to such treatment approaches.

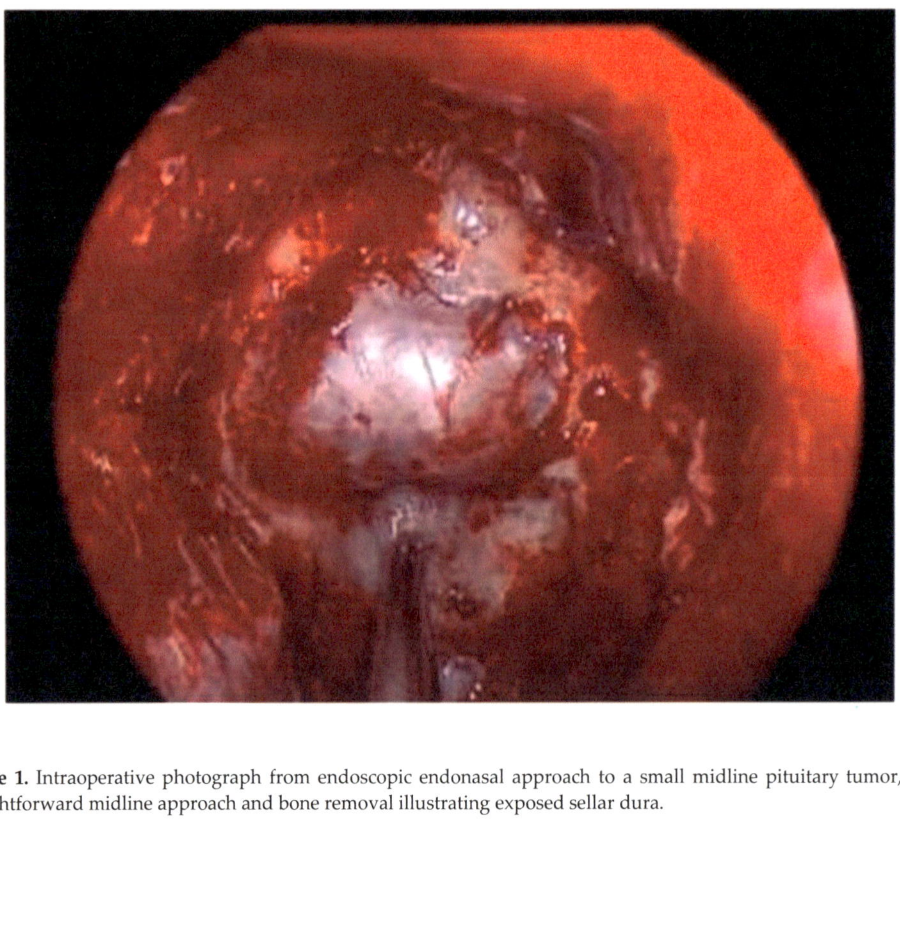

**Figure 1.** Intraoperative photograph from endoscopic endonasal approach to a small midline pituitary tumor, after straightforward midline approach and bone removal illustrating exposed sellar dura.

Lesions from the crista galli all the way down to the body of C2 can be treated with different variations of this approach[1,2,6,8-11]. Superiorly the medial orbits serve as a lateral limit on exposure [6]; however, more advanced techniques utilizing an oculoplastic surgeon and a small conjunctival incision can even expand this border (figure 2.). Traditionally the carotid arteries served as the lateral extent at the level of the sella [6,10]; however more advanced techniques now allow lateral exposure all the way to the infratemporal fossa [2,5].

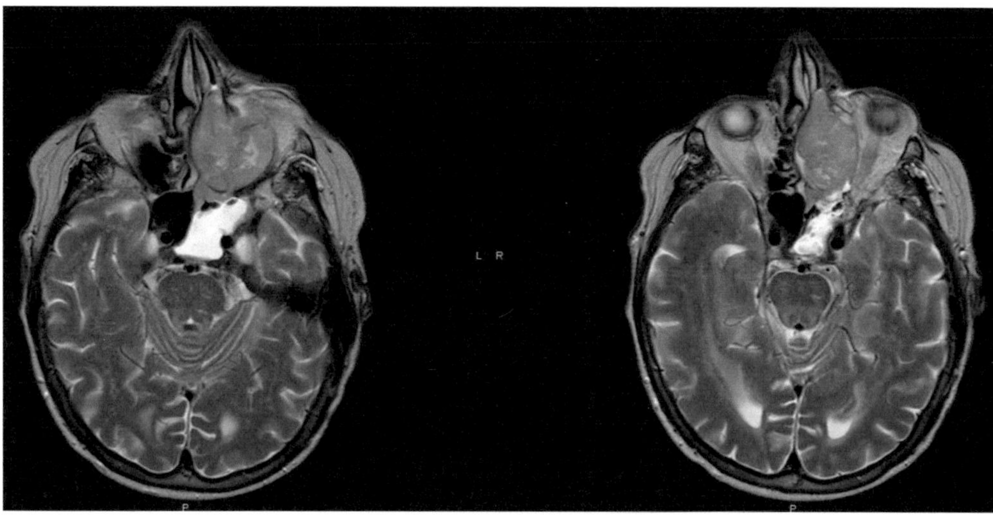


**Figure 2.** Preoperative axial T2-wieghted preoperative MRI showing primary sinus melanoma with left orbital compression in an 86 year old gentleman. Patient underwent endoscopic removal with aide of a small subconjunctival incision for palliative debulking of the lesion without globe removal.

Studies comparing endoscopic techniques with more traditional transcranial procedures have found either equivalent or superior results with endoscopic approaches[7,8]. However, limitations with endoscopic techniques continue to exist. These include anatomical constraints that may place major neural or vascular structures ventral to the pathology and thus increase the surgical risks and minimize utility. Limitations in visualization have been overcome with newer endoscopic lighting and camera systems. The 2 dimensional view with endoscopic techniques may create some challenges; however, experienced surgeons have learned to accommodate to these limitations. Newer 3D systems will soon become readily commercially available and as these systems evolve will likely overcome this limitation all together. Hemostasis and repair of postoperative CSF leaks have been the two most challenging aspects of these procedures [1,2,6,8,10,12]. Various commercially available products and surgical nuances can be used to overcome many of the challenges with hemostasis. In addition, vascular lesions are approached from the ventral side of dural involvement thus allowing devascularization of the lesion prior to any tumor manipulation or debulking. Control of postoperative CSF leaks deserves special mention and will be discussed below. Finally, the method of tumor removal must be modified to safely perform these techniques. While en bloc resection may be possible for small midline lesions this is not safely feasible for the majority of tumors. This becomes especially important in the realm of malignant tumor management where the historical standard has always been en bloc resection with negative margins. Even though this may be the goal, studies have shown that this in actually only obtained in 70% of cases of "open" resections for these lesions [13,14]. There is no convincing evidence to prove that a less invasive piecemeal resection portends to a worse prognosis and studies in this area are lacking [8].

## 3. Complications associated with EEA

Major neurological complications following this type of procedure are rare. They are typically related to either damage to major vascular structures or perforating vessels, optic nerve and chiasm or cranial nerves [1,2,4-8]. New or worsening visual symptoms are rare and their occurrence varies considerably based on pathology. Intraoperative monitoring of cranial nerve 3, 4, 6 may minimize the risk of damage to these structures.

Unlike transcranial approaches there is no skin incision or autologous bone flap, thus the risk of wound infection is almost entirely eliminated [7]. During the early experience with this exposure the concern for operating through a contaminated nasal corridor and the associated risk of meningitis or intracranial abscess was an enormous concern; however, experience has shown that this risk is minimal and usually limited to the setting of postoperative CSF leakage. In fact most authors recommend standard perioperative gram positive antibiotic coverage (cefazolin, clindamycin, vancomycin) for 24-48 hours [1,2,4,7]. In addition, because the pathological process is approached from the ventral bone interface, brain retraction and manipulation is minimal in these procedures. Therefore the risk of postoperative seizures, cognitive or other detrimental neurological changes from brain retraction and manipulation are almost entirely eliminated.

### 3.1. Postoperative CSF leaks

The creation of postoperative CSF fistulas has been one of the most challenging limitations to overcome with these techniques. Direct repair with suturing is not possible because of the deep surgical corridor and limited lateral exposure. Rates of postoperative CSF leakage vary between (0%-30%)[15-19]; and most surgeons have shown a direct relationship to experience with higher rates early on in their series despite progressing to more complex and invasive modifications of this procedure as their experience grew [1,2,4,6-8].

To try to prevent the occurrence of these events numerous reconstructive procedures have been attempted. These include the use of various autologous, allogenic and synthetic substrates from abdominal fat, fascia lata, nasal mucosa or turbinates, temporalis muscle, pericardium, and synthetic dural substitutes. In addition, bone reconstruction has been attempted with various autologous and synthetic commercial substances. These implants may be inserted as inlay or onlay grafts as well as the "gasket seal" techniques [20]. The addition of biological sealants such as Tisseal (Baxter Bioscience, Deerfield, IL) and DuraSeal (Integra, Plainsboro, NJ) are often commonly used as well.

A recent advancement has been the use of vascularized nasoseptal flaps [1,2,6,7,10,12]. These flaps which are typically developed at the beginning of the procedure prior to bone removal to reduce the risk of damage to the vascularity, have significantly decreased the risk of postoperative CSF leaks in cases where opening of the dura and arachnoid is anticipated [6]. A complete understanding of the vascular anatomy of this region is required to ensure that adequate vascularized tissue is available for reconstruction at the end of the procedure. Harvesting of such grafts lengthens surgical times only slightly but does increase postoperative nasal crusting and discomfort. Typically the septum is remucosalized by 3 months [6].

## 4. Combination of endoscopic techniques with advanced imaging technology

Despite the fact that endoscopic techniques may actually improve illumination and visualization over conventional microsurgical techniques there are many instances where it may be difficult to determine whether or not the surgical goals have been obtained. The use of angled (30, 45, 70 degree) telescopes can help surgeons evaluate around corners but not through objects. The surgical goals vary from case to case and depend on patient age, comorbidities, preoperative neurological status and pathology. While gross total resection may be the goal for most procedures in some lesion debulking for symptom control followed by stereotactic radiosurgery to the capsule may be the safest approach to minimize surgical morbidity (figure 3).

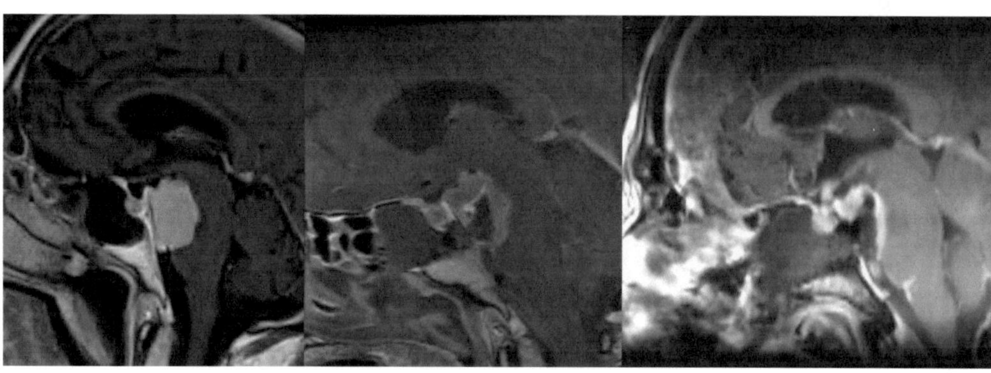

**Figure 3.** Sagittal T1-weighted post contrast preoperative, first intraoperative and second intraoperative MRI in 78 year old myelopathic gentleman with clival meningioma with significant brainstem compression. The surgical goal was to debulk the lesion leaving a small capsule however endoscopically it was difficult to determine how much residual tumor persisted behind the pituitary gland which is clearly seen on the middle image. On the final image the capsule can be seen falling away from the diencephalon and chiasmatic region.

O-Arm (Medtronic, Minneapolis, MN) and similar technologies may be useful in defining bone anatomy during some very complex procedures. The lack of tissue differentiation makes this technology very limiting for determining the extent of tumor removal for most cases. We have found this extremely useful in verifying adequate surgical results in cases of basilar invagination treated with the EEA. Following what is felt to be complete resection of the compressive pathology imaging can be obtained to verify the actual surgical results (figure 4). In addition, this technology can also be used in cases where more lateral temporal bone removal is required to verify actual bone removal prior to dural opening and tumor resection.

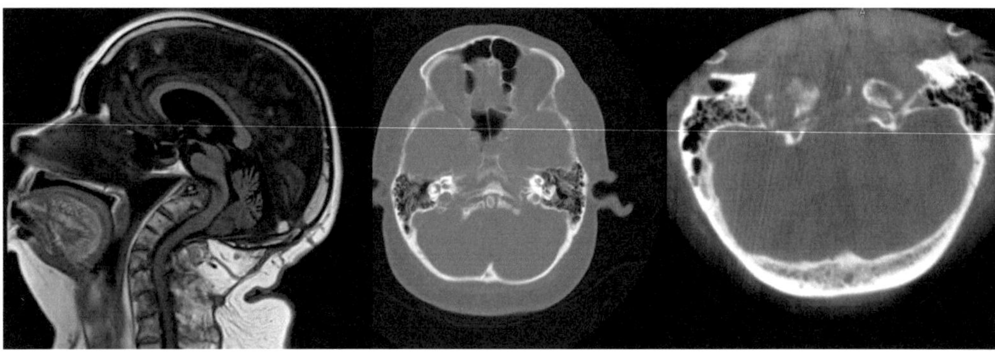

**Figure 4.** Preoperative Sagittal T1-weighted MRI and axial CT scan; and axial post midline decompression O-Arm image (sagittal reformatted images show complete decompression from clivus to C2/3 level) in 44 year old myelopathic female with platybasia and basilar invagination with brainstem compression, treated via endoscopic approach with O-Arm assisted navigation.

Another more common technology is the use of Intraoperative MRI. This technology has been extensively utilized for endoscopic removal of pituitary tumors for more than ten years [3,21]. We have found this exceptionally helpful in cases of giant pituitary tumors (figure 5) and other skull base cases such as meningiomas and craniopharyngiomas (figure 6). Following completion of resection imaging can be performed and then additional tumor resection can occur if significant residual is appreciated on these scans. Extreme care must be used in interpreting these results as surgical induced changes on peritumoral structures or capsule can mimic significant residual tumor in some instances.

We have found intraoperative imaging helpful in cases of large pituitary macroademonas where the capsule/diaphragm fails to prolapse into the field (figure 7). Imaging can be performed to determine the degree of residual tumor and decide whether opening the capsule and proceeding with extracapsular dissection is warranted. Finally, in cases where surgical debulking may be the primary goal intraoperative imaging can be performed to ensure that adequate results are obtained.

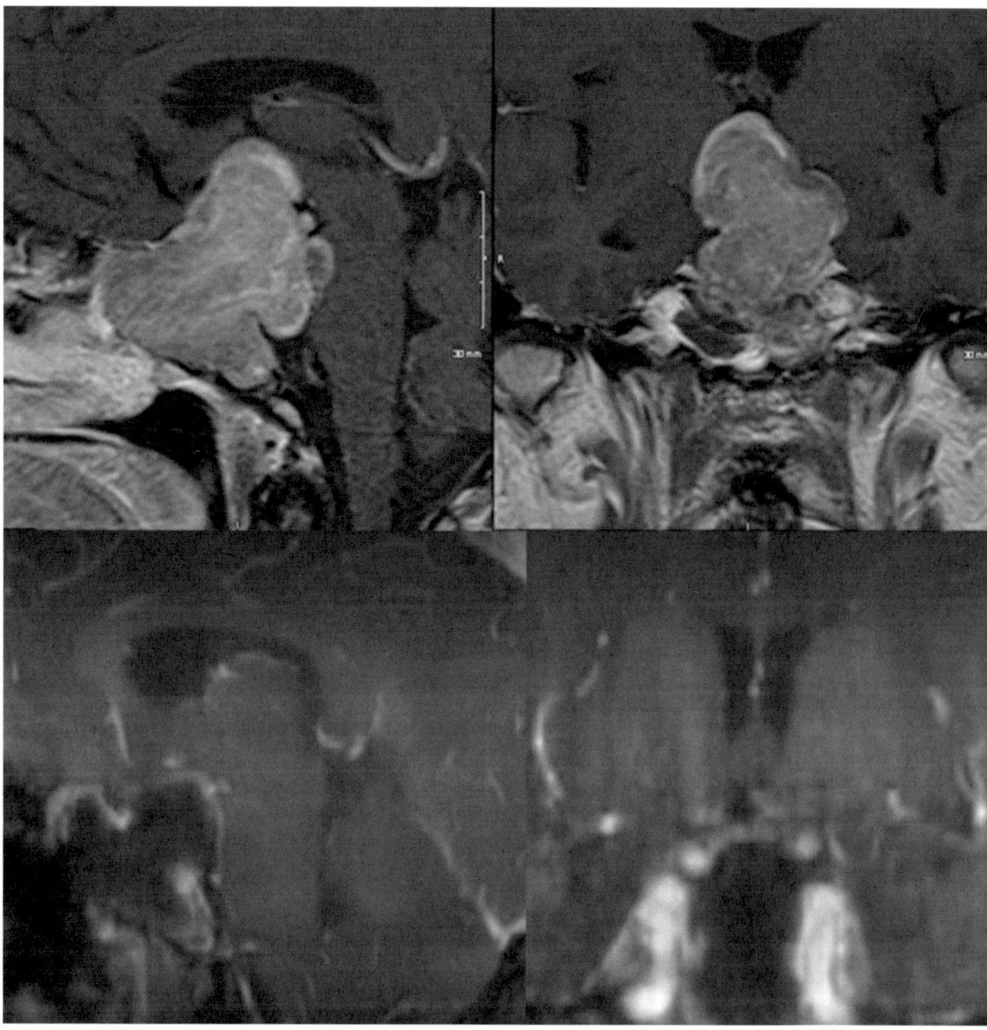

**Figure 5.** Post contrast T1-weighted sagittal and coronal preoperative (upper) and intraoperative (lower) images from a patient with a giant pituitary macroadenoma.

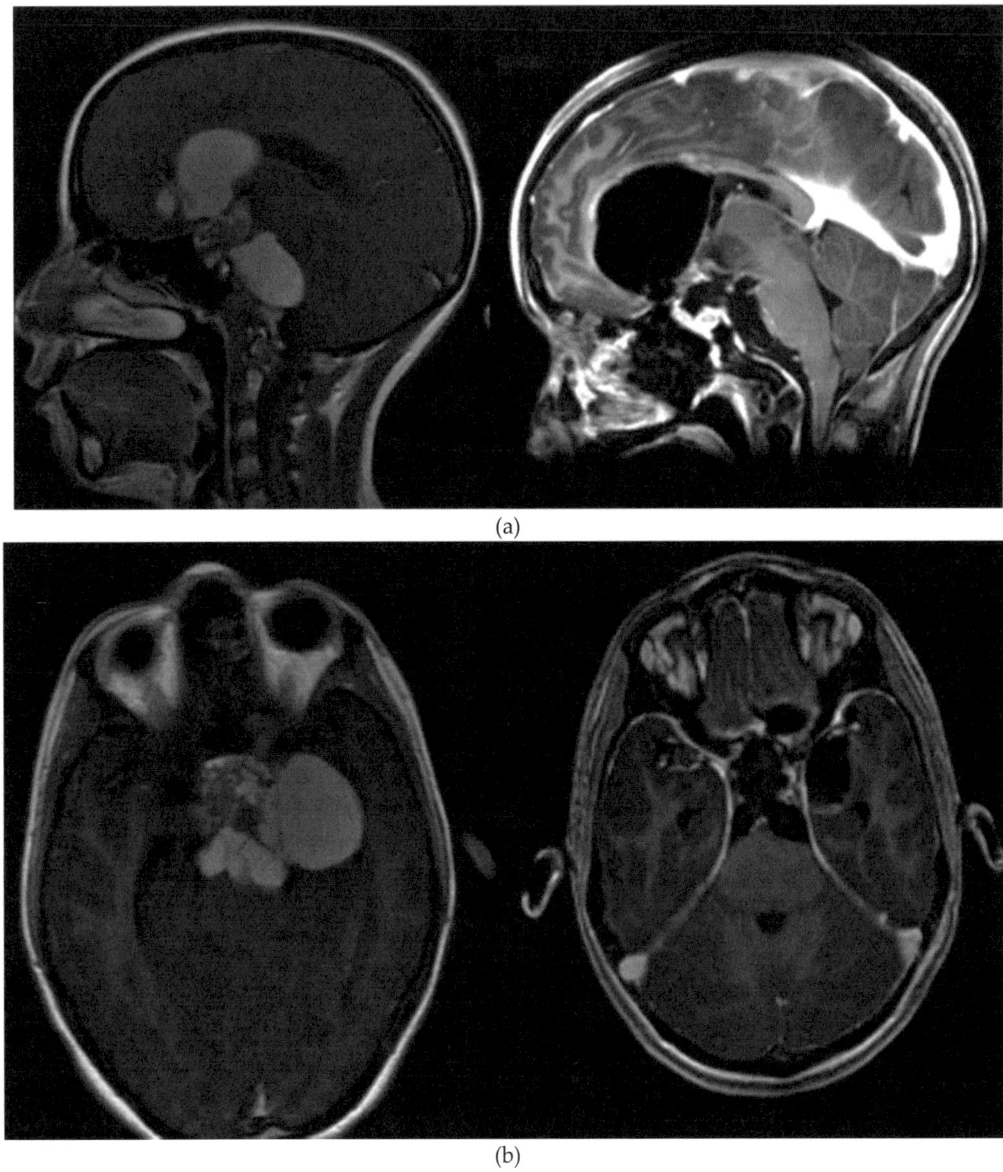

**Figure 6.** Post contrast T1-weighted preoperative and intraoperative Sagittal (a.) and axial (b.) images in 12 year old female with giant polycystic Craniopharyngioma with 2 cm enhancing nodule. iMRI was helpful in determining complete removal of enhancing nodule and drainage of all major cyst compartments following endoscopic midline approach from posterior ethmoids to clivus, working above and below pituitary gland, air visualized on intraoperative images was irrigated out of ventricles prior to closure.

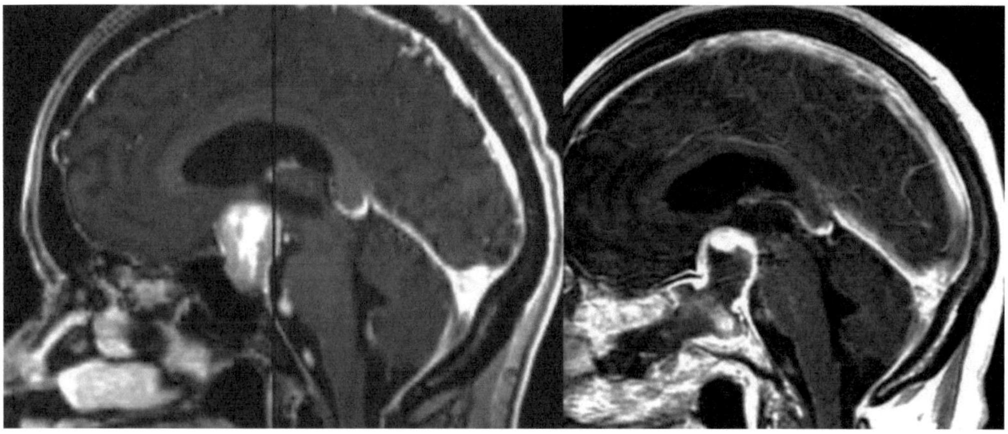

**Figure 7.** Post contrast sagittal preoperative and intraoperative sagittal MRI scans for a 76 year old female with a large pituitary macroadenoma, tumor capsule failed to prolapse into field during resection, visual inspection following imaging showed mostly blood products with a small amount of residual tumor along the superior aspect, given the patients age and preoperative visual status it was decided that a more aggressive resection was not in the patients best interest.

## Author details

Kaveh Asadi-Moghaddam[1], Joseph C. Taylor[2] and Todd W. Vitaz[1*]

*Address all correspondence to: todd.vitaz@spectrumhealth.org

1 Department of Clinical Neurosciences Spectrum Health Medical Group, and College of Human Medicine Michigan State University, Grand Rapids, MI, USA

2 Grand Rapids Ear Nose and Throat, Grand Rapids, MI, USA

## References

[1] Kassam AB, Snyderman CH, Mintz A, Gardner P, Carrau RL. Expanded endonasal approach: the rostrocaudal axis. Part I. Crista Galli to the sella turcica. Neurosurgical Focus 2005;19(E3): 1-12.

[2] Kassam AB, Gardner P, Snyderman C, Mintz A, Carrau R. Expanded endonasal approach: fully endoscopic, completely transnasal approach to the middle third of the clivus, petrous bone, middle cranial fossa, and infratemporal fossa. Neurosurgical Focus 2005;19(E3): 1-10.

[3] Anand VK, Schwartz TH, Hiltzik DH, Kacker A. Endoscopic transphenoidal pituitary surgery with real-time intraoperative magnetic resonance imaging. American Journal of Rhinology 2006;20: 401-405.

[4] Ensenat J, de Notaris M, Sanchez M, Fernandez C, Ferrer E, Bernal-Sprekelsen M, Alobid I. Endoscopic Endonasal surgery for skull base tumours: technique and preliminary results in a consecutive case series report. Rhinology 2013;51: 37-46.

[5] Ceylan S, Koc K, Anik I. endoscopic endonasal transsphenoidal approach for pituitary adenomas invading the cavernous sinus. Journal of Neurosurgery 2010;112: 99-107.

[6] Verillaud B, Bresson D, Sauvaget E, Mandonnet E, Georges B, Kania R, Herman P. Endoscopic endonasal skull base surgery. European Annals of Otorhinolaryngology, Head and Neck Diseases 2012;129: 190-196.

[7] Komotar RJ, Starke RM, Raper DM, Anand VK, Schwartz TH. Endoscopic endonasal compared with microscopic transcranial resection of craniopharyngiomas. World Neurosurgery 2012;77(2): 329-341.

[8] Greenfield JP, Anand VK, Kacker A, Seibert MJ, Singh A, Brown SM, Schwartz TH. Endoscopic endonasal transethmoidal transcribriform transfoveal ethmoidalis approach to the anterior cranial fossa skull base. Neurosurgery 2010;66: 883-892.

[9] Visocchi M, Doglietto F, Della Pepa GM, Esposito G, La Rocca G, Di Rocca C, Maira G, Fernandez E. Endoscope-assisted microsurgical transoral approach to the anterior craniovertebral junction compressive pathologies. European Spine Journal 2011;20: 1518-1525.

[10] Abuzayed B, Tanriover N, Gazioglu N, Sanus G, Ozlen F,Biceroglu H et al. Endoscopic endonasal anatomy and approaches to the anterior skull base: a neurosurgeon's perspective. The Journal of Craniofacial Surgery 2010;21(2): 529-537.

[11] Catapano D, Sloffer C, Frank G, Pasquini E, D'Angelo V, Lanzino G. Comparison between the microscope and endoscope in direct endonasal extended transsphenoidal approach: anatomical study. Journal of Neurosurgery 2006;104: 419-425.

[12] Cavallo LM, Messina A, Esposito F, De Vivitiis O, Dal Fabbro M, De Divittiis E, Cappabianca P. Skull base reconstruction in the extended endoscopic transsphenoidal approach for suprasellar lesions. Journal of Neurosurgery 2007;107: 713-720.

[13] Patel SG, Singh B, Polluri A, Bridger PG, Cantu G, Cheesman AD, et al. Craniofacial surgery for malignant skull base tumours: report of an international collaborative study. Cancer 2003;98: 1179-1187.

[14] Ganly I, Patel SG, Singh B, Kraus DH, Bridger PG, Cantu G, et al. Craniofacial resection for malignant paranasal sinus tumours: report of an international collaborative study. Head and Neck 2005;27: 575-584.

http://dx.doi.org/10.5772/59051

[15] de Vivitiis E, Cappabianca P, Cavallo LM, Esposito F, de Divitiis O, Messina A. Extended endoscopic transsphenoidal approach for extrasellar craniopharyngiomas. Neurosurgery 2007; 61: 219-228.

[16] Frank G, Pasquini E, Doglietto F, Mazzatenta D, Sciarretta V, Farneti G, Calbucci F. The endoscopic extended transsphenoidal approach for craniopharyngiomas. Neurosurgery 2006;59: 75-83.

[17] Jane Jr JA, Kiehna E, Payne SC, Early SV, Laws Jr ER. Early outcomes of endoscopic transsphenoidal surgery for adult craniopharyngiomas. Neurosurgical Focus 2010;28: E9.

[18] Leng LZ, Greenfield JP, Souweidane MM, Anand VK, Schwartz TH. Endoscopic resection of craniopharyngiomas: analysis of outcome including extent of resection, cerebrospinal fluid leak, return to preoperative productivity, and body mass index. Neurosurgery 2012;70: 110-123.

[19] Stamm AC, Vellutin E, Harvey RJ, Nogeir Jr JF, Herman DR. Endoscopic transnasal craniotomy and the resection of Craniopharyngioma. Laryngoscope 2008;118: 1142-1148.

[20] Leng LZ, Brown S, Anand K, Schwartz TH. "Gasket-seal" watertight closure in minimal-access endoscopic cranial base surgery. Neurosurgery 2008;62: 342-342.

[21] Vitaz TW, Inkabi KE, Carruba CJ. Intraoperative MRI for transphenoidal procedures: short-term outcome for 100 consecutive cases. Clinical Neurology and Neurosurgery 2011;113: 731-735.

Chapter 10

# Techniques to Improve the Extent of Brain Tumor Resection — Awake Speech and Motor Mapping, and Intraoperative MRI

Todd W. Vitaz

Additional information is available at the end of the chapter

http://dx.doi.org/10.5772/58977

## 1. Introduction

It has long been believed by many neurosurgeons that maximizing tumor resection improved patient outcome for patients with high-grade gliomas. Over the past decade the impact of maximizing tumor resection has been clearly shown to be a favorable prognostic factor in the treatment of many types of brain tumors in clinical studies [1-11]. This holds true not only for GBM and other high-grade gliomas but also for lower grade lesions as well [11-13]. In addition, complete tumor resection has also been long known to be potentially curative for many "benign" intracranial lesions such as meningiomas and pituitary tumors with much higher rates of progression free survival for these types of lesions when complete resection has been performed [14].

Even for the most experienced surgeon visual inspection and surgical judgment are not enough to determine when complete resection has been obtained [3,15,16]. Too little resection increases the chances for earlier recurrence and disease progression and overly aggressive resection leads to an increased risk of potential neurological and cognitive deficits. As a result of this many technological advances have been developed to try to assist the surgeon with determining when complete resection has been obtained. These developments included intraoperative ultrasound, frame based and frameless navigation systems, intraoperative MRI, and intraoperative fluorescence with 5-aminolevulinic acid (5-ALA).

In addition, the utilization of awake mapping procedures also allows surgeons to maximize tumor resection by enabling them to monitor the patient's neurological status (motor or speech) throughout a resection. This real-time feedback enables surgeons to maximize tumor resection in lesions near eloquent cortex while minimizing the development of neurological deficits [17].

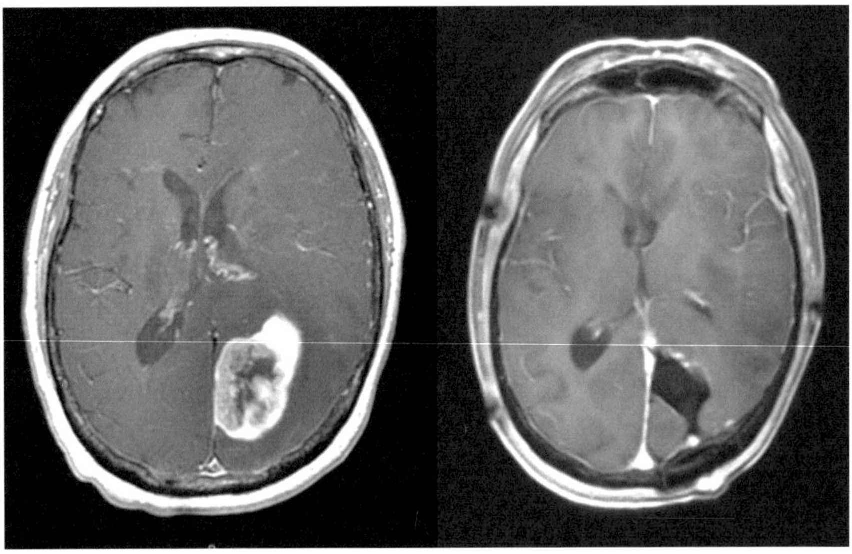

**Figure 1.** T1 Weighted post contrast preoperative and intraoperative MRI scans illustrating complete resection of a left parietal GBM

## 2. Literature review of positive prognostic effect for extent of resection (EOR)

One of the original studies to clearly show a survival advantage for extent of resection was a large retrospective endeavor by LaCroix and the MD Anderson Group [1]. They showed a survival advantage for extent of resection greater than 90% and an even greater advantage when resection was over 97%. A 2012 review by Sanai found five studies which used volumetric imaging to compare pre and postoperative MRIs for the EOR of contrast enhancement for patients undergoing surgical treatment of primary GBM. Three of these studies showed a survival advantage of between 2-8 months for patients undergoing complete resections compared to subtotal resections [18]. He also found that seventeen out of twenty eight nonvolumetric studies also found a survival advantage for extent of resection on univariate analysis [18]. Fourteen of these twenty eight studies also performed multivariate analysis to attempt to control for patient age, KPS and other factors. All fourteen of these papers found extent of resection to be a positive prognostic factor using this type of analysis [18].

In 2011 Sanai et al. [2] published a retrospective review evaluating extent of resection from a retrospective series of 500 consecutive newly diagnosed GBM patients treated at the University of California San Francisco Brain Tumor Center. Not only did they find a survival advantage based on extent of resection; but they also showed that a resection threshold greater than 78% was associated with a significant survival advantage. Although this study was retrospective in nature, the large patient volume adds significantly to its importance and illustrates that even in cases where complete resection may not be deemed safe that a significant debulking of greater than 78% likely conveys a survival advantage versus less aggressive resections [2].

Finally Marko et al. [19] recently published another retrospective review of 721 primary GBM patients treated at MD Anderson. They used an Accelerated Failure Time computer modeling system to evaluate the effects of various parameters on patient outcome. They once again showed a significant survival advantage for patients based on extent of resection. Unlike previous studies they felt that there was an advantage across all levels compared to biopsy alone and therefore felt that surgery should not be withheld based on preoperative assumptions of only obtaining a subtotal resection. In addition, they also showed the strength of such systems in reliably modelling outcome based on numerous patient and treatment parameters and suggest possible uses for this system in determining personalized outcome models as well as more appropriately stratifying patients for future clinical studies [19].

## 3. Elderly patients with GBM

At many institutions older patients with GBMs are not treated as aggressively as their younger counterparts. Part of this problem is associated with higher rates of medical comorbidities which may make more aggressive surgical interventions riskier. However, another bias is the belief that elderly patients will not tolerate more aggressive procedures and subsequent adjuvant treatments. Osvald et al. [20] performed a retrospective review of a large prospectively collected database to evaluate the impact of patient age on treatment. They found that 72% of patients younger than 65 were treated with resection vs. 55% of the older patients ($p<0.001$). Elderly patients had lower KPS and significantly more medical comorbidities. However, of the patients undergoing resection there was no statistical difference in the percent that had gross total resection when the two groups were compared. Elderly patients had a significantly decreased overall survival (9.1 months vs. 14.9 months), but subgroup analysis of patients undergoing resection showed no difference in overall survival based on age (13.0 months for elderly vs. 13.3 months in younger patients) [20].

Grossman et al. [21] evaluated the effect of age on a group of patients undergoing awake craniotomy for high-grade gliomas. They found perioperative morbidity (3.3% vs 0.59%) as well as length of stay (6.6 vs 4.9 days) higher in the elderly group (age >65 years). The EOR was not significantly different between the two groups (77.25 vs 81.9%).

## 4. Recurrent GBM

The value of extent of resection for patients with recurrent GBM is even more difficult to determine. Part of the issue in evaluating these patients is secondary to the bias created in evaluating patients who are candidates for surgery, as less than 30% of patients are typically deemed candidates for additional surgery. Factors in determining surgical eligibility include patient performance, tolerance to previous treatments, patient wishes, and tumor factors such as timing, size and location of recurrence [2,22-26].

Subgroup analysis of the Lacroix [1] paper showed a survival advantage for patients with recurrent GBM who had maximal tumor resection at time of recurrence. In addition Bloch et al. [7] evaluated the importance of extent of resection at the time of repeat surgery on a group of 107 patients who underwent multiple resections at USCF. They found that if patients had gross total resection at time of initial surgery than the extent of resection at recurrence did not affect outcome; however, in patients who had subtotal resections at time of initial surgery than the extent of resection at time of recurrence did impact overall survival. In addition, they found that in patients who had an initial subtotal resection had a complete resection at recurrence than there was no difference between them and patients who had complete resection initially and were candidates for additional surgery regardless of extent of resection [7].

Oppenlander et al. [22] published results of 170 patients who were treated with recurrent GBM at Barrow Neurological Institute. They found a distinct survival advantage based on an extent of resection of 80% or greater in these patients. The median interval between initial and subsequent surgery was 8.6 months (range 1.1-93.1 months) [22]. While these data do once again show level 3 data of a survival advantage for these patients it is important to approach this subgroup of patients with great care. First of all, early recurrence (less than 4-6 months) should be approached with great hesitancy. Many of these patients harbor "treatment effect" or pseudo-progression which can be managed medically in most of these patients. Secondly patients who have true progression in this very short time frame often have very aggressive tumor subtypes and are likely to progress despite further surgical interventions. My personal practice is to typically withhold additional cytoreductive surgery in patients who have disease progression prior to 6 months unless surgery is planned as a salvage intervention for symptom management in an otherwise healthy individual, for tissue diagnosis, or to obtain tissue for enrollment in a clinical trial. Finally, the incidence of wound healing and neurological complications is much higher in this patient population. The Barrow group [22] reported preoperative motor and language deficits in 33 and 31% respectively. Additionally they found new or worsened deficits in 19% and 13% postoperatively at one week which only decreased to 15% and 9% at one month [22]. These lesions are not curable and thus patient quality of life is of paramount importance. Every effort should be made to minimize neurological worsening in this patient population and thus judicious evaluation should be performed when determining who is a candidate for additional cytoreductive surgery.

http://dx.doi.org/10.5772/58977

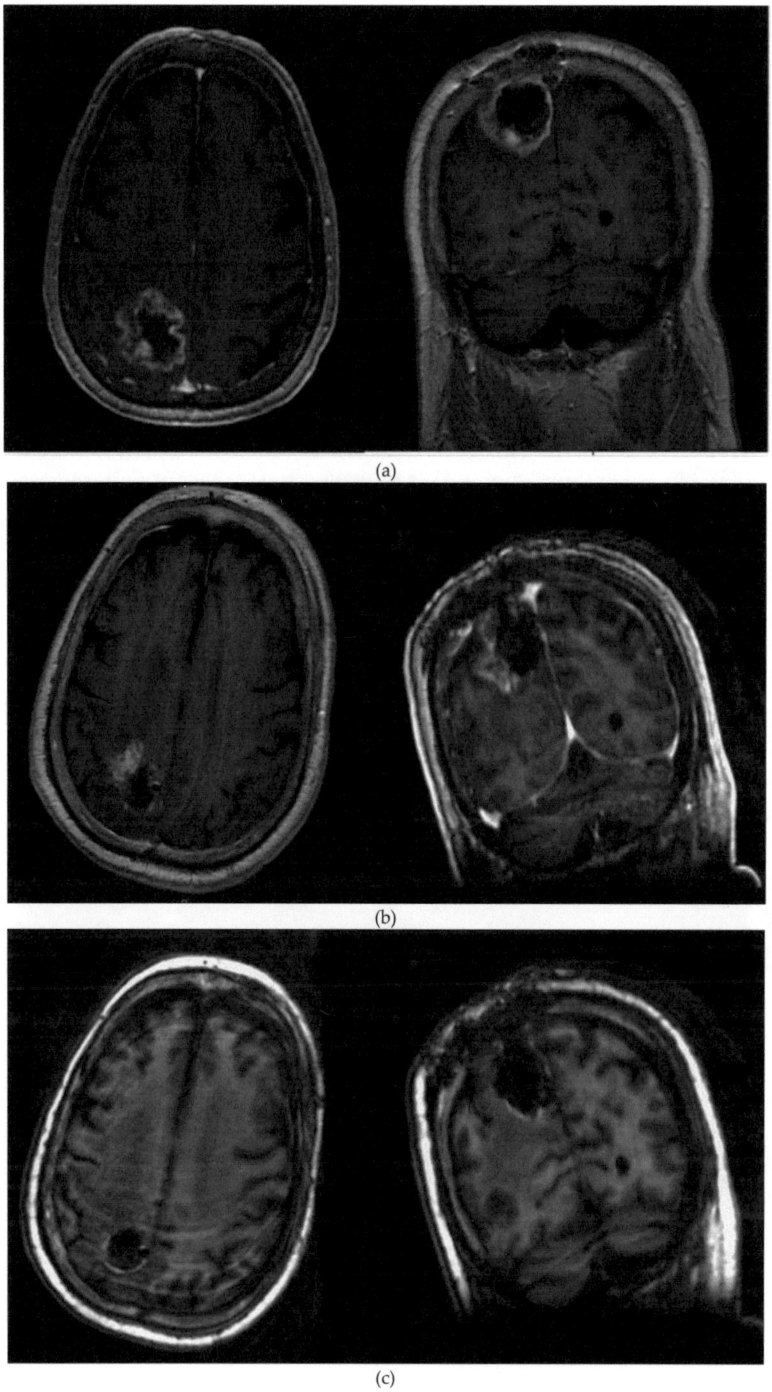


**Figure 2.** Post contrast axial and coronal T1-weighted images of recurrent GBM, A. Preoperative; B. First intraoperative (showing residual tumor along the lateral wall); C. Second intraoperative MRI scans

## 5. Low grade gliomas

Once again in Sanai's 2012 review [18] he found three papers which evaluated EOR for low grade gliomas using volumetric analysis and all three of these showed a significant increase in 5 year survival. He also reviewed eight nonvolumetric studies and once again found an advantage in five year survival in 7 of these 8 studies. Five year survival was shown to increase from 50-70% in cases with subtotal resection to 80-95% in total resections.

Several recent studies have also shown that increasing the extent of resection in low grade gliomas may also decrease the rate of malignant transformation in these tumors. Typically only pilocytic gliomas and other infrequent subtypes such as Ganglioglioma can be cured with complete surgical resection. For the remainder of these lesions recurrence and often progression to a higher grade lesion is the norm. Smith et al. [11] in their review of 216 low grade lesions found that increased EOR was associated with increased malignant progression free survival (MPFS). However, Snyder et al [12] reviewed the impact of EOR on overall survival and MPFS in 93 pure grade II oligodendrogliomas treated at their institution. They found that an increased EOR was associated with an improved OS but did not influence the rate or timing of progression in these patients as MPFS was not influenced by EOR [12].

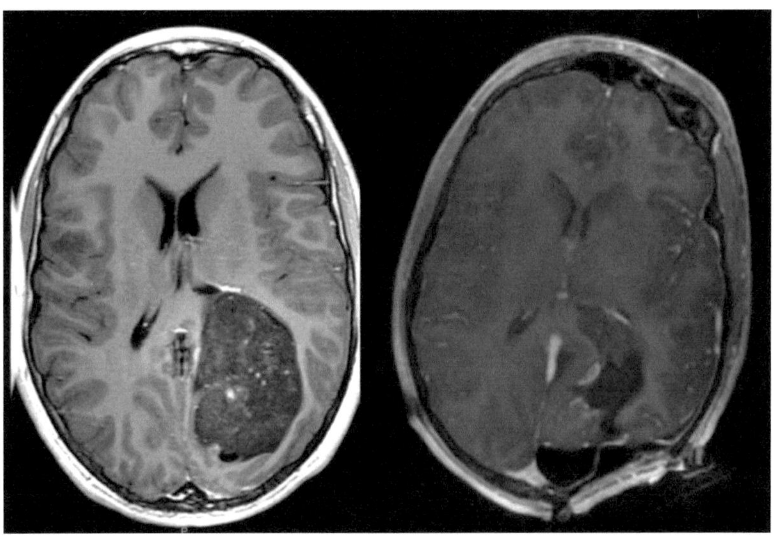

**Figure 3.** Axial T1-weighted preoperative and intraoperative scans showing low-grade non-enhancing tumor with residual tumor positioned next to atrium on intraoperative scan, that was subsequently resected.

## 6. Methods to increase extent of resection

Despite the growing body of evidence leaning towards significant survival advantage in both low and high grade gliomas, complete resection is often only obtained between 17-47% of cases

[1,27-33]. Numerous intraoperative adjuncts have been trialed to help increase the EOR in these procedures. Intraoperative frameless navigation is a mainstay in most North American Brain Tumor Centers. This technology which is based on a preoperatively obtained imaging set has been shown to be ineffective in increasing the EOR in a prospective randomized trial [34]. Upon opening the dura and proceeding with CSF drainage and tumor resection considerable brain shift can occur which makes the information obtained from preoperative datasets inaccurate (figure 4)[35].

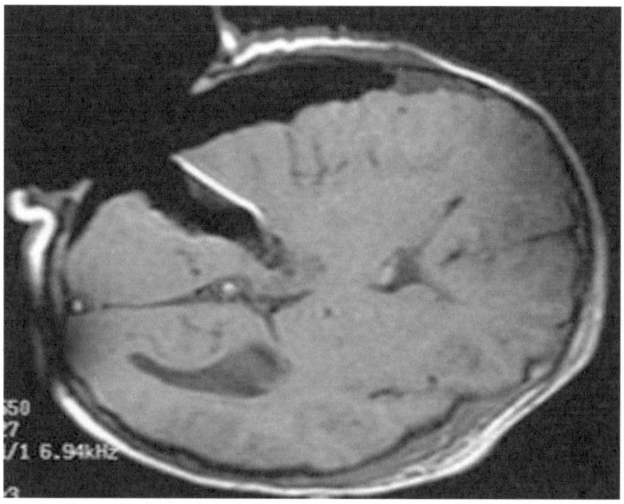

**Figure 4.** Axial T1 weighted intraoperative MRI scan illustrating the extreme degree of brain shift that can occur with opening the dura, drainage of CSF and tumor resection.

Orringer et al. [27] evaluated patient and tumor characteristics that might effect EOR in GBM patients. Interestingly they found that based on postoperative MRI scans complete resection was obtained in only 17% of cases despite the surgeon's belief that GTR had been obtained based on intraoperative assessments. They also found that larger tumors, lesions touching the ventricles and lesions in or near eloquent cortex were associated with lower extent of resection [27]. Of the 17 cases where complete resection was felt to be possible based on blinded review of two experienced surgeons this was only obtained in four patients (23%)[27]. This study clearly shows that the surgeon's impression alone is not enough to maximize tumor resections for these patients.

### 6.1. Ultrasound

Ultrasound was introduced as a surgical tool in the 1960s. This technology which typically utilized low frequencies was extremely limited secondary to poor image resolution and cumbersome intraoperative probes. The sensitivity and specificity of findings was limited especially for highlighting small tumor remnants or differentiating tumor from edematous brain. In addition, it was even more difficult to differentiate tumor from surrounding normal brain in low grade gliomas [36,37]. However, newer developments in ultrasound technology; with the use of higher frequency devices, has created a recent resurgence in this technology. New smaller light-weight probes can be placed within a resection cavity and give a much better spatial resolution of surrounding areas. The use of higher frequencies improves image resolution however this has a tradeoff of lower tissue penetration [38]. Serra et al. [38] performed a retrospective review of 22 patients with high grade lesions (mixed pathology) who they felt to be good candidates for gross total resection based on preoperative imaging findings. High frequency intraoperative ultrasound was used for all patients. They found that 21 of the 22 patients had gross total resection of the enhancing lesion on postoperative imaging; however, as the study was retrospective they were unable to determine how many patients underwent additional imaging based on ultrasound findings.

### 6.2. Fluorescence guided resections

5-aminolevulinic acid (5-ALA) is an orally administered pro-drug which is metabolized intracellularly to protoporphyrin IX which gives off a red-violet fluorescent signal to blue light. This agent preferentially accumulates in certain tumor types and thus can be used to help differentiate tumor from normal surrounding brain tissue [39]. The oral agent is administered 3 hours prior to surgery and then the operative field can be intermittently interrogated for evidence of fluorescence throughout the procedure by switching back and forth between white and blue light on the operative microscope.

Several prospective studies have been performed evaluating the benefits of 5-ALA in patients undergoing surgical resection of high-grade gliomas [39]. Stummer et al [40] performed a phase IIIa prospective study evaluating the impact of this technology on patients with high-grade gliomas. The study was terminated early because interim analysis showed a significant benefit in the study arm. Gross total resection was seen in 65% of patients in the 5-ALA arm vs. 36% in the control group [40]. The utility of this technology only seems beneficial in patients with high-grade lesions as significant accumulation has not been shown to occur in low grade gliomas [41,42].

### 6.3. Intraoperative MRI

Intraoperative MRI (iMRI) was first used in Boston in the mid 1990's. Since then numerous revisions and variations of the technology have been performed. While significant expansion in the number of centers with this technology has occurred in the past decade, cost is still the limiting factor. The current technology can be divided into two categories based on magnet strength. Low field systems such as the original 0.5 Tesla GE Signa SP (GE Medical Systems, Milwaukee, WI) the 0.12 Tesla Odin Polestar table mounted system (Odin Technologies, Yokneam, Israel); versus high-field systems which consist of 1.5 or 3.0 Tesla magnets. The high-field systems all require cessation of the surgical procedure for imaging. Two subgroups exist in this category. One in which the magnet is moved from a storage facility into the operating theater via an overhead crane system (IMRIS Inc., Winnipeg Canada) and the other in which the patient is moved from the operating theater into an adjacent ferrous free imaging zone (figure 5). This use of this technology allows for intraoperative imaging for evaluation and confirmation of the anticipated surgical results. In addition, it also allows for intraoperative updating of the navigation system to offset the changes that result from tumor resection and brain shift. Each system has its own advantages and tradeoffs in terms of cost, ease of use and image resolution [43].

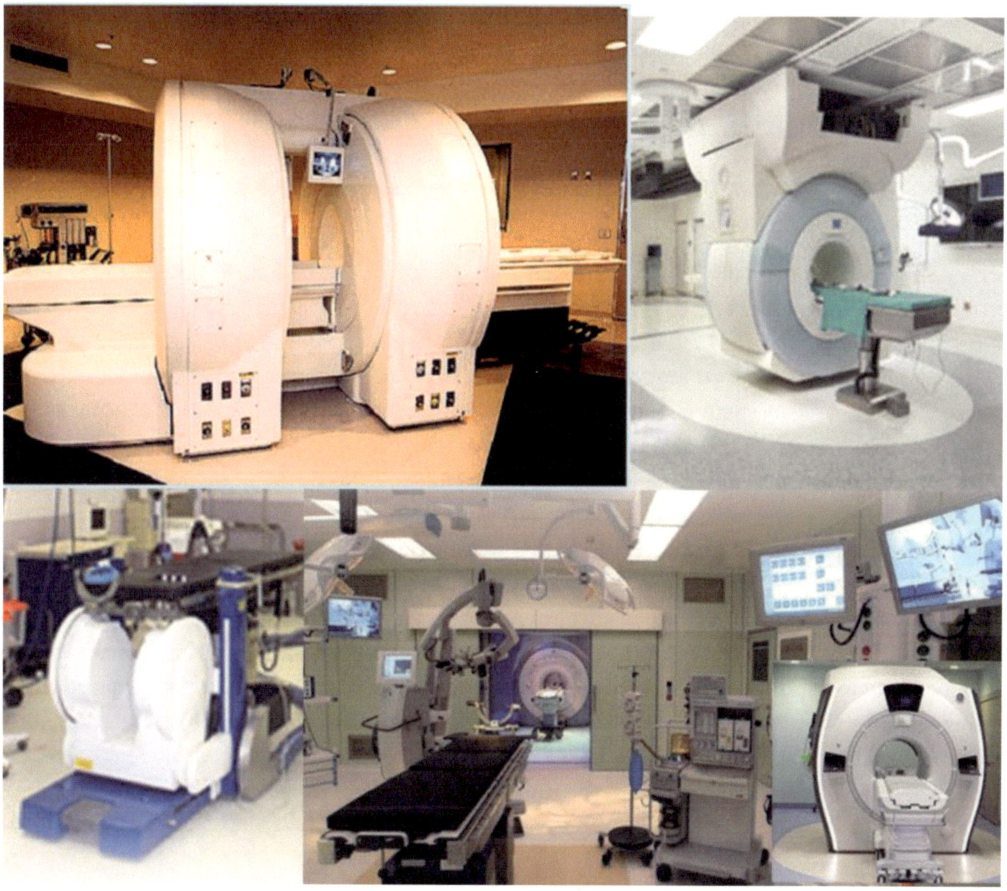

**Figure 5.** Various Intraoperative MRI concepts (clockwise from top left: GE Signa SP double doughnut, IMRIS mobile ceiling mounted system (scanner moves to patient), GE hybrid OR concept (inset shows close up of scanner; patient moves to scanner), Odin table mounted system.

I [44] previously reviewed the results for treatment of GBM using the older GE Signa SP system at Norton Healthcare (Louisville, KY) and found that additional surgical resection was performed in 71.4% of cases based on intraoperative imaging results. The average EOR in this patient group was 93.7% and was limited secondary to tumor location and vascular anatomy in cases where EOR was less than 95%. Numerous other authors have shown the value of such systems in increasing EOR [15,16,45-50].

Senft [6] performed a randomized controlled study looking at the utility of iMRI for treatment of gliomas. All patients were felt to be candidates for complete resection based on preoperative imaging findings. Patients were randomized to undergo surgery with conventional microsurgical techniques vs iMRI using the Odin Polestar system. In the study group the use of iMRI led to additional tumor resection in 33% of patients with 96% of patients in the iMRI group obtaining complete resection vs 68% in the control arm. Six month progression free survival was 67% in the iMRI group compared to 36% in the control arm ($p<0.05$).

Roder et al. [51] compared a group of 117 patients treated with iMRI (IMRIS Visius System) vs. a control arm treated with microsurgical techniques plus 5-ALA in some patients. 5-ALA was used in 70% of iMRI patients and 60% of patients in the control arm. Complete tumor resection was seen in 74% of the iMRI group vs 34% for the conventional group. Subgroup analysis of the control group showed that complete resection in the conventional group increased to 45% and mean residual volume decreased for patients who had 5-ALA fluorescence as part of their procedure.

These studies all show a significant advantage for the use of this technology not only for high-grade gliomas as outlined above but also for low-grade gliomas and pituitary tumors [16,43,52-54]. However, despite the use of this technology complete resection is sometimes still not possible. This can be secondary to tumor location in or near eloquent cortex, tumor adjacent to the ventricle or tumor extending into deep or midline structures or associated around major vascular structures[27,35,55,56]. Image interpretation during intraoperative procedures can also lead to its own challenges. Tissue can become distorted and damaged secondary to surgical trauma. This can lead to a disruption of the blood-brain barrier and thus increased contrast enhancement. In addition, blood products and air in the surgical cavity can also distort the imaging findings [35,43,44]. Finally the administration of contrast agents for preoperative navigational studies the morning of surgery can also affect intraoperative imaging results. As a result of these issues we routinely review all intraoperative imaging scans alongside an experienced neuroradiologist in the iMRI control room during all procedures. Intraoperative scans are directly compared to preoperative studies and when necessary any areas of questionable residual tumor are directly investigated after the new dataset is downloaded to the navigation system. Careful review of the imaging findings are necessary as overly aggressive resections can lead to increased risk of new neurological deficits.

## 7. Awake mapping techniques

Regardless of the surgical techniques used for tumor resection the goal for extensive tumor removal must always be tempered with the potential risk of inducing new or worsened neurological injuries, as the patients postoperative neurological status is strongly correlated with overall outcome. For lesions located in or near motor or speech centers intraoperative mapping via electro-cortical stimulation can effectively identify these eloquent areas.

Newer developments in preoperative imaging such as functional MRI (fMRI) and diffusion tensor imaging based fiber tracking (DTI-FT) can help to grossly localize the location of eloquent cortex and their corresponding deep white matter tracts; however the accuracy of exact localization is more reliably determined with intraoperative cortical and subcortical mapping techniques [57-64]. A meta-analysis of over 8000 patients who underwent craniotomy for resection of intracranial glioma showed that patients who underwent intraoperative mapping had a greater than two fold reduction in permanent neurological deficits [65].

Motor mapping can be performed either with the patient awake or under general anesthesia (without muscle paralysis) while speech mapping requires the use of an awake anesthesia technique at least during the mapping portion. Remifentanil and propofol or dexmetomidate infusions are often used for these procedures as they have very short half-lives [17,55]. The use of longer acting narcotics should be minimized as patients can become agitated and uncooperative with the over use of sedatives or narcotics. In addition an extensive local field block of all regional nerves with a combination of a short and long-acting local anesthetic also helps significantly with patient comfort and cooperation [17]. Patient selection is of paramount importance as patients with severe edema, or significant pulmonary or airway issues may not tolerate such a procedure. Time should be taken with the patient preoperatively to address and concerns and thus minimize anxiety as well as to prepare the patient for their involvement for the procedure. Complete details regarding the anesthesia for this technique are available elsewhere [17,55]. I prefer to conduct all of my mapping procedures with an awake technique regardless of whether speech function is being interrogated as having the ability to converse with the patient and readily assess their neurological function is as important as localizing the area of eloquent cortex. I have my anesthesiologist or operating room nurse regularly assess the patients motor function throughout tumor resection, if speech cortex is involved we routinely employ the assistance of a trained speech and language therapist who also assists the patient in carrying on a conversation during tumor resection after mapping and stimulation have been completed.

Mapping is routinely performed using a bipolar stimulation probe with 5 mm spacing between the electrodes. Stimulation is performed at increasing amplitudes until a positive result in encountered or after discharges are seen on electrocorticography or a upper threshold limit is reached. The use of surface EEG is of great importance as it can minimize the risk of generalized seizure activity induced by the stimulation and can verify that the stimulation system in functioning adequately. A constant current generator is used to provide square biphasic wave pulses for 1-4 seconds at 60Hz frequency (figure 6) [17,55,66]. Unlike epilepsy surgery where positive stimulation results are almost always obtained the growing trend among tumor surgeons is to perform smaller more tailored craniotomies for these cases. In these instances negative stimulation results (with appropriate artifact on surface recordings) can be interpreted as absence of eloquent tissue [18]. Most authors recommend keeping a border of at least 0.8-1.0 cm of tissue between resection site and any site showing positive stimulation results [17,18,55,66].

Subcortical stimulation can be performed using the same equipment and settings. The surgeon must frequently alternate between deep white matter tract stimulation and tumor resection. Resection is continued until either positive stimulation results are obtained or complete tumor resection has been achieved. Higher rates of postoperative neurological deficits have been shown in cases where positive motor stimulation is obtained during subcortical mapping, likely secondary to manipulation in close proximity of these pathways [55,67].

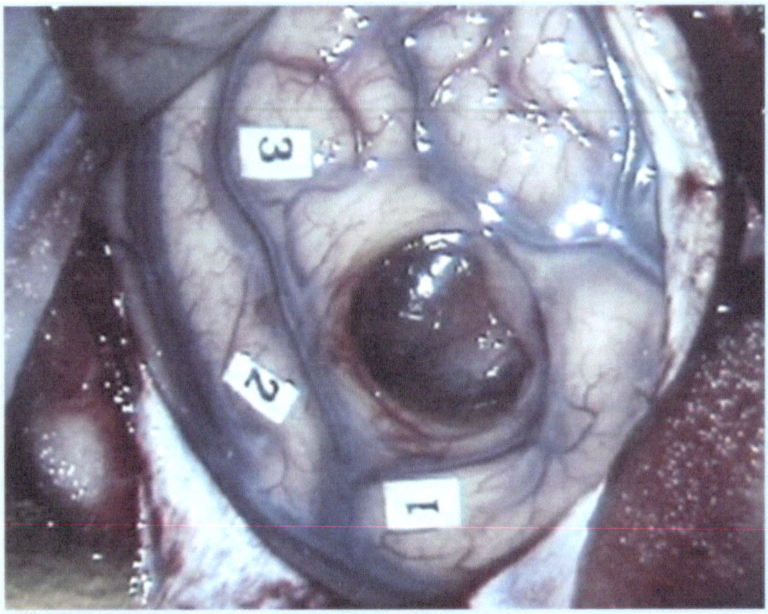

**Figure 6.** Picture of intraoperative mapping case; #1 corresponds to area of lower extremity stimulation, #2 hand stimulation, #3 face stimulation, lesion is seen just anterior to #2 on surface of the brain.

In appropriately selected patients awake mapping procedures can be performed safely with minimal patient anxiety or discomfort. The information obtained from mapping and intraoperative neurological assessment allows the surgeon to make a well informed decision regarding the safety of continued resection vs. the risk of inducing new neurological deficits (figure 7).

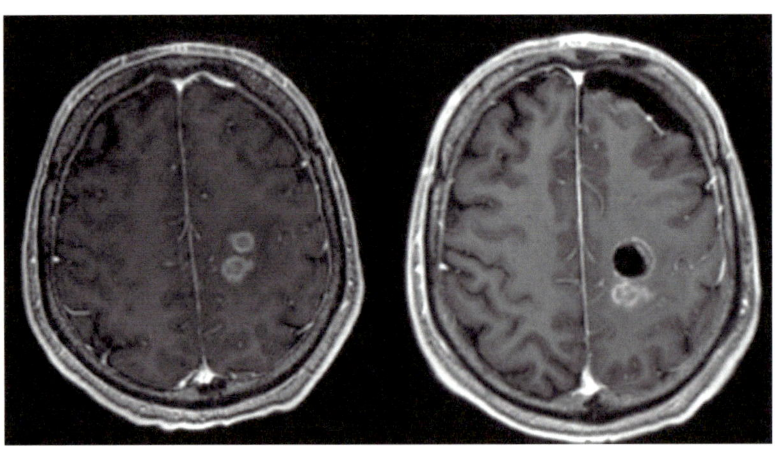

**Figure 7.** Preoperative and intraoperative axial T1-weighted post contrast scans; subcortical stimulation was positive along the lateral and posterior border of the resection cavity thus a portion of the tumor was not resected.

## 8. Conclusion: Combining technologies to obtain maximal safest results

I and several other authors have had experience combining several of these advanced technologies together for the treatment of high risk patients undergoing treatment of intracranial gliomas [44,45,56,68]. Select patients with lesions near or in eloquent cortex can undergo awake mapping procedures with frequent neurological assessment to ensure the absence of generating new neurological deficits. Intraoperative imaging can be performed once maximal tumor resection has been performed to verify that the anticipated results have been obtained (figure 8). If significant residual tumors remains than the surgeon can immediately determine whether further resection is deemed safe and continue with additional tumor removal while constantly assessing the patients function or evaluating subcortical stimulation results. In cases where the patient may be sedated but not intubated than transport of the patient into the scanner does carry additional risks as the anesthesiologist has even more limited access to the patient and their airway during imaging; however, I am unaware of any serious complications as a result of performing iMRI on a mildly sedated non-intubated patient.

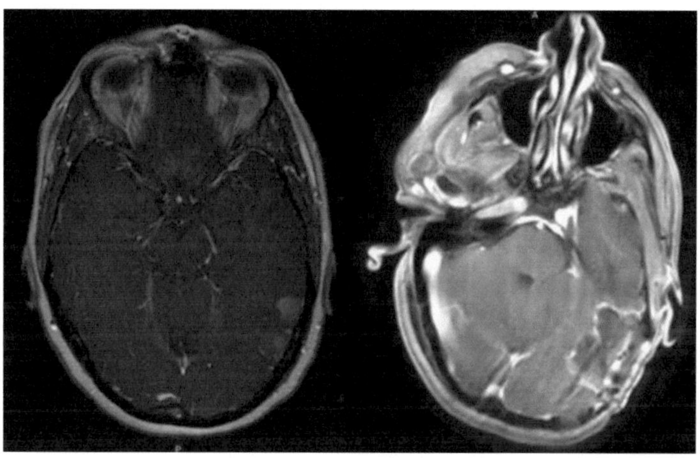

**Figure 8.** Preoperative and intraoperative axial T1-weighted post contrast images showing complete resection of a posterior left temporal lesion that was removed using an awake mapping technique in the intraoperative MRI.

One of the main drawbacks of the current high-field iMRI systems is the time required for patient transport and scanning. For a majority of our cases we conduct only a single intraoperative scan, typically if any residual tumor exists than further resection is performed based off of updated neuronavigation results. In a minority of cases, typically those with large volumes of residual tumor on the first scan, than a second confirmatory scan is performed. The use of 5-ALA plus iMRI in patients with high-grade gliomas can further decrease the need for additional scans. By maximizing the EOR based on the intraoperative fluorescence findings, there is a higher likelihood of satisfactory results on the first scan, thus eliminating the need for subsequent imaging. Any small or deep areas of residual tumor not appreciated with 5-ALA can be seen on the iMRI images and resected with updated neuronavigation [51].

## Author details

Todd W. Vitaz*

Address all correspondence to: todd.vitaz@spectrumhealth.org

Department of Clinical Neurosciences Spectrum Health Medical Group, and College of Human Medicine, Michigan State University, Grand Rapids, Michigan, USA

## References

[1] Lacroix M, Abi-Said D, Fourney DR, Gokaslan ZL, Shi W, DeMonte F, et al. A multivariate analysis of 416 patients with glioblastoma multiforme: prognosis, extent of resection, and survival. Journal of Neurosurgery 2001;95: 190-198.

[2] Sanai, N, Mei-Yin P, McDermott MW, Parsa AT, Berger MS. An extent of resection threshold for newly diagnosed glioblastomas. Journal of Neurosurgery 2011;115: 3-8.

[3] Senft C, Franz K, Blasel S, Osvald A, Rather J, Seifert V, Gasser T. Influence of iMRI-guidance on the extent of resection and survival of patients with glioblastoma multiforme. Technology in Cancer Research and Treatment 2010;9: 339-346.

[4] Hassaneen W, Levine NB, Suki D, Salaskar AL, de Moura Lima, McCutcheon IE, et al. Multiple craniotomies in the management of multifocal and multicentric glioblastoma. Journal of Neurosurgery 2011;114: 576-584.

[5] De Bonis P, Anile C, Pompucci A, Fiorentino A, Balducci M, Chiesa S, et al. The influence of surgery on recurrence pattern of glioblastoma. Clinical Neurology and Neurosurgery 2013;115: 37-43.

[6] Senft C, Bink A, Franz K, Vatter H, Gasser T, Seifert V. Intraoperative MRI guidance and extent of resection in glioma surgery: a randomized, controlled trial. The Lancet Oncology 2011;12: 997-1003.

[7] Bloch O, Han SJ, Cha S, Sun M, Aghi MK, McDermott MW et al. Impact of extent of resection for recurrent glioblastoma on overall survival. Journal of Neurosurgery 2012;117: 1032-1038.

[8] McGirt MJ, Chaichana KL, Gathinji M, Attenello FJ, Than K, Olivi A et al. Independent association of extent of resection with survival in patients with malignant brain astrocytoma. Journal of Neurosurgery 2009;110: 156-162.

[9] Laws ER, Parney IF, Huang W, Anderson F, Morris AM, Asher A, et al. Survival following surgery and prognostic factors for recently diagnosed malignant glioma: data from the glioma outcomes project. Journal Neurosurgery 2003;99: 467-473.

[10] Murkami R, Hirai T, Nakamura H, Furusawa M, Nakaguchi Y, Uetani H, et al. Recurrence patterns of glioblastoma treated with postoperative radiation therapy: relationship between extent of resection and progression-free survival. Japanese Journal of Radiology 2012;30: 193-197.

[11] Smith JS, Chang EF, Lamborn KR, Chang SM, Prados MD, Cha S, et al. Role of extent of resection in the long-term outcome of low-grade hemispheric gliomas. Journal of Clinical Oncology 2008;26:1338-1345.

[12] Snyder LA, Wolf AB, Oppenlander ME, Bina R, Wilson JR, Ashby L, et al. The impact of extent of resection on malignant transformation of pure oligodendrogliomas. Journal of Neurosurgery 2014;120: 309-314.

[13] Yordanova YN, Moritz-Gasser S, Duffau H. Awake surgery for WHO grade II gliomas within "noneloquent" areas in the left dominant hemisphere: toward a "supratotal" resection. Journal of Neurosurgery 2011;115:232-239.

[14] Bumrungrachpukdee P, Pruphetkaew N, Phukaoloun M, Pheunpathom N. Recurrence of intracranial meningioma after surgery: analysis of influencing factors and outcome. Journal of the Medical Association of Thailand 2014;97(4): 399-406.

[15] Schneider JP, Trantakis C, Rubach M, Schulz T, Dietrich J, Winkler D, et al. Intraoperative MRI to guide the resection of primary supratentorial glioblastoma multiforme-a quantitative radiological analysis. Neuroradiology 2005;47: 489-500.

[16] Bohinski RJ, Kokkino AK, Warnick RE, Gaskill-Shipley MF, Kormos DW, Lukin RR, et al. Glioma resection in a shared resource magnetic resonance operating room after optimal image guided frameless stereotactic resection. Neurosurgery 2001;48: 731-742.

[17] Vitaz TW, Marx W, Victor JD, Gutin PH. Comparison of conscious sedation and general anesthesia for motor mapping and resection of tumors located near motor cortex. Neurosurgical Focus 2003;15: article 8.

[18] Sanai N. Emerging operative strategies in neurosurgical oncology. Current Opinion in Neurology 2012;25: 756-766.

[19] Marko NF, Weil RJ, Schroeder JL, Lang FF, Suki D, Sawaya RE. Extent of resection of glioblastoma revisited: personalized survival modeling facilitates more accurate survival prediction and supports a maximum-safe-resection approach to surgery. Journal of Clinical Oncology 2014;32: 774-782.

[20] Osvald A, Guresir E, Setzer M, Vatter H, Senft C, Seifert V, Franz K. Glioblastoma therapy in the elderly and the importance of the extent of resection regardless of age. Journal Neurosurgery 2012;116:357-364.

[21] Grossman R, Nossek E, Sitt R, Hayat D, Shahar T, Barzilai O, et al. Outcome of elderly patients undergoing awake-craniotomy for tumor resection. Annals of Surgical Oncology 2013;20: 1722-1728.

[22] Oppenlander ME, Wolf AB, Snyder LA, Bina R, Wilson JR, Coons SW, et al. An extent of resection threshold for recurrent glioblastoma and its risk for neurological morbidity. Journal of Neurosurgery 2014; 120:846-853.

[23] Barker FG, Chang SM, Gutin PH, Malec MK, McDermott MW, Prados MD, et al. Survival and functional status after resection of recurrent glioblastoma multiforme. Neurosurgery 1998;42:709-723.

[24] Chaichana KL, Zadnik P, Weingart JD, Olivi A, Gallia GL, Blakeley J, et al. Multiple resections for patients with glioblastoma: prolonging survival. Journal of Neurosurgery 2013;118: 812-820.

[25] Helseth R, Helseth E, JohannesenTB, Langberg CW,Lote K, Ronning P, et al. Overall survival, prognostic factors, and repeated surgery in a consecutive series of 516 patients with glioblastoma multiforme. Acta Neurologica Scandinavia 2010;122: 159-167.

[26] Zinn PO, Colen RR, Kasper EM, Burkhardt JK. Extent of resection and radiotherapy in GBM: a 1973 to 2007 surveillance, epidemiology and end results analysis of 21,783 patients. International Journal of Oncology 2013;42: 929-934.

[27] Orringer D, Lau D, Khatri S, Zamora-Berridi GJ, Zhang K, Wu C et al. Extent of resection in patients with glioblastoma: limiting factors, perception of resectability, and effect on survival. Journal Neurosurgery 2012;117: 851-859.

[28] Chen X, Xu BN, Meng X, Zhang J, Yu X, Zhou D. Dual-room 1.5T intraoperative magnetic resonance imaging suite with a movable magnet: implementation and preliminary experience. Neurosurgical Review 2012;35: 95-109.

[29] Senft C, Seifert V, Hermann E, Franz K, Gasser T. Usefulness of intraoperative ultra-low-field magnetic resonance imaging in glioma surgery. Neurosurgery 2008;63: 257.

[30] Kuhnt D, Becker A, Ganslandt O, Bauer M, Buchfelder M, Nimsky C. Correlation of the extent of tumor volume resection and patient survival in surgery of glioblastoma multiforme with high-field intraoperative MRI guidance. Neuro Oncology 2011;13: 1339-1348.

[31] Chicoine MR, Lim CC, Evans JA, Singla A, Zipfel GJ, Rich KM, et al. Implementation and preliminary clinical experience with the use of ceiling mounted mobile high-field intraoperative magnetic resonance imaging between two operating rooms. Intraoperative Imaging. Acta Neurochirgica Supplemental 2011;109: 97-102.

[32] Nimsky C, Fujita A, Ganslandt O, Von Keller B, Fahlbusch R. Volumetric assessment of glioma removal by intraoperative high-field magnetic resonance imaging. Neurosurgery 2004;55: 358-370.

[33] Hatiboglu MA, Weinberg JS, Suki D, Rao G, Prabhu SS, Shah K, et al. Impact of intraoperative high-field magnetic resonance imaging guidance on glioma surgery: a prospective volumetric analysis. Neurosurgery 2009;64: 1073-1081.

[34] Willems PWA, Taphoorn MJB, Burger H, van der Sprenkel JWB, Tulleken CAF. Effectiveness of neuronavigation in resecting solitary intracerebral contrast-enhancing tumors: a randomized controlled trial. Journal of Neurosurgery 2006;104: 360-368.

[35] Kubben PL, terMeulen KJ, Schijns OEMG, ter Laak-Poor MP, van Ovenbeeke JJ, van Santbrink H. Intraoperative MRI-guided resection of glioblastoma multiforme: a systemic review. Lancet Oncology 2011;12:1062-1070.

[36] Erdogan N, Tucer B, Mavili E, Menkü A, Kurtsoy A. Ultrasound guidance in intracranial tumor resection: correlation with postoperative magnetic resonance findings. Acta Radiology 2005;46: 743-749.

[37] Gerganov VM, Samii A, Akbarian A, Stieglitz L, Samii M, Fahlbusch R. Reliability of intraoperative high-resolution 2D ultrasound as an alternative to high-field strength MR imaging for tumor resection control: a prospective comparative study. Journal of Neurosurgery 2009;111: 512-519

[38] Serra C, Stauffer A, Actor B, Burkhardt JK, Ulrich NH, Bernays RL, Bozinov O. Intraoperative high frequency ultrasound in intracerebral high-grade tumors. Ultrasound in Medicine 2012;33: 306-312.

[39] Tykocki T, Michalik R, Bonicki W, Nauman P. Fluorescence-guided resection of primary and recurrent malignant gliomas with 5-aminolevulinic acid. Preliminary results. Neurology and Neurosurgery Poland 2012;46: 47-51.

[40] Stummer W, Pichlmeier U, Meinel T, Wiestler OD, Zanella F, Reulen HJ, et al. Fluorescence-guided surgery with 5-aminolevulinic acid for resection of malignant glioma: a randomized controlled multicenter phase III trial. Lancet Oncology 2006;7: 392-401.

[41] Ishihara R, Katayama Y, Watanabe T, Yoshino A, Fukushima T, Sakatani K. Quantitative spectroscopic analysis of 5-aminolevulinic acid-induced protoporphyrin IX fluorescence intensity in diffusely infiltrating astrocytomas. Neurologia medicochirurgica 2007;47: 53-57.

[42] Floeth FW, Sabel M, Ewelt C, Stummer W, Felsberg J, Reifenberger G, et al. Comparison of (18)F-FET PET and 5-ALA fluorescence in cerebral gliomas European Journal of Medical Molecular Imaging 2011;38: 731-417.

[43] Ram Z, Hadani M. Intraoperative imaging-MRI. Acta Neurchirgica Supplemental 2003;88: 1-4.

[44] Lenaburg HJ, Inkabi KE, Vitaz TW. The use of intraoperative MRI for the treatment of glioblastoma multiforme. Technology in Cancer Research and Treatment 2009;8: 159-162.

[45] Senft C, Forster MT, Bink A, Mittelbronn M, Franz K, Seifert V, Szelenyi A. Optimizing the extent of resection in eloquently located gliomas by combining intraoperative

MRI guidance with intraoperative neurophysiological monitoring. Journal Neurooncology 2012;109: 81-90.

[46] Black PMcL, Moriarty T, Alexander ER, Stieg P, Woodard EJ, Gleason PL, et al. Development and implementation of intraoperative magnetic resonance imaging and its neurosurgical applications. Neurosurgery 1997;41: 831-842.

[47] Sutherland GR, Kaibara T, Louw D, Hoult DI, Tomanek B, Saunders J. A mobile high-field magnetic resonance imaging system for neurosurgery. Neurosurgical Focus 1999;6: article 6.

[48] Hirschberg H, Samset E, Hol PK, Tillung T, Lote K. Impact of intraoperative MRI on the surgical results for high-grade gliomas. Minimally invasive Neurosurgery 2005;48: 77-84.

[49] Schulder M, Carmel PW. Intraoperative magnetic resonance imaging: impact on brain tumor surgery. Cancer Control 2003;10: 115-124.

[50] Nimsky C, Fujita A, Ganslandt O, Von Keller B, Fahlbusch R. Volumetric assessment of glioma removal by intraoperative high-field magnetic resonance imaging. Neurosurgery 2004;55: 358-370.

[51] RoderC, Bisdas S, Ebner FH, Honegger J, Naegel T,Ernemann U, Tatagiba M. Maximizing the extent of resection and survival benefit of patients in glioblastoma surgery: High-field iMRI versus conventional and 5-ALA-assisted surgery. European Journal of Surgical Oncology 2014;40: 297-304.

[52] Vitaz TW, Inkabi KE, Carruba CJ. Intraoperative MRI for transphenoidal procedures: short-term outcome for 100 consecutive cases. Clinical Neurology and Neurosurgery 2011;113: 731-735.

[53] Anand VK, Schwartz TH, Hiltzik DH, Kacker A. Endoscopic transphenoidal pituitary surgery with real-time intraoperative magnetic resonance imaging. American Journal of Rhinology 2006;20: 401-405.

[54] Lu J, Wu J, Yao C, Zhang D, Qiu T, Hu X et al. Awake language mapping and 3-Tesla intraoperative MRI-guided volumetric resection for gliomas in language areas. Journal of Clinical Neuroscience 2013;20: 1280-1287.

[55] Carrabba G, Fava E, Giussani C, Acerbi F, Portaluri F, Songa V, et al. Cortical and subcortical motor mapping in rolandic and perirolandic glioma surgery: impact on postoperative morbidity and extent of resection.

[56] Sanai N, Berber MS. Extent of Resection influences outcome for patients with gliomas. Neurology Review 2011;167: 648-654.

[57] Vassal F, Schneider F, Nuti C. Intraoperative use of diffusion tensor imaging-based tractography for resection of gliomas located near the pyramidal tract: comparison

with subcortical stimulation mapping and contribution to surgical outcomes. British Journal of Neurosurgery 2013;27: 668-75.

[58] Roux FE, Ibarrola D, Tremoulet M, Lazorthes Y, Henry P, Sol JC, Berry I. Methodological and technical issues for integrating functional magnetic resonance imaging data in a neuronavigational system. Neurosurgery 2001;49: 1145-1156.

[59] Sunaert S. Presurgical planning for tumor resection. Journal Magnetic Resonance Imaging 2006;23: 887-905.

[60] Vlieger EJ, Majoie CB, Leenstra S, den Heeten GJ. Functional magnetic resonance imaging for neurosurgical planning in neurooncology. European Journal of Radiology 2004;14: 1143-1153.

[61] Berman JI, Berger MS, Mukherjee P, Henry RG. Diffusion tensor imaging-guided tracking of fibers of the pyramidal tract combined with intraoperative cortical stimulation mapping in patients with gliomas. Journal Neurosurgery 2004;101: 66-72.

[62] Clark CA, Barrick TR, Murphy MM, Bell BA. White matter fiver tracking in patients with space-occupying lesions of the brain: a new technique for neurosurgical planning? Neurological Imaging 2003;20: 1601-1608.

[63] Hendler T, Pianka P, Sigal M, Kafri M, Ben-Bashat D, Constantini S, et al. Delineating gray and white matter involvement in brain lesions: three-dimensional alignment of functional magnetic resonance and diffusion-tensor imaging. Journal Neurosurgery 2003;99: 1018-1027.

[64] Nimsky C, Ganslandt O, Hastreiter P, Wang R, Benner T, Sorensen AG, Fahlbusch R. Preoperative and intraoperative diffusion tensor imaging-based fiber tracking in glioma surgery. Neurosurgery 2005;56: 130-137.

[65] De Witt Hamer PC, Gil Robles S, Zwinderman AH, Duffau H, Berger MS. Impact of intraoperative stimulation brain mapping on glioma surgery outcome: a meta-analysis. Journal Clinical Oncology 2012;10: 2559-2565.

[66] Sanai N, Berger MS. Operative Techniques for gliomas and the value of extent of resection. Neurotherapeutics 2009;6:478-486.

[67] Keles GE, Lundin DA, Lamborn KR, Chang EF, Ojemann G, Berger MS. Intraoperative subcortical stimulation mapping for hemispherical perirolandic gliomas located within or adjacent to the descending motor pathways: evaluation of morbidity and assessment of functional outcome in 294 patients. Journal Neurosurgery 2004;100: 369-375.

[68] Hatiboglu MA, Weinberg JS, Suki D, Tummala S, Rao G, Sawaya R, Prabhu S. Utilization of intraoperative motor mapping in glioma surgery with high-field intraoperative magnetic resonance imaging. Stereotactic and Functional Neurosurgery 2009;88: 345-352.

Chapter 11

# Seizures in Children with Brain Tumours — Epidemiology, Significance, Management, and Outcomes

Adrianna Ranger and David Diosy

Additional information is available at the end of the chapter

http://dx.doi.org/10.5772/58961

## 1. Introduction

Cancer is the most frequently diagnosed disease-related cause of death among children and adolescents [1], and malignancies involving the brain are collectively the most common solid tumour [2, 3]. They are also either first or second in incidence overall (second only to leukaemia) in the United States (USA) [1, 4,7], Canada [8], and Mexico [9]. The *American Brain Tumour Association* has estimated that approximately 4,200 American children younger than age 20 would be diagnosed with a primary brain tumour in the year 2012, of whom three in four would be under the age of 15 years [10]. However, the overall prognosis for brain malignancies is much better in children than in adults, with up to half of paediatric brain cancer patients surviving long-term [11]. The reason for this enhanced survival in youths is that children and adolescents are much more likely than adults to have low-grade astrocytomas, in particular pilocytic astrocytomas and other low-grade gliomas that are almost never fatal and often cured, depending upon their location and surgical accessibility, rather than the grade III and IV astrocytomas that account for the majority of tumours among adults [12-14].

Long-term survival, even in the setting of cure, is not without problems, however, with empirical evidence accumulating that paediatric brain cancer survivors continue to suffer from significant morbidity [15-20] and, sometimes, early death [15]. Among the more common long-term sequelae of brain cancer and brain cancer treatment in children are seizures, which can be quite disabling and, at times, life-threatening in themselves [15, 21-30]. In one study, seizures were the number one predictor of disability in long-term brain cancer survivors [24, 25]. Seizures even increase a paediatric survivor's risk of suicide into adulthood [31]. In addition, there is a subset of children, up to 50% [32], whose low-grade brain cancer presents as seizures [26, 32-42]. Though the vast majority of epileptogenic tumours are supratentorial, some are not, especially among children in whom infratentorial tumours generally comprise the majority [43, 44], and in less typical locations like the thalamus and hypothalamus [38, 45-47]. Among thalamic tumours, for example, up to one third of paediatric patients present with seizures [38]. As such, and because even low-grade gliomas can nonetheless be infiltrative into high-function brain tissue [19, 48-50], while some of these lesions are totally resectable, others are not [51-54]. This creates dilemmas as to how aggressive to be, and therefore how much risk to take in their resection [55]. As well, the return of seizures at some distant time post-operatively may indicate tumour growth or relapse [28, 30, 56-66], transformation into a more aggressive lesion [28, 60, 65, 67, 68], or even the emergence of a secondary (e.g., radiation-induced) tumour [64].

Why seizures occur in patients with brain tumours is not entirely clear [27, 69-71], and several conjectures have been made, including alterations in regional metabolism and pH, immunologic activity, disordered neuronal function, altered vascular supply and permeability, the release of altered tumoral amino acids, proteins and enzymes, and abnormal protein transport and binding to receptors [27, 44, 69, 71-74]. Even genetic predispositions for tumour-related seizures have been postulated [71, 75]. A recent excellent review of current theories and empirical evidence on the pathogenesis of tumour-related epilepsy has been published by You et al. [74] Discussing the relative merits of each theory is a paper in itself, and beyond the scope of the current review.

Interestingly, tumour size has a somewhat paradoxical relationship with seizure occurrence, in that, though the opposite is true of low-grade lesions, high-grade gliomas that present with seizures tend to be smaller than those that present with other symptoms [76]. Moreover, high-grade lesions that present with seizures tend to have a better prognosis than lesions of the same size that present otherwise [77]. What this suggests is that the aggressiveness of the tumour might have an effect upon seizure development. This being said, low-grade lesions comprise the majority of epileptogenic tumours, both in children and adults [78]; and some tumour types — like gangliogliomas and dysembryoplastic neuroepithelial tumours (DNET) — are more likely to induce seizures than others [28].

In this chapter, we will thoroughly review the literature on seizures in paediatric brain cancer patients, looking at them (1) as a presenting symptom; (2) in the early tumour management/ peri-operative period; and (3) long-term. Specific questions to be addressed in each of these sections are: How common are they? What is their history? How do they impact patients' lives, both short-and long-term, and in terms of management and prognosis? How do they effect management of the underlying tumour? How are seizures managed themselves? As much as possible, these questions will be answered by examining empirical evidence across a number of studies to provide, if not definitive answers, at least conclusions that are supported by published research.

## 2. Seizures as a presenting symptom of a brain tumour

### 2.1. How seizures present

A brain tumour is ultimately discovered in between one and three percent of children who present with new-onset seizures [40, 42], though a slightly higher percentage has been reported in children presenting with partial versus generalized seizures [79], and percentages as high as 20% have been reported in children undergoing epilepsy surgery [80]. From the reverse perspective, somewhere between 10 and 50% of brain tumours present with seizures as a symptom [69, 74, 81-83], and sometimes as the only symptom [32, 41, 84-86], with supratentorial and especially temporal lesions the most likely to be epileptogenic [44, 66, 78, 86-88]. In one study that compared children with supra-and infratentorial tumours, for example, among those with supratentorial lesions, 42% experienced vomiting as their first symptom, followed by seizures in 37%, and headache in 31% [43]. Meanwhile, 62% of children with an infratentorial lesion experienced headaches as their first symptom, with vomiting and ataxia accounting for most of the remainder, and seizures not observed in a single case.

Because children are more likely than adults to have infra-versus supratentorial lesions, the percentage of children presenting with seizures may be somewhat less than among adults, closer to the 10-20% than the 30-50% range [51, 89, 90], though 50% or more has been reported in some series [32, 35]. As in adults, of these epileptic tumours, the vast majority are supratentorial. For example, in their series of 157 children presenting to the hospital with brain tumour-related seizures, of mean age 3.3 years, Khan et al. found that 81% of the tumours were supratentorial and just 19% within the posterior fossa [82]. Meanwhile, Ianelli et al. reported that 80% of their 37 paediatric patients presenting with a temporal lobe malignancy had seizures as a presenting symptom [86]. Another excellent study on new-onset seizures presenting in children with brain cancers was published by Shady et al. [32] who analyzed 98 paediatric brain tumour patients and found that 50% percent of the children had seizures as part of their presentation, and 30% as their only presenting phenomenon; complex (55%) and simple (28%) partial seizures were the most common types, accounting for more than three quarters of all cases. Pre-operative electroencephalography (EEG) accurately lateralized to the tumour side in 88% of the cases and to the correct lobe in 56%. In addition, tumours involving cerebral cortex were much more likely than non-cortical lesions to present with seizures (59% vs. 15% of patients, respectively), with temporal and frontal lobe lesions exhibiting the highest incidence of seizures. Moreover, whereas 88% of gangliogliomas and 86% of oligoastrocytomas were associated with seizures, seizures were noted in just 21% of the patients with an anaplastic astrocytoma. Finally, as described elsewhere [32, 77], patients with seizures at presentation had a better prognosis than those without ($p=0.02$) [32].

Virtually every possible tumour type has been reported presenting as seizures, especially low-grade gliomas [27, 30, 32, 34, 37, 39, 70-72, 75, 76, 78, 91-93] and glioneuronal tumours like ganglioglioma and dysembryoplastic neuroepithelial tumour [28, 44, 62, 73, 88, 89, 91, 94, 95]; but including oligodendroglioma [77, 96, 97], cortical ependymoma [98], medulloblastoma

[47], subependymal giant cell astrocytoma (SEGA) [99], meningioma [10][0], thalamic and cerebellar glioma [38, 46], and a variety of atypical, systemic and metastatic tumours, like primary meningeal osteosarcoma [84], acute lymphoblastic leukemia [101], anaplastic large cell lymphoma [102], neuroblastoma [103], melanoma [104], various sarcomas [105, 106], Ewing's sarcoma [107], malignant germ cell tumours [108], and others [16, 109].

There is no stereotypical seizure presenting as an early symptom of a brain tumour. Early seizures may be generalized, simple partial, complex partial, or mixed, depending upon the tumour's size, location, level of aggressiveness, and other factors [24, 26, 27, 33, 34, 37, 70, 74, 77, 82, 87, 110-115]. This being said, among children, seizures as a presenting symptom of brain tumour are most commonly complex or simple partial, versus generalized, with complex partial seizures generally accounting for from 50% to as high as 85% of all new-onset seizures [32, 63, 69, 86, 115-117]. The lone series in which this was not true was that reported by Hirsch et al., in which complex and simple partial seizures together only accounted for half of all cases [118]. The percentages generally reported for children and adolescents are somewhat different than for adults, in whom tumour-associated seizures tend to be more evenly distributed across the four most typical seizure types [58]. Other atypical and, therefore, less well recognized forms of seizure have been described in children as well, including gelastic seizures, characterized by uncontrolled fits of inappropriate laughter [45], tics and Tourrette-like symptoms [119], and sympathetic storms in a 7-year old with a midbrain glioma [120]. In addition, especially in the paediatric population, tumors may arise in the setting of a variety of familial syndromes such as neurofibromatosis types 1 [121] and 2 [122], and tuberous sclerosis [123]. Seizures in these conditions are often blong-standing, frequent, and intractable because of the numerous non-neoplastic lesions that can involve the CNS [55, 124, 125]. In such patients, the diagnosis of a new neoplastic lesion can be especially challenging [124, 126].

The diagnosis of brain tumour does not always quickly follow the onset of seizures. In one study reported by Ibrahim et al., for example, the time from seizure onset to tumour diagnosis among ten children presenting with seizures ranged from two weeks to two years, averaging six months [37]. A wide range of opinions and practices exist regarding how aggressive to pursue diagnostic imaging in children presenting with seizures [36, 41, 51, 79, 80, 100, 127-133]. For example, in one series of eighteen patients between the ages of 1 month and 13 years who presented with seizures and were discovered to have DNETs between January 1992 and December 2004, the preoperative evaluation included magnetic resonance (MR) imaging and interictal scalp electro-encephalography (EEG) in all patients, but functional MR imaging also was performed in eight patients, video monitoring with scalp EEG during seizures in 12 patients, interictal single-photon emission computerized tomography (SPECT) scanning in one patient, and ictal SPECT scanning in two patients [132]. Meanwhile, in their 2010 review of eleven clinical trials for anti-epileptic drugs (AEDs) conducted over the preceding two years, Jansky et al. noted that none of the trials required MRI as part of the patient enrollment protocol [128]. Increasingly, with advances in imaging and the recognition that the resection of epileptogenic lesions is both safe and effective for many patients, there seems to be growing opinion that the initial work-up of new-onset non-febrile seizures in children should include both an EEG and MRI, despite the likelihood that the majority of imaging studies will be either normal or inconclusive [134, 135]. As discussed in the next section, mounting evidence suggests that new-onset seizures in the setting of a tumour, and conversely, tumours in the setting of new-onset seizures both have therapeutic and prognostic implications.

## 2.2. Implications of brain-tumour induced seizures

Having a child's brain tumour present as seizures adds therapeutic complexity with respect to how the patient is initially managed, since peri-operative control of seizures is obviously considered of extreme clinical importance. The type of seizure a patient has also may have prognostic significance, both in terms of patient survival [65, 136] and how easily the seizures are controlled with anti-epilepsy drugs (AED), both peri-operatively and long-term. How well AEDs work, in turn, may have implications relating to how aggressive surgical resection should be.

Although no reliable data have been published for children, adults who present with seizures as their sole symptom tend to have less aggressive or advanced lesions than those who present with symptoms or signs of increased intracranial pressure like papilloedema, headaches [65], neurological or cognitive deficits [65, 136]. Although this intrinsically makes sense — the fewer the symptoms, the less aggressive or advanced the disease — extrapolating these findings to children must be done with caution, because a disproportionate number of paediatric lesions tend to be brainstem tumours that, though usually low-grade and non-epileptogenic, often are non-resectable because of their location and proximity to function-rich neural tissue [2, 3, 137-139]. Nonetheless, especially among supratentorial lesions, it makes sense that having seizures present before all other symptoms develop is a hopeful prognostic sign, given that low-grade gliomas and other so-called benign lesions tend to be associated with much higher seizure rates than high-grade lesions [32, 87, 91, 113, 140, 141].

Having seizures in the presence of a tumour has implications with respect to management of the seizures as well, in that studies have shown that such seizures tend to be more resistant to AEDs than idiopathic seizures [133, 142]. This appears to be especially true for patients who present with a history of numerous seizures [142]. This likelihood of *drug resistance*, which has been formally defined as *"the failure of adequate trials of two tolerated, appropriately-chosen and used antiepileptic drug schedules (whether as monotherapies or in combination) to achieve sustained seizure freedom"* [143], may play a role in determining the aggressiveness of surgery for tumour resection. For example, given the clear superiority of epilepsy surgery over medical management alone, in terms of achieving freedom from seizures in patients with intractable seizures (65% vs. 8% in one relatively recent meta-analysis [144]), a decision might be made to pursue more aggressive resection in a patient with repeated new-onset seizures upon initial work-up of seizures and diagnosis of their brain tumour, versus the patient who presents with a single seizure prior to tumour detection. Moreover, for many epileptogenic lesions, surgical resection often leads to either complete resolution of seizures, sometimes without the need for continued AEDs, or to a marked reduction in their frequency, as will be elaborated upon next.

### 2.3. General principles of management

How tumor-induced seizures are managed largely depends upon the aggressiveness and location, and therefore, the prognosis of the underlying tumour. In patients with invariably terminal forms of cancer, including primary brain neoplasms like glioblastoma multiforme (GBM), and metastatic spread to brain, the goal usually is to prolong life over months to, at most, a few years, while preserving as high a quality of life as possible. In both adult and paediatric patients with high-grade astrocytomas like GBM, even partial resection of terminal lesions has been shown both to prolong life and reduce the frequency and severity of seizures [145-147]. Clearly, such surgery needs to be performed as soon after diagnosis of the lesion as possible to have any effect upon outcome. Such is not the case in many patients with low-grade tumours like stage I and II gliomas and gangliogliomas, in whom progression of the tumour may be so slow as to be virtually undetectable, and patients can live for years without apparent disease progression, so that any decision to surgically remove the offending lesion may be delayed for years [58, 93, 148, 149]. This being said, there has been increasing emphasis on surgically resecting low-grade tumours early in the course of disease [131] for a multiplicity of reasons. Among these reasons are that anywhere from 20% to roughly one third of low-grade gliomas (LGG) fail to respond to anti-epileptic medications [72, 150], and many that do respond require more than a single AED [150], placing patients, and especially children, at risk for long-term drug toxicities [23, 24, 59, 71, 151-153]. Among the various documented toxicities of AEDs are wide-ranging adverse effects on cognitive function [23, 153], which already may be impaired because of the tumour itself and the radiation therapy sometimes administered to treat it [18, 20, 154-156]. Moreover, surgical resection of LGG has been shown to enhance long-term survival [19] and to significantly improve the likelihood of seizure control [27, 70].

Though the data are not definitive, there is some evidence suggesting that, among the various seizure types, partial seizures, either simple or complex, may be less likely to respond to anti-epileptic drugs than generalized or mixed seizures [93, 157, 158]. This resistance may be noted initially, so that seizure control is never achieved; but it also may develop over time, so that seizure control is lost and never regained [158, 159]. In such patients, therefore, there may even be an increased incentive to pursue surgical resection of the tumour+/-any adjacent epileptogenic foci, if the lesion can be accessed with no undue risk.

Several studies have shown that radical removal of an epileptogenic brain tumour is a strong, and likely the strongest, predictor of seizure freedom [127]. However, additional predictors include the type of seizure, the histopathology of the tumour, the age of the patient at the time of surgery, and the duration of epilepsy [127]. Among the various tumour histologies, tumours that are non-resectable due to infiltration, like high-grade astrocytomas, can be problematic over the patient's relatively brief period of survival [160]. However, as stated earlier, such high-grade lesions tend to be less often epileptogenic than their low-grade counterparts [32, 87, 91, 113, 140, 141]. In long-term brain cancer survivors, glioneuronal tumours, and particularly low-grade gliomas, gangliogliomas and dysembryoplastic neuroepithelial tumours (DNETs), often produce quite drug-resistant epilepsy in children, so that complete surgical resection of the tumour is typically considered the primary focus of treatment [28, 61-63, 88, 94, 116, 132].

In such patients, post-operative seizure-freedom rates often approach or exceed 80% [35, 48, 51, 58, 66, 86, 88, 90, 93, 115, 157, 161-169].

Traditionally, there has been some concern about being too aggressive with younger children with brain tumours, because of the risk of long-term adverse effects on neurological development, the risk of secondary neoplasms, and other neurological sequelae [155]. That such risks exist is certainly true of radiation therapy [18, 20, 64, 153-156], but it also is true of surgery [170]. However, recent studies have shown that surgery to resect epileptogenic brain tumours is both effective and safe for the vast majority of infants and toddlers [35, 55, 171]. In one large survey, for example, data were collected retrospectively on 116 patients less than 3-years old from eight centers across Canada from January 1987 to September 2005 who had undergone epilepsy surgery [171]. Among the various seizure aetiologies were malformations of cortical development (n=57), tumours (22), Sturge-Weber syndrome (19), and infarcts (8), with 10 cases either of unknown or some other cause. Seizure onset was in the first year of life in 82%, and the mean age at the time of the initial surgery was 15.8 months (range: 1-35 months). Second surgeries were performed in 27 patients, with six patients requiring a third surgical procedure. Among the initial 116 procedures performed were 40 hemispheric operations, 33 cortical resections, 35 lesionectomies, 7 temporal lobectomies, and one callosotomy. Of the 151 operations, including the 27 second and six third procedures, only one resulted in a surgery-related death. The most common surgical complications were infection, in 17 patients, and aseptic meningitis in 13. Of 107 patients assessed more than one year postoperatively, 72 (67.3%) were seizure free (Engel I), 15(14%) had experienced at least a 90% reduction in seizures (Engel II), and 12 had at least a 50% reduction (Engel III), with only eight exhibiting no benefit (Engel IV). Moreover, 55.3% of the children exhibited signs of improved development post-operatively [171].

Consequently, regardless of patient age, the focus for most patients with low-grade lesions has become, whenever possible without the undue risk of peri-operative death or long-term adverse neurological sequelae, to attempt total or at least subtotal tumor resection earlier rather than later in the course of disease. Debate rages, however, as to how aggressive to be achieving this goal, whether or not resecting the lesion alone is enough, and what intra-operative technologies to use to aid in identifying tumour margins and other epileptogenic foci. Moreover, not all patients will be eligible for surgery and will have to rely on non-neurosurgical treatments alone, most notably anti-epileptic drugs (AEDs) and radiation therapy. The next section briefly discusses the benefits, risks and utilization of AEDs both prior to and in lieu of surgery.

## 3. Anti-Epileptic Drugs (AEDs)

An extensive review paper could be written discussing the various advantages and disadvantages, indications and contra-indications, and drug-drug interactions that exist for the extensive list of anti-epileptic drugs that now are available for use in patients with brain tumour-induced epilepsy, all of which is beyond the scope of the current review. Here, we briefly describe the roles of AEDs, both in prophylaxis against and control of tumour-induced seizures, some of the risks of prolonged use, and at least the theoretical advantages of the new class of non-enzyme inducing drugs.

### 3.1. AEDs for seizure prophylaxis

In three recent surveys of neurosurgeons, including one survey specifically of members of the *American Association of Neurologic Surgeons* (AANS), the majority (up to 70%) of respondents reported prophylactically initiating AEDs in brain tumour patients who had not yet experienced a seizure [172-174]. This practice of prescribing AEDs prophylactically in brain tumour patients with no seizure history persists, even though empirical evidence addressing this practice is inconclusive at best [78, 81, 127, 140, 172]. Moreover, many authors and the most current *American Association of Neurology* practice parameters argue against it [113, 140, 172, 175, 176]. The argument of AED detractors is that both meta-analyses published since 2000 to address this issue failed to provide sufficient evidence to promote their prophylactic use in brain-tumour patients without seizures [173, 177]. The first meta-analysis, published in 2000 by Glantz et al. [173], analyzed 12 studies, of which four were randomized controlled trials and eight were considered to be "well-designed observational studies with concurrent controls", sufficient to be classified as class II evidence. Not one of these twelve studies demonstrated a statistical advantage of the AED being studied (phenytoin, depakote, or phenobarbital) over placebo [173]. The second, somewhat more stringent meta-analysis, published in 2004 by Sirven et al [177], only included five RCTs, assessing the prophylactic use of either phenobarbital, phenytoin, or valproic acid. Of the five trials, four identified no statistical benefit of AED use for peri-operative seizure prophylaxis. The one exception was a 1983 study published by North et al [178], in which not only patients with brain tumours, but patients who had undergone craniotomies for aneurisms and head injuries were included. A closer, empirical look at these data reveals no advantage at all when brain tumours are considered alone: seizures occurred in 9/42 on phenytoin, and in 5/39 on placebo (OR=1.11, 95% CI=0.58, 2.12). Further considering just those patients with glial tumours (versus meningiomas, sellar tumours, and metastases), seizures occurred in three of 16 on phenytoin versus just one of 16 on placebo (1.15; 0.42, 3.19) [178]. Overall meta-analysis across the five RCT confirmed the lack of any AED benefit at both one week (OR, 0.91; 95% confidence interval [CI], 0.45-1.83) and six months (OR, 1.01; 95% CI, 0.51-1.98) of follow-up. The AEDs also exhibited no effect on seizure prevention for specific tumours, including primary glial tumors (OR, 3.46; 95% CI, 0.32-37.47), cerebral metastases (OR, 2.50; 95% CI, 0.25-24.72), and meningiomas (OR, 0.62; 95% CI, 0.10-3.85) [177].

More recently, in a review published in 2011, Kargiotis et al. non-statistically examined published evidence on more currently-used AED, including the newer non-enzyme inducing drugs, and concluded that, among patients with either brain metastases or primary brain tumors who have never experienced seizures, prophylactic anticonvulsant treatment might be justified, but only for up to six months postoperatively after surgical excision of the cerebral tumour, since most of these patients will never experience seizures, and the anti-epileptic drugs may cause toxicity and adverse interactions with chemotherapeutic treatments administered to control the neoplasm itself [109]. For such prophylaxis, the authors argued that newer antiepileptic drugs like levetiracetam and oxcarbazepine are preferable to older agents like phenytoin and carbamazepine [109]. To date, however, no hard evidence supports any of these recommendations, and certainly not in children.

In a study by Hardesty et al., only 7.4% of 223 paediatric patients with brain tumours but no history of seizures experienced even a single seizure during their surgical admission, even though only 4.4% of patients had been started on a prophylactic AED [179]. This percentage is similar to the 8.0% observed among those on placebo in a controlled study in which 127 patients awaiting brain tumour surgery, ranging in age from 16 to 84 years, were randomized to receive either phenytoin 15mg/kg intravenously in the operating room, followed by 100 mg three times daily, either by mouth or intravenously, for seven days or placebo [180]. Thereafter, the dose of each was tapered. The 30-day incidence of seizures actually was higher in the phenytoin group (10.0%) than in controls (8.0%), albeit not statistically so. Moreover, the rate of complications was 18.0% versus 0% in the treatment versus placebo group, respectively ($p < 0.001$).

In the Hardesty study on youths [179], dependent factors associated with peri-operative seizures included a supratentorial tumour, patient age less than two years, and the presence of post-operative hyponatraemia due to either the syndrome of inappropriate antidiuretic hormone (SIADH) or cerebral salt wasting. No other factor was independently predictive of incident seizures, including tumour type, the lobe of the brain affected, the amount of operative blood loss, and the length of surgery [179]. Consequently, though children and adolescents who are awaiting brain-tumour resection and have recurrent seizures might warrant the initiation of an AED pre-operatively, and perhaps also children under age two years with a supratentorial tumour and those with highly-epileptogenic tumours like DNETs, even in the absence of seizures, the prophylactic use of these drugs is far from empirically justified. What is more prudent is to monitor all patients carefully throughout the peri-operative period to identify clinical factors that might place the child at risk, like electrolyte imbalances and fever.

### 3.2. AEDs for seizure control

Although in some small series of patients, seizures have been found to occur in up to 50% of paediatric patients with a brain tumour [170], in most populations, the overall incidence of seizures in this patient population is considerably lower, in the 10-20% range [51, 89, 90]. This is largely due to the infratentorial location of the majority of paediatric tumours, where very few are epileptogenic [37]. As such, only a small minority of children and adolescents with a brain tumour will likely ever require an AED, and almost all will have a supratentorial lesion. For example, from a database of 334 patients up to 21-years old, Sogawa et al. only identified 32 (10%) who had been started on an AED [83]; 94% of these 32 tumours were supratentorial, and 78% were glial [83]. Similarly, in their series of 280 patients between the ages of two months and 18 years of age, Khan et al. identified only 55 (20%) patients who had required an AED, among whom 49 (89%) had a supratentorial lesion [90]. This being said, over a 20-year period at a single institution, Khan et al. followed 157 patients who had presented with seizures and a brain tumour during childhood or adolescence, all of whom had been on at least one AED at some point [82]. Of these patients, phenytoin was the first AED used for 52 patients, carbamazepine for 38 patients, gabapentin for 31, and phenobarbitol for 14. Sixty-two of these patients ultimately were taken off all AEDs; but 17 of these 62 (27%) suffered seizure recurrence [181].

DNETs and gangliogliomas, which typically become manifest during childhood, adolescence or young adulthood, represent only a small percentage of CNS tumours in either youths or adults [6]. However, these tumours are almost always associated with seizures. Consequently, they comprise a disproportionate percentage of tumour-associated epilepsy cases [28, 44, 62, 73, 88, 89, 91, 94, 95]. Moreover, DNETs tend to be extremely resistant to AED therapy [62, 182-186]. Consequently, though AEDs generally are initiated in such patients, the majority ultimately will require surgical resection.

There is virtually no debate that AEDs are of use in treating brain tumour patients with seizures, in patients with repeated seizures awaiting surgery, in patients in whom tumour resection is infeasible, and in those whose seizures remain refractory despite surgery. However, there is concern about the risks of their long-term use, especially in patients who require on-going chemotherapy for their brain malignancy due to drug interactions and mutually-shared toxicities [81, 83, 127, 140, 151, 159, 172, 176], 187]; and significant debate regarding when and how AEDs should be discontinued post-operatively.

One of the biggest issues relating to AEDs is their potential interactions with anti-neoplastic drugs administered to control tumours and prolong survival. In a paper reviewing anti-epileptic drugs, Kargiotis et al. [109] listed 25 chemotherapeutic medications that interact with AEDs, most commonly carbamazepine, phenobarbitol, phenytoin and primidone, but also valproic acid. Common interactions are the AED accelerating metabolism of the chemotherapeutic drug, and the chemotherapeutic drug reducing serum levels of the AED [109], two results that potentially accentuate each other — when AED levels fall, AED doses must be increased to achieve seizure control, which will further increase metabolism of the chemotherapeutic drug, resulting in its doses needing to be increased, and so on. Included on their list of 25 drugs were 13 drugs often selected for the treatment of brain metastases, as well as nine drugs currently used to treat glioblastomas, six drugs to treat medulloblastomas, and five to treat malignant meningiomas.

In the current paper, Table 1 lists these interactions in reverse, indicating those anti-neoplastic drugs used for CNS malignancies that have had documented interactions with each of the five AEDs listed above. What is clear from this table is that all but valproic acid interacts with almost all of the chemo-therapeutic drugs typically used for CNS cancers.

The only drug on the list published by Kargiotis et al. [109] this is not considered to interact with AEDs is temozolomide (TMZ), a less toxic and more-easily tolerated orally-administered drug that effectively crosses the blood-brain barrier [188] and is now commonly used for both high-grade [189] and low-grade [190, 191] gliomas, as well as for brain metastases [192] and melanomas, often in combination with radiation therapy. There also is evidence that TMZ itself reduces the frequency of seizures, independent of AED dose. In one study in which 39 patients receiving TMZ (mean age 46.0 years) were followed for a mean 39 months and compared with 30 patients not on TMZ (mean age 41.5 years), patients on TMZ experienced a 59% reduction in seizure frequency versus just 13% in controls ($p < 0.001$) [150]. However, for reasons that are not entirely understood, TMZ appears to be less effective in children [193]. For this reason, other anti-neoplastic drugs typically are prescribed in children and adolescents, particularly multiple-drug regimens that include carboplatin and vincristine [193-195], two drugs both documented to interact with the older, cytochrome P450-inducing anti-eptileptics [109] (Table 1).

Meanwhile, evidence continues to mount documenting both the effectiveness and safety of newer-generation AEDS, like levetiracetam, oxcarbazepine and pregabalin [152, 196-204]. Though direct comparisons against the older drugs are generally lacking, theoretical advantages include the lack of any effect on cytochrome P450, and the fact that these drugs generally target specific risk factors for tumour-induced seizures [81]. Recently, in a survey of 32 paediatric brain-tumour patients requiring AEDs for seizure control, Sogawa et al. found that patients who had been started on any the newer–generation drugs (levetiracetam, oxcarbazepine and lamotrigine) were three times as likely to remain on these drugs than those started on one of the older drugs like valproic acid, phenytoin, and phenobarbitol (73% vs. 28%, respectively, $p=0.04$) [83]. Although the sample was small, there also was evidence of increased toxicity with the older drugs, with five versus just two adverse events resulting in drug discontinuation [83].

Of course, the treatment of brain tumours is anything but a static field. In attempts to reduce tumour progression and prolong survival, newer chemotherapeutic drugs are continuously being tested. Some, like nimotuzumab [205]and bevacizumab [206], both of them antibodies against epithelial growth factor receptors (EGFR), have been demonstrating considerable promise, and this may have implications for which AEDs are best tolerated as interactions and mutual toxicities become clearer. What is evident is that AEDs, in themselves, are usually inadequate to control seizures in most patients with epileptogenic brain tumours. And while novel treatments like stereotactic radiosurgery [154], vagus nerve stimulation [207], and ionizing radiation [208] are emerging, at this time optimal management of a child or adolescent with epilepsy caused by a brain tumour almost always necessitates resection of the lesion itself.

## 4. Surgical resection of epileptogenic brain tumours

### 4.1. The benefits and risks of surgery

In recent years, there has been a trend towards earlier surgical intervention in young patients with low-grade epileptogenic tumours; but is this justified? One potential justification is the risk of malignant transformation of low-grade tumours which, even though uncommon, has been described for virtually all tumour types and often is catastrophic [60, 64, 65, 67, 68, 97, 112, 131, 209-213]. A second justification pertains to improved seizure control and the decreased reliance on AEDs, with some patients potentially able to discontinue anti-epileptic medications altogether[59], [61, 181, 185]. But how successful is tumour resection in terms of controlling or eliminating seizures?

Table 2 lists 26 studies [35, 51, [61-63, 86, 90, 94, 96, 132, 148, 149, 168, 182, 184, 185, 214-223] published over the past two decades in which seizure outcomes in children and adolescents undergoing surgery to remove epileptogenic brain neoplasms were examined. Across these 26 studies are 741 patients, ranging in age from one month to 21 years of age, with a mean age of 9.1 years and a mean duration of post-operative follow-up of more than four years (overall mean=52 months, with individual study means ranging from 12 to 148 months). Though one study [86] included six paediatric patients with high-grade gliomas (either GBM or grade III astrocytoma), and another indicated 11 patients with either grade III or grade IV lesions [35], almost all of the remaining 724 patients had low-grade (grade I or II) lesions, including various low-grade gliomas and glioneuronal tumours, and less typically epileptogenic tumours like craniopharyngiomas and a dysplastic cyst. Spanning these studies, surgical approaches clearly differed, with some surgeons either largely or exclusively performing lesionectomies alone, others performing further procedures like partial lobectomies [86, 148] and amygdylohypocampectomies [182], and still others using various intra-operative mapping technologies like electrocortography (ECoG) [63, 132, 184, 214] to identify and ultimately resect extra-tumoral epileptogenic tissue. However, the ubiquitous goal was total tumour resection, whenever possible, an objective that was achieved in roughly two-thirds of cases.

Overall, the series with the lowest total resection rates were those that included a number of oligodendrogliomas (ODG), with resection rates ranging from 30% in a study exclusively of ODG and ODG-mixed lesions [96] and 40% in an older study in which half the patients had ODG [219], to 58% and 61% in studies in which the proportion of ODG was considerably lower [90, 220]. This discovery is not unexpected, given the highly infiltrative nature of these tumours [77, 96, 97, 191].

The outcomes of surgery otherwise were impressive, with almost four out of every five patients (77.7%) seizure free at the time of the final follow-up assessment, and 92.6% experiencing a significant improvement in their seizures from baseline, to Engel class 1, 2 or 3. Examining these data further reveals moderately strong, borderline statistically-significant correlations between the percentage of total resections achieved within any given series and the rate of seizure freedom ($r=0.37$, $p=0.08$), and between the percentage of total resections and the percentage of patients whose seizures were improved post-operatively ($r=0.36$, $p=0.09$). However, no correlation is apparent between the duration of follow-up and either outcome ($r=0.06$, $p=0.78$ and $r=0.26$, $p=0.22$, respectively), suggesting that it was the surgical procedure, rather than post-operative management, that influenced seizure outcomes.

There also were no peri-operative deaths among the 741 patients, some of whom even underwent second procedures to resect residual tumour detected by imaging after the first procedure. The overall operative complication rate, adjusted for missing data, was 11.7%, with the vast majority of complications and new neurological deficits transient and completely resolved within weeks to months of the procedure. As stated above, a small number of patients required repeat surgeries to achieve seizure control, sometimes associated with total tumour resection. For example, in one series a second surgery was required in three of 29 paediatric patients with supratentorial gangliogliomas, and all became seizure free after the second operation [216].

The studies by Jo et al. [223] and Gaggero et al. [35] are of special note because all the patients were infants, under the age of 5 and 3 years, respectively. In the first small series of 14 patients of mean age 2.7 years (32 months) [223], total resection of the epileptogenic lesion was achieved in 71%, as was total seizure freedom an average of 35 months post-operatively. In addition, all 14 infants experienced a significant reduction in seizure frequency, either being totally seizure free or having seizures limited to auras alone [223]. There also were no deaths and no reported operative complications. In the second study, which included 20 infants under age 3 years (mean age 1.5 years), eleven of the 20 children had either a grade III or grade IV neoplasm, including four choroid plexus carcinomas, one anaplastic oligodendroglioma, one anaplastic ependymoma, one immature teratoma, two glioblastoma multiforme, one PNET and one neuroblastoma [35]. Despite this, total resection was achieved in 70% of the children, seizure freedom beyond four years in 55%, and seizure improvement in 90%. Interestingly, all 20 patients lived beyond four years, and 17 remained alive at eight years of follow-up [35]. These two studies that imply both the effectiveness and safety of aggressive brain tumour resection in infants is counter to another study on 18 infants under one year of age who had a variety of grade I through IV lesions [170]. In this series, there was only one peri-operative death, due to massive brain haemorrhage in an 8-month old child with a deep, right parieto-occipital ganglioglioma. However, three patients had new-onset seizures following surgery, and an additional three had worsened neurological deficits. Of the nine patients who had pre-operative seizures, three improved, five did not improve, and one died. Overall, as of the paper's publication, only eight of the twenty patients had survived beyond infancy, with five now into adulthood (ages 18 – 26) [170]; two of the adult survivors were severely disabled at the time of the report, both having a Karnofsky score [224] of just 40%.

Also worth noting from Table 2 are the six studies in which only patients with dysembryoplastic neuroepithelial tumours (DNETs) were included (Table 3) [61, 62, 94, 132, 182, 184]. These six studies encompass 132 patients, of mean age 9.7 years, amongst whom total tumour resection was achieved in almost 82%, seizure freedom in 87%, and seizure improvement in all but a single patient (99%). However, the adjusted surgical complication rate was slightly higher than that noted across all 26 studies.

Table 4 lists four additional studies of note. Among these four additional studies, three were excluded from the previous table and its summation totals because vascular and other non-neoplastic lesions were intermingled with non-vascular lesions, with no data provided to distinguish between them; and the fourth was excluded because all the patients had tuberous sclerosis, in which brain tubors often cause uncontrolled seizures [225, 226]. The fifteen patients in this fourth study all had subependymal giant cell astrocytomas (SEGA), a tumour that is found in between five and fifteen percent of TS patients [123], typically developing in the region of the foramen of Monro, where it frequently causes obstructive hydrocephalus. Seizures primarily result from a broad array of intra-cerebral tumors, which include the cortical tubers mentioned above, and subependymal nodules, in addition to SEGA [225, 226]. The long-term prognosis therefore is poor, with death primarily resulting from intractable seizures or SEGA-induced obstructive hydrocephalus [225, 226]. As such, it is not unexpected that Cuccia et al. [99] failed to achieve either seizure freedom or any meaningful clinical improvement in seizure frequency in any of their patients. The inherent complexities of SEGA removal, given the relative inaccessibility of these tumours, also could account for the high complication rate (6 of 15, 40%).

The three remaining studies [117, 227, 228] involved a high proportion of non-neoplastic lesions that were not analyzed distinctly from neoplastic cases. Mean seizure free rates across the three studies ranged from a low of 56% to a high of 81%, with seizure improvement noted in 81.3% and 92.4% in the two studies in which this outcome was reported [117, 227]. Although no deaths were reported, almost one in four patients (73 of 320, 22.8%) had a significant post-operative complication, likely due to the highly vascular nature of many of the lesions and the increased risk of intracranial bleeding.

### 4.2. Post-operative management

According to the 30 studies (26+4) analysed above, the rate of post-operative complications among patients with epileptogenic brain tumours is low, likely somewhere between 10 and 20 percent, depending upon the nature of the tumour resected, its location, and perhaps other factors as well. The risk of peri-operative mortality also appears to be exceedingly low, with not a single surgery-related death reported among those 873 patients.

Few papers have been published on the post-operative management of paediatric brain tumour patients. What has been reported is that youths tend to experience different intra-operative and post-operative complications than adults, and that these complications affect both short and long-term outcomes, including disability, mortality and hospital and PICU lengths of stay and, hence, direct health care costs [229, 230]. Among the various risk factors for complications are fluid and electrolyte imbalances, which may be especially significant in children. One also must consider that volume of blood loss is all relative to the age and size of the child, given that a human's total blood volume varies dramatically relative to their age and size: falling from roughly 85 to 90 ml per kg in term neonates, to roughly 85 ml/kg in infants, 80 ml/kg in children under age 10, 70-75 ml in children > 10 and adolescents, and 70ml/kg in adults [231, 232]. Clearly then, 100 ml of blood loss may mean nothing to an adult, but may represent 25% or more of the total blood volume of a newborn.

In general, the most common fluid and electrolyte abnormalities observed after brain surgery in children relate to serum sodium levels, with hyponatraemia secondary to either the syndrome of inappropriate diuretic hormone (SIADH) secretion or cerebral salt wasting syndrome, and hypernatraemia caused by diabetes insipidis (DI) [233-236]. In one series of 79 children, for example, water and sodium disorders were noted in 36 (46%): 23 (29%) with DI, 12 (15%) with SIADH, and a single patient with cerebral salt wasting [236]. Why this is especially important in the paediatric patient in whom an epileptogenic brain tumour has been resected is that sodium disturbances are a significant risk factor for seizures. In one study involving 223 paediatric patients with epileptic brain tumours undergoing 229 surgical procedures, post-operative hyponatraemia — due to either SIADH or cerebral salt wasting — was one of just three independent factors associated with peri-operative seizures, the other two being a supratentorial tumour and patient age less than two years [179].

In another study of 105 paediatric patients post brain tumor resection admitted to the PICU, patients required an average of 0.7 unexpected intensive care unit interventions, mostly secondary to sodium abnormalities, followed by new neurologic deficits, paresis, and seizures

[237]. Interestingly, however, 68% of the patients were stable enough to be transferred out of the PICI within 24 hours of surgery.

With respect to anti-epileptic drugs, the same applies post-operatively as pre-operatively, in that there is generally no need to initiate AEDs in patients who have not yet experienced seizures, given the lack of evidence documenting any benefit of prophylaxis [180, 238]. This being said, there are no clear guidelines as to when and how to discontinue AEDs if they have been initiated pre-operatively, and there is always the potential risk of withdrawal-induced seizures [59]. In one study of 332 mostly adult patients, but including some as young as age 16, among those with AEDs that had been initiated to treat seizures pre-operatively, patients with a longer history of seizures ($p<0.001$) and those with simple partial seizures ($p=0.004$) were found to be especially likely to continue to have seizures in the immediate post-operative period, as well as poorer control long-term [58]. If AEDs are started post-operatively to reduce the risk of seizures following the trauma of surgery in a patient who otherwise has not had seizures, they generally should be administered short-term [239].

## 5. When seizures persist or recur

In virtually every series we have reviewed, patients were described who underwent resection of their epileptogenic brain tumour, with apparently successful removal of the tumour, yet no achieved control of seizures. Additional patients were noted to suffer from the post-operative onset of new seizures [170]. And still others had complete control of their seizures, only to relapse later, either while still on an anti-epileptic drug or after all AEDs had been withdrawn. Each of these three scenarios has implications with respect to patient prognosis and management.

### 5.1. Implications of post-operative seizures

The clinical implications of seizures that either start or re-start months or years after the initial resection of tumour are somewhat different than seizures that start immediately post-operatively or that started pre-operatively and failed to resolve with surgery. The major concern with the latter two scenarios is that tumour resection either was incomplete, or that extra-tumoral epileptogenic tissue was not removed. Over the years, attempts have been made to optimize the resection of epileptogenic lesions by both better delineating their margins and identifying extra-tumoral epileptogenic tissue, using intra-operative tools like electrocorticography (ECoG) to identify potential seizure-inducing tissue irregularities like cortical dysplasia [63, 77, 93, 132, [1] [6][3], 184, 214, 216, 240, 241]. This has led to debate regarding the relative benefits and safety of performing epilepsy surgery rather than just lesionectomies in patients with tumour-triggered seizures [242]; though, in fact, many surgeons have been utilizing additional surgical steps like lobectomies, amygdylohypocampectomies and, in extreme cases, hemispherectomies for decades [63, 86, 94, 117, 132, 148, 149, 168, 182, 185, 214, 217, 218, 222, 227, 243]. To date, almost no direct empirical comparisons have been undertaken. In perhaps the most methodologically sound study, Gelinas et al. retrospectively compared

34 patients who underwent ECoG-aided epilepsy surgery and 33 patients who had undergone simple lesionectomies without ECoG, all between the ages of 3 months and 16 years, in Vancouver, Canada [214]. One year post-operatively, the two treatment arms were virtually identical, with roughly 80% of patients in each group seizure free. However, at a mean follow-up of 5.8 years, there was a trend towards improved seizure freedom in patients in the ECoG group, with 79% versus 61% patients still seizure free (p=0.08). The investigators also noted no increase in neurological morbidity among patients who had undergone the more extensive ECoG-guided cortical resection, and that these patients were less likely to require repeat epilepsy surgery [214]. Why this has implications post-operatively relates to the potential need for re-operation, as discussed in the next section.

If the major concern of continued seizures is residual tumour or other epileptogenic tissue, the major concerns with later tumour recurrence are multiple. They include the possibility: (1) that the tumour itself is re-growing, having never been fully resected; (2) that the tumour has undergone malignant transformation; or (3) that some secondary tumour has started to develop, perhaps as a consequence of brain irradiation, chemotherapy, or some other cause. The risk of second brain malignancies is especially high in patients with CNS tumour-associated familial syndromes like neurofibromatosis types 1 [121] and 2 [122], tuberous sclerosis [123], von Hippel Lindau disease [244, 245], and basal cell nevus syndrome [246], with some of these tumours originating within the brain and others the result of metastatic spread from some extra-cranial site. All of the above-mentioned scenarios warrant investigation, which will include diagnostic imaging, due to their potentially dire consequences

Re-growth of tumour is anticipated among children with high-grade lesions, especially glioblastomas [81, 146, 247]. However, although long-term prognoses remain dismal, small improvements in survival times are being reported even among patients with GBMs, relating to advanced surgical techniques, the introduction of real-time, intra-operative imaging and brain mapping, and combining TMZ with radiation therapy [147, 189, 247-250]. Recall that in one study in which eleven of the 20 children had either a grade III or grade IV lesion, including two GBMs, a grade IV PNET, and a grade IV neuroblastoma, all 20 patients lived beyond four years [35]. Nonetheless, when the return of seizures leads to the discovery of grade IV tumour progression, surgery is almost never indicated. Instead, radiation therapy, chemotherapy, or both can be used and may be effective at reducing seizures [81, 208]. The recurrence of seizures does not necessarily indicate tumour progression, however. Sometimes, intrinsic changes within the tumour itself render AEDs less effective, so that switching or combining drugs may be beneficial [72]. As mentioned in Section 3, in such cases, care must be taken to avoid interactions between chemotherapeutic and anti-epileptic drugs [109].

Tumour re-growth also in anticipated in many low-grade gliomas and other neuroglial tumours when total resection is not achieved, and this can be manifested by the recurrence or worsening of seizures. This being said, malignant transformation has been documented with virtually every form of low-grade brain tumour, especially low-grade gliomas [65, 68, 112, 131], but also traditionally-benign lesions like DNETS [64, 67, 209-211], gangliogliomas [209, 212], meningiomas [251, 252], vestibular schwannomas [251], pituitary adenomas [251], and haemangioblastomas [251], among others. Glioblastomas have even been documented to arise at the site of previously totally-resected tumours [253]. Previously-controlled seizures generally are harder to control once malignant-transformation has occurred, even independent of tumour size or rate of progression [78]. Identification of such transformation therefore has implications in terms of patient prognosis, and management of both the tumour and the seizures.

Finally, the late recurrence of seizures can represent the formation of a secondary tumour, perhaps induced by brain irradiation or chemotherapy [251].

### 5.2. Surgical management of persistent and recurrent seizures

Whether seizures start immediately after surgery, later along in follow-up, or never fully remit, in all three scenarios, some patients will have seizures that remain uncontrolled despite the use of AEDs. In our review of the 26 studies listed in Table 2, as well as in various other case series and case studies, we found that, occasionally, patients undergo second or even third resections to remove either residual tumour that is now identified on post-operative imaging, or a residual or newly-identified epileptogenic focus. Though sometimes prolonged attempts are made to control the seizures with medication prior to the second surgery, in some cases, surgery is almost immediate, even within a few days of the initial procedure [254]. In one multi-centre survey that involved 116 children under age 3 undergoing epilepsy surgery for a variety of causes, 27 children were brought into the operating room for a second procedure, and six of these for a third procedure to control seizures [171]. Both the approaches and results of these second operations are mixed. In terms of the former, attempts are usually made to resect any residual or newly-discovered tumour, as well as to identify and resect other epileptogenic foci. Approaches range from simple lesionectomies to lobectomies and, in the most severe cases, hemispherectomies [243].

Table 5 summarizes ten studies we identified, published over the past two decades, in which second operative procedures were performed [46, 77, 157, [1] [6][2], 171, 216, 242, 254-256]. Half of these studies were exclusive to paediatric patients, while the other half included children, adolescents and adults. The study by Steinbok et al. was restricted to infants under the age of 3 years at the time of their initial surgery [171]. In this study, six of the patients required a third surgical procedure prior to achieving their final seizure outcome. Follow-up for most of these studies was approximately two years, but sometimes not reported. Overall, slightly less than half of the patients (46%) achieved seizure freedom, with roughly half the remainder (where reported) achieving at least a significant reduction in seizures. As with the first procedures, operative mortality was low, with only one death in 132 patients and 138 procedures.

## 6. Conclusions

A brain tumour is identified in one to three percent of non-febrile seizures that occur in a child. Meanwhile, seizures occur in between one in ten and one in five paediatric patients with a brain tumour, often as a presenting symptom. Most are associated with low-grade gliomas, like pilocytic astrocytoma, or with neuroglial tumours like ganglioglioma or dysembryoplastic neuroectodermal tumour (DNET). There is no empirical justification for initiating an anti-epileptic drug in a brain tumour patient without seizures, and some would restrict their use to those patients who experience at least two ictal episodes.

The cornerstone of management in most patients with a low-grade lesion is surgical resection, both because doing so often prolongs survival and reduces or eliminates seizures. Overall, almost 80% of children who undergo surgery to for resection of an epileptogenic brain tumour will attain prolonged seizure-freedom, and more than 90% will experience at least some meaningful clinical improvement, associated with a negligible risk of death in experienced surgical hands. Risks may be greater and results poorer in very small infants (under one year of age), but most-preschool children can undergo epilepsy-lesion resections safely and with benefit. Significant surgical complications occur in 10-20% of patients and include fluid and electrolyte imbalances, as well as typically short-lived neurological deficits in most patients, so that vigilant post-operative monitoring is essential.

Late post-operative seizure recurrence is an ominous sign that can be a harbinger of tumour recurrence, progression, or malignant transformation, as well as the appearance of new tumours, especially in patients with familial tumour syndromes like neurofibromatosis and tuberous sclerosis, and those who have received brain irradiation. When low-grade tumours recur and cause seizures, second resections may be effective at again controlling seizures.

These claims must be interpreted with caution, however, given that many essential questions remain unanswered — like whether more extensive epilepsy surgery is more effective or as safe as lesionectomy alone; and what factors best predict outcomes. In addition, with the emergence of new anti-epileptics, new anti-neoplastic treatments, and new surgical technologies, the management of epilepsy in children and adolescents with brain tumours appears to be rapidly changing.

| AED | Interactions with |
|---|---|
| Phenytoin | carboplain, cisplatin, cyclophosphamide, dacarbazine, erlotinib, etoposide, fluorouracil, ifosfamide, imatanib, irinotecan, carmustine, lomustine, paclitaxel, procarbazine, tegafur, teniposide, thiotepa, topotecan, vincristine |
| Carbamazepine | cisplatin, cyclophosphamide, erlotinib, etoposide, ifosfamide, imatinib, irinotecan, carmustine, lomustine, palitaxel, procarbazine*, teniposide, thiotepa, topotecan, vincristine |
| Phenobarbitol | cyclophosphamide, erlotinib, etoposide, ifosfamide, imatinib, irinotecan, carmustine, lomustine, paclitaxel, procarbazine, teniposide, thiotepa, topotecan, vincristine |
| Primidone | cyclophosphamide, erlotinib, etoposide, ifosfamide, imatinib, irinotecan, carmustine, lomustine, paclitaxel, procarbazine, teniposide, thiotepa, topotecan, vincristine |
| Valproic Acid | cisplatin, cyclophosphamide, vorinostat |

*Carbamazepine is contraindicated in patients on procarbazine

**Table 1.** Anti-epileptic drugs (AED) and their interactions with CNS anti-neoplastic drugs

| First Author | Year Published | # Subjects | Mean Age (y) | Age Range | Tumour Types | Surgical Procedure | # Total Resection | % Total Resection | Mean FU (mo) | # Seizure Free | % Seizure Free | # Improved | % Improved | # Peri-Op Deaths | # Surgical Compl. |
|---|---|---|---|---|---|---|---|---|---|---|---|---|---|---|---|
| Ramantani | 2014 | 29 | 11.7 | 2y - 17y | GG, DNET | L+E | 16 | 55.2% | 148 | 22 | 75.9% | 29 | 100.0% | 0 | 2 |
| Consales | 2013 | 22 | 6.5 | 10m - 16y | GG, DNET | L | 15 | 68.2% | 12 | 20 | 90.9% | 22 | 100.0% | 0 | 0 |
| Babini | 2013 | 30 | 12.1 | 3y - 18y | GG, DNET, PGNT | L, L+E | 30 | 100.0% | 85 | 26 | 86.7% | 30 | 100.0% | 0 | 1 |
| Fattal-Valevski* | 2013 | 54 | 7.1 | 1m - 19y | LGG, DNET | ? | ? | ? | 24 | 38 | 77.6% | 51 | 94.4% | 0 | 4 |
| Jo | 2013 | 9 | 2.7 | 6m - 5y | GG(2), AC(2), ODG, DNT, PNET, CPP, CP | L | 7 | 77.8% | 63 | 7 | 77.8% | 9 | 100.0% | 0 | 0 |
| Uliel-Sibony | 2011 | 41 | 8.2 | 1y - 18y | LGG, DNET | L, L+A | 35 | 85.4% | 62 | 34 | 82.9% | 36 | 87.8% | 0 | 2 |
| Gelinas | 2011 | 67 | 9.1 | 3m - 16y | 43 LGG, 11 DNET; 14 other | L vs. L=ECoG | 65 | 97.0% | 12 | 52 | 77.6% | ? | ? | 0 | 13 |
| Spalice | 2010 | 13 | 6.7 | 1y - 14y | DNET | L+E | 12 | 92.3% | 78 | 13 | 100.0% | 13 | 100.0% | 0 | 1 |
| Ogiwara | 2010 | 30 | 8.6 | 9m - 16y | GG | L, L+E | 29 | 96.7% | 62 | 27 | 90.0% | 30 | 100.0% | 0 | 2 |
| Bilginer | 2009 | 29 | 10.7 | 3y - 21y | DNET | TL ± AHC | ? | ? | 52 | 27 | 93.1% | 29 | 100.0% | 0 | ? |
| Lee | 2009 | 22 | 12.4 | 3y - 18y | DNET | L ± L | 22 | 100.0% | 44 | 20 | 90.9% | 22 | 100.0% | 0 | 1 |
| Gaggero | 2009 | 20 | 1.5 | 1m - 3y | Grade I(5), II(4), III(7), IV(4) | L | 14 | 70.0% | 48 | 11 | 55.0% | 18 | 90.0% | 0 | ? |
| Minkin | 2008 | 24 | 8.9 | 1y - 15y | DNET | L | 21 | 87.5% | 80 | 20 | 83.3% | 24 | 100.0% | 0 | 9 |
| Kan*** | 2008 | 16 | ? | 2y - 21y | GG, DNET, LGG | L+E | ? | ? | (1 - 8 y) | 13 | 81.3% | 15 | 93.8% | 0 | ? |
| Khan | 2006 | 55 | 9.3 | 2m - 18y | LGG, DNET, ODG | L | 32 | 58.2% | 54 | 46 | 83.6% | 50 | 90.9% | 0 | ? |
| Cataltepe | 2005 | 29 | 10.5 | 2y - 18y | GG, DNET, AC (T) | L, L+L+A, L+L | 18 | 62.1% | 31 | 20 | 69.0% | 24 | 82.8% | 0 | 5 |
| Sandberg | 2005 | 18 | 9.6 | 1m - 13y | DNET | L ± mapping | 18 | 100.0% | 19 | 18 | 100.0% | 18 | 100.0% | 0 | 1 |
| Giulioni | 2005 | 15 | 12.6 | 3y - 18y | GG, DNET | L | 13 | 86.7% | 67 | 13 | 86.7% | 15 | 100.0% | 0 | 2 |
| Nolan | 2004 | 26 | 10.0 | 4y - 18y | DNET | ? | 11 | 42.3% | 52 | 16 | 61.5% | 25 | 96.2% | 0 | ? |
| Im** | 2002 | 18 | 9.2 | 1y - 16y | GG | L | 14 | 77.8% | 43 | 15 | 83.3% | 18 | 100.0% | 0 | ? |
| Kim | 2001 | 23 | 7.9 | 8m - 15y | DNET, ODG, GG | L, L+E | 14 | 60.9% | 43 | 16 | 69.6% | 21 | 91.3% | 0 | 7 |
| Ianelli* | 2000 | 37 | 9.1 | 1y - 15y | LGG (31), HGG (6) | L, L+A, L+L | 22 | 59.5% | 72 | 26 | 81.3% | 37 | 100.0% | 0 | 3 |
| Khajavi | 1999 | 34 | 12.6 | 1.5y - 18y | GG, LGG, DNET | L, lobectomy | 28 | 82.4% | 43 | 25 | 73.5% | 29 | 85.3% | 0 | 5 |
| Razach | 1998 | 10 | 11.2 | 1y - 16y | ODG/mixed ODG/AC | L | 3 | 30.0% | 40 | ? | ? | 3 | 30.0% | 0 | ? |
| Kim | 1995 | 10 | 9.8 | 1y - 15y | 5 ODG, 3 LGG, PNET, vasc | L | 4 | 40.0% | 40 | 6 | 60.0% | 9 | 90.0% | 0 | ? |
| Packer | 1994 | 60 | 10.6 | 1y - 20y | LGG, GG | L, L+E | 47 | 78.3% | 24 | 45 | 75.0% | 47 | 78.3% | 0 | ? |
| TOTALS | | 741 | 9.1 | 1m - 19y | | | 490 | 66.1% | 51.9 | 576 | 77.7% | 624 | 92.6% | 0 | 58 |
| | | | | | | | | | | | | | | 0.0% | 7.8% |
| | | | | | | | | | | | | | | Adjusted = | 11.7% |

* some patients died before final seizure assessment; ** three patients underwent a second resection; *** these 16 patients part of a larger series with other seizure aetiologies included

GG = ganglioglioma; DNET = dysembryoplastic neuroepithelial tumour; PGNT = papillary glioneuronal tumour; LGG = low-grade glioma; ODG = oligodendroglioma; AC = astrocytoma; CPP = choroid plexus papilloma; CP = craniopharyngioma

L = lesionectomy; L+E = lesionectomy + additional resection of adjacent epileptogenic tissue; L+A = lesionectomy + amygdylohypocampectomy; L+L = lesionectomy + lobectomy;

TL = temporal lobectomy; L+L+A = lesionectomy + lobectomy + amygdylohypocampectomy; AHC = amygdylohypocampectomy; (T) = all temporal lesions

? = missing data

* Some patients died before final seizure assessment; ** Three patients underwent a second reaction; *** These 16 patients part of a larger series with other seizure aetiologies included

GG=ganglioglioma; DNET=dysembryoplastic neuroepithelial tumor; PGNT=papillary glioneuronal tumor; LGG=low-grade glioma; ODG=oligodendroglioma; AC=astrocytoma; CPP=choroid plexus papilloma; CP=craniopharyngioma; L=lesionectomy; L+E=lesionectomy+additional resection of adjacent epileptogenic tissue; L+A=lesionectomy+amygdylohypocampectomy; L+L=lesionectomy+lobectomy; TL=temporal lobectomy; L+L+A=lesionectomy+lobectomy+amygdylohypocampectomy; AHC=amygdylohypocampectomy; (T)=all temporal lesions

**Table 2.** Seizure response to surgical resection of epileptogenic tumor

| First Author | Year Published | # Subjects | Mean Age (y) | Age Range | Tumour Types | Surgical Procedure | # Total Resection | % Total Resection | Mean FU (mo) | # Seizure Free | % Seizure Free | # Improved | % Improved | # Peri-Op Deaths | # Surgical Compl. |
|---|---|---|---|---|---|---|---|---|---|---|---|---|---|---|---|
| Spalice | 2010 | 13 | 6.7 | 1y - 14y | DNET | L+E | 12 | 92.3% | 78 | 13 | 100.0% | 13 | 100.0% | 0 | 1 |
| Bilginer | 2009 | 29 | 10.7 | 3y - 21y | DNET | TL ± AHC | ? | ? | 52 | 27 | 93.1% | 29 | 100.0% | 0 | ? |
| Lee | 2009 | 22 | 12.4 | 3y - 18y | DNET | L ± L | 22 | 100.0% | 44 | 20 | 90.9% | 22 | 100.0% | 0 | 1 |
| Minkin | 2008 | 24 | 8.9 | 1y - 15y | DNET | L | 21 | 87.5% | 80 | 20 | 83.3% | 24 | 100.0% | 0 | 9 |
| Sandberg | 2005 | 18 | 9.6 | 1m - 13y | DNET | L ± mapping | 18 | 100.0% | 19 | 18 | 100.0% | 18 | 100.0% | 0 | 1 |
| Nolan | 2004 | 26 | 10.0 | 4y - 18y | DNET | ? | 11 | 42.3% | 52 | 16 | 61.5% | 25 | 96.2% | 0 | ? |
| | | 132 | 9.7 | | | | 84 | 81.6% | 54.2 | 114 | 86.4% | 131 | 99.2% | 0 | 12 |
| | | | | | | | | | | | | | | | 15.6% |

**Table 3.** Seizure response to surgical resection of dysembroplastic neuroectodermal tumors

| First Author | Year Published | # Subjects | Mean Age (y) | Age Range | Tumour Types | Surgical Procedure | # Total Resection | % Total Resection | Mean FU (mo) | # Seizure Free | % Seizure Free | # Improved | % Improved | # Peri-Op Deaths | # Surgical Compl. |
|---|---|---|---|---|---|---|---|---|---|---|---|---|---|---|---|
| Kim | 2008 | 134 | 8.5 | 8m - 18y | various, incl. vasc. | various | ? | ? | 62 | 93 | 69.4% | 109 | 81.3% | 0 | 23 |
| Cuccia | 2003 | 15 | 10.5 | 4.5y - 19y | SEGA (+TS) | L | 12 | 80.0% | 52 | 0 | 0.0% | 0 | 0.0% | 0 | 6 |
| Sonderkaer | 2003 | 18 | ? | ? | various | ? | ? | #VALUE! | 128 | 10 | 55.6% | ? | ? | ? | ? |
| Borgeois | 1999 | 171 | 8.3 | 10m - 15y | ~40 vascular, etc | various | ? | ? | 62 | 139 | 81.3% | 158 | 92.4% | 0 | 44 |

vasc. = vascular lesion; SEGA = subependymal giant cell astrocytoma; TS = tuberous sclerosis; FU = follow-up

Vasc=vascular lesions; SEGA=subependymal cell astrocytoma; TS=tuberous sclerosis; FU=follow-up

**Table 4.** Seizure response to surgical resection of epileptogenic tumor – studies including vascular lesions

| First | Year | # | Mean | # |
|---|---|---|---|---|
| Author | Published | Subjects | Age (y)* | Seizure Free |
| Benifla | 2006 | 12 | 13.5 | 7 |
| Chae | 2001 | 1 | 0.3 | 1 |
| Gonzalez-Martinez | 2007 | 57 | 24.7 | 22 |
| Im | 2002 | 3 | 16.5 | 3 |
| Jooma | 1995 | 8 | 24.0 | 5 |
| Lombardi | 1997 | 1 | ? | 1 |
| Ojemann | 2012 | 4 | 8.5 | 2 |
| Steinbok | 2009 | 24 | 1.5 | 12 |
| Tian | 2011 | 9 | 13.7 | 3 |
| Whittle | 1995 | 4 | 36.0 | 0 |
| Totals | | 123 | | 56 |
| Mean | | | 15.4 | |
| Percentages | | | | 45.5% |

**Table 5.** Seizure response to a second surgical resection

## Author details

Adrianna Ranger[1*] and David Diosy[2]

*Address all correspondence to: aranger@uwo.ca

1 Department of Clinical Neurological Sciences, Division of Neurosurgery, Children's Hospital-London Health Sciences Center, Western University, London, Ontario, Canada

2 Department of Clinical Neurological Sciences, Division of Neurology, London Health Sciences Center, Western University, London, Ontario, Canada

## References

[1] Centers for Disease Control and Prevention (CDC). Trends in childhood cancer mortality--United States, 1990-2004. *MMWR Morb Mortal Wkly Rep.* 2007;56:1257-1261.

[2] Centers for Disease Control and Prevention (CDC): Trends in childhood cancer mortality--United States, 1990-2004. *MMWR Morb Mortal Wkly Rep.* 2007;56:1257-1261.

[3] Ellison LF, De P, Mery LS, Grundy PE. Canadian Cancer Society's Steering Committee for Canadian Cancer Statistics.: Canadian cancer statistics at a glance: cancer in children. *CMAJ.* 2009;180:422-424.

[4] Linet MS, Ries LA, Smith MA, Tarone RE, Devesa SS. Cancer surveillance series: recent trends in childhood cancer incidence and mortality in the United States. *J Natl Cancer Inst.* 1999;91:1051-1058.

[5] Bunin GR, Feuer EJ, Witman PA, Meadows AT. Increasing incidence of childhood cancer: report of 20 years experience from the greater Delaware Valley Pediatric Tumor Registry. *Paediatr Perinat Epidemiol.* 1996;10:319-338.

[6] Gurney, J. G., Smith, M. A., and Bunin, G. R. CNS and miscellaneous intra-cranial and intraspinal neoplasms. SEER Pediatric Monograph, National Cancer Institute, 51-63. 2001. Ref Type: Serial (Book,Monograph)

[7] National Cancer Institute. A Snapshot of Pediatric Cancers: Incidence on Mortality Rate Trends. 2011. Ref Type: Report

[8] Ellison LF, De P, Mery LS, Grundy PE, Canadian Cancer Society's Steering Committee for Canadian Cancer Statistics. Canadian cancer statistics at a glance: cancer in children. *CMAJ 2009 Feb 17;180(4):422-4.* 2009;180:422-424.

[9] Rendón-Macías ME, Ramos-Becerril C, Bernardez-Zapata I, Iglesias-Leboreiro J. [Cancer epidemiology in children and adolescents at private health care (1995-2004)] [Article in Spanish]. *Rev Med Inst Mex Seguro Soc.* 2008;46:353-360.

[10] Brain Tumor Facts. American Brain Tumor Association. 2012. Ref Type: Electronic Citation

[11] Dolecek TA, Propp JM, Stroup NE, Kruchko C. CBTRUS statistical report: primary brain and central nervous system tumors diagnosed in the United States in 2005-2009. *Neuro Oncol.* 2012;14:1-49.

[12] Sievert AJ, Fisher MJ. Pediatric low-grade gliomas. *J Child Neurol.* 2009;24:1397-1408.

[13] Qaddoumi I, Sultan I, Gajjar A. Outcome and prognostic features in pediatric gliomas: a review of 6212 cases from the Surveillance, Epidemiology, and End Results database. *Cancer.* 2009;115:5761-5770.

[14] Taylor MD, Sanford RA, Boop FA. Cerebellar pilocytic astrocytomas. In: Albright AL, Pollack IF, Adelson PD, eds. *Principles and Practice of Pediatric Neurosurgery.* New York: Thieme Medical pUBLISHERS, iNC.; 2008:655-67.

[15] Sato I, Higuchi A, Yanagisawa T et al. Impact of Late Effects on Health-Related Quality of Life in Survivors of Pediatric Brain Tumors: Motility Disturbance of Limb(s), Seizure, Ocular/Visual Impairment, Endocrine Abnormality, and Higher Brain Dysfunction. *Cancer Nurs 2014 Mar 13 [Epub ahead of print].* 2014.

[16] Huang LT, Hsiao CC, Weng HH, Lui CC. Neurologic complications of pediatric systemic malignancies. *J Formos Med Assoc.* 1996;95:209-212.

[17] Lovely MP. Symptom management of brain tumor patients. *Semin Oncol Nurs.* 2004;20:273-283.

[18] Packer RJ, Gurney JG, Punyko JA et al. Long-term neurologic and neurosensory sequelae in adult survivors of a childhood brain tumor: childhood cancer survivor study. *J Clin Oncol.* 2003;21:3255-3261.

[19] Shields LB, Choucair AK. Management of Low-Grade Gliomas: A Review of Patient-Perceived Quality of Life and Neurocognitive Outcome. *World Neurosurg 2014 Feb 19 pii: S1878-8750(14)00164-8 doi: 10 1016/j wneu 2014 02 033 [Epub ahead of print].* 2014.

[20] Vargo M. Brain tumor rehabilitation. *Am J Phys Med Rehabil.* 2011;90:S50-S62.

[21] Sato I, Higuchi A, Yanagisawa T et al. Impact of Late Effects on Health-Related Quality of Life in Survivors of Pediatric Brain Tumors: Motility Disturbance of Limb(s), Seizure, Ocular/Visual Impairment, Endocrine Abnormality, and Higher Brain Dysfunction. *Cancer Nurs [Epub ahead of print].* 2014.

[22] Armstrong GT. Long-term survivors of childhood central nervous system malignancies: the experience of the Childhood Cancer Survivor Study. *Eur J Paediatr Neurol.* 2010;14:298-303.

[23] Klein M, Engelberts NH, van der Ploeg HM et al. Epilepsy in low-grade gliomas: the impact on cognitive function and quality of life. *Ann Neurol.* 2003;54:514-520.

[24] Maschio M, Dinapoli L. Patients with brain tumor-related epilepsy. *J Neurooncol.* 2012;109:1-6.

[25] Maschio M, Sperati F, Dinapoli L et al. Weight of epilepsy in brain tumor patients. *J Neurooncol.* 2014;118:385-393.

[26] Riva M. Brain tumoral epilepsy: a review. *Neurol Sci.* 2005;26 Suppl 1:S42.

[27] Ruda R, Trevisan E, Soffietti R. Epilepsy and brain tumors. *Curr Opin Oncol.* 2010;22:611-620.

[28] Thom M, Blumcke I, Aronica E. Long-term epilepsy-associated tumors. *Brain Pathol.* 2012;22:350-379.

[29] Ullrich NJ. Neurologic sequelae of brain tumors in children. *J Child Neurol.* 2009;24:1446-1454.

[30] Wells EM, Gaillard WD, Packer RJ. Pediatric brain tumors and epilepsy. *Semin Pediatr Neurol.* 2012;19:3-8.

[31] Brinkman TM, Liptak CC, Delaney BL, Chordas CA, Muriel AC, Manley PE. Suicide ideation in pediatric and adult survivors of childhood brain tumors. *J Neurooncol.* 2013;113:425-432.

[32] Shady JA, Black PM, Kupsky WJ et al. Seizures in children with supratentorial astroglial neoplasms. *Pediatr Neurosurg.* 1994;21:23-30.

[33] Backus RE, Millichap JP. The seizure as a manifestation of intracranial tumor in childhood. *Pediatrics.* 1962;29:978-984.

[34] Blume WT, Girvin JP, Kaufmann JC. Childhood brain tumors presenting as chronic uncontrolled focal seizure disorders. *Ann Neurol.* 1982;12:538-541.

[35] Gaggero R, Consales A, Fazzini F et al. Epilepsy associated with supratentorial brain tumors under 3 years of life. *Epilepsy Res.* 2009;87:184-189.

[36] Gaillard WD, Chiron C, Cross JH et al. Guidelines for imaging infants and children with recent-onset epilepsy. *Epilepsia.* 2009;50:2147-2153.

[37] Ibrahim K, Appleton R. Seizures as the presenting symptom of brain tumours in children. *Seizure.* 2004;13:108-112.

[38] Martinez-Lage JF, Perez-Espejo MA, Esteban JA, Poza M. Thalamic tumors: clinical presentation. *Childs Nerv Syst.* 2002;18:405-411.

[39] Rutledge SL, Snead OC3, Morawetz R, Chandra-Sekar B. Brain tumors presenting as a seizure disorder in infants. *J Child Neurol.* 1987;2:214-219.

[40] Sjors K, Blennow G, Lantz G. Seizures as the presenting symptom of brain tumors in children. *Acta Paediatr.* 1993;82:66-70.

[41] Sun DC, Shen EY, Wong TT. Epilepsy as the sole manifestation of brain tumor--report of two cases. *Zhonghua Min Guo Xiao Er Ke Yi Xue Hui Za Zhi.* 1995;36:142-145.

[42] Williams BA, Abbott KJ, Manson JI. Cerebral tumors in children presenting with epilepsy. *J Child Neurol.* 1992;7:291-294.

[43] Klitbo DM, Nielsen R, Illum NO, Wehner PS, Carlsen N. Symptoms and time to diagnosis in children with brain tumours. *Dan Med Bull.* 2011;58:A4285.

[44] Shamji MF, Fric-Shamji EC, Benoit BG. Brain tumors and epilepsy: pathophysiology of peritumoral changes. *Neurosurg Rev.* 2009;32:275-284.

[45] Coppola G, Spagnoli D, Sciscio N, Russo F, Villani RM. Gelastic seizures and low-grade hypothalamic astrocytoma: a case report. *Brain Dev.* 2002;24:183-186.

[46] Chae JH, Kim SK, Wang KC, Kim KJ, Hwang YS, Cho BK. Hemifacial seizure of cerebellar ganglioglioma origin: seizure control by tumor resection. *Epilepsia.* 2001;42:1204-1247.

[47] Ho CH, Chen SJ, Juan CJ, Lee HS, Tsai SH, Fan HC. Sudden death due to medulloblastoma: a case report. *Acta Neurol Taiwan.* 2013;22:76-80.

[48] Berger MS, Ghatan S, Geyer JR, Keles GE, Ojemann GA. Seizure outcome in children with hemispheric tumors and associated intractable epilepsy: the role of tumor removal combined with seizure foci resection. *Pediatr Neurosurg.* 1991;17:185-191.

[49] Berger MS. Functional mapping-guided resection of low-grade gliomas. *Clin Neurosurg.* 1995;42:437-452.

[50] Chang EF, Clark A, Smith JS et al. Functional mapping-guided resection of low-grade gliomas in eloquent areas of the brain: improvement of long-term survival. Clinical article. *J Neurosurg.* 2011;114:566-573.

[51] Fattal-Valevski A, Nissan N, Kramer U, Constantini S. Seizures as the clinical presenting symptom in children with brain tumors. *J Child Neurol.* 2013;28:292-296.

[52] Consales A, Striano P, Nozza P et al. Glioneuronal tumors and epilepsy in children: seizure outcome related to lesionectomy. *Minerva Pediatr.* 2013;65:609-616.

[53] Gump WC, Skjei KL, Karkare SN. Seizure control after subtotal lesional resection. *Neurosurg Focus.* 2013;34:E1.

[54] Babini M, Giulioni M, Galassi E et al. Seizure outcome of surgical treatment of focal epilepsy associated with low-grade tumors in children. *J Neurosurg Pediatr.* 2013;11:214-223.

[55] Jo KI, Shin HJ, Hong SC. Seizure outcomes of lesionectomy in pediatric lesional epilepsy with brain tumor--single institute experience. *Brain Dev.* 2013;35:810-815.

[56] Kim YH, Park CK, Kim TH et al. Seizures during the management of high-grade gliomas: clinical relevance to disease progression. *J Neurooncol.* 2013;113:101-109.

[57] Chaichana KL, Parker SL, Oliva A, Quinones-Hinojosa A. Long-term seizure outcomes in adult patients undergoing primary resection of malignant brain astrocytomas. Clinical article. *J Neurosurg.* 2009;111:282-292.

[58] Chang EF, Potts MB, Keles GE et al. Seizure characteristics and control following resection in 332 patients with low-grade gliomas. *J Neurosurg.* 2008;108:227-235.

[59] Das RR, Artsy E, Hurwitz S et al. Outcomes after discontinuation of antiepileptic drugs after surgery in patients with low grade brain tumors and meningiomas. *J Neurooncol.* 2012;107:565-570.

[60] Luyken C, Blumcke I, Fimmers R et al. The spectrum of long-term epilepsy-associated tumors: long-term seizure and tumor outcome and neurosurgical aspects. *Epilepsia.* 2003;44:822-830.

[61] Minkin K, Klein O, Mancini J, Lena G. Surgical strategies and seizure control in pediatric patients with dysembryoplastic neuroepithelial tumors: a single-institution experience. *J Neurosurg Pediatr.* 2008;1:206-210.

[62] Nolan MA, Sakuta R, Chuang N et al. Dysembryoplastic neuroepithelial tumors in childhood: long-term outcome and prognostic features. *Neurology.* 2004;62:2270-2276.

[63] Ogiwara H, Nordi DR, DiPatri AJ, Alden TD, Bowman RM, Tomita T. Pediatric epileptogenic gangliogliomas: seizure outcome and surgical results. *J Neurosurg Pediatr.* 2010;5:271-276.

[64] Ray WZ, Blackburn SL, Casavilca-Zambrano S et al. Clinicopathologic features of recurrent dysembryoplastic neuroepithelial tumor and rare malignant transformation: a report of 5 cases and review of the literature. *J Neurooncol.* 2009;94:283-292.

[65] Smits A, Duffau H. Seizures and the natural history of World Health Organization Grade II gliomas: a review. *Neurosurgery.* 2011;68:1326-1333.

[66] Tandon N, Esquenazi Y. Resection strategies in tumoral epilepsy: is a lesionectomy enough? *Epilepsia.* 2013;54:72-78.

[67] Hammond RR, Duggal N, Woulfe JM, Girvin JP. Malignant transformation of a dysembryoplastic neuroepithelial tumor. Case report. *J Neurosurg.* 2000;92:722-725.

[68] Unal E, Koksal Y, Cimen O, Paksoy Y, Tavli L. Malignant glioblastomatous transformation of a low-grade glioma in a child. *Childs Nerv Syst.* 2008;24:1385-1389.

[69] Schaller B, Ruegg SJ. Brain tumor and seizures: pathophysiology and its implications for treatment revisited. *Epilepsia.* 2003;44:1223-1232.

[70] Ruda R, Bello L, Duffau H, Soffietti R. Seizures in low-grade gliomas: natural history, pathogenesis, and outcome after treatments. *Neuro Oncol.* 2012;14:iv55-iv64.

[71] van Breemen M, Wilms EB, Vecht CJ. Epilepsy in patients with brain tumours: epidemiology, mechanisms, and management. *Lancet Neurol.* 2007;6:421-430.

[72] Calatozzolo C, Pollo B, Botturi A et al. Multidrug resistance proteins expression in glioma patients with epilepsy. *J Neurooncol.* 2012;110:129-135.

[73] Alkonyi B, Mittal S, Zitron I et al. Increased tryptophan transport in epileptogenic dysembryoplastic neuroepithelial tumors. *J Neurooncol.* 2012;107:365-372.

[74] You G, Sha Z, Jiang T. The pathogenesis of tumor-related epilepsy and its implications for clinical treatment. *Seizure.* 2012;21:153-159.

[75] Berntsson SG, Malmer B, Bondy ML, Qu M, Smits A. Tumor-associated epilepsy and glioma: are there common genetic pathways? *Acta Oncol.* 2009;48:955-963.

[76] Lee JW, Wen PY, Hurwitz S et al. Morphological characteristics of brain tumors causing seizures. *Arch Neurol.* 2010;67:336-342.

[77] Whittle IR, Beaumont A. Seizures in patients with supratentorial oligodendroglial tumours. Clinicopathological features and management considerations. *Acta Neurochir (Wien).* 1995;135:19-24.

[78] Rosati A, Tomassini A, Pollo B et al. Epilepsy in cerebral glioma: timing of appearance and histological correlations. *J Neurooncol.* 2009;93:395-400.

[79] Kramer U, Nevo Y, Reider-Groswasser I et al. Neuroimaging of children with partial seizures. *Seizure.* 1998;7:115-118.

[80] Harvey AS, Cross JH, Shinnar S, Mathern GW, ILAE Pediatric Epilepsy Surgery Survey Taskforce. Defining the spectrum of international practice in pediatric epilepsy surgery patients. *Epilepsia.* 2008;49:146-155.

[81] Perucca E. Optimizing antiepileptic drug treatment in tumoral epilepsy. *Epilepsia.* 2013;54:97-104.

[82] Khan RB, Hunt DL, Boop FA et al. Seizures in children with primary brain tumors: incidence and long-term outcome. *Epilepsy Res.* 2005;64:85-91.

[83] Sogawa Y, Kan L, Levy AS, Maytal J, Shinnar S. The use of antiepileptic drugs in pediatric brain tumor patients. *Pediatr Neurol.* 2009;41:192-194.

[84] Dagcinar A, Bayrakli F, Yapicier O, Ozek M. Primary meningeal osteosarcoma of the brain during childhood. Case report. *J Neurosurg Pediatr.* 2008;1:325-329.

[85] Fulton SP, Clarke DF, Wheless JW, Ellison DW, Ogg R, Boop FA. Angiocentric glioma-induced seizures in a 2-year-old child. *J Child Neurol.* 2009;24:852-856.

[86] Iannelli A, Guzzetta F, Battaglia D, Iuvone L, Di Rocco C. Surgical treatment of temporal tumors associated with epilepsy in children. *Pediatr Neurosurg.* 2000;32:248-254.

[87] Bromfield EB. Epilepsy in patients with brain tumors and other cancers. *Rev Neurol Dis.* 2004;1:S27-S33.

[88] Wallace D, Ruban D, Kanner A et al. Temporal lobe gangliogliomas associated with chronic epilepsy: long-term surgical outcomes. *Clin Neurol Neurosurg.* 2013;115:472-476.

[89] Shamji MF, Vassilyada M, Lam CH, Montes JL, Farmer JP. Congenital tumors of the central nervous system: the MCH experience. *Pediatr Neurosurg.* 2009;45:368-374.

[90] Khan RB, Boop FA, Onar A, Sanford RA. Seizures in children with low-grade tumors: outcome after tumor resection and risk factors for uncontrolled seizures. *J Neurosurg.* 2006;104:377-382.

[91] Lynam LM, Lyons MK, Drazkowski JF et al. Frequency of seizures in patients with newly diagnosed brain tumors: a retrospective review. *Clin Neurol Neurosurg.* 2007;109:634-638.

[92] Ruda R, Trevisan E, Soffietti R. Low-grade gliomas. *Handb Clin Neurol.* 2012;105:437-450.

[93] Englot DJ, Berger MS, Barbaro NM, Chang EF. Predictors of seizure freedom after resection of supratentorial low-grade gliomas. A review. *J Neurosurg.* 2011;115:240-244.

[94] Spalice A, Ruggieri M, Grosso S et al. Dysembryoplastic neuroepithelial tumors: a prospective clinicopathologic and outcome study of 13 children. *Pediatr Neurol.* 2010;43:395-402.

[95] Karremann M, Pietsch T, Janssen G, Kramm CM, Wolff JE. Anaplastic ganglioglioma in children. *J Neurooncol.* 2009;92:157-163.

[96] Razack N, Baumgartner J, Bruner J. Pediatric oligodendrogliomas. *Pediatr Neurosurg.* 1998;28:121-129.

[97] Wang KC, Chi JG, Cho BK. Oligodendroglioma in childhood. *J Korean Med Sci.* 1993;8:110-116.

[98] Lehman NL, Jordan MA, Huhn SL et al. Cortical ependymoma. A case report and review. *Pediatr Neurosurg.* 2003;39:50-54.

[99] Cuccia V, Zuccaro G, Sosa F, Monges J, Lubienieky F, Taratuto AL. Subependymal giant cell astrocytoma in children with tuberous sclerosis. *Childs Nerv Syst.* 2003;19:232-243.

[100] Amirjamshidi A, Mehrazin M, Abbassioun K. Meningiomas of the central nervous system occurring below the age of 17: report of 24 cases not associated with neurofibromatosis and review of literature. *Childs Nerv Syst.* 2000;16:406-416.

[101] Goldsby RE, Liu Q, Nathan PC et al. Late-occurring neurologic sequelae in adult survivors of childhood acute lymphoblastic leukemia: a report from the Childhood Cancer Survivor Study. *J Clin Oncol.* 2010;28:324-331.

[102] Karikari O, Thomas KK, Lagoo A, Cummings TJ, George TM. Primary cerebral ALK-1-positive anaplastic large cell lymphoma in a child. Case report and literature review. *Pediatr Neurosurg.* 2007;43:516-521.

[103] Astigarraga I, Lejarretta R, Navajas A, Fernandez-Teijeiro A, Imaz I, Bezanilla JL. Secondary central nervous system metastases in children with neuroblastoma. *Med Pediatr Oncol.* 1996;27:529-533.

[104] Lopez-Castilla J, Diaz-Fernandez F, Soult JA, Munoz M, Barriga R. Primary leptomeningeal melanoma in a child. *Pediatr Neurol.* 2001;24:390-392.

[105] Postovsky S, Ash S, Ramu IN et al. Central nervous system involvement in children with sarcoma. *Oncology.* 2003;65:118-124.

[106] Postovsky S, Moaed B, Krivoy E, Ofir R, Ben Arush MW. Practice of palliative sedation in children with brain tumors and sarcomas at the end of life. *Pediatr Hematol Oncol.* 2007;24:409-415.

[107] Shuper A, Cohen IJ, Mor C, Ash S, Kornreich L, Zaizov R. Metastatic brain involvement in Ewing family of tumors in children. *Neurology.* 1998;51:1336-1338.

[108] Spunt SL, Walsh MF, Krasin MJ et al. Brain metastases of malignant germ cell tumors in children and adolescents. *Cancer.* 2004;101:620-626.

[109] Kargiotis O, Markoula S, Kyritsis AP. Epilepsy in the cancer patient. *Cancer Chemother Pharmacol.* 2011;67:489-501.

[110] Hughlings-Jackson J. Localised convulsions from tumour of the brain. *Brain.* 1882;5:364-374.

[111] Jackson JH. Localized convulsions from tumors of the brain. *Brain.* 1882;36:4-374.

[112] Loiacono G, Cirillo C, Chiarelli F, Verrotti A. Focal epilepsy associated with glioneuronal tumors. *ISRN Neurol 2011:867503 doi: 10 5402/2011/867503 Epub 2011 Jul 7.* 2011.

[113] Rossetti AO, Stupp R. Epilepsy in brain tumor patients. *Curr Opin Neurol.* 2010;23:603-609.

[114] White JC, Liu CT, Mixter WJ. Focal epilepsy; a statistical study of its causes and the results of surgical treatment; epilepsy secondary to intracranial tumors. *N Engl J Med.* 1948;238:891-899.

[115] Zaatreh MM, Firlik KS, Spencer DD, Spencer SS. Temporal lobe tumoral epilepsy: characteristics and predictors of surgical outcome. *Neurology.* 2003;61:636-641.

[116] Consales A, Striano P, Nozza P et al. Glioneuronal tumors and epilepsy inchildren:seizureoutcome related to lesionectomy. *Minerva Pediatr.* 2013;65:609-616.

[117] Kim SK, Wang KC, Hwang YS et al. Epilepsy surgery in children: outcomes and complications. *J Neurosurg Pediatr.* 2008;1:277-283.

[118] Hirsch JF, Sainte Rose C, Pierre-Kahn A, Pfister A, Hoppe-Hirsch E. Benign astrocytic and oligodendrocytic tumors of the cerebral hemispheres in children. *J Neurosurg.* 1989;70:568-572.

[119] Luat AF, Behen ME, Juhasz C, Sood S, Chugani HT. Secondary tics or tourettism associated with a brain tumor. *Pediatr Neurol.* 2009;41:457-460.

[120] Goh KY, Conway EJ, DaRosso RC, Muszynski CA, Epstein FJ. Sympathetic storms in a child with a midbrain glioma: a variant of diencephalic seizures. *Pediatr Neurol.* 1999;21:742-744.

[121] Hottinger AF, Khakoo Y. Neuro-oncology of Neurofibromatosis Type 1. *Curr Treat Options Neurol.* 2009;11:306-314.

[122] Lu-Emerson C, Plotkin SR. The neurofibromatoses. Part 2: NF2 and schwannomatosis. *Rev Neurol Dis.* 2009;6:E81-E86.

[123] Goh S, Butler W, Thiele EA. Subependymal giant cell tumors in tuberous sclerosis complex. *Neurology.* 2004;63:1457-1461.

[124] Ferner RE, Huson SM, Thomas N et al. Guidelines for the diagnosis and management of individuals with neurofibromatosis 1. *J Med Genet.* 2007;44:81-8.

[125] Hou JW, Wang PJ, Wang TR. Tuberous sclerosis in children. *Zhonghua Min Guo Xiao Er Ke Yi Xue Hui Za Zhi.* 1994;35:102-107.

[126] Roaches ES, Gomez MR, Northrup H. Tuberous sclerosis complex consensus conference: revised clinical diagnostic criteria. *J Child Neurol.* 1998;13:624-628.

[127] Guerrini R, Rosati A, Giordano F, Genitori L, Barba C. The medical and surgical treatment of tumoral seizures: current and future perspectives. *Epilepsia.* 2013;54:84-90.

[128] Jansky J, Kovacs N, Gyimesi C, Fogarasi A, Doczi T, Wiebe S. Epilepsy surgery, antiepileptic drug trials, and the role of evidence. *Epilepsia.* 2010;51:1004-1009.

[129] Kumar A, Juhasz C, Asano E, Sood S, Muzik O, Chugani HT. Objective detection of epileptic foci by 18F-FDG PET in children undergoing epilepsy surgery. *J Nucl Med.* 2010;51:1901-1907.

[130] Maytal J, Krauss JM, Novak G, Nagelberg J, Patel M. The role of brain computed tomography in evaluating children with new onset of seizures in the emergency department. *Epilepsia.* 2000;41:950-954.

[131] Prabhu VC, Khaldi A, Barton KP et al. Management of diffuse low-grade cerebral gliomas. *Neurol Clin.* 2010;28:1037-1059.

[132] Sandberg DI, Ragheb J, Dunoyer C, Bhatia S, Olavarria G, Morrison G. Surgical outcomes and seizure control rates after resection of dysembryoplastic neuroepithelial tumors. *Neurosurg Focus.* 2005;18:E5.

[133] Spooner CG, Berkovic SF, Mitchell LA, Wrennal JA, Harvey AS. New-onset temporal lobe epilepsy in children: lesion on MRI predicts poor seizure outcome. *Neurology.* 2006;67:2147-2153.

[134] Taheri MR, Krauthamer A, Otjen J, Khanna PC, Ishak GE. Neuroimaging of migrational disorders in pediatric epilepsy. *Curr Probl Diagn Radiol.* 2012;41:11-19.

[135] Hardasmalani MD, Saber M. Yield of diagnostic studies in children presenting with complex febrile seizures. *Pediatr Emerg Care.* 2012;28:789-791.

[136] Lote K, Egeland T, Hager B et al. Survival, prognostic factors, and therapeutic efficacy in low-grade glioma: a retrospective study in 379 patients. *J Clin Oncol.* 1997;15:3129-3140.

[137] Recinos PF, Sciubba DM, Jallo GI. Brainstem tumors: where are we today? *Pediatr Neurosurg.* 2007;43:192-201.

[138] Shuper A, Kornreich L, Loven D, Michowitz S, Schwartz S, Cohen IJ. Diffuse brain stem gliomas. Are we improving outcome? *Childs Nerv Syst.* 1998;14:578-581.

[139] Freeman CR, Farmer JP. Pediatric brain stem gliomas: a review. *Int J Radiat Oncol Biol Phys.* 1998;40:265-271.

[140] van Breeman MS, Vecht CJ. Optimal seizure management in brain tumor patients. *Curr Neurol Neurosci Rep.* 2005;5:207-213.

[141] Vecht CJ, Wilms EB. Seizures in low-and high-grade gliomas: current management and future outlook. *Expert Rev Anticancer Ther.* 2010;10:663-669.

[142] Kwan P, Brodie MJ. Early identification of refractory epilepsy. *N Engl J Med.* 2000;342:314-319.

[143] Kwan P, Arzimanoglou A, Berg AT et al. Definition of drug resistant epilepsy: consensus proposal by the ad hoc Task Force of the ILAE Commission on Therapeutic Strategies. *Epilepsia.* 2010;51:1069-1077.

[144] Wiebe S. Effectiveness and safety of epilepsy surgery: what is the evidence? *CNS Spectr.* 2004;9:120-122.

[145] Kim YH, Park CK, Kim TM et al. Seizures during the management of high-grade gliomas: clinical relevance to disease progression. *J Neurooncol.* 2013;113:101-109.

[146] Verla T, Babu R, Agarwal V, Halvorson KG, Adamson DC. Treatment outcomes and prognostic factors of pediatric glioblastoma multiforme. *Neurosurgery.* 2014;61:217-218.

[147] Napolitino M, Vaz G, Lawson TM et al. Glioblastoma surgery with and without intraoperative MRI at 3.0T. *Neurochirurgie 2014 Jun 26 pii: S0028-3770(14)00064-2 doi: 10 1016/j neuchi 2014 03 010 [Epub ahead of print].* 2014.

[148] Cataltepe O, Turanli G, Yalnizoglu D, Topcu M, Akalan N. Surgical management of temporal lobe tumor-related epilepsy in children. *J Neurosurg.* 2005;102:280-287.

[149] Uliel-Sibony S, Kramer U, Fried I, Fattal-Valevski A, Constantini S. Pediatric temporal low-grade glial tumors: epilepsy outcome following resection in 48 children. *Childs Nerv Syst.* 2011;27:1413-1418.

[150] Sherman JH, Moldovan K, Yeoh HK et al. Impact of temozolomide chemotherapy on seizure frequency in patients with low-grade gliomas. *J Neurosurg.* 2011;114:1617-1621.

[151] Cramer JA, Mintzer S, Wheless J, Mattson RH. Adverse effects of antiepileptic drugs: a brief overview of important issues. *Expert Rev Neurother.* 2010;10:885-891.

[152] Maschio M, Dinapoli L. Lecture: profile of risks and benefits of new antiepileptic drugs in brain tumor-related epilepsy. *Neurol Sci.* 2011;32:S259-S262.

[153] Taphoorm MJ. Neurocognitive sequelae in the treatment of low-grade gliomas. *Semin Oncol.* 2003;30:45-48.

[154] Chang EF, Quigg M, Oh DC et al. Predictors of efficacy after stereotactic radiosurgery for medial temporal lobe epilepsy. *Neurology*. 2010;74:165-172.

[155] Grenier Y, Tomita T, Marymont MH, Byrd S, Burrowes DM. Late postirradiation occlusive vasculopathy in childhood medulloblastoma. Report of two cases. *J Neurosurg*. 1998;89:460-464.

[156] Shuper A, Yaniv Y, Michowitz S et al. Epilepsy associated with pediatric brain tumors: the neuro-oncologic perspective. *Pediatr Neurol*. 2003;29:232-235.

[157] Jooma R, Yeh HS, Privitera MD, Gartner M. Lesionectomy versus electrophysiologically guided resection for temporal lobe tumors manifesting with complex partial seizures. *J Neurosurg*. 1995;83:231-236.

[158] Siegel AM. Presurgical evaluation and surgical treatment of medically refractory epilepsy. *Neurosurg Rev*. 2004;27:1-18.

[159] Pati S, Alexopoulos AV. Pharmacoresistant epilepsy: from pathogenesis to current and emerging therapies. *Cleve Clin J Med*. 2010;77:457-467.

[160] Riva M, Salmaggi A, Marchioni E et al. Tumour-associated epilepsy: clinical impact and the role of referring centres in a cohort of glioblastoma patients. A multicentre study from the Lombardia Neurooncology Group. *Neurol Sci*. 2006;27:345-351.

[161] Alexiou GA, Varela M, Sfakianos G, Prodromou N. Benign lesions accompanied by intractable epilepsy in children. *J Child Neurol*. 2009;24:697-700.

[162] Benifla M, Otsubo H, Ochi A et al. Temporal lobe surgery for intractable epilepsy in children: an analysis of outcomes in 126 children. *Neurosurgery*. 2006;59:1203-1213.

[163] Berger MS, Ghatan S, Haglund MM, Dobbins J, Ojemann GA. Low-grade gliomas associated with intractable epilepsy: seizure outcome utilizing electrocorticography during tumor resection. *J Neurosurg*. 1993;79:62-69.

[164] Chang EF, Christis C, Sullivan JE et al. Seizure control outcomes after resection of dysembryoplastic neuroepithelial tumor in 50 patients. *J Neurosurg Pediatr*. 2010;5:123-130.

[165] Duffau H, Capelle L, Lopes M, Bitar.A., Sichez JP, van Effenterre R. Medically intractable epilepsy from insular low-grade gliomas: improvement after an extended lesionectomy. *Acta Neurochir (Wien)*. 2002;144:563-572.

[166] Fried I, Kim JH, Spencer DD. Limbic and neocortical gliomas associated with intractable seizures: a distinct clinicopathological group. *Neurosurgery*. 1994;34:815-823.

[167] Giuloni M, Rubboli G, Marucci G et al. Seizure outcome of epilepsy surgery in focal epilepsies associated with temporomesial glioneuronal tumors: lesionectomy compared with tailored resection. *J Neurosurg*. 2009;111:1275-1282.

[168] Packer RJ, Sutton LN, Patel KM et al. Seizure control following tumor surgery for childhood cortical low-grade gliomas. *J Neurosurg.* 1994;80:998-1003.

[169] Zentner J, Hufnagel A, Wolf HK et al. Surgical treatment of neoplasms associated with medically intractable epilepsy. *Neurosurgery.* 1997;41:378-386.

[170] Mehrotra N, Shamji MF, Vassilyada M, Ventureyra EC. Intracranial tumors in first year of life: the CHEO experience. *Childs Nerv Syst.* 2009;25:1563-1569.

[171] Steinbok P, Gan PY, Connolly MB et al. Epilepsy surgery in the first 3 years of life: a Canadian survey. *Epilepsia.* 2009;50:1442-1449.

[172] Stevens GH. Antiepileptic therapy in patients with central nervous system malignancies. *Curr Neurol Neurosci Rep.* 2006;6:311-318.

[173] Glantz MJ, Cole BF, Forsyth PA et al. Practice parameter: anticonvulsant prophylaxis in patients with newly diagnosed brain tumors. Report of the Quality Standards Subcommittee of the American Academy of Neurology. *Neurology.* 2000;54:1886-1893.

[174] Siomin V, Angelov L, Li L, Vogelbaum MA. Results of a survey of neurosurgical practice patterns regarding the prophylactic use of anti-epilepsy drugs in patients with brain tumors. *J Neurooncol.* 2005;74:211-215.

[175] van Breeman M, Wilms EB, Vecht CJ. Epilepsy in patients with brain tumours: epidemiology, mechanisms, and management. *Lancet Neurol.* 2007;6:421-430.

[176] Vecht CJ, van Breeman M. Optimizing therapy of seizures in patients with brain tumors. *Neurology.* 2006;67:S10-S13.

[177] Sirven JI, Wingerchuk DM, Drazkowski JF, Lyons MK, Zimmerman RS. Seizure prophylaxis in patients with brain tumors: a meta-analysis. *Mayo Clin Proc.* 2004;79:1489-1494.

[178] North JB, Penhall RK, Hanieh A, Frewin DB, Taylor WB. Phenytoin and postoperative epilepsy. A double-blind study. *J Neurosurg.* 1983;58:672-677.

[179] Hardesty DA, Sanborn MR, Parker WE, Storm PB. Perioperative seizure incidence and risk factors in 223 pediatric brain tumor patients without prior seizures. *J Neurosurg Pediatr.* 2011;7:609-615.

[180] Wu AS, Trinh VT, Suki D et al. A prospective randomized trial of perioperative seizure prophylaxis in patients with intraparenchymal brain tumors. *J Neurosurg.* 2013;118:873-883.

[181] Khan RB, Onar A. Seizure recurrence and risk factors after antiepilepsy drug withdrawal in children with brain tumors. *Epilepsia.* 2006;47:375-379.

[182] Bilginer B, Yalnizoglu D, Soylemezoglu F et al. Surgery for epilepsy in children with dysembryoplastic neuroepithelial tumor: clinical spectrum, seizure outcome, neuroradiology, and pathology. *Childs Nerv Syst.* 2009;25:485-491.

[183] Chan CH, Bittar RG, Davis GA, Kalnins RM, Fabinyi GC. Long-term seizure outcome following surgery for dysembryoplastic neuroepithelial tumor. *J Neurosurg.* 2006;104:62-69.

[184] Lee J, Lee BL, Joo EY et al. Dysembryoplastic neuroepithelial tumors in pediatric patients. *Brain Dev.* 2009;31:671-681.

[185] Ramantani G, Kadish NE, Anastasopoulos C et al. Epilepsy surgery for glioneuronal tumors in childhood: avoid loss of time. *Neurosurgery.* 2014;74:648-657.

[186] Chassoux F, Daumas-Duport C. Dysembryoplastic neuroepithelial tumors: where are we now?Chassoux F1, Daumas-Duport C. *Epilepsia.* 2013;54:129-134.

[187] Ruggiero A, Rizzo D, Mastrangelo S, Battaglia D, Attina G, Riccardi R. Interactions between antiepileptic and chemotherapeutic drugs in children with brain tumors: is it time to change treatment? *Pediatr Blood Cancer.* 2010;54:193-198.

[188] Baker SD, Wirth M, Statkevich P et al. Absorption, metabolism, and excretion of 14C-temozolomide following oral administration to patients with advanced cancer. *Clin Cancer Res.* 1999;5:309-317.

[189] Yang LJ, Zhou CF, Lin ZX. Temozolomide and radiotherapy for newly diagnosed glioblastoma multiforme: a systematic review. *Cancer Invest.* 2014;32:31-36.

[190] Pouratian N, Schiff D. Management of low-grade glioma. *Curr Neurol Neurosci Rep.* 2010;10:224-231.

[191] van den Bent MJ, Snijders TJ, Bromberg JE. Current treatment of low grade gliomas. *Memo.* 2012;5:223-227.

[192] Zhu W, Zhou L, Qian JQ, Qiu TZ, Shu YQ, Liu P. Temozolomide for treatment of brain metastases: A review of 21 clinical trials. *World J Clin Oncol.* 2014;5:19-27.

[193] Hummel TR, Chow LM, Fouladi M, Franz D. Pharmacotherapeutic management of pediatric gliomas : current and upcoming strategies. *Paediatr Drugs.* 2013;15:29-42.

[194] Packer RJ, Lange B, Ater J et al. Carboplatin and vincristine for recurrent and newly diagnosed low-grade gliomas of childhood. *J Clin Oncol.* 1993;11:850-856.

[195] Packer RJ, Ater J, Allen J et al. Carboplatin and vincristine chemotherapy for children with newly diagnosed progressive low-grade gliomas. *J Neurosurg.* 1997;86:747-754.

[196] Maschio M, Dinapoli L, Saveriano F et al. Efficacy and tolerability of zonisamide as add-on in brain tumor-related epilepsy: preliminary report. *Acta Neurol Scand.* 2009;120:210-212.

[197] Maschio M, Dinapoli L, Mingoia M et al. Lacosamide as add-on in brain tumor-related epilepsy: preliminary report on efficacy and tolerability. *J Neurol.* 2011;258:2100-2104.

[198] Maschio M, Dinapoli L, Sperati F et al. Levetiracetam monotherapy in patients with brain tumor-related epilepsy: seizure control, safety, and quality of life. *J Neurooncol.* 2011;104:205-214.

[199] Maschio M, Dinapoli L, Sperati F et al. Effect of pregabalin add-on treatment on seizure control, quality of life, and anxiety in patients with brain tumour-related epilepsy: a pilot study. *Epileptic Disord.* 2012;14:388-397.

[200] Maschio M, Dinapoli L, Sperati F et al. Oxcarbazepine monotherapy in patients with brain tumor-related epilepsy: open-label pilot study for assessing the efficacy, tolerability and impact on quality of life. *J Neurooncol.* 2012;106:651-656.

[201] Newton HB, Goldlust SA, Pearl D. Retrospective analysis of the efficacy and tolerability of levetiracetam in brain tumor patients. *J Neurooncol.* 2006;78:99-102.

[202] Newton HB, Dalton J, Goldlust SA, Pearl D. Retrospective analysis of the efficacy and tolerability of levetiracetam in patients with metastatic brain tumors. *J Neurooncol.* 2007;84:293-296.

[203] Novy.J., Stupp R, Rossetti AO. Pregabalin in patients with primary brain tumors and seizures: a preliminary observation. *Clin Neurol Neurosurg.* 2009;111:171-173.

[204] Rossetti AO, Jeckelmann S, Novy.J., Roth P, Weller M, Stupp R. Levetiracetam and pregabalin for antiepileptic monotherapy in patients with primary brain tumors. A phase II randomized study. *Neuro Oncol.* 2014;16:584-588.

[205] Cabanas R, Saurez G, Alert J et al. Prolonged use of nimotuzumab in children with central nervous system tumors: safety and feasibility. *Cancer Biother Radiopharm.* 2014;29:173-178.

[206] Narayana A, Kunnakkat S, Chacko-Mathew J et al. Bevacizumab in recurrent high-grade pediatric gliomas. *Neuro Oncol.* 2010;12:985-990.

[207] Boon P, Raedt R, de Herdt V, Wyckhuys T, Vonck K. Electrical stimulation for the treatment of epilepsy. *Neurotherapeutics.* 2009;6:218-227.

[208] Chalifoux R, Elisevich K. Effect of ionizing radiation on partial seizures attributable to malignant cerebral tumors. *Stereotact Funct Neurosurg.* 1996;67:169-182.

[209] Aronica E, Leenstra S, van Veelen CW et al. Glioneuronal tumors and medically intractable epilepsy: a clinical study with long-term follow-up of seizure outcome after surgery. *Epilepsy Res.* 2001;43:179-191.

[210] Chuang NA, Yoon JM, Newbury RO, Crawford JR. Glioblastoma Multiforme Arising From Dysembryoplastic Neuroepithelial Tumor in a Child in the Absence of Therapy. *J Pediatr Hematol Oncol 2013 Dec 4 [Epub ahead of print].* 2013.

[211] Moazzam AA, Wagle N, Shiroishi MS. Malignant transformation of DNETs: a case report and literature review. *Neuroreport.* 2014;25:894-899.

[212] Moreno A, de Felipe J, Garcia Sola R, Navarro A, Ramon y Cajal S. Neuronal and mixed neuronal glial tumors associated to epilepsy. A heterogeneous and related group of tumours. *Histol Histopathol.* 2001;16:613-622.

[213] Yang T, Pruthi S, Geyer JR, Ojemann JG. MRI changes associated with vigabatrin treatment mimicking tumor progression. *Pediatr Blood Cancer.* 2010;55:1221-1223.

[214] Gelinas JN, Battison AW, Smith S, Connolly MB, Steinbok P. Electrocorticography and seizure outcomes in children with lesional epilepsy. *Childs Nerv Syst.* 2011;27:381-390.

[215] Giulioni M, Galassi E, Zucchelli M, Volpi L. Seizure outcome of lesionectomy in glioneuronal tumors associated with epilepsy in children. *J Neurosurg Ped.* 2005;102:288-293.

[216] Im SH, Chung CK, Cho BK, Lee SK. Supratentorial ganglioglioma and epilepsy: postoperative seizure outcome. *J Neurooncol.* 2002;57:59-66.

[217] Kan P, Van Orman C, Kestle JR. Outcomes after surgery for focal epilepsy in children. *Childs Nerv Syst.* 2008;24:587-591.

[218] Khajavi K, Comair YG, Wyllie E, Palmer J, Morris HH, Hahn JF. Surgical management of pediatric tumor-associated epilepsy. *J Child Neurol.* 1999;14:15-25.

[219] Kim SK, Wang KC, Cho BK. Intractable seizures associated with brain tumor in childhood: lesionectomy and seizure outcome. *Childs Nerv Syst.* 1995;11:634-638.

[220] Kim SK, Wang KC, Hwang YS, Kim KJ, Cho BK. Intractable epilepsy associated with brain tumors in children: surgical modality and outcome. *Childs Nerv Syst.* 2001;17:445-452.

[221] Consales A, Striano P, Nozza P et al. Glioneuronal tumors and epilepsy inchildren:seizureoutcome related to lesionectomy. *Minerva Pediatr.* 2013;65:609-616.

[222] Babini M, Giulioni M, Galassi E et al. Seizure outcome of surgical treatment of focal epilepsy associated with low-grade tumors in children. *J Neurosurg Pediatr.* 2013;11:214-223.

[223] Jo KI, Chung SB, Jo KW, Kong DS, Seol HJ, Shin HJ. Microsurgical resection of deep-seated lesions using transparent tubular retractor: pediatric case series. *Childs Nerv Syst.* 2011;27:1989-1994.

[224] Karnofsky DA, Burchenal JH. The Clinical Evaluation of Chemotherapeutic Agents in Cancer. In: MacLeod CM, ed. *Evaluation of Chemotherapeutic Agents*. New York, NY: Columbia University Press; 1949:196.

[225] Grajkowska W, Kotulska K, Jurkiewicz E, Matyja E. Brain lesions in tuberous sclerosis complex. Review. *Folia Neuropathol.* 2010;48:139-149.

[226] Orlova KA, Crino PB. The tuberous sclerosis complex. *Ann N Y Acad Sci.* 2010;1184:87-105.

[227] Bourgeois M, Sainte-Rose C, Lellouch-Tubiana A et al. Surgery of epilepsy associated with focal lesions in childhood. *J Neurosurg.* 1999;90:833-842.

[228] Sonderkaer S, Schmiegelow M, Carstensen H, Nielsen LB, Muller J, Schmiegelow K. Long-term neurological outcome of childhood brain tumors treated by surgery only. *J Clin Oncol.* 2003;21:1347-1351.

[229] Mekitarian Filho E, Brunow de Carvalho W, Cavalheiro S, Horigoshi NK, Freddi NA. Perioperative factors associated with prolonged intensive care unit and hospital length of stay after pediatric neurosurgery. *Pediatr Neurosurg.* 2011;47:423-429.

[230] Drake JM, Riva-Cambrin J, Jea A, Auguste K, Tamber M, Lamberti-Pasculli M. Prospective surveillance of complications in a pediatric neurosurgery unit. *J Neurosurg Pediatr.* 2010;5:544-548.

[231] Graham GR. Blood volume in children. *Ann R Coll Surg Engl.* 1963;33:149-158.

[232] Guidance: Blood Draw Guidelines. University of Michigan Medical School. 2013. Ref Type: Electronic Citation

[233] Lobel DA. Pediatric Intensive Care Unit Management of Neurosurgical Diseases. In: Lobel DA, Lee MR, Duhaime A-C, eds. *The Central Nervous System in Pediatric Critical Illness and Injury*. London: Springer; 2009:1-10.

[234] Hammer GB, Krane EJ. Perioperative care of the child with acute neurological disease. In: Hammer GB, Andrews BT, eds. *Pediatric Neurosurgical Intensive Care*. Park Ridge, IL: American Association of Neurological Surgeons (AANS); 1997:25-36.

[235] Segura Matute S, Balaguer Gargallo M, Cambra Lasaosa FJ, Zambudio Sert S, Martin Rodrigo JM, Palomeque Rico A. [Fluid and electrolyte disorders following surgery for brain tumors]. [Article in Spanish]. *An Pediatr (Barc).* 2007;67:225-230.

[236] Hiranrat P, Katavetin P, Supornsilchai V, Wacharasindhu S, Srivuthana S. Water and sodium disorders in children undergoing surgical treatment of brain tumors. *J Med Assoc Thai.* 2003;86:S152-S159.

[237] Spentzas T, Escue JE, Patters AB, Varelas PN. Brain tumor resection in children: neurointensive care unit course and resource utilization. *Pediatr Crit Care Med.* 2010;11:718-722.

[238] Pruitt AA. Treatment of Medical Complications in Patients with Brain Tumors. *Curr Treat Options Neurol.* 2005;7:323-336.

[239] Michelucci R. Optimizing therapy of seizures in neurosurgery. *Neurology.* 2006;67:S14-S18.

[240] Asano E, Benedek K, Shah A et al. Is intraoperative electrocorticography reliable in children with intractable neocortical epilepsy? *Epilepsia.* 2004;45:1091-1099.

[241] Wennberg R, Quesney LF, Lozano A, Olivier A, Rasmussen T. Role of electrocorticography at surgery for lesion-related frontal lobe epilepsy. *Can J Neurol Sci.* 1999;26:33-39.

[242] Lombardi D, Marsh R, de Tribolet N. Low grade glioma in intractable epilepsy: lesionectomy versus epilepsy surgery. *Acta Neurochir Suppl.* 1997;68:70-74.

[243] Terra-Bustamante VC, Inuzuka LM, Fernandes RM et al. Outcome of hemispheric surgeries for refractory epilepsy in pediatric patients. *Childs Nerv Syst.* 2007;23:321-326.

[244] Butman JA, Linehan WM, Lonser RR. Neurologic manifestations of von Hippel-Lindau disease. *JAMA.* 2008;300:1334-1342.

[245] Richard S, Campello C, Taillandier L, Parker F, Resche F. Haemangioblastoma of the central nervous system in von Hippel-Lindau disease. French VHL Study Group. *J Intern Med.* 1998;243:547-553.

[246] Shanley S, Ratcliffe J, Hockey A, et al. Nevoid basal cell carcinoma syndrome: review of 118 affected individuals. *Am J MedGenet.* 1994;50:282-290.

[247] Yang T, Temkin N, Barber J et al. Gross total resection correlates with long-term survival in pediatric patients with glioblastoma. *World Neurosurg.* 2013;79:537-544.

[248] Hart MG, Garside R, Rogers G, Stein K, Grant R. Temozolomide for high grade glioma. *Cochrane Database Syst Rev 2013 Apr 30;4:CD007415 doi: 10 1002/14651858 CD007415 pub2.* 2013.

[249] Ho RHVK, Reijneveld JC, Enting et al. Changing incidence and improved survival of gliomas. *Eur J Cancer 2014 Jun 24 pii: S0959-8049(14)00718-7 doi: 10 1016/j ejca 2014 05 019 [Epub ahead of print].* 2014.

[250] Weller M, Gorlia T, Cairncross JG et al. Prolonged survival with valproic acid use in the EORTC/NCIC temozolomide trial for glioblastoma. *Neurology.* 2011;77:1156-1164.

[251] Evans DG, Birch JM, Ramsden RT, Sharif S, Baser ME. Malignant transformation and new primary tumours after therapeutic radiation for benign disease: substantial risks in certain tumour prone syndromes. *J Med Genet.* 2006;43:289-294.

[252] Osipov V, Ho KC, Krouwer HG, Meyer G, Shidham VB. Post-radiation dedifferentiation of meningioma into osteosarcoma. *BMC Cancer.* 2002;2:34.

[253] Pereira EA, Dabbous B, Qureshi HU, Ansorge O, Bojanic S. Rapid development of glioblastoma at the site of atypical meningioma resection. *Br J* Neurosurg. 2010;24:471-473.

[254] Gonzalez-Martinez JA, Srikijvilaikul T, Nair D, Bingaman WE. Long-term seizure outcome in reoperation after failure of epilepsy surgery. Neurosurgery. 2007;60:873-880.

[255] Ojemann JG, Hersonskey TY, Abeshaus S et al. Epilepsy surgery after treatment of pediatric malignant brain tumors. Seizure. 2012;21:624-630.

[256] Tian AG, Edwards MS, Williams AJ, Olson DM. Epilepsy surgery following brain tumor resection in children. J Neurosurg Pediatr. 2011;7:229-234.

Chapter 12

# Imaging of Brain Tumours

Mike Fay, Chris Bell, Nick Dowson,
Simon Puttick and Stephen Rose

Additional information is available at the end of the chapter

http://dx.doi.org/10.5772/59981

## 1. Introduction

The last 20 years have seen a dramatic and rapid improvement in imaging technology. Developments in magnetic resonance (MR) imaging and more recently in positron emission tomography (PET) have allowed unique insights into tumour biology. Although careful evaluation this technology's clinical value is still being undertaken, improved imaging techniques have potential to assist many of the difficult problems currently faced in neuro-oncology. [1, 2]

One of the most significant clinical issues following treatment for high grade glioma is injury to the blood-brain barrier; so called pseudoprogression. [3] This results in oedema and apparent deterioration in the CT and MRI images, often associated with increased steroid dose. Brandes et al have highlighted the need for better imaging biomarkers for the problem of pseudo-progression. [1]

There are two potential outcomes of improved medical imaging for conventional imaging techniques currently adopted in the clinic. Firstly, treating clinicians may abandon treatment if imaging shows it to have an apparent negative impact. Secondly, if imaging shows that treatment regimes are not working, clinicians can decide whether or not to continue the current regime given the opportunity cost and risk of the treatment to the patient. As the number of treatment options slowly increase; the impact of this opportunity cost grows. In addition, data from a study by Stupp et al suggests the survival with glioblastoma treated with temozolomide is 14.6 months; [4] allowing clinicians little time to change treatment course.

Further insights into tumour biology could be gained from a better understanding of treatment efficacy. There is a need for better ways to choose patients for treatment, assess when these treatments are working and move onto something else when they are not. As an example, the benefit of temozolomide has been obscured to some degree by overestimating progression when MRI alone is considered. [5]

Increasingly, radiotherapy (RT) technology, often combined with new drug treatments, is allowing clinicians to treat more aggressively than could have been the case in the past. Modern radiotherapy is a complex chain of procedures. [6] If the tumour is poorly delineated; the risks of geographic misses increase. If the volume of treatment is too large, the toxicity increases and limits the dose that can be achieved.

Clinical trials involving brain tumour imaging face a number of difficulties. Brain tumours are relatively rare (excluding skin tumours; glioblastoma accounts for about 1% of tumours diagnosed in Australia), often making patient recruitment difficult. There are also difficulties with patient consent, as patients have frequent cognitive problems; especially when it comes to salvage treatment regimes. Imaging trials are difficult to perform - requiring blinded comparison of current best practice methods with and without the new modality. Finally, patients may require multiple imaging sessions on separate machines, requiring a significant amount of organisation. With each significant advance in imaging the studies may have to be repeated. It is no surprise that progress has been slow.

The Cancer Genome Atlas has shown us a vast amount about the complex biology of brain tumours such as glioblastoma. We are gaining "a window into its mutational landscape". [7] However, the more we know, the more complex the situation appears. U87, a commonly studied glioma cell line, has at least 512 homozygously mutated genes. [7] Targeted therapies are a last bearing fruit; as evidenced by CML treatment with imatinib or non-small cell lung cancer with EGFR inhibitors. We are moving from a single drug to the era of the rationally designed therapeutic regimen. Traditional response measures used in the chemotherapy era are much less successful when the response is cytostatic – as it is with many targeted agents. [8] The challenge is how to assess and integrate new agents within existing protocols.

## 2. Current imaging techniques

Computed Tomography (CT) provides good delineation of bony anatomy, can show haemorrage or hydrocephalus and can be useful in planning resection of lesions. In combination with PET; CT provides both improved anatomical localisation and improved PET images by allowing attenuation correction. Although CT is often the initial imaging modality used, it has a relatively small role in the investigation of brain tumours and has not been shown to be useful in response assessment or to accurately delineate tumour outlines. [9]

In radiation oncology practice; a planning CT is routinely used to define the shape of the patient and to provide an electron density map to allow modelling of the dose deposited by the radiotherapy beam. The tumour itself, however, is usually delineated on a contrast enhanced MRI fused to a non-contrast planning CT. MRI provides much greater anatomic detail of the structures within the brain. Additionally, with increased magnet strength and better design of coils, images obtained have steadily improved. MRI is routinely used for delineation of the tumour both in neurosurgical and radiation oncology practice. [10]

http://dx.doi.org/10.5772/59981

A contrast agent containing gadolinium is usually added to assist with interpretation. While it is has been established that MRI can identify oedema and necrosis along with tumour microstructure in great anatomical detail, as well as regions displaying dysfunction of the blood-brain barrier (BBB). However, it is often the case that these regions do not correlate with areas of infiltration or other neoplastic molecular events. [11] This is particularly concerning in low-grade gliomas, where the blood brain barrier may not be disrupted.

Recently the growth in the use of MRI has stimulated a body of research aimed at estimating electron density from the MR data and using this alone for radiotherapy planning. This avoids the necessity for a CT, reducing both treatment costs and patient radiation burden. [12]

A variety of MR sequences are usually obtained – T1/ T2/ DCE and spin echo. The detailed evaluation of a glioma patient usually involves about 45 minutes on the scanner for the patient and would usually be repeated about every 3 months.

Diffusion weighted imaging (DWI), or the more elaborate Diffusion Tensor Imaging (DTI), are developments of MRI based on the diffusion of water molecules. This diffusion occurs preferentially down the axons rather than across cell membranes. DTI post-processing can identify white matter fibre tracts within the brain, allowing ablative therapies (such as radiosurgery) to eloquent areas to be avoided. [10]

Spectroscopy can be useful in certain clinical scenarios, particularly when radionecrosis is suspected post radiotherapy. It is most commonly undertaken using proton nuclei on commercial scanners. [13] Ratios of choline to N-acetyl aspartate (NAA) have been found to correlate with tumour tissue. [13] NAA, associated with mature neuronal cell density, [14] is decreased in tumours, while choline, involved in cell membrane turnover, [14] is increased, leading to an increase in the ratio of choline/NAA. [13] However, Horska makes the point that spectroscopy looks very different depending on the zone of the tumour being examined (necrotic core, actively growing tumour or peritumoural oedema) [13]. In clinical practice, spectroscopy is complicated by the need for large voxels; limiting the resolution and application in small lesions. There have been attempts to incorporate wider field MRS in radiotherapy planning; even using whole brain acquisition. [14] With the limitation of difficulty in the anterior cranial fossa and prolonged scan time; it looks potentially useful. Spectroscopy's clinical role currently is to provide confirmatory information to other modalities.

The issue of response assessment is critical to development in neuro-oncology, from early phase testing of drugs through to community oncology clinics delivering care to patients. The traditional approach to tumour response has been to base assessment on the change in size of the lesion. Volumetric criteria perform poorly in slowly growing lesions such as low grade glioma. [15] Initially, response assessment was based on two dimensional imaging (MacDonald criteria) of high grade lesions but it was appreciated that these criteria did not account for non-enhancing progression and so Response Assessment for Neuro-Oncology (RANO) criteria were developed. [9, 15]

CT and MRI are not sensitive for early malignant transformation – a significant problem with low grade glioma. The usual clinical situation is – has the patient progressed? The MRI is very difficult to interpret for the 3 months post chemo-radiotherapy. Limitations of both CT and

MRI have led to the increased interest and development of functional imaging. [16-18] Combined PET-MR scanners are finding their way into the clinical setting and may become more than the sum of their parts. It is clear to us that the skill set required for development runs across chemistry, medical physics, pharmacology, computational informatics, radiology, nuclear medicine and clinical oncology. [19] This chapter will concentrate on the clinical applications across a number of entities and review where advanced imaging may help us improve treatment.

## 3. Metabolic imaging of the brain

PET imaging involves injection of a radioactive tracer, which undergoes decay, with positron emission. Positrons collide with electrons, resulting in positron annihilation and the emission two photons at 180 degrees, detected by the scanner's detector ring. Following the acquisition, detected events are reconstructed into an image. PET scanning can be performed in static or dynamic mode. In static mode, a single PET image is acquired which is a sum of all events detected during the period of the scan. From this, a measure of tumour-to-background contrast can be used to provide both qualitative and quantitative results. In dynamic mode, the scan is divided up into temporal segments, allowing an insight into the pharmacokinetics and temporal path of the tracer, with kinetic modelling offering quantitative measures that can provide insights into tumour biology. Although dynamic imaging has been shown to provide more information, static acquisitions are still considered the norm in the clinical setting largely due to time and data storage constraints.

### 3.1. PET radiotracers

A large number of radiotracers have been developed for clinical imaging with many investigated for brain tumours. Selection of an appropriate radiotracer is critical for the investigation being performed, as many target a specific molecular process. A list of common radiotracers used for brain tumour imaging is presented in Table 1.

| Radiotracer | Abbreviation | Molecular Target |
|---|---|---|
| [$^{18}$F]Fluorodeoxyglucose | $^{18}$F-FDG | Glycolysis |
| 6-[$^{18}$F]fluoro-dihydroxy-l-phenylalanine | $^{18}$F-FDOPA | Dopamine / Amino acid transport |
| [$^{18}$F]fluoromisonidazole | $^{18}$F-FMISO | Hypoxia |
| [$^{11}$C]-L-methionine | $^{11}$C-MET | Amino Acid Transport |
| O-(2-[$^{18}$F]fluoroethyl)-l-tyrosine | $^{18}$F-FET | Amino Acid Transport |
| 3-deoxy-3-[$^{18}$F]fluorothymidine | $^{18}$F-FLT | Thymidine Kinase Enzyme |

**Table 1.** Common radiotracers used for imaging of brain tumours.

It should be remembered that the difficulty in synthesis and half-life of many of these tracers varies greatly. This can limit their availability, especially in areas with a widely dispersed population. The ultimate utility of an imaging molecule depends on a combination of cost, benefit over other modalities, availability and half-life of the tracer.

### 3.2. $^{18}$F-Flurodeoxyglucose (FDG)

Tumours such as glioma have a predisposition for increased proliferation and metabolism and there is a wealth of literature investigating the clinical applications of FDG,. These include comparison to MRI [20], detection of glioma [21-28], tumour grading [29-36], choice of biopsy site and radiotherapy planning [37-39], detecting tumour progression [40], recurrence and necrosis [41-53], predicting prognosis and survival [54-58], and patient follow up [59]. FDG PET has the advantage that it is available in most centres due to its wide, relatively simple synthesis and low cost of production. However, the literature highlights numerous limitations in application to brain tumours. The brain is an obligate metaboliser of glucose,. This results in a higher tracer uptake in normal brain tissue. While high-grade gliomas such as glioblastoma are still detectable over background uptake, low-grade and slow progressing tumours often show uptake equal to that of surrounding normal tissue. Other pathologies such as inflammatory diseases can cause tracer up regulation, [60] leading to false positive diagnoses. More sensitive scanner technology has improved this to some degree but a number of studies have been performed exploring alternative radiotracers that may be more useful in brain tumour imaging, such as [$^{11}$C]-L-methionine (MET), 6- [$^{18}$F]fluoro-dihydroxy-l-phenylalanine (FDOPA), O-(2- [$^{18}$F]fluoroethyl)-l-tyrosine (FET) and 3-deoxy-3- [$^{18}$F]fluorothymidine (FLT).

### 3.3. [$^{11}$C]-L-Methionine (MET)

MET is an amino acid. MET has advantages over FDG due to both its low cortical uptake and high uptake in neoplastic tissues. (i.e better signal to noise ratio) Methionine is involved in protein synthesis, energy production. I t is clear that MET is a powerful diagnostic tool for the detection of primary [61-66] and recurrent [42, 52, 62, 66-70] glioma, as well as having some benefit in prediction of survival. [30, 55, 71-74] Numerous investigations have been performed comparing the diagnostic accuracy of FDG and MET, with reported findings clearly showing the superiority ot MET in detection [21, 30, 75] and grading [30, 31] of primary glioma. Conflicting reports have been published, however, regarding the benefit of MET in detection of recurrent glioma. [20, 21, 41, 42, 47, 52]

The ability to provide complimentary information to that of MRI is a key strength of PET, assisting in diagnosis and treatment planning where differential diagnosis on MRI alone is difficult. However, while findings have been published showing the superiority of MET over standard MRI protocols for both primary [61] and recurrent [76] glioma, dynamic susceptibility contrast-enhanced magnetic resonance imaging (DSCE MRI) [77] and perfusion MRI [45, 78] have been shown to be superior to MET PET for tumour detection.

Conflicting findings have been reported for the use of MET PET for grading gliomas. Ceyssens et al [74] and Moulin-Romsee et al [79] reported that MET could not differentiate between glioma grades. However, Singhal et al [30] found that MET could discriminate between high and low-grade gliomas and Miyake et al [31] and Santoni et al [62] found the tracer could discriminate between grades II and IV and grades II, III and IV, respectively.

While the literature does support the integration of MET PET into the clinical setting, there remain two significant caveats for the tracer. The half-life of $^{11}C$ isotopes such as MET is considerably short at 20.3 minutes, limiting this isotope and its tracers to centres with onsite production capabilities. Finally, similar to FDG, MET accumulates in inflammatory lesions, complicating differential diagnosis.

### 3.4. 6- [$^{18}$F]fluoro-dihydroxy-l-phenylalanine (FDOPA)

An alternative to MET is 6- [$^{18}$F]fluoro-dihydroxy-l-phenylalanine (FDOPA), a tracer that is commonly used for the assessment of Parkinson's Disease and other neurodegenerative diseases. However, a case study was published in 1996 by Heiss et al [80] revealed the tracer's potential application to brain tumour imaging. While investigating a patient with suspected Parkinson's disease, F-DOPA uptake was visualized in a small region of the brain later pathologically confirmed to be a low-grade glioma. This discovery generated significant interest in FDOPA, with the subsequent literature showing that it provides complimentary information to that of MRI, assisting in diagnosis, prognosis and guiding treatment in primary and recurrent glioma patients.

Studies by Ledezma et al [81] and Karunanithi et al [82] have shown the potential for FDOPA to provide information complementary to that of MRI. Ledezma et al showed that using FDOPA PET along with MRI provided a good mechanism for detecting lesions in primary and recurrent glioma. Karunanithi et al compared the two modalities, finding that FDOPA PET was able to detect tumour recurrence in more cases that MRI. Hence, while MRI is currently implemented in the diagnosis and treatment of glioma, these studies support the potential of FDOPA as modality for complimentary assessment to MRI. Specifically, $^{18}$F-FDOPA could have utility where the MRI findings are negative in primary/recurrent tumours or inconclusive in recurrent tumours.

A number of studies have been performed comparing the efficacy of FDOPA PET to that of other radiotracers such as FDG, FLT, FET, Ammonia (NH3) and MET. Investigations performed by Chen et al [50], Tripathi et al [28], Jora et al [27] and Jacob et al [83] all reported that FDOPA PET was more specific and sensitive to detecting primary and recurrent lesions than FDG. Tripathi et al and Jacob et al also showed that FDOPA PET was more sensitive than FLT and ammonia, respectively.

Given the aforementioned drawbacks of MET, Becherer et al [84] investigated FDOPA as a potential alternative, finding that both tracers had similar standard uptake values (SUVs) and almost identical patterns of spatial uptake.

Many factors are considered in determining prognosis of patients including Karnovsky performance status (KPS), age, tumour size, extent of surgery and tumour grade and histology. In addition, Karunanithi et al [85] have shown that numerous indices derived from FDOPA PET were independent predictors of survival, with Dowson et al further corroborating these findings by showing that the uptake changes in the most treatment resistant region of tumour post-treatment are predictive of survival.

Another potential application of glioma PET imaging currently under investigation is tumour grading. Confirmation of a glioma diagnosis generally involves surgical biopsy or resection followed by a pathological assessment to determine tumour microvascularity. [86] There are some limitations to performing biopsies. Firstly, biopsy is an invasive procedure, sometimes not possible due to the anatomic location of the tumour, or the condition of the patient. Secondly, as biopsy tissue samples often represent only a small part of the entire tumour, there is a chance that the true tumour grade will be underestimated, as different tumour regions may be of a different grade. [74] Finally, surgery of certain regions may involve surrounding normal brain tissue, exacerbating the prognosis by causing additional neurological morbidity or dysfunction. [87] While FDG has been investigated for glioma grading, alternatives to biopsy methods are yet to be widely implemented in the clinical environment.

Numerous investigations have been performed in an attempt to discriminate high-grade gliomas from low-grade using FDOPA. However, reports are conflicting. Studies by Fueger et al [88], Pafundi et al [89] and Nioche et al [90] reported that FDOPA PET could discriminate between high and low-grade primary glioma. However, as part of their study, Chen et al found no significant difference in FDOPA uptake between the two classes. For recurrent glioma, only Nioche et al was able to discriminate between high and low-grade, while neither Fueger et al nor Kratochwil et al could differentiate the grades in their cohorts. While these studies do suggest that FDOPA has the potential to discriminate between tumour grades in newly diagnosed gliomas, further investigation is needed, especially for recurrent tumours.

While there are clear clinical benefits to using FDOPA for the assessment and management of patients with glioma, this tracer comes with its own set of caveats. The main drawback of FDOPA is synthesis. The most widely used method for FDOPA synthesis uses an electrophilic approach, based on a two-step process. [91, 92] A fully automated method for synthesis of FDOPA is now also available. [93, 94] However, there are limitations with this approach, such as the requirement of additional equipment, precautions for dealing with $^{18}$F in gaseous form, and the low radiotracer production rate. [95, 96] Recent developments have seen the introduction of nucleophilic approaches. [97, 98] In contrast to electrophilic, nucleophilic pipelines produce $^{18}$F in liquid form. In addition, nucleophilic methods for production of FDOPA are similar to that of FDG and thus require less additional equipment than electrophilic-based synthesis. Finally, the recent availability of single-use synthesis cassettes for FDOPA could make it more readily available..

### 3.5. O-(2- [$^{18}$F]fluoroethyl)-l-tyrosine (FET)

O-(2- [$^{18}$F]fluoroethyl)-l-tyrosine (FET) has also been widely investigated for imaging of brain tumours. FET is one of the first amino acid radiotracers that can be synthesised in large amounts for clinical purposes. Unlike MET and FDG, it has been shown in animal models that FET exhibits low uptake in inflammatory lesions.

A number of studies have been performed investigating FET in brain tumour imaging, with findings strongly supporting the use of the tracer for detecting both primary [99-10][4] and recurrent [52, 100, 105-108] glioma and showing superiority in detection, [25] treatment planning [24] and biopsy planning [24, 38] to that of FDG PET.

A key strength of FET PET is its apparent ability to differentiate between different grades of glioma. While some studies report that static imaging alone can provide the information necessary to grade tumours in vivo, [109-111] kinetic analysis from dynamic imaging appears to be superior for both primary [102, 110, 112, 113] and recurrent [114] cases. A combination of MRI, DWI and FET PET indices has also been investigated for grading tumours, providing promising results. [115]

In addition, like other radiotracers, FET PET has been investigated as a possible tool for predicting prognosis, [71, 100, 116-120] treatment planning, [121] and monitoring treatment response [122-124] with findings from all studies supporting its use.

Compared to FDG and MET, FET is a relatively new radiotracer, with the first human experiments performed in the late 1990s. It has been shown to be a cost effective tracer for adoption into the clinic, [123, 125] and future studies could see this tracer being brought closer towards clinical translation.

### 3.6. 3-deoxy-3- [$^{18}$F]fluorothymidine (FLT)

3-deoxy-3- [$^{18}$F]fluorothymidine (FLT) is another recently developed amino acid radiotracer that has been investigated for imaging of brain tumour proliferation. [126-131] FLT is an analogue of the thymidine nucleoside, altered to prevent it from following the full biochemical pathway of the nucleoside. Once the tracer is diffused into the cells by active transport, it is phosphorylated but not incorporated into the DNA, thus it becomes trapped within the cell.

FLT has been shown to effectively detect both primary [28, 132] and recurrent [22], [49, 127, 130, 133, 134] tumours, with a large body of work supporting it as a prognostic factor in both cases. [101, 135-141]

Further research has investigated FLT PET as a tool for assessing treatment response [142-145] as well as tumour grading. [129, 132, 134] A study by Jeong et al also found that FLT PET uptake in recurrent glioma correlated with the initial grade of the tumour.

However, despite the body of work supporting FLT as a surrogate biomarker for proliferation, [126-129] its use remains controversial [131, 146] and further studies are warranted to fully elucidate the role of FLT in future clinical practice.

### 3.7. Hypoxia and $^{18}$F-Flouromisonidazole (FMISO)

Hypoxia has been shown to have a significant effect on treatment outcome for patients diagnosed with glioma. Low oxygen tension correlates with radioresistance, resulting in the development of local recurrence or metastasis. [147-149] It is well known that hypoxic tumour cells are significantly more resistant to radiation than normoxic cells, as the lack of oxygen inhibits permanent DNA damage. In fact, it has been shown that up to three times the radiation dose is required to kill hypoxic cells. [150] While cell hypoxia is rare in normal tissue, it is a common occurrence in many solid tumours; [41, 42] classified as acute, chronic or anaemic.

Cells become acutely hypoxic when they are temporarily deprived of oxygen due to the closure or disruption of blood vessels, often caused by the hostile nature and abnormalities within the tumour environment. The abrupt changes in vasculature prevent the supply of oxygen and other nutrients to the cells. Upon return of oxygen to the cells, often due to angiogenesis or vasculogenesis, cells become normoxic again. Chronically hypoxic cells on the other hand, are cells that will remain hypoxic until they become necrotic, often due to the tumour outgrowing its blood supply or proliferation pressure forcing cells away from blood vessels. [151] In fact, necrosis is a requirement for the diagnosis of glioblastoma; as the highly proliferative nature of the tumour forces it to outgrow the blood supply in areas, resulting in a necrotic core usually visible from MRI. Anaemic hypoxia results from low oxygen concentrations within the blood supply and can be due to either pathology or the treatment itself.

There are numerous methods available for measuring hypoxia, both in vivo and in vitro, with the polarographic needle electrode regarded at the gold standard. While this method has been used extensively to assess hypoxia, [39, 44, 49-55] there are concerns with this approach. [74] Firstly, since the needle is invasive, not only is it uncomfortable for the patient, but there also exists a risk that it may cause trauma to the sample site, resulting in exacerbation of injury. Secondly, since only a small sample of the tumour is assessed, there is a risk of underestimating the level of hypoxia. Other, non-invasive methods exist for hypoxia assessment, including phosphorescent imaging, [152-154] which exploits the oxygen-depending quenching of phosphorescence, blood oxygen level dependent (BOLD) MRI, which is able to identify hypoxic vasculature using paramagnetic properties of deoxyheamaglobin, $^{19}$F MRI, [155] which utilizes the linear relationship between $^{19}$F and tissue oxygen concentration, and near infrared spectroscopy (NIRS), [156-159] which exploits the low absorption of near infrared wavelengths by tissue chromophores.

In addition to the above methods, there is now significant interest in the use of PET radiotracers for assessing tumour hypoxia. Many radiotracers exist for investigating tumour hypoxia [160-170], including $^{18}$F-HX4, $^{18}$F-FAZA, $^{18}$F-EF5, [124]I-IAZA, [123]/ [125]I-IAZP, $^{64}$Cu–ATSM, $^{18}$F-FENI, $^{62}$Cu-diacetyl-bis(N$^{4}$-methylthiosemicarbazone), $^{18}$F-FETA, $^{18}$F-EF1 and [$^{18}$F]fluoroerythronitroimidazole. However, $^{18}$F-Fluoromisonidazole (FMISO) PET is clearly the most widely used, as it provides the best compromise between sensitivity, specificity and invasiveness.

FMISO is a derivative of nitroimidazole, which is metabolized by intracellular nitroreductases at low oxygen concentrations. They form covalent bonds with macromolecules and become biochemically trapped within these hypoxic cells. [171] This has been shown to occur in oxygen concentrations below 10mmHg [70], [71]. Nitroimidazole metabolism relies on active enzymes and thus does not get absorbed by necrotic tissue.

The first to investigate FMISO as a potential hypoxia imaging agent was Valk et al, [172] who elegantly showed that high-grade gliomas were clearly delineable 40 minutes post-injection of the tracer. Since this pioneering work, many studies have been performed on both humans and animal models, bringing this tracer closer to clinical translation.

Further research has compared FMISO PET to other imaging modalities such as MRI and FDG PET. MR imaging sequences such as FLAIR, $T_2$ and contrast enhanced $T_1$ are regularly used in the diagnosis, treatment planning and treatment evaluation of glioma. However, there are limitations with MRI as described above, especially for low-grade glioma, due to the invasive nature of glioma beyond areas of BBB disruption. Hypoxia has been shown to promote neovascularization through the angiogenic cascade and other molecular signalling events, leading to leakage of the blood-brain barrier. [173, 174] Hence, an understanding of the relationship between hypoxia, as assessed by FMISO PET and MR imaging may lead to an improved understanding of tumour physiology.

Studies by Spence et al, [175] Swanson et al [176], Szeto et al [177] and Kawai et al [178] have confirmed that a relationship does in fact exist between the two imaging modalities. Spence et al showed that hypoxic regions delineated using FMISO PET correlated with contrast enhanced $T_1$ defined regions. This result was verified by Swanson et al, who reported on two important findings in their study on pre- and post- operative glioma patients: regions of hypoxia correlated with MRI defined volumes; and regions of hypoxia were not restricted to inside MRI defined volumes. Further corroboration came from Kawai et al, who found that individual hypoxic volumes significantly correlated with volumes defined on contrast enhanced $T_1$. Finally, Szeto et al used a mathematical model adopted from Swanson et al to show that regions of hypoxia correlated with quantitative measures of tumour aggressiveness and sphericity.

It is well established that hypoxic cells can increase their glycolysis to maintain energy levels, suggesting that a relationship between hypoxia and glycolysis does exist. However, proliferation is considerably inhibited in chronic hypoxia, significantly reducing glycolysis. [179-181] This suggests that a complex relationship may exist, the understanding of which may lead to a more comprehensive understanding of the tumour microenvironment.

Investigations by Rejendran et al, [182] Hatano et al [183] and Cher et al [184] have confirmed that any relationship that may exist between the two microbiological processes is complex. While Rejendran et al and Hatano et al found little to no correlation between FMISO and FDG Uptake, Cher et al found that a correlation did exist within individual tumour grades. These results suggest that complementary information can be obtained from FDG and FMISO imaging. However, further studies are warranted to fully elucidate any relationship between the two tracers.

Accurate grading of glioma cases is imperative for both patient prognosis and treatment planning, as patients diagnosed with higher-grade glioma fair significantly worse compared those with lower grade. While necrosis, usually visualized with MRI, is a key requirement for diagnosis of glioblastoma, the most widely accepted method for grading is pathological assessment from biopsy. However as described previously, there are concerns with this approach: Biopsy is not always possible due to tumour location; where biopsy is possible, further neurological dysfunction is a risk with such an invasive procedure; and the sample only represents a small section of the tumour volume, possibly resulting in an underestimation of the tumour grade.

However, studies into FMISO PET have found that tracer uptake correlates very well with tumour grade, offering up a non-invasive method for tumour grading. Cher et al, [184] Hirata et al, [185] Yamamoto et al [186] and Kawai et al [187] all reported a higher uptake of $^{18}$F-FMISO in glioblastoma patients than all other grades. While Cher et al and Hirata et al reported no tracer uptake in lower-grade tumours compared to normal tissue, Yamamoto et al and Kawai et al reported higher uptake in grade III than surrounding cortex. These results suggest that, at the very least, FMISO PET could be used to confirm a diagnosis of high-grade (grade III-IV) glioma. However, further studies are needed to conclude distinction between grade III and IV cases.

Probably the most fascinating property of hypoxia is its apparent strong negative correlation with patient prognosis, which has been investigated since the development of the polarographic electrode needle. Cher et al [184] and Hirata et al [185] both reported FMISO PET defined hypoxia as a significant negative prognostic factor, with Cher et al able to predict the site of recurrence in two patients from $^{18}$F-FMISO images. Spence et al was also able to correlate FMISO PET images with time-to-tumour-progression (TTP), survival and KPS. Finally, Swanson et al was able to negatively correlate FMISO PET images with patient survival in pre-operative cases of glioblastoma. These studies add to the growing body of evidence that suggests hypoxia is a key factor in treatment success and patient survival.

Finally, Valable et al [188] performed an investigation into hypoxia and the anti-angiogenic treatment sunitinib. Anti-angiogenic treatments were proposed as a possible cancer therapy, as they target VEGF pathways, leading to a decrease in tumour vasculature. However, treatment results were disappointing, with treatment benefits being temporary, leading to a short increase in time to progression at best. However, the concept of vascular normalisation rekindled the idea of anti-angiogenic treatments, whereby therapy improves tumours vasculature, reducing tumour hypoxia and improving the efficacy of radiotherapy. Valable et al showed in a mouse model that tumours treated with sunitinib had a significant decrease in FMISO PET after 7 days, suggesting that the use of anti-angiogenic treatments may be viable to improve tumour oxygenation and therefore radiotherapy treatments.

The body of work surrounding hypoxia strongly suggests that important information can be obtained from F-MISO PET imaging of glioma and, while more needs to be done to fully elucidate tumour biology, it is clear that hypoxia is an important aspect of future treatment for patients diagnosed with glioma.

### 3.8. Dual-tracer imaging (multiplexing)

The current literature strongly supports the idea that, given the complex and heterogeneous nature of glioma, knowledge of multiple biological characteristics is needed for effective patient treatment. For example, amino acid activity from FDOPA PET, proliferation from FLT PET and hypoxia from FMISO PET. Currently, however, the physical limitations of PET imaging prevents ascertaining information from two radiotracers simultaneously. Thus, to acquire the necessary biological information, PET acquisitions must be performed on separate days, allowing the first radiotracer to decay.

Unfortunately, however, there are many disadvantages to this approach. Firstly, performing multiple PET acquisitions requires that the patient be prepared multiple times, significantly increases the scanner time and increases the associated costs. Secondly, performing acquisitions on separate days introduces spatial uncertainty in two ways: Tumour evolution between scans can be significant, especially given the aggressive nature of glioma. In addition, registration of the images introduces uncertainty due to change in patient positions and image artefacts. This, however, can be mitigated provided there is enough mutual anatomical information available between the two scans.

With the need to image multiple biological characteristics becoming evident, and the obvious inherent logistical limitations in performing multiple scans, the field of dual-tracer imaging is gaining momentum.

Dual-tracer imaging, or multiplexing, allows for imaging of multiple PET radiotracers within a single scanning session by employing novel post-processing techniques to separate the two tracer signals. This approach trades-off tracer signal fidelity for logistics, circumventing some of these issues encountered when performing multiple acquisitions: The patient need only be prepared for scanning once; the required scanning time is shorter than that of two individual acquisitions; tumour evolution between the two images is negligible; and, provided the patient does not move during the scan, registration is no longer required.

However, this technique has one major logistical limitation, requiring that multiple radiotracers be synthesized and available at the same time. This is a difficult task in most centres, as simultaneous synthesis of two $^{18}$F radiotracers, for example, would be impossible without two cyclotrons. This limitation may be mitigated, however, by either using radiotracers with differing isotopes and/or synthesis methods, or using radiotracers with sufficiently long half-lives that allow the two tracers to be synthesized consecutively before application.

Since dual-tracer imaging was first proposed by Huang et al, [189] a number of methods have been proposed and can be loosely grouped by their method for signal separation. Methods that allow both tracers to be injected simultaneously reduce the scanning time but require that both tracers have different half-lives, with signal separation performed by exploiting the difference in tracer decay rates. Such methods include those by Huang et al, [189] who investigated $^{13}$N, $^{18}$F, $^{68}$Ga and $^{64}$Cu isotopes in phantoms, Figueiras et al, [190] who investigated FDG and ammonia in both phantoms and an ischemic rat model, and Kadrmas et al, [191] who exploited differing decay rates in conjunction with differing kinetics and distribution for FDG, ATSM and PTSM. Other methods, such as those by Koeppe et al [192] and Kadrmas et al, [193] employ a staggered injection that allows for the discrimination of tracer signals with the same half-life, increasing the selection of available radiotracers that can be used. Both methods rely on kinetic modeling to separate the two signals. In addition, Verhaeghe et al [194] and Ikoma et al [195] proposed methods that exploit differing tracer half-lives in addition to a staggered injection interval and kinetic analysis to separate tracer signals.

http://dx.doi.org/10.5772/59981

The above studies propose methods that require scanning to be initiated at the injection of the first tracer. To reduce the required scanning time further, a study by Bell et al [196] investigated separation of two $^{18}F$ radiotracers by staggering the injection interval and initiating the PET acquisition once the first tracer had reached steady state. Using this method, scanning time was only increased by 10 to 20 minutes over a standard PET acquisition.

Finally, two studies have been performed investigating performing signal separation at the reconstruction level. Gao et al [197] and Cheng et al [198] incorperate kinetic modelling into the reconstruction process to separate tracer information.

Dual-tracer imaging offers a viable alternative to performing multiple PET acquisitions, with the above methods illustrating its potential in future research practices. However, further studies are required to fully develop the concept of simultaneous multiplexing, with particular attention to circumventing the logistical issue of simultaneous radiotracer synthesis.

## 4. Clinical applications

Medical imaging is important at many junctures during the course of the treatment path for glioma patients, from the initial diagnosis and grading of the disease to planning and assessing response to therapy. MRI is the gold standard for obtaining morphological information on tumours, but has some limitations as mentioned previously. One role of imaging is in establishing a continually updated prognosis at all stages during treatment. So in addition to detecting and localising tumours, the differentiation of treatment induced pseudo-progression from recurrence is important. The latter is a particular challenge, as is establishing the grade of diffuse tumours and the late identification of recurrence. [199]

Non-structural MR modalities can assist in overcoming the difficulties of differentiating recurrence from post treatment radiation effect. A previous study [200] examined the use of relative cerebral blood volume, and measured a sensitivity of 92% with a specificity of 100%. Relative cerebral blood volume (rCBV) has shown superior abilities in distinguishing recurrence from radiation necrosis than either FDG or MET-PET. [45]

The sensitivity of molecular imaging techniques such as PET can be used to surmount some limitations of MRI, [16] for instance FDG, the most widely used PET tracer, can predict anaplastic transformation in low-grade gliomas. However PET should be used in conjunction with anatomical imaging as greater sensitivity and specificity is demonstrated when PET is combined with MRI. [16] In clinical practice, PET is considered useful for resolving ambiguities between recurrence and treatment induced changes. [201] It is broadly acknowledged that the augmentation of MRI and CT with other modalities such as PET, SPECT and diffusion imaging may assist in differentiating treatment effects from progression, but more research is needed, [202, 203] and efforts have been made to standardize assessments when considering metabolic imaging modalities, at least when using FDG. [204] As mentioned however, although FDG has demonstrated efficacy for many oncologic applications, it is of less utility in cortical regions where healthy tissue has high FDG-avidity preventing the unambiguous differentiation of normal and neoplastic tissue. FDG retains some utility for glioma applications, for instance in a study of 19 patients changes in glucose metabolism measured using FDG-PET predicted response to temozolomide, but not when combined with radiotherapy. [205]

Amino acid tracers, such as MET and F-DOPA. are more sensitive for imaging recurrent tumours, especially LGG, [16] as amino acid transport is up-regulated in malignant lesions. [206] Some debate exists around the relative efficacy of different amino-acid tracers, with a number of tracers examined in the literature. [52] MET is popular choice due it its relative ease of synthesis [207] MET-PET is a better prognostic predictor and improves inter-observer consistency compared to FDG, [42] although it is noted combining FDG with MET further improves prognostic predictions. However, the aforementioned limitations with the half life of MET have seen FDOPA to be a viable alternative to MET, which more accessible in the clinic due to its longer half-life. [84]

FDOPA precisely localizes tumours as verified on MRI [81] and can also identify tumour not visible on MRI. FDOPA has also been shown to better identify regions of higher density disease than MRI on a study examining 23 biopsy specimens from 10 patients. [89] When evaluating 28 of 30 patients on anti-angiogenic therapy, the absolute volume based on FDOPA two weeks after initiation of therapy, was the most significant predictor of overall survival. [208] This slightly out-performed MRI, possibly implying that the overall tumour burden is a factor in survival, and that metabolic images potentially provide better estimates of disease burden. Such early yet accurate predictions of treatment response offer the potential to select more appropriate therapeutic strategies.

FLT has also been examined as an alternative to FDG for the purposes of estimating tumour margins, and in a study of 25 patients, FLT demonstrated greater with Ki-67 proliferation index. [127] FLT demonstrated superior performance to MET in the grading and assessment of proliferation in 41 newly diagnosed glioma of different grade, [132] with no complimentary information being observed. In comparison to FDOPA, the kinetic parameters of FLT were more predictive of overall survival in 126 glioma patients treated with Bevacizumab-Irinotecan, [145] although combining the modalities further improved predictive performance. However, for low grade glioma FDOPA offers better visualisation than either FLT or FDG for primary and recurrent low grade glioma. [28]

Considering low grade glioma in particular, FET has demonstrated efficacy. [209] In a retrospective study of 59 patients [210] found that the presence of FET uptake was not predictive of outcome, but in the subset of 30 patients with abnormal uptake and dynamic data, a decrease in FET was significantly predictive of outcome. FET PET has also accurately predicted antiangiogenic treatment failure in 11 patients, predicting treatment failure earlier than MRI alone. [211] However changes in FET was found to only be prognostic in astrocytic tumours and not for oligodendral tumours in a cohort of 83 patients. [212]

However, in addition to assessing glioma at the various stages of treatment, functional imaging has a role to play in the treatment of the disease by supplying metabolic information during the planning of surgery and of radiotherapy. The augmentation of MRI with PET to assist surgical planning, has demonstrated the potential to improve cost effectiveness for two scenarios of varying disease severity. [213] Recently, a fluorescent biological markers that is tumour specific, 5-Aminolevulinic Acid (5-ALA), is becoming available following its proposal and the improvement in progression free survival in stage III trials. [214] 5-ALA is efficacious not only because tumour remains easily identifiable despite tissue movement, but because anaplastic foci are not always detectable on MRI. However 5-ALA is less sensitive than FET for low grade glioma, [215] although for high grade glioma regions of high FET uptake also fluoresce. Even so there is some motivation for the use of PET during surgical planning even when in-vivo biomarkers are available, especially since the greater tumour extent made visible by FDOPA imaging compared to MRI has been revealed by biopsies to be pathological in almost all cases. [89] The latter result also has implications for radiotherapy planning.

The availability of PET imaging influences the definition of GTV when it is used to augment MR images, which has the benefit of reducing inter-observer variability and better sparing normal tissues, at least for some oncology applications. [216] A further study [121] examined patterns of failure in a cohort of 10 patients, and found that treatment failures are generally in the central region, but that neither FET-PET nor MRI optimally predicted recurrence, and that the two modalities were complementary. However inadequate coverage of GTVs as defined by increased MET-PET activity in 5 of 34 patients were associated with an increased risk of treatment failure. [217] Such contradictions mean that although the potential of PET to assist radiotherapy planning is acknowledged, more research is required before consensus is reached on what strategy should be used to define treatment volumes. [218]

Although increased metabolic activity is useful to establishing target volumes, the margins added for infiltration and patient movement to respectively obtain clinical and planned target volumes are probably sufficient to prevent geographic misses, and focal radio-resistance plays a larger role in recurrence. A recent study [219] showed that the uptake in focal regions was a better predictor of recurrence, than uptake over the tumour as a whole, highlighting the importance of intra-tumour heterogeneity. The importance of heterogeneity was confirmed for FDOPA in a study examining high-grade gliomas, [220]where focal uptake was significantly correlated with survival time while tumour-global uptake was not. At the intra-tumour scale, patterns of FET kinetic parameters have been correlated with histopathology in suspected grade II gliomas, and focal regions of anaplastic change were identified. [103]

Given the large treatment volumes, the fact that treatment failure is typically focal, and that the radio-resistance associated with local hypoxia is a contender for the cause of treatment failures, the imaging of hypoxia in conjuction with MRI could have greater efficacy than imaging using amino-acid tracers. FMISO is a PET tracer that can be used to identify hypoxic regions.

Typically only static PET images are analysed, but PET is intrinsically a dynamic modality and kinetic analysis of the dynamic data contained by PET images can reveal supplementary biological factors that are of clinical relevance. Hence, the kinetic analysis of PET data is of increasing interest, for instance Pyka et al [219] demonstrated that recurrence can be best predicted using parameters derived from dynamic data in cohort of 34 patients, and static uptake had a lower significance for low grade gliomas. The kinetics of PET uptake have been investigated for some time. Kinetic parameters derived from FDOPA demonstrated the potential to distinguishing between low and high grade gliomas for 37 patients. [221] Ellingson et al [222] have also proposed using parametric response maps to evaluate treatment response, especially for slow growing tumours. FET-PET has been shown to predict recurrence on a cohort of 14 patients with a sensitivity of 83% and a specificity 88% [219], when using the relative slope of FET uptake. Parameters derived from dynamic PET appear to offer advantages over the analysis static PET images for FET, when applied to grading gliomas. [114]

The role of medical imaging varies depending on type and grade of tumour in addition to the clinical application. When planning the surgery of low grade glioma, the intrinsic plasticity of the brain can be established using fMRI and diffusion imaging to better trade-off the resection of tumour tissue with the prevention of damage to eloquent areas. [223] PET has applicability in a wide range of clinical settings including biopsy guidance, estimating the true extent of tumours, establishing a prognosis, planning resections, detecting recurrence and monitoring therapy, [224] but benefits fewer patients for radiotherapy planning. [225] For low grade glioma the most promising PET tracers appear to be the amino acid markers FET and MET. [224] Examples of the complementary nature of PET to MRI have been noted by Berntsson et al, [226] where no correlation between tumour metabolism (MET uptake) and vascularity was found, and Rahm et al [227] where no agreement between FET uptake and anisotropic diffusion occurred. The pattern of MET uptake has also been found to differ from the pattern of neuronal cell loss and membrane proliferation shown by Cho/NAA ratios obtained from MRS and should potentially be taken into account when planning biopsies. [228]

FDOPA was found to be prognostic of low grade gliomas with non-enhancing T2 changes on MRI in a cohort of 93 patients by Rangan et al. [229] FET was also found to be prognostic in 59 patients by Jansen et al, [210] who found a rapid roll-off uptake dynamics to be predictive of shortened progression free survival although lack of uptake was not indicate of indolent disease. The pattern of uptake MRI uptake (circumscribed versus diffuse) augmented with FET PET has been found to significantly predict malignant transformation in 33 patients. [230] FET has also been used to establish whether brain lesions are neo-plastic. [111]

Static FET uptake when normalized to background is useful for predicting the malignant transformations, as is the dynamic parameter time-to-peak, [112] although the repeated PET scans suggested to detect malignant transformation early might not be possible in general clinical practice.

PET has potential utility in radiotherapy planning for recurrent and high-grade glioma. In a study of 39 patients with high-grade glioma MET defined gross tumour volumes exceeded those of MRI defined volumes in 74% of cases. [68] For the re-irradiation of recurrent high-grade glioma, in a cohort of 44 patients, patients planned using metabolic imaging (MET-PET and IMT-SPECT) had a significantly longer survival time than those planned using anatomical images alone. [231] However, Hutterer et al [232] note that the specificity of PET may be limited by passive tracer influx through the disrupted blood brain barrier and non-neoplastic lesions. The utility of PET for surgical planning for high-grade glioma has also been demonstrated, where 66 patients whose tumours were completely resected according to PET images used in planning had a prolonged survival. [233] In terms of response measurement, FET PET uptake has been demonstrated to be better than MRI at predicting the failure of Bevacizumab-

Irotocenin treatment. [234]Galldiks et al [122] also found tumour to background ratio (both mean and max) to be significant and independent predictors of progression free survival and overall survival.

For meningioma, the use of MET-PET was shown to improve inter-observer consistency for delineating margins of neoplasticity compared to MRI/CT alone in a study of 10 patients. [235] Another tracer, DOTATOC has also been used to delineate the extent of infracranial invasion [236] and has more recently been incorporated into radiotherapy planning. [237] Notably there were some masses that only DOTA could adequately identify. Cornelius et al [238] has highlighted the efficacy of PET for planning the surgery of meningioma as compliment to MRI and 5-ALA. [239]

Such observations motivate for the use of PET/MR during the planning of radiotherapy and surgery; initial experiences in the clinic have found few drawbacks for such systems in comparison to standard PET/CT and separate MRI systems. [240-242] While MRI will remain the standard baseline modality, PET has demonstrated applicability for several types of brain tumour. Applications include grading of tumours, detecting conversion to an aggressive phenotype, establishing a prognosis, planning surgery and planning radiotherapy. The enhanced sensitivity and specificity of metabolic imaging could assist in further delaying progression and improving survival time by reducing the risk of geographic misses and by identifying regions of infiltration that are occult to MRI, but only when used in concert with structural MRI. The increased availability and use of PET/MR scanners will be key to realising such ambitions.

## 5. Future developments in PET

### 5.1. Macromolecular imaging

Molecular imaging, in particular nuclear imaging, has been integral to the development and growth of the field of nanomedicine [243, 244]. The development of nanomedicines occurs over several stages, from materials development, characterisation and understanding at a molecular level to in vitro testing and eventually into in vivo models in the preclinical environment. Molecular imaging techniques have become the cornerstone of in vivo investigations in nanomedicine development and this, in turn, has led to the development of macromolecular imaging agents. The birth of the field of theranostics [245], therapeutic delivery and diagnostic reporter combined in the same molecule, has highlighted the potential of macromolecular imaging agents, which has translated into the field of neuro-oncology. The shift from a highly specific targeting molecule such as an antibody, fragment antibody, peptide or synthetic polymer to an imaging agent has become achievable with the development of facile and commercially available chemistries for the attachment of chelating ligands specific to radiometals [246]. Essentially, the library of nuclear imaging agents has expanded to the almost infinite library of specific biomolecules that have been developed over the past 40 years in the biotechnology field. The power of this approach in the imaging of brain tumours is yet to be fully realised in the clinical environment. However, an increasing number of preclinical studies are beginning to show the potential of the approach [243, 244, 247-257]. The attraction of a macromolecular imaging agent is very similar to the attractions of antibody-based therapeutics. Whereas with a targeted therapeutic the desired effect is increased anti-tumour efficacy with decreased toxicity, the advantage of an imaging agent is greater contrast between diseased and healthy tissue leading to a lower risk of misinterpretation. Additional benefits lie in the half-life of the radionuclides used to label macromolecules. Radiometals commonly used in labelling macromolecules are $^{68}$Ga (68 minute half-life), $^{64}$Cu (762.06 minute half-life) and $^{89}$Zr (4704.6 minute half-life) each offering distinct advantages over the commonly used $^{11}$C (half life = 20.3 minutes) and $^{18}$F (half-life = 109.8 minutes). Due to the short half-life, a prerequisite for using $^{11}$C and $^{18}$F tracers is access to a cyclotron and radiochemistry facilities. The enormous expense of installation of these facilities often limits the use of PET based brain tumour imaging. The long half-life of $^{64}$Cu and $^{89}$Zr allows production of the isotope at one location, shipment overnight and conjugation to the macromolecular imaging agent at the imaging facility without significant loss of tracer activity. Although the short half-life of $^{68}$Ga excludes this approach, $^{68}$Ga is produced from a generator and not by cyclotron methods, which are comparatively inexpensive and have small footprints, leading to relative ease of installation in the majority of facilities [258].

### 5.2. Macromolecular theranostics

As the chelators used to conjugate imaging nuclides can also be used to conjugate therapeutics, beta emitting nuclides such as $^{90}$Y and $^{177}$Lu the use of highly specific labelled macromolecules leads to a unique solution for personalised medicine. Essentially, what you see is what you treat. Imaging with a radiolabelled macromolecule will give the clinician a quantitative map of macromolecule tracer within the body. This can be used to either recommend the patient for treatment with the diagnostic analogue of the tracer, or rule out the patient as a successful candidate and recommend another course of treatment. The potential of this approach can be evidenced with translation of materials and regimes to the clinic. The family of octreotate peptides specific to the somatostatin family of receptors are used with increasing success in the management of neuroendocrine tumours [259-261]. A $^{68}$Ga labelled version of the peptide can be used for diagnosis and treatment planning and, if the patient is likely to display a response, a $^{177}$Lu labelled version of the peptide is administered as the treatment.

### 5.3. Molecular imaging switches

Further potential for macromolecular imaging lies in switchable imaging agents. Hardware developments in MRI have led to the possibility of multinuclear MRI. $^{19}$F (not to be confused with $^{18}$F) MRI shows great promise as a molecular imaging modality and is being investigated for a number of applications [262-269]. The gyromagnetic ratio of $^{19}$F is very close to that of $^{1}$H ($^{19}$F = 40.052, $^{1}$H = 42.576), the natural abundance of $^{19}$F is 100 % and the only endogenous $^{19}$F in the body is in the bones and the teeth. Essentially this means that $^{19}$F can be imaged on most clinical MRI scanners with the addition of a $^{19}$F radiofrequency coil, providing a higher resolution molecular imaging modality. The use of $^{19}$F MRI is most predominant in cell tracking and many cell types have been labelled with highly fluorinated polyether emulsions. Both

http://dx.doi.org/10.5772/59981

preclinical [269] and clinical [269, 270] trials have shown that imaging labelled cells in vivo is feasible at sub millimetre resolution, enough to visualise $10^3 – 10^5$ cells. [269] $^{19}F$ MRI however comes with an additional bonus: the signal can be switched on and off in response to a biological signal. There have been several reports of $^{19}F$ containing molecules that can be imaged in vivo and are sensitive to pH changes [271-275], temperature [276] and enzyme activity [277]. This is largely achieved through changes to the $T_2$ relaxation rate induced by a physical change to the environment of the polymer. The potential of this approach is high as, in theory, the same mechanism could be used to monitor the release of a drug from a nano-medicine. In this way, and with multimodal imaging platforms such as PET/MRI, key questions surrounding the efficacy of targeted therapeutics, 'how much reaches the target?', 'how fast is it cleared from the target?', 'is the drug delivered to the target?' and 'what is the response to the therapy?' can be answered by molecular imaging.

## 6. Conclusions

CT and MR imaging are currently considered the gold standard when treating patients diagnosed with a brain tumour but these techniques are much harder to interpret after treatment has commenced. Developing new therapies and improving care in the clinic will depend on overcoming these shortcomings. The introduction of PET offers the ability to gain complimentary information to that of MR and CT imaging, with many radiotracers developed for investigating tumour microbiology. While each radiotracer has its own set of caveats, there are continuing advances in tracer development and synthesis.

Hypoxia has been shown to significantly affect treatment outcomes, and although many radiotracers have been developed for imaging hypoxia, FMISO continues to be the most applicable. In addition, hypoxia has been shown to provide information on patient prognosis, tumour grading and response to therapy. Multiplexing PET imaging may provide further advances in treatment regimes, offering the ability to image with multiple radiotracers within a single acquisition, although further investigations will need to be performed to bring the technique towards clinical translation.

PET imaging has shown application far beyond the detection of tumours, including tumour grading, detecting transformation to a more aggressive phenotype, predicting outcome, planning surgery and radiotherapy. It's application to surgery and radiotherapy planning offers the potential to improve treatment by reducing the risk of geographic misses and by identifying regions of infiltration that are not seen on MRI.

Future developments in PET technology as well as radiopharmaceutical developments should see the wide adoption of theranostics, providing qualitative and quantitative measures of therapeutic efficacy. With the incorporation of molecular imaging switches in conjunction with newly developed PET/MR technology, the ability to answer vital questions about therapeutic delivery to the tumour can be answered, significantly advancing treatment development for the treatment of glioma.

## Acronyms

PET - Positron emission tomography

MRI - Magnetic resonance imaging

FET - [18F]-fluoroethyl-L-tyrosine

FDG - [18F]-Flurodeoxyglucose

FLT - [18F]fluorothymidine

LGG - Low grade glioma

FDOPA - [18F]fluoro-L-dihydroxyphenylalanine

MET - Methyl- [11C]-l-methionine

GTV - Gross tumour volume

IMT - 123I-$\alpha$-methyl-tyrosine

5-ALA - 5-Aminolevulinic acid

DOTA - 68-Ga-DOTATOC-PET

SUV - Standard uptake value

KPS - Karnofsky performance status

NAA – N-acetyl asparte

MRS - Magnetic resonance spectroscopy

BOLD MRI - Blood oxygen level dependant magnetic resonance imaging

NIRS - near infrared spectroscopy

FLAIR - Fluid attenuated inversion recovery

MVD – Microvessel density

VEGF - Vascular endothelial growth factor

HIF-1$\alpha$ - Hypoxia inducible factor-1$\alpha$

TTP - Time to tumour progression

DSCE MRI - Dynamic susceptibility contrast-enhanced magnetic resonance imaging

BBB - Blood brain barrier

RANO – Response Assessment for Neuro-Oncology

CT - computed tomography

http://dx.doi.org/10.5772/59981

## Author details

Mike Fay[1,2,3], Chris Bell[4], Nick Dowson[4], Simon Puttick[5] and Stephen Rose[4,6]

1 University of Queensland School of Medicine, Brisbane, Australia

2 Genesis Cancer Care NSW, Newcastle, Australia

3 Royal Brisbane and Women's Hospital, Queensland Health, Brisbane, Australia

4 The Australian e-Health Research Centre, CSIRO Digital Productivity & Services Flagship, Royal Brisbane and Women's Hospital, Brisbane, Australia

5 AIBN, University of Queensland, Brisbane, Australia

6 University of Queensland Centre for Clinical Research (UQCCR) Brisbane, Australia

## References

[1] Brandes AA, Tosoni A, Spagnolli F, et al. Disease progression or pseudoprogression after concomitant radiochemotherapy treatment: pitfalls in neurooncology. Neuro Oncol 2008;10:361-367.

[2] Curran SD, Muellner AU, Schwartz LH. Imaging response assessment in oncology. Cancer Imaging 2006;6:S126-130.

[3] Holdhoff M, Grossman SA. Controversies in the adjuvant therapy of high-grade gliomas. Oncologist 2011;16:351-358.

[4] Stupp R, Mason WP, van den Bent MJ, et al. Radiotherapy plus concomitant and adjuvant temozolomide for glioblastoma. N Engl J Med 2005;352:987-996.

[5] Brandes AA, Franceschi E, Tosoni A, et al. MGMT promoter methylation status can predict the incidence and outcome of pseudoprogression after concomitant radiochemotherapy in newly diagnosed glioblastoma patients. J Clin Oncol 2008;26:2192-2197.

[6] Peters LJ, O'Sullivan B, Giralt J, et al. Critical impact of radiotherapy protocol compliance and quality in the treatment of advanced head and neck cancer: results from TROG 02.02. J Clin Oncol 2010;28:2996-3001.

[7] Cloughesy TF, Mischel PS. New strategies in the molecular targeting of glioblastoma: how do you hit a moving target? Clin Cancer Res 2011;17:6-11.

[8] Matthews PM, Rabiner EA, Passchier J, Gunn RN. Positron emission tomography molecular imaging for drug development. Br J Clin Pharmacol 2012;73:175-186.

[9] Ahmed R, Oborski MJ, Hwang M, Lieberman FS, Mountz JM. Malignant gliomas: current perspectives in diagnosis, treatment, and early response assessment using advanced quantitative imaging methods. Cancer Manag Res 2014;6:149-170.

[10] Sundgren PC, Dong Q, Gomez-Hassan D, Mukherji SK, Maly P, Welsh R. Diffusion tensor imaging of the brain: review of clinical applications. Neuroradiology 2004;46:339-350.

[11] Chan JL, Lee SW, Fraass BA, et al. Survival and failure patterns of high-grade gliomas after three-dimensional conformal radiotherapy. J Clin Oncol 2002;20:1635-1642.

[12] Prabhakar R, Julka PK, Ganesh T, Munshi A, Joshi RC, Rath GK. Feasibility of using MRI alone for 3D radiation treatment planning in brain tumors. Jpn J Clin Oncol 2007;37:405-411.

[13] Horska A, Barker PB. Imaging of brain tumors: MR spectroscopy and metabolic imaging. Neuroimaging Clin N Am 2010;20:293-310.

[14] Parra NA, Maudsley AA, Gupta RK, et al. Volumetric Spectroscopic Imaging of Glioblastoma Multiforme Radiation Treatment Volumes. Int J Radiat Oncol Biol Phys 2014.

[15] van den Bent MJ, Wefel JS, Schiff D, et al. Response assessment in neuro-oncology (a report of the RANO group): assessment of outcome in trials of diffuse low-grade gliomas. Lancet Oncol 2011;12:583-593.

[16] Chen W. Clinical applications of PET in brain tumors. J Nucl Med 2007;48:1468-1481.

[17] Schiepers C, Dahlbom M, Chen W, et al. Kinetics of 3'-deoxy-3'-18F-fluorothymidine during treatment monitoring of recurrent high-grade glioma. J Nucl Med 2010;51:720-727.

[18] Timmers HJ, Chen CC, Carrasquillo JA, et al. Comparison of 18F-fluoro-L-DOPA, 18F-fluoro-deoxyglucose, and 18F-fluorodopamine PET and 123I-MIBG scintigraphy in the localization of pheochromocytoma and paraganglioma. J Clin Endocrinol Metab 2009;94:4757-4767.

[19] Fay MF, Martin JH, Rose S. New imaging techniques for more effective treatment in glioblastoma. Internal Medicine Journal 2014;44:5-6.

[20] Wang X, Hu X, Xie P, Li W, Li X, Ma L. Comparison of magnetic resonance spectroscopy and positron emission tomography in detection of tumor recurrence in post-treatment of glioma: A diagnostic meta-analysis. Asia Pac J Clin Oncol 2014.

[21] Li DL, Xu YK, Wang QS, Wu HB, Li HS. (1)(1)C-methionine and (1)(8)F-fluorodeoxyglucose positron emission tomography/CT in the evaluation of patients with suspected primary and residual/recurrent gliomas. Chin Med J (Engl) 2012;125:91-96.

[22] Spence AM, Muzi M, Mankoff DA, et al. 18F-FDG PET of gliomas at delayed intervals: improved distinction between tumor and normal gray matter. J Nucl Med 2004;45:1653-1659.

[23] Prieto E, Marti-Climent JM, Dominguez-Prado I, et al. Voxel-based analysis of dual-time-point 18F-FDG PET images for brain tumor identification and delineation. J Nucl Med 2011;52:865-872.

[24] Pauleit D, Stoffels G, Bachofner A, et al. Comparison of (18)F-FET and (18)F-FDG PET in brain tumors. Nucl Med Biol 2009;36:779-787.

[25] Lau EW, Drummond KJ, Ware RE, et al. Comparative PET study using F-18 FET and F-18 FDG for the evaluation of patients with suspected brain tumour. J Clin Neurosci 2010;17:43-49.

[26] Das K, Mittal BR, Vasistha RK, Singh P, Mathuriya SN. Role of (18)F-fluorodeoxyglucose Positron Emission Tomography scan in differentiating enhancing brain tumors. Indian J Nucl Med 2011;26:171-176.

[27] Jora C, Mattakarottu JJ, Aniruddha PG, et al. Comparative evaluation of 18F-FDOPA, 13N-AMMONIA, 18F-FDG PET/CT and MRI in primary brain tumors - A pilot study. Indian J Nucl Med 2011;26:78-81.

[28] Tripathi M, Sharma R, D'Souza M, et al. Comparative evaluation of F-18 FDOPA, F-18 FDG, and F-18 FLT-PET/CT for metabolic imaging of low grade gliomas. Clin Nucl Med 2009;34:878-883.

[29] Yoon JH, Kim JH, Kang WJ, et al. Grading of cerebral glioma with multiparametric MR imaging and 18F-FDG-PET: concordance and accuracy. Eur Radiol 2014;24:380-389.

[30] Singhal T, Narayanan TK, Jacobs MP, Bal C, Mantil JC. 11C-methionine PET for grading and prognostication in gliomas: a comparison study with 18F-FDG PET and contrast enhancement on MRI. J Nucl Med 2012;53:1709-1715.

[31] Miyake K, Shinomiya A, Okada M, Hatakeyama T, Kawai N, Tamiya T. Usefulness of FDG, MET and FLT-PET studies for the management of human gliomas. J Biomed Biotechnol 2012;2012:205818.

[32] Tsuchida T, Takeuchi H, Okazawa H, Tsujikawa T, Fujibayashi Y. Grading of brain glioma with 1-11C-acetate PET: comparison with 18F-FDG PET. Nucl Med Biol 2008;35:171-176.

[33] Derlon JM, Chapon F, Noel MH, et al. Non-invasive grading of oligodendrogliomas: correlation between in vivo metabolic pattern and histopathology. Eur J Nucl Med 2000;27:778-787.

[34] Kim CK, Alavi JB, Alavi A, Reivich M. New grading system of cerebral gliomas using positron emission tomography with F-18 fluorodeoxyglucose. J Neurooncol 1991;10:85-91.

[35] Mertens K, Acou M, Van Hauwe J, et al. Validation of 18F-FDG PET at conventional and delayed intervals for the discrimination of high-grade from low-grade gliomas: a stereotactic PET and MRI study. Clin Nucl Med 2013;38:495-500.

[36] Shi X, Liu Y, Zhang X, et al. The comparison of 13N-ammonia and 18F-FDG in the evaluation of untreated gliomas. Clin Nucl Med 2013;38:522-526.

[37] Lammering G, De Ruysscher D, van Baardwijk A, et al. The use of FDG-PET to target tumors by radiotherapy. Strahlenther Onkol 2010;186:471-481.

[38] Plotkin M, Blechschmidt C, Auf G, et al. Comparison of F-18 FET-PET with F-18 FDG-PET for biopsy planning of non-contrast-enhancing gliomas. Eur Radiol 2010;20:2496-2502.

[39] Pirotte B, Goldman S, Massager N, et al. Comparison of 18F-FDG and 11C-methionine for PET-guided stereotactic brain biopsy of gliomas. J Nucl Med 2004;45:1293-1298.

[40] Imani F, Boada FE, Lieberman FS, Davis DK, Mountz JM. Molecular and metabolic pattern classification for detection of brain glioma progression. Eur J Radiol 2014;83:e100-105.

[41] Takenaka S, Asano Y, Shinoda J, et al. Comparison of (11)C-methionine, (11)C-choline, and (18)F-fluorodeoxyglucose-PET for distinguishing glioma recurrence from radiation necrosis. Neurol Med Chir (Tokyo) 2014;54:280-289.

[42] Van Laere K, Ceyssens S, Van Calenbergh F, et al. Direct comparison of 18F-FDG and 11C-methionine PET in suspected recurrence of glioma: sensitivity, inter-observer variability and prognostic value. Eur J Nucl Med Mol Imaging 2005;32:39-51.

[43] Ozsunar Y, Mullins ME, Kwong K, et al. Glioma recurrence versus radiation necrosis? A pilot comparison of arterial spin-labeled, dynamic susceptibility contrast enhanced MRI, and FDG-PET imaging. Acad Radiol 2010;17:282-290.

[44] Gomez-Rio M, Rodriguez-Fernandez A, Ramos-Font C, Lopez-Ramirez E, Llamas-Elvira JM. Diagnostic accuracy of 201Thallium-SPECT and 18F-FDG-PET in the clinical assessment of glioma recurrence. Eur J Nucl Med Mol Imaging 2008;35:966-975.

[45] Kim YH, Oh SW, Lim YJ, et al. Differentiating radiation necrosis from tumor recurrence in high-grade gliomas: assessing the efficacy of 18F-FDG PET, 11C-methionine PET and perfusion MRI. Clin Neurol Neurosurg 2010;112:758-765.

[46] Santra A, Kumar R, Sharma P, et al. F-18 FDG PET-CT in patients with recurrent glioma: comparison with contrast enhanced MRI. Eur J Radiol 2012;81:508-513.

http://dx.doi.org/10.5772/59981

[47] Tripathi M, Sharma R, Varshney R, et al. Comparison of F-18 FDG and C-11 methionine PET/CT for the evaluation of recurrent primary brain tumors. Clin Nucl Med 2012;37:158-163.

[48] Santra A, Kumar R, Sharma P, Bal C, Julka PK, Malhotra A. Detection of recurrence in glioma: a comparative prospective study between Tc-99m GHA SPECT and F-18 FDG PET/CT. Clin Nucl Med 2011;36:650-655.

[49] Enslow MS, Zollinger LV, Morton KA, et al. Comparison of 18F-fluorodeoxyglucose and 18F-fluorothymidine PET in differentiating radiation necrosis from recurrent glioma. Clin Nucl Med 2012;37:854-861.

[50] Chen W, Silverman DH, Delaloye S, et al. 18F-FDOPA PET imaging of brain tumors: comparison study with 18F-FDG PET and evaluation of diagnostic accuracy. J Nucl Med 2006;47:904-911.

[51] Karunanithi S, Sharma P, Kumar A, et al. 18F-FDOPA PET/CT for detection of recurrence in patients with glioma: prospective comparison with 18F-FDG PET/CT. Eur J Nucl Med Mol Imaging 2013;40:1025-1035.

[52] Nihashi T, Dahabreh IJ, Terasawa T. Diagnostic accuracy of PET for recurrent glioma diagnosis: a meta-analysis. AJNR Am J Neuroradiol 2013;34:944-950, S941-911.

[53] Santra A, Kumar R, Sharma P, Bal C, Julka PK, Malhotra A. F-18 FDG PET-CT for predicting survival in patients with recurrent glioma: a prospective study. Neuroradiology 2011;53:1017-1024.

[54] De Witte O, Lefranc F, Levivier M, Salmon I, Brotchi J, Goldman S. FDG-PET as a prognostic factor in high-grade astrocytoma. J Neurooncol 2000;49:157-163.

[55] Kim S, Chung JK, Im SH, et al. 11C-methionine PET as a prognostic marker in patients with glioma: comparison with 18F-FDG PET. Eur J Nucl Med Mol Imaging 2005;32:52-59.

[56] Pardo FS, Aronen HJ, Fitzek M, et al. Correlation of FDG-PET interpretation with survival in a cohort of glioma patients. Anticancer Res 2004;24:2359-2365.

[57] Colavolpe C, Chinot O, Metellus P, et al. FDG-PET predicts survival in recurrent high-grade gliomas treated with bevacizumab and irinotecan. Neuro Oncol 2012;14:649-657.

[58] Padma MV, Said S, Jacobs M, et al. Prediction of pathology and survival by FDG PET in gliomas. J Neurooncol 2003;64:227-237.

[59] Potzi C, Becherer A, Marosi C, et al. [11C] methionine and [18F] fluorodeoxyglucose PET in the follow-up of glioblastoma multiforme. J Neurooncol 2007;84:305-314.

[60] van Waarde A, Cobben DC, Suurmeijer AJ, et al. Selectivity of 18F-FLT and 18F-FDG for differentiating tumor from inflammation in a rodent model. J Nucl Med 2004;45:695-700.

[61] Galldiks N, Kracht LW, Dunkl V, et al. Imaging of non- or very subtle contrast-enhancing malignant gliomas with [(1)(1)C]-methionine positron emission tomography. Mol Imaging 2011;10:453-459.

[62] Santoni M, Nanni C, Bittoni A, et al. [(11) C]-methionine positron emission tomography in the postoperative imaging and followup of patients with primary and recurrent gliomas. ISRN Oncol 2014;2014:463152.

[63] Kracht LW, Miletic H, Busch S, et al. Delineation of brain tumor extent with [11C]L-methionine positron emission tomography: local comparison with stereotactic histopathology. Clin Cancer Res 2004;10:7163-7170.

[64] Okada Y, Nihashi T, Fujii M, et al. Differentiation of newly diagnosed glioblastoma multiforme and intracranial diffuse large B-cell Lymphoma using (11)C-methionine and (18)F-FDG PET. Clin Nucl Med 2012;37:843-849.

[65] Gumprecht H, Grosu AL, Souvatsoglou M, Dzewas B, Weber WA, Lumenta CB. 11C-Methionine positron emission tomography for preoperative evaluation of suggestive low-grade gliomas. Zentralbl Neurochir 2007;68:19-23.

[66] Yamane T, Sakamoto S, Senda M. Clinical impact of (11)C-methionine PET on expected management of patients with brain neoplasm. Eur J Nucl Med Mol Imaging 2010;37:685-690.

[67] Terakawa Y, Tsuyuguchi N, Iwai Y, et al. Diagnostic accuracy of 11C-methionine PET for differentiation of recurrent brain tumors from radiation necrosis after radiotherapy. J Nucl Med 2008;49:694-699.

[68] Grosu AL, Weber WA, Riedel E, et al. L-(methyl-11C) methionine positron emission tomography for target delineation in resected high-grade gliomas before radiotherapy. Int J Radiat Oncol Biol Phys 2005;63:64-74.

[69] Tsuyuguchi N, Takami T, Sunada I, et al. Methionine positron emission tomography for differentiation of recurrent brain tumor and radiation necrosis after stereotactic radiosurgery--in malignant glioma. Ann Nucl Med 2004;18:291-296.

[70] Ullrich RT, Kracht L, Brunn A, et al. Methyl-L-11C-methionine PET as a diagnostic marker for malignant progression in patients with glioma. J Nucl Med 2009;50:1962-1968.

[71] Galldiks N, Dunkl V, Kracht LW, et al. Volumetry of [(1)(1)C]-methionine positron emission tomographic uptake as a prognostic marker before treatment of patients with malignant glioma. Mol Imaging 2012;11:516-527.

[72] Smits A, Westerberg E, Ribom D. Adding 11C-methionine PET to the EORTC prognostic factors in grade 2 gliomas. Eur J Nucl Med Mol Imaging 2008;35:65-71.

[73] Nuutinen J, Sonninen P, Lehikoinen P, et al. Radiotherapy treatment planning and long-term follow-up with [(11)C]methionine PET in patients with low-grade astrocytoma. Int J Radiat Oncol Biol Phys 2000;48:43-52.

[74] Ceyssens S, Van Laere K, de Groot T, Goffin J, Bormans G, Mortelmans L. [11C]methionine PET, histopathology, and survival in primary brain tumors and recurrence. AJNR Am J Neuroradiol 2006;27:1432-1437.

[75] Yamamoto Y, Nishiyama Y, Kimura N, et al. 11C-acetate PET in the evaluation of brain glioma: comparison with 11C-methionine and 18F-FDG-PET. Mol Imaging Biol 2008;10:281-287.

[76] Galldiks N, Ullrich R, Schroeter M, Fink GR, Jacobs AH, Kracht LW. Volumetry of [(11)C]-methionine PET uptake and MRI contrast enhancement in patients with recurrent glioblastoma multiforme. Eur J Nucl Med Mol Imaging 2010;37:84-92.

[77] Deng SM, Zhang B, Wu YW, Zhang W, Chen YY. Detection of glioma recurrence by (1)(1)C-methionine positron emission tomography and dynamic susceptibility contrast-enhanced magnetic resonance imaging: a meta-analysis. Nucl Med Commun 2013;34:758-766.

[78] Dandois V, Rommel D, Renard L, Jamart J, Cosnard G. Substitution of 11C-methionine PET by perfusion MRI during the follow-up of treated high-grade gliomas: preliminary results in clinical practice. J Neuroradiol 2010;37:89-97.

[79] Moulin-Romsee G, D'Hondt E, de Groot T, et al. Non-invasive grading of brain tumours using dynamic amino acid PET imaging: does it work for 11C-methionine? Eur J Nucl Med Mol Imaging 2007;34:2082-2087.

[80] Heiss WD, Wienhard K, Wagner R, et al. F-Dopa as an amino acid tracer to detect brain tumors. J Nucl Med 1996;37:1180-1182.

[81] Ledezma CJ, Chen W, Sai V, et al. 18F-FDOPA PET/MRI fusion in patients with primary/recurrent gliomas: initial experience. Eur J Radiol 2009;71:242-248.

[82] Karunanithi S, Sharma P, Kumar A, et al. Comparative diagnostic accuracy of contrast-enhanced MRI and (18)F-FDOPA PET-CT in recurrent glioma. Eur Radiol 2013;23:2628-2635.

[83] Jacob MJ, Pandit AG, Jora C, Mudalsha R, Sharma A, Pathak HC. Comparative study of (18)F-DOPA, (13)N-Ammonia and F18-FDG PET/CT in primary brain tumors. Indian J Nucl Med 2011;26:139-143.

[84] Becherer A, Karanikas G, Szabo M, et al. Brain tumour imaging with PET: a comparison between [18F]fluorodopa and [11C]methionine. Eur J Nucl Med Mol Imaging 2003;30:1561-1567.

[85] Karunanithi S, Sharma P, Kumar A, et al. Can F-FDOPA PET/CT predict survival in patients with suspected recurrent glioma? A prospective study. Eur J Radiol 2013.

[86] Behin A, Hoang-Xuan K, Carpentier AF, Delattre JY. Primary brain tumours in adults. Lancet 2003;361:323-331.

[87] Spetzler RF, Martin NA. A proposed grading system for arteriovenous malformations. J Neurosurg 1986;65:476-483.

[88] Fueger BJ, Czernin J, Cloughesy T, et al. Correlation of 6-18F-fluoro-L-dopa PET uptake with proliferation and tumor grade in newly diagnosed and recurrent gliomas. J Nucl Med 2010;51:1532-1538.

[89] Pafundi DH, Laack NN, Youland RS, et al. Biopsy validation of 18F-DOPA PET and biodistribution in gliomas for neurosurgical planning and radiotherapy target delineation: results of a prospective pilot study. Neuro Oncol 2013;15:1058-1067.

[90] Nioche C, Soret M, Gontier E, et al. Evaluation of quantitative criteria for glioma grading with static and dynamic 18F-FDopa PET/CT. Clin Nucl Med 2013;38:81-87.

[91] Dolle F, Demphel S. 6- [18F]Fluoro-L-DOPA by radiofluorodestannylation: a short and simple synthesis of a new labelling precursor. Journal of Labelled ,Ä 1998.

[92] Namavari M, Bishop A, Satyamurthy N, Bida G, Barrio JR. Regioselective radiofluorodestannylation with [18F]F2 and [18F]CH3COOF: a high yield synthesis of 6-[18F]Fluoro-L-dopa. Int J Rad Appl Instrum A 1992;43:989-996.

[93] Kao C-HK, Hsu W-L, Xie H-L, Lin M-C, Lan W-C, Chao H-Y. GMP production of [18F]FDOPA and issues concerning its quality analyses as in USP "Fluorodopa F 18 Injection". Annals of nuclear medicine 2011;25:309-316.

[94] Vries EFJD, Luurtsema G, Bru M, Elsinga PH, Vaalburg W. Fully automated synthesis module for the high yield one- pot preparation of 6- [18 F] Ø uoro- L -DOPA. 1999;51.

[95] Behnam Azad B, Chirakal R, Schrobilgen GJ. Trifluoromethanesulfonic acid, an alternative solvent medium for the direct electrophilic fluorination of DOPA: new syntheses of 6- [18F]fluoro-L-DOPA and 6- [18F]fluoro-D-DOPA. Journal of Labelled Compounds and Radiopharmaceuticals 2007;50:1236-1242.

[96] Forsback S, Eskola O, Haaparanta M, Bergmann Jr, Solin O. Electrophilic synthesis of 6- [18F]fluoro-L-DOPA using post-target produced [18F]F2. Radiochimica Acta 2008;96:845-848.

[97] Lemaire C, Gillet S, Guillouet Sp, Plenevaux A, Aerts Jl, Luxen A. Highly Enantioselective Synthesis of No-Carrier-Added 6- [18F]Fluoro-L-dopa by Chiral Phase-Transfer Alkylation. European Journal of Organic Chemistry 2004;2004:2899-2904.

[98] Wagner FM, Ermert J, Coenen HH. Three-step, "one-pot" radiosynthesis of 6-fluoro-3,4-dihydroxy-L-phenylalanine by isotopic exchange. Journal of nuclear medicine : official publication, Society of Nuclear Medicine 2009;50:1724-1729.

[99] Benouaich-Amiel A, Lubrano V, Tafani M, et al. Evaluation of O-(2- [18F]-Fluoroethyl)-L-Tyrosine in the Diagnosis of Glioblastoma. Arch Neurol 2010;67:370-372.

[100] Floeth FW, Pauleit D, Wittsack HJ, et al. Multimodal metabolic imaging of cerebral gliomas: positron emission tomography with [18F]fluoroethyl-L-tyrosine and magnetic resonance spectroscopy. J Neurosurg 2005;102:318-327.

[101] Jeong SY, Lim SM. Comparison of 3'-deoxy-3'- [18F]fluorothymidine PET and O-(2-[18F]fluoroethyl)-L-tyrosine PET in patients with newly diagnosed glioma. Nucl Med Biol 2012;39:977-981.

[102] Kratochwil C, Combs SE, Leotta K, et al. Intra-individual comparison of 18F-FET and 18F-DOPA in PET imaging of recurrent brain tumors. Neuro-oncology 2013:1-7.

[103] Kunz M, Thon N, Eigenbrod S, et al. Hot spots in dynamic (18)FET-PET delineate malignant tumor parts within suspected WHO grade II gliomas. Neuro Oncol 2011;13:307-316.

[104] Pauleit D, Floeth F, Hamacher K, et al. O-(2- [18F]fluoroethyl)-L-tyrosine PET combined with MRI improves the diagnostic assessment of cerebral gliomas. Brain 2005;128:678-687.

[105] Grosu AL, Astner ST, Riedel E, et al. An interindividual comparison of O-(2- [18F]fluoroethyl)-L-tyrosine (FET)- and L- [methyl-11C]methionine (MET)-PET in patients with brain gliomas and metastases. Int J Radiat Oncol Biol Phys 2011;81:1049-1058.

[106] Mehrkens JH, Popperl G, Rachinger W, et al. The positive predictive value of O-(2-[18F]fluoroethyl)-L-tyrosine (FET) PET in the diagnosis of a glioma recurrence after multimodal treatment. J Neurooncol 2008;88:27-35.

[107] Popperl G, Gotz C, Rachinger W, Gildehaus FJ, Tonn JC, Tatsch K. Value of O-(2-[18F]fluoroethyl)- L-tyrosine PET for the diagnosis of recurrent glioma. Eur J Nucl Med Mol Imaging 2004;31:1464-1470.

[108] Rachinger W, Goetz C, Popperl G, et al. Positron emission tomography with O-(2-[18F]fluorocthyl)-l-tyrosine versus magnetic resonance imaging in the diagnosis of recurrent gliomas. Neurosurgery 2005;57:505-511; discussion 505-511.

[109] Calcagni ML, Galli G, Giordano A, et al. Dynamic O-(2- [18F]fluoroethyl)-L-tyrosine (F-18 FET) PET for glioma grading: assessment of individual probability of malignancy. Clin Nucl Med 2011;36:841-847.

[110] Popperl G, Kreth FW, Mehrkens JH, et al. FET PET for the evaluation of untreated gliomas: correlation of FET uptake and uptake kinetics with tumour grading. Eur J Nucl Med Mol Imaging 2007;34:1933-1942.

[111] Rapp M, Heinzel A, Galldiks N, et al. Diagnostic performance of 18F-FET PET in newly diagnosed cerebral lesions suggestive of glioma. J Nucl Med 2013;54:229-235.

[112] Galldiks N, Stoffels G, Ruge MI, et al. Role of O-(2-18F-fluoroethyl)-L-tyrosine PET as a diagnostic tool for detection of malignant progression in patients with low-grade glioma. J Nucl Med 2013;54:2046-2054.

[113] Jansen NL, Graute V, Armbruster L, et al. MRI-suspected low-grade glioma: is there a need to perform dynamic FET PET? Eur J Nucl Med Mol Imaging 2012;39:1021-1029.

[114] Popperl G, Kreth FW, Herms J, et al. Analysis of 18F-FET PET for grading of recurrent gliomas: is evaluation of uptake kinetics superior to standard methods? J Nucl Med 2006;47:393-403.

[115] Dunet V, Maeder P, Nicod-Lalonde M, et al. Combination of MRI and dynamic FET PET for initial glioma grading. Nuklearmedizin 2014;53.

[116] Niyazi M, Jansen N, Ganswindt U, et al. Re-irradiation in recurrent malignant glioma: prognostic value of [18F]FET-PET. J Neurooncol 2012;110:389-395.

[117] Piroth MD, Holy R, Pinkawa M, et al. Prognostic impact of postoperative, pre-irradiation (18)F-fluoroethyl-l-tyrosine uptake in glioblastoma patients treated with radiochemotherapy. Radiother Oncol 2011;99:218-224.

[118] Piroth MD, Pinkawa M, Holy R, et al. Prognostic value of early [18F]fluoroethyltyrosine positron emission tomography after radiochemotherapy in glioblastoma multiforme. Int J Radiat Oncol Biol Phys 2011;80:176-184.

[119] Sweeney R, Polat B, Samnick S, Reiners C, Flentje M, Verburg FA. O-(2- [(18)F]fluoroethyl)-L-tyrosine uptake is an independent prognostic determinant in patients with glioma referred for radiation therapy. Ann Nucl Med 2014;28:154-162.

[120] Thiele F, Ehmer J, Piroth MD, et al. The quantification of dynamic FET PET imaging and correlation with the clinical outcome in patients with glioblastoma. Phys Med Biol 2009;54:5525-5539.

[121] Weber DC, Casanova N, Zilli T, et al. Recurrence pattern after [(18)F]fluoroethyltyrosine-positron emission tomography-guided radiotherapy for high-grade glioma: a prospective study. Radiother Oncol 2009;93:586-592.

[122] Galldiks N, Langen KJ, Holy R, et al. Assessment of treatment response in patients with glioblastoma using O-(2-18F-fluoroethyl)-L-tyrosine PET in comparison to MRI. J Nucl Med 2012;53:1048-1057.

[123] Heinzel A, Muller D, Langen KJ, et al. The use of O-(2-18F-fluoroethyl)-L-tyrosine PET for treatment management of bevacizumab and irinotecan in patients with recurrent high-grade glioma: a cost-effectiveness analysis. J Nucl Med 2013;54:1217-1222.

[124] Popperl G, Goldbrunner R, Gildehaus FJ, et al. O-(2- [18F]fluoroethyl)-L-tyrosine PET for monitoring the effects of convection-enhanced delivery of paclitaxel in patients with recurrent glioblastoma. Eur J Nucl Med Mol Imaging 2005;32:1018-1025.

[125] Heinzel A, Stock S, Langen KJ, Muller D. Cost-effectiveness analysis of FET PET-guided target selection for the diagnosis of gliomas. Eur J Nucl Med Mol Imaging 2012;39:1089-1096.

[126] Backes H, Ullrich R, Neumaier B, Kracht L, Wienhard K, Jacobs AH. Noninvasive quantification of 18F-FLT human brain PET for the assessment of tumour proliferation in patients with high-grade glioma. Eur J Nucl Med Mol Imaging 2009;36:1960-1967.

[127] Chen W, Cloughesy T, Kamdar N, et al. Imaging proliferation in brain tumors with 18F-FLT PET: comparison with 18F-FDG. J Nucl Med 2005;46:945-952.

[128] Price SJ, Fryer TD, Cleij MC, et al. Imaging regional variation of cellular proliferation in gliomas using 3'-deoxy-3'- [18F]fluorothymidine positron-emission tomography: an image-guided biopsy study. Clin Radiol 2009;64:52-63.

[129] Saga T, Kawashima H, Araki N, et al. Evaluation of primary brain tumors with FLT-PET: usefulness and limitations. Clin Nucl Med 2006;31:774-780.

[130] Shishido H, Kawai N, Miyake K, Yamamoto Y, Nishiyama Y, Tamiya T. Diagnostic Value of 11C-Methionine (MET) and 18F-Fluorothymidine (FLT) Positron Emission Tomography in Recurrent High-Grade Gliomas; Differentiation from Treatment-Induced Tissue Necrosis. Cancers (Basel) 2012;4:244-256.

[131] Ullrich R, Backes H, Li H, et al. Glioma proliferation as assessed by 3'-fluoro-3'-deoxy-L-thymidine positron emission tomography in patients with newly diagnosed high-grade glioma. Clin Cancer Res 2008;14:2049-2055.

[132] Hatakeyama T, Kawai N, Nishiyama Y, et al. 11C-methionine (MET) and 18F-fluorothymidine (FLT) PET in patients with newly diagnosed glioma. Eur J Nucl Med Mol Imaging 2008;35:2009-2017.

[133] Spence AM, Muzi M, Link JM, et al. NCI-sponsored trial for the evaluation of safety and preliminary efficacy of 3'-deoxy-3'- [18F]fluorothymidine (FLT) as a marker of proliferation in patients with recurrent gliomas: preliminary efficacy studies. Mol Imaging Biol 2009;11:343-355.

[134] Yamamoto Y, Wong TZ, Turkington TG, Hawk TC, Reardon DA, Coleman RE. 3'-Deoxy-3'- [F-18]fluorothymidine positron emission tomography in patients with recurrent glioblastoma multiforme: comparison with Gd-DTPA enhanced magnetic resonance imaging. Mol Imaging Biol 2006;8:340-347.

[135] Belohlavek O, Fencl P, Majovsky M, Jaruskova M, Benes V. FLT-PET in previously untreated patients with low-grade glioma can predict their overall survival. Nucl Med Rev Cent East Eur 2014;17:7-12.

[136] Chen W, Delaloye S, Silverman DH, et al. Predicting treatment response of malignant gliomas to bevacizumab and irinotecan by imaging proliferation with [18F] fluorothymidine positron emission tomography: a pilot study. J Clin Oncol 2007;25:4714-4721.

[137] Harris RJ, Cloughesy TF, Pope WB, et al. 18F-FDOPA and 18F-FLT positron emission tomography parametric response maps predict response in recurrent malignant gliomas treated with bevacizumab. Neuro Oncol 2012;14:1079-1089.

[138] Idema AJ, Hoffmann AL, Boogaarts HD, et al. 3'-Deoxy-3'-18F-fluorothymidine PET-derived proliferative volume predicts overall survival in high-grade glioma patients. J Nucl Med 2012;53:1904-1910.

[139] Schwarzenberg J, Czernin J, Cloughesy TF, et al. 3'-deoxy-3'-18F-fluorothymidine PET and MRI for early survival predictions in patients with recurrent malignant glioma treated with bevacizumab. J Nucl Med 2012;53:29-36.

[140] Wardak M, Schiepers C, Dahlbom M, et al. Discriminant analysis of (1)(8)F-fluorothymidine kinetic parameters to predict survival in patients with recurrent high-grade glioma. Clin Cancer Res 2011;17:6553-6562.

[141] Zhao F, Cui Y, Li M, et al. Prognostic value of 3'-Deoxy-3'-18F-Fluorothymidine ( [F] FLT PET) in patients with recurrent malignant gliomas. Nucl Med Biol 2014;41:710-715.

[142] Laymon CM, Oborski MJ, Lee VK, et al. Combined imaging biomarkers for therapy evaluation in glioblastoma multiforme: correlating sodium MRI and F-18 FLT PET on a voxel-wise basis. Magn Reson Imaging 2012;30:1268-1278.

[143] Sanghera B, Wong WL, Sonoda LI, et al. FLT PET-CT in evaluation of treatment response. Indian J Nucl Med 2014;29:65-73.

[144] Viel T, Schelhaas S, Wagner S, et al. Early assessment of the efficacy of temozolomide chemotherapy in experimental glioblastoma using [18F]FLT-PET imaging. PLoS One 2013;8:e67911.

[145] Wardak M, Schiepers C, Cloughesy TF, Dahlbom M, Phelps ME, Huang SC. (1)(8)F-FLT and (1)(8)F-FDOPA PET kinetics in recurrent brain tumors. Eur J Nucl Med Mol Imaging 2014;41:1199-1209.

[146] Shinomiya A, Kawai N, Okada M, et al. Evaluation of 3'-deoxy-3'- [18F]-fluorothymidine (18F-FLT) kinetics correlated with thymidine kinase-1 expression and cell proliferation in newly diagnosed gliomas. Eur J Nucl Med Mol Imaging 2013;40:175-185.

[147] Brizel DM, Dodge RK, Clough RW, Dewhirst MW. Oxygenation of head and neck cancer: changes during radiotherapy and impact on treatment outcome. Radiother Oncol 1999;53:113-117.

http://dx.doi.org/10.5772/59981

[148] Gatenby RA, Kessler HB, Rosenblum JS, et al. Oxygen distribution in squamous cell carcinoma metastases and its relationship to outcome of radiation therapy. Int J Radiat Oncol Biol Phys 1988;14:831-838.

[149] Kolstad P. Intercapillary distance, oxygen tension and local recurrence in cervix cancer. Scand J Clin Lab Invest Suppl 1968;106:145-157.

[150] Hall EJ. Radiobiology for the Radiologist, 4 ed. Philadelphia, PA: JB Lippincott Company, 1994.

[151] Rampling R, Cruickshank G, Lewis AD, Fitzsimmons SA, Workman P. Direct measurement of pO2 distribution and bioreductive enzymes in human malignant brain tumors. Int J Radiat Oncol Biol Phys 1994;29:427-431.

[152] Rumsey WL, Vanderkooi JM, Wilson DF. Imaging of phosphorescence: a novel method for measuring oxygen distribution in perfused tissue. Science 1988;241:1649-1651.

[153] Vinogradov SA, Grosul P, Rozhkov V, et al. Oxygen distributions in tissue measured by phosphorescence quenching. Adv Exp Med Biol 2003;510:181-185.

[154] Zhang S, Hosaka M, Yoshihara T, et al. Phosphorescent light-emitting iridium complexes serve as a hypoxia-sensing probe for tumor imaging in living animals. Cancer Res 2010;70:4490-4498.

[155] Foo SS, Abbott DF, Lawrentschuk N, Scott AM. Functional imaging of intratumoral hypoxia. Mol Imaging Biol 2004;6:291-305.

[156] Kitai T, Tanaka A, Tokuka A, et al. Quantitative detection of hemoglobin saturation in the liver with near-infrared spectroscopy. Hepatology 1993;18:926-936.

[157] Hull EL, Conover DL, Foster TH. Carbogen-induced changes in rat mammary tumour oxygenation reported by near infrared spectroscopy. Br J Cancer 1999;79:1709-1716.

[158] Jobsis FF. Non-invasive, infra-red monitoring of cerebral O2 sufficiency, bloodvolume, HbO2-Hb shifts and bloodflow. Acta Neurol Scand Suppl 1977;64:452-453.

[159] Pennekamp CW, Bots ML, Kappelle LJ, Moll FL, de Borst GJ. The value of near-infrared spectroscopy measured cerebral oximetry during carotid endarterectomy in perioperative stroke prevention. A review. Eur J Vasc Endovasc Surg 2009;38:539-545.

[160] Jette DC, Wiebe LI, Flanagan RJ, Lee J, Chapman JD. Iodoazomycin riboside (1-(5'-iodo-5'-deoxyribofuranosyl)-2-nitroimidazole), a hypoxic cell marker. I. Synthesis and in vitro characterization. Radiat Res 1986;105:169-179.

[161] Mannan RH, Somayaji VV, Lee J, Mercer JR, Chapman JD, Wiebe LI. Radioiodinated 1-(5-iodo-5-deoxy-beta-D-arabinofuranosyl)-2-nitroimidazole (iodoazomycin arabinoside: IAZA): a novel marker of tissue hypoxia. J Nucl Med 1991;32:1764-1770.

[162] Mannan RH, Mercer JR, Wiebe LI, Kumar P, Somayaji VV, Chapman JD. Radioiodinated azomycin pyranoside (IAZP): a novel non-invasive marker for the assessment of tumor hypoxia. J Nucl Biol Med 1992;36:60-67.

[163] Hustinx R, Eck SL, Alavi A. Potential applications of PET imaging in developing novel cancer therapies. J Nucl Med 1999;40:995-1002.

[164] Sorger D, Patt M, Kumar P, et al. [18F]Fluoroazomycinarabinofuranoside (18FAZA) and [18F]Fluoromisonidazole (18FMISO): a comparative study of their selective uptake in hypoxic cells and PET imaging in experimental rat tumors. Nucl Med Biol 2003;30:317-326.

[165] Koch CJ, Scheuermann JS, Divgi C, et al. Biodistribution and dosimetry of (18)F-EF5 in cancer patients with preliminary comparison of (18)F-EF5 uptake versus EF5 binding in human glioblastoma. Eur J Nucl Med Mol Imaging 2010;37:2048-2059.

[166] Rasey JS, Hofstrand PD, Chin LK, Tewson TJ. Characterization of [18F]fluoroetanidazole, a new radiopharmaceutical for detecting tumor hypoxia. J Nucl Med 1999;40:1072-1079.

[167] Hwang DR, Dence CS, Bonasera TA, Welch MJ. No-carrier-added synthesis of 3-[18F]fluoro-1-(2-nitro-1-imidazolyl)-2-propanol. A potential PET agent for detecting hypoxic but viable tissues. Int J Rad Appl Instrum A 1989;40:117-126.

[168] Kachur AV, Dolbier Jr WR, Evans SM, et al. Synthesis of new hypoxia markers EF1 and [18F]-EF1. Appl Radiat Isot 1999;51:643-650.

[169] Wada H, Iwata R, Ido T, Takai Y. Synthesis of 1- [2- [18F]fluoro-1-(hydroxymethyl)-ethoxy]methyl-2-nitroimidazole ( [18F]FENI), a potential agent for imaging hypoxic tissues by PET. Journal of Labelled Compounds and Radiopharmaceuticals 2000;43:785-793.

[170] Yang DJ, Wallace S, Cherif A, et al. Development of F-18-labeled fluoroerythronitroimidazole as a PET agent for imaging tumor hypoxia. Radiology 1995;194:795-800.

[171] Koh WJ, Rasey JS, Evans ML, et al. Imaging of hypoxia in human tumors with [F-18]fluoromisonidazole. Int J Radiat Oncol Biol Phys 1992;22:199-212.

[172] Valk PE, Mathis CA, Prados MD, Gilbert JC, Budinger TF. Hypoxia in human gliomas: demonstration by PET with fluorine-18-fluoromisonidazole. J Nucl Med 1992;33:2133-2137.

[173] Dunn IF, Heese O, Black PM. Growth factors in glioma angiogenesis: FGFs, PDGF, EGF, and TGFs. J Neurooncol 2000;50:121-137.

[174] Fischer I, Gagner JP, Law M, Newcomb EW, Zagzag D. Angiogenesis in gliomas: biology and molecular pathophysiology. Brain Pathol 2005;15:297-310.

[175] Spence AM, Muzi M, Swanson KR, et al. Regional hypoxia in glioblastoma multiforme quantified with [18F]fluoromisonidazole positron emission tomography be-

fore radiotherapy: correlation with time to progression and survival. Clin Cancer Res 2008;14:2623-2630.

[176] Swanson KR, Chakraborty G, Wang CH, et al. Complementary but distinct roles for MRI and 18F-fluoromisonidazole PET in the assessment of human glioblastomas. J Nucl Med 2009;50:36-44.

[177] Szeto MD, Chakraborty G, Hadley J, et al. Quantitative metrics of net proliferation and invasion link biological aggressiveness assessed by MRI with hypoxia assessed by FMISO-PET in newly diagnosed glioblastomas. Cancer Res 2009;69:4502-4509.

[178] Kawai N, Maeda Y, Kudomi N, et al. Correlation of biological aggressiveness assessed by 11C-methionine PET and hypoxic burden assessed by 18F-fluoromisonidazole PET in newly diagnosed glioblastoma. Eur J Nucl Med Mol Imaging 2011;38:441-450.

[179] Bos R, van Der Hoeven JJ, van Der Wall E, et al. Biologic correlates of (18)fluorodeoxyglucose uptake in human breast cancer measured by positron emission tomography. J Clin Oncol 2002;20:379-387.

[180] Clavo AC, Wahl RL. Effects of hypoxia on the uptake of tritiated thymidine, L-leucine, L-methionine and FDG in cultured cancer cells. J Nucl Med 1996;37:502-506.

[181] Evans SM, Hahn SM, Magarelli DP, Koch CJ. Hypoxic heterogeneity in human tumors: EF5 binding, vasculature, necrosis, and proliferation. Am J Clin Oncol 2001;24:467-472.

[182] Rajendran JG, Mankoff DA, O'Sullivan F, et al. Hypoxia and glucose metabolism in malignant tumors: evaluation by [18F]fluoromisonidazole and [18F]fluorodeoxyglucose positron emission tomography imaging. Clin Cancer Res 2004;10:2245-2252.

[183] Hatano T, Zhao S, Zhao Y, et al. Biological characteristics of intratumoral [F-18]fluoromisonidazole distribution in a rodent model of glioma. Int J Oncol 2013;42:823-830.

[184] Cher LM, Murone C, Lawrentschuk N, et al. Correlation of hypoxic cell fraction and angiogenesis with glucose metabolic rate in gliomas using 18F-fluoromisonidazole, 18F-FDG PET, and immunohistochemical studies. J Nucl Med 2006;47:410-418.

[185] Hirata K, Terasaka S, Shiga T, et al. (1)(8)F-Fluoromisonidazole positron emission tomography may differentiate glioblastoma multiforme from less malignant gliomas. Eur J Nucl Med Mol Imaging 2012;39:760-770.

[186] Yamamoto Y, Maeda Y, Kawai N, et al. Hypoxia assessed by 18F-fluoromisonidazole positron emission tomography in newly diagnosed gliomas. Nucl Med Commun 2012;33:621-625.

[187] Kawai N, Lin W, Cao WD, et al. Correlation between F-fluoromisonidazole PET and expression of HIF-1alpha and VEGF in newly diagnosed and recurrent malignant gliomas. Eur J Nucl Med Mol Imaging 2014.

[188] Valable S, Petit E, Roussel S, et al. Complementary information from magnetic resonance imaging and (18)F-fluoromisonidazole positron emission tomography in the assessment of the response to an antiangiogenic treatment in a rat brain tumor model. Nucl Med Biol 2011;38:781-793.

[189] Huang SC, Carson RE, Hoffman EJ, Kuhl DE, Phelps ME. An investigation of a double-tracer technique for positron computerized tomography. J Nucl Med 1982;23:816-822.

[190] Figueiras FP, Jimnez X, Pareto D, et al. Simultaneous dual-tracer PET imaging of the rat brain and its application in the study of cerebral ischemia. Molecular imaging and biology : MIB : the official publication of the Academy of Molecular Imaging 2011;13:500-510.

[191] Kadrmas DJ, Rust TC. Feasibility of rapid multitracer PET tumor imaging. Nuclear Science, IEEE Transactions on 2005;52:1341-1347.

[192] Koeppe RA, Raffel DM, Snyder SE, Ficaro EP, Kilbourn MR, Kuhl DE. Dual-[11C]tracer single-acquisition positron emission tomography studies. J Cereb Blood Flow Metab 2001;21:1480-1492.

[193] Kadrmas DJ, Rust TC, Hoffman JM. Single-scan dual-tracer FLT+FDG PET tumor characterization. Phys Med Biol 2013;58:429-449.

[194] Verhaeghe J, Reader AJ. Simultaneous water activation and glucose metabolic rate imaging with PET. Physics in medicine and biology 2013;58:393-411.

[195] Ikoma Y, Toyama H, Uemura K, Uchiyama A. Evaluation of the reliability in kinetic analysis for dual tracer injection of FDG and flumazenil PET study. In; 2001 2001, 2001: 2054-2057.

[196] Bell C, Rose S, Puttick S, et al. Dual acquisition of (18)F-FMISO and (18)F-FDOPA. Phys Med Biol 2014;59:3925-3949.

[197] Gao F, Liu H, Jian Y, Shi P. Dynamic dual-tracer PET reconstruction. Inf Process Med Imaging 2009;21:38-49.

[198] Cheng X, Navab N, Ziegler S, Shi K. Direct Parametric Image Reconstruction of Rapid Multi-tracer PET. In: Mori K, Sakuma I, Sato Y, Barillot C, Navab N, eds.: Springer Berlin Heidelberg, 2013: 155-162.

[199] Heiss WD, Raab P, Lanfermann H. Multimodality assessment of brain tumors and tumor recurrence. J Nucl Med 2011;52:1585-1600.

[200] Hu LS, Baxter LC, Smith KA, et al. Relative cerebral blood volume values to differentiate high-grade glioma recurrence from posttreatment radiation effect: direct correlation between image-guided tissue histopathology and localized dynamic susceptibility-weighted contrast-enhanced perfusion MR imaging measurements. AJNR Am J Neuroradiol 2009;30:552-558.

[201] Stupp R, Brada M, van den Bent MJ, Tonn JC, Pentheroudakis G. High-grade glioma: ESMO Clinical Practice Guidelines for diagnosis, treatment and follow-up. Ann Oncol 2014.

[202] Chaskis C, Neyns B, Michotte A, De Ridder M, Everaert H. Pseudoprogression after radiotherapy with concurrent temozolomide for high-grade glioma: clinical observations and working recommendations. Surg Neurol 2009;72:423-428.

[203] Wen PY, Macdonald DR, Reardon DA, et al. Updated response assessment criteria for high-grade gliomas: response assessment in neuro-oncology working group. J Clin Oncol 2010;28:1963-1972.

[204] Wahl RL, Jacene H, Kasamon Y, Lodge MA. From RECIST to PERCIST: Evolving Considerations for PET response criteria in solid tumors. J Nucl Med 2009;50 Suppl 1:122S-150S.

[205] Charnley N, West CM, Barnett CM, et al. Early change in glucose metabolic rate measured using FDG-PET in patients with high-grade glioma predicts response to temozolomide but not temozolomide plus radiotherapy. Int J Radiat Oncol Biol Phys 2006;66:331-338.

[206] Jager PL, Vaalburg W, Pruim J, de Vries EG, Langen KJ, Piers DA. Radiolabeled amino acids: basic aspects and clinical applications in oncology. J Nucl Med 2001;42:432-445.

[207] Langstrom B, Antoni G, Gullberg P, et al. Synthesis of L- and D- [methyl-11C]methionine. J Nucl Med 1987;28:1037-1040.

[208] Schwarzenberg J, Czernin J, Cloughesy TF, et al. Treatment Response Evaluation Using 18F-FDOPA PET in Patients with Recurrent Malignant Glioma on Bevacizumab Therapy. Clin Cancer Res 2014;20:3550-3559.

[209] Rapp M, Floeth FW, Felsberg J, et al. Clinical value of O-(2- [(18)F]-fluoroethyl)-L-tyrosine positron emission tomography in patients with low-grade glioma. Neurosurg Focus 2013;34:E3.

[210] Jansen NL, Suchorska B, Wenter V, et al. Dynamic 18F-FET PET in newly diagnosed astrocytic low-grade glioma identifies high-risk patients. J Nucl Med 2014;55:198-203.

[211] Hutterer M, Nowosielski M, Putzer D, et al. O-(2-18F-fluoroethyl)-L-tyrosine PET predicts failure of antiangiogenic treatment in patients with recurrent high-grade glioma. J Nucl Med 2011;52:856-864.

[212] Jansen N, Suchorska B, Wenter V, et al. Prognostic value of [F-18]FET-PET in newly diagnosed low grade glioma. Society of Nuclear Medicine Annual Meeting Abstracts 2013;54:355.

[213] Heinzel A, Stock S, Langen KJ, Muller D. Cost-effectiveness analysis of amino acid PET-guided surgery for supratentorial high-grade gliomas. J Nucl Med 2012;53:552-558.

[214] Stummer W, Pichlmeier U, Meinel T, Wiestler OD, Zanella F, Reulen HJ. Fluorescence-guided surgery with 5-aminolevulinic acid for resection of malignant glioma: a randomised controlled multicentre phase III trial. Lancet Oncol 2006;7:392-401.

[215] Ewelt C, Floeth FW, Felsberg J, et al. Finding the anaplastic focus in diffuse gliomas: the value of Gd-DTPA enhanced MRI, FET-PET, and intraoperative, ALA-derived tissue fluorescence. Clin Neurol Neurosurg 2011;113:541-547.

[216] van Baardwijk A, Baumert BG, Bosmans G, et al. The current status of FDG-PET in tumour volume definition in radiotherapy treatment planning. Cancer Treat Rev 2006;32:245-260.

[217] Lee IH, Piert M, Gomez-Hassan D, et al. Association of 11C-methionine PET uptake with site of failure after concurrent temozolomide and radiation for primary glioblastoma multiforme. Int J Radiat Oncol Biol Phys 2009;73:479-485.

[218] Vees H, Senthamizhchelvan S, Miralbell R, Weber DC, Ratib O, Zaidi H. Assessment of various strategies for 18F-FET PET-guided delineation of target volumes in high-grade glioma patients. Eur J Nucl Med Mol Imaging 2009;36:182-193.

[219] Pyka T, Gempt J, Ringel F, et al. Prediction of Glioma Recurrence Using Dynamic 18F-Fluoroethyltyrosine PET. AJNR Am J Neuroradiol 2014.

[220] Dowson N, Thomas P, Fay M, et al. Early prediction of treatment response in advanced gliomas with (18)F-dopa positron-emission tomography. Curr Oncol 2014;21:e172-178.

[221] Schiepers C, Chen W, Cloughesy T, Dahlbom M, Huang SC. 18F-FDOPA kinetics in brain tumors. J Nucl Med 2007;48:1651-1661.

[222] Ellingson BM, Chen W, Harris RJ, et al. PET Parametric Response Mapping for Clinical Monitoring and Treatment Response Evaluation in Brain Tumors. PET Clinics 2013;8:201-217.

[223] Duffau H. Lessons from brain mapping in surgery for low-grade glioma: insights into associations between tumour and brain plasticity. Lancet Neurol 2005;4:476-486.

[224] Duffau H. Diffuse Low-Grade Gliomas in Adults. London: Springer London, 2013.

[225] Grosu AL, Weber WA. PET for radiation treatment planning of brain tumours. Radiother Oncol 2010;96:325-327.

[226] Berntsson SG, Falk A, Savitcheva I, et al. Perfusion and diffusion MRI combined with (1)(1)C-methionine PET in the preoperative evaluation of suspected adult low-grade gliomas. J Neurooncol 2013;114:241-249.

[227] Rahm V, Boxheimer L, Bruehlmeier M, et al. Focal changes in diffusivity on apparent diffusion coefficient MR imaging and amino acid uptake on PET do not colocalize in nonenhancing low-grade gliomas. J Nucl Med 2014;55:546-550.

[228] Bisdas S, Ritz R, Bender B, et al. Metabolic mapping of gliomas using hybrid MR-PET imaging: feasibility of the method and spatial distribution of metabolic changes. Invest Radiol 2013;48:295-301.

[229] Rangan A, al e. Prognostic value of 18F-FDOPA PET in treated low-grade gliomas with non-enhancing T2 changes on MRI. Society of Nuclear Medicine Annual Meeting Abstracts, 2013;54(Supplement 2):359.

[230] Floeth FW, Pauleit D, Sabel M, et al. Prognostic value of O-(2-18F-fluoroethyl)-L-tyrosine PET and MRI in low-grade glioma. J Nucl Med 2007;48:519-527.

[231] Grosu AL, Weber WA, Franz M, et al. Reirradiation of recurrent high-grade gliomas using amino acid PET (SPECT)/CT/MRI image fusion to determine gross tumor volume for stereotactic fractionated radiotherapy. Int J Radiat Oncol Biol Phys 2005;63:511-519.

[232] Hutterer M, Nowosielski M, Putzer D, et al. [18F]-fluoro-ethyl-L-tyrosine PET: a valuable diagnostic tool in neuro-oncology, but not all that glitters is glioma. Neuro Oncol 2013;15:341-351.

[233] Pirotte BJ, Levivier M, Goldman S, et al. Positron emission tomography-guided volumetric resection of supratentorial high-grade gliomas: a survival analysis in 66 consecutive patients. Neurosurgery 2009;64:471-481; discussion 481.

[234] Galldiks N, Rapp M, Stoffels G, et al. Response assessment of bevacizumab in patients with recurrent malignant glioma using [18F]Fluoroethyl-L-tyrosine PET in comparison to MRI. Eur J Nucl Med Mol Imaging 2013;40:22-33.

[235] Grosu AL, Weber WA, Astner ST, et al. 11C-methionine PET improves the target volume delineation of meningiomas treated with stereotactic fractionated radiotherapy. Int J Radiat Oncol Biol Phys 2006;66:339-344.

[236] Graf R, Plotkin M, Steffen IG, et al. Magnetic resonance imaging, computed tomography, and 68Ga-DOTATOC positron emission tomography for imaging skull base meningiomas with infracranial extension treated with stereotactic radiotherapy--a case series. Head Face Med 2012;8:1.

[237] Thorwarth D, Muller AC, Pfannenberg C, Beyer T. Combined PET/MR imaging using (68)Ga-DOTATOC for radiotherapy treatment planning in meningioma patients. Recent Results Cancer Res 2013;194:425-439.

[238] Cornelius JF, Langen KJ, Stoffels G, Hanggi D, Sabel M, Jakob Steiger H. Positron emission tomography imaging of meningioma in clinical practice: review of literature and future directions. Neurosurgery 2012;70:1033-1041; discussion 1042.

[239] Cornelius JF, Slotty PJ, Stoffels G, Galldiks N, Langen KJ, Steiger HJ. 5-Aminolevulinic Acid and (18)F-FET-PET as Metabolic Imaging Tools for Surgery of a Recurrent Skull Base Meningioma. J Neurol Surg B Skull Base 2013;74:211-216.

[240] Bisdas S, Nagele T, Schlemmer HP, et al. Switching on the lights for real-time multimodality tumor neuroimaging: The integrated positron-emission tomography/MR imaging system. AJNR Am J Neuroradiol 2010;31:610-614.

[241] Boss A, Bisdas S, Kolb A, et al. Hybrid PET/MRI of intracranial masses: initial experiences and comparison to PET/CT. J Nucl Med 2010;51:1198-1205.

[242] Schwenzer NF, Stegger L, Bisdas S, et al. Simultaneous PET/MR imaging in a human brain PET/MR system in 50 patients--current state of image quality. Eur J Radiol 2012;81:3472-3478.

[243] Jarzabek MA, Sweeney KJ, Evans RL, et al. Molecular imaging in the development of a novel treatment paradigm for glioblastoma (GBM): an integrated multidisciplinary commentary. Drug Discov Today 2013;18:1052-1066.

[244] James ML, Gambhir SS. A Molecular Imaging Primer: Modalities, Imaging Agents, and Applications. Physiol Rev 2012;92:897-965.

[245] Kelkar SS, Reineke TM. Theranostics: Combining Imaging and Therapy. Bioconjugate Chem 2011;22:1879-1903.

[246] Cutler CS, Hennkens HM, Sisay N, Huclier-Markai S, Jurisson SS. Radiometals for Combined Imaging and Therapy. Chem Rev 2013;113:858-883.

[247] Boase NRB, Blakey I, Thurecht KJ. Molecular imaging with polymers. Polym Chem-Uk 2012;3:1384-1389.

[248] M. S, G. T. PET imaging using radiolabelled antibodies: future direction in tumor diagnois and correlate applications. Research and Reports in Nuclear Medicine 2013;3:9-17.

[249] Stockhofe K, Postema J, Schieferstein H, Ross T. Radiolabeling of Nanoparticles and Polymers for PET Imaging. Pharmaceuticals 2014;7:392-418.

[250] Accardo A, Tesauro D, Morelli G. Peptide-based targeting strategies for simultaneous imaging and therapy with nanovectors. Polym J 2013;45:481-493.

[251] Zhu Q, Qiu F, Zhu BS, Zhu XY. Hyperbranched polymers for bioimaging. Rsc Adv 2013;3:2071-2083.

[252] Boase NRB, Blakey I, Rolfe BE, Mardon K, Thurecht KJ. Synthesis of a multimodal molecular imaging probe based on a hyperbranched polymer architecture. Polymer Chemistry 2014;5:4450-4458.

[253] Wehrenberg-Klee E, Redjal N, Leece A, et al. A F(ab)'2-based EGFR targeted PET probe for glioma imaging. J NUCL MED MEETING ABSTRACTS 2014;55:1793-.

[254] Petrulli JR, Sullivan JM, Zheng MQ, et al. Quantitative Analysis of [C-11]-Erlotinib PET Demonstrates Specific Binding for Activating Mutations of the EGFR Kinase Domain. Neoplasia 2013;15:1347-1353.

[255] Olafsen T, Betting D, Kenanova VE, et al. Recombinant Anti-CD20 Antibody Fragments for Small-Animal PET Imaging of B-Cell Lymphomas. J Nucl Med 2009;50:1500-1508.

[256] Natarajan A, Hackel BJ, Gambhir SS. A Novel Engineered Anti-CD20 Tracer Enables Early Time PET Imaging in a Humanized Transgenic Mouse Model of B-cell Non-Hodgkins Lymphoma. Clin Cancer Res 2013;19:6820-6829.

[257] Cai WB, Ebrahimnejad A, Chen K, et al. Quantitative radioimmunoPET imaging of EphA2 in tumor-bearing mice. Eur J Nucl Med Mol I 2007;34:2024-2036.

[258] Rosch F. Past, present and future of Ge-68/Ga-68 generators. Appl Radiat Isotopes 2013;76:24-30.

[259] Hofman MS, Kong G, Neels OC, Eu P, Hong E, Hicks RJ. High management impact of Ga-68 DOTATATE (GaTate) PET/CT for imaging neuroendocrine and other somatostatin expressing tumours. J Med Imag Radiat On 2012;56:40-47.

[260] Hofman MS, Hicks RJ. Changing Paradigms with Molecular Imaging of Neuroendocrine Tumors. Discov Med 2012;74:71-81.

[261] Al-Nahhas A, Win Z, Szyszko T, et al. Gallium-68 PET: A new frontier in receptor cancer imaging. Anticancer Res 2007;27:4087-4094.

[262] Thurecht KJ, Blakey I, Peng H, et al. Functional Hyperbranched Polymers: Toward Targeted in Vivo F-19 Magnetic Resonance Imaging Using Designed Macromolecules. J Am Chem Soc 2010;132:5336-+.

[263] Rolfe BE, Blakey I, Squires O, et al. Multimodal Polymer Nanoparticles with Combined F-19 Magnetic Resonance and Optical Detection for Tunable, Targeted, Multimodal Imaging in Vivo. J Am Chem Soc 2014;136:2413-2419.

[264] Srinivas M, Heerschap A, Ahrens ET, Figdor CG, de Vries IJM. F-19 MRI for quantitative in vivo cell tracking. Trends Biotechnol 2010;28:363-370.

[265] Ruiz-Cabello J, Barnett BP, Bottomley PA, Bulte JWM. Fluorine (F-19) MRS and MRI in biomedicine. Nmr Biomed 2011;24:114-129.

[266] Ahrens ET, Flores R, Xu HY, Morel PA. In vivo imaging platform for tracking immunotherapeutic cells. Nat Biotechnol 2005;23:983-987.

[267] Du WJ, Nystrom AM, Zhang L, et al. Amphiphilic Hyperbranched Fluoropolymers as Nanoscopic (19)F Magnetic Resonance Imaging Agent Assemblies. Biomacromolecules 2008;9:2826-2833.

[268] Peng H, Blakey I, Dargaville B, Rasoul F, Rose S, Whittaker AK. Synthesis and evaluation of partly fluorinated block copolymers as MRI imaging agents. Biomacromolecules 2009;10:374-381.

[269] Ahrens ET, Bulte JWM. Tracking immune cells in vivo using magnetic resonance imaging. Nat Rev Immunol 2013;13:755-763.

[270] Ahrens ET, Schwartzman D, inventors; Univ Carnegie Mellon (UYCM-C) Univ Pittsburgh Commonwealth System High (UPIT-C) Ahrens E T (AHRE-Individual) Schwartzman D (SCHW-Individual), assignee. Image-guided treatment for condition associated with inflammatory response in internal organ by administering fluorine-19 MRI fluorocarbon imaging reagent, identifying internal organ and administering medicament patent WO2014043677-A2; US2014093452-A1 WO2014043677-A2 20 Mar 2014 A61K-049/06 201425.

[271] Oishi M, Sumitani S, Nagasaki Y. On-off regulation of F-19 magnetic resonance signals based on pH-Sensitive PEGylated nanogels for potential tumor-specific smart F-19 MRI probes. Bioconjugate Chem 2007;18:1379-1382.

[272] Criscione JM, Le BL, Stern E, et al. Self-assembly of pH-responsive fluorinated dendrimer-based particulates for drug delivery and noninvasive imaging. Biomaterials 2009;30:3946-3955.

[273] Nurmi L, Peng H, Seppala J, Haddleton DM, Blakey I, Whittaker AK. Synthesis and evaluation of partly fluorinated polyelectrolytes as components in F-19 MRI-detectable nanoparticles. Polym Chem-Uk 2010;1:1039-1047.

[274] Wang KW, Peng H, Thurecht KJ, Puttick S, Whittaker AK. pH-responsive star polymer nanoparticles: potential F-19 MRI contrast agents for tumour-selective imaging. Polym Chem-Uk 2013;4:4480-4489.

[275] Wang KW, Peng H, Thurecht KJ, Puttick S, Whittaker AK. Biodegradable core crosslinked star polymer nanoparticles as F-19 MRI contrast agents for selective imaging. Polym Chem-Uk 2014;5:1760-1771.

[276] Langereis S, Keupp J, van Velthoven JLJ, et al. A Temperature-Sensitive Liposomal H-1 CEST and F-19 Contrast Agent for MR Image-Guided Drug Delivery. J Am Chem Soc 2009;131:1380-+.

[277] Mizukami S, Takikawa R, Sugihara F, Shirakawa M, Kikuchi K. Dual-Function Probe to Detect Protease Activity for Fluorescence Measurement and F-19 MRI. Angew Chem Int Edit 2009;48:3641-3643.

Chapter 13

# Clinical Trials in Glioblastoma — Designs and Challenges

Helen Madsen, Justin E. Hellwinkel and
Michael W. Graner

Additional information is available at the end of the chapter

http://dx.doi.org/10.5772/58973

## 1. Introduction

High-grade gliomas are the most common and aggressive group of primary central nervous system tumors, and are characterized by grim prognoses. The glioma with the worst associated survival is Glioblastoma Multiforme (GBM), otherwise known as anaplastic astrocytoma grade IV. The median survival of patients diagnosed with GBM is just 12 to 15 months. After recurrence, only 9-15% of patients are alive and progression free at 6 months (APF6), with a median survival of 9 months.

Advances in surgical techniques and neuroimaging have proven important, but nonetheless have done little to improve survival. The standard treatment for newly diagnosed GBM remains an aggressive tripartite strategy of surgery, radiation therapy (RT), and chemotherapy with adjuvant and concurrent temozolomide (TMZ), and yet GBM almost inevitably recurs. TMZ was added to the standard of care after Stupp et al. published results in 2005 showing that TMZ extended survival by 2.5 months [1]. Other FDA approved treatments for GBM include the nitrosoureas lomustine and carmustine, as well as gliadel wafers that release carmustine and are placed during surgery. The use of these agents has been controversial and not standard, despite the fact that they have a similar effect on survival as TMZ. Upon recurrence, the treatment options for GBM are drastically diminished. Therapy is varied, and can include re-irradiation or surgery for some patients, and drug treatments. Only recently has the anti-angiogenic drug, bevacizumab, been added to the therapeutic regimen for recurrent tumors, although its impact on survival is debated [2]. NovoTTF, an electric current therapy, is also approved for use in recurrent GBM.

Current treatment for GBM is not without toxicity. None of the GBM treatments considerably extend survival or improve quality of life, and consequently the risk-benefit ratio in treating GBM is not greatly tipped towards beneficial. Indeed, individual prognostic factors of each patient, including 06-Methylguanine-DNA methyltransferase (MGMT) methylation status, presence of mutant epidermal growth factor variant III (EGFRvIII), baseline performance status, age, and extent of surgical resection, usually have a better correlation to survival than available treatments [3]. Younger age, MGMT methylation, IDH1 mutation, gross total surgical resection, and a higher performance status as measured by Karnofsky Performance Score (KPS) are positive predictors of survival [4-7].

The lack of effective treatments can be largely attributed to the biology of this glioma making it elusive to treatment. GBM is largely infiltrative of the surrounding brain tissue, so separation for surgical and radiation treatment is essentially impossible, thwarting efforts to prevent recurrence. Drugs may fail to impact GBM because of their inability to cross the blood-brain-barrier (BBB). Although it has been argued that the BBB becomes permeable due to a GBM, it is likely that many cancerous cells remain in areas with an intact BBB [8]. Additionally, the ubiquitous mutations and redundant biologic pathways in GBM allow the tumor to easily escape many therapies. Upon recurrence, GBM often mutates and takes on new genetic abnormalities, conferring resistance to treatment that previously achieved some success. Combination therapy approaches are likely the best solution to GBM's escape and resistance mechanisms[9]. New therapies, possibly combined with older ones, are sorely needed to see remarkable advancements in the treatment of GBM. Only a handful of agents have been FDA approved for GBM in the last four decades, and these include: nitrosoureas, gliadel wafers, TMZ, bevacizumab, and Novo-TTF. As such, clinical trials remain as vital as ever.

Clinical trials of innovative treatments are the avenue for progress in GBM treatment, but serious obstacles plague trials and discourage advancements. Enrollment of patients and success of investigational agents is sub-par. Only 5% of adults with cancer enter clinical trials, and a mere 6% of the agents that go into trials are ultimately FDA approved.

A major barrier to developing new treatments has been the relative infrequency of GBM. The incidence of GBM is 11,000 diagnoses and a prevalence of 25,000 each year [10]. Although it gained some notoriety in the media when Senator Edward Kennedy passed away as a result of the disease in 2009, GBM is still seen as an orphan disease. Its rarity contributes to a paucity of funding, and makes innovative drug development through clinical trial research slow and frustrating as a result of low patient accrual. With just 3% of patients who receive standard of care surviving past 5 years, new clinical trials will shape the future of this diagnosis, but presently, a very small handful of GBM patients participate in clinical trials. The world of clinical trials is fraught with ethical debates, frustrating lack of standardization across trial parameters, and low funding. The efficacy of new treatments is obscured by poorly designed trials with insufficient stratification by individual prognostic factors or ill-chosen end-point analyses. However, as researchers continue to elucidate the molecular mechanisms of GBM, innovative, targeted treatments have gained promise as the new possible solution. These include immunotherapies, anti-angiogenic drugs, and therapies against target molecules like EGFR. Well-designed clinical trials involving these agents are necessary for finding progress for the low survival rate of GBM.

Although it has been debated whether or not clinical trial research should be conducted on terminally ill patients who may not reap a survival benefit, two recent studies have shown that clinical trials unequivocally help patients, irrespective of the trial's occurrence before or after standard of care advances, including the addition of TMZ. Shahar et al [11] discovered a significant survival benefit for GBM patients who participated in clinical trials, regardless of their placement in the control or experimental arm, and independent of baseline performance scores or age. This important finding was corroborated by Field et al whose group showed that patients in clinical trials had improved outcomes, once again regardless of assigned trial arm, age, or performance status [12]. Clinical trials are valuable to academic and medical communities, and now it would appear, they can be to the patient. Patients in both arms of a trial could exhibit better outcomes because of the additional close surveillance by medical teams that offer psychological and physical support. The act of following a rigid protocol, placebo effect, and/or a change in the physician patient relationship as a result of both being observed may also suffice as explanations [12]. A disconcerting question is provoked from these results, if patients on the control arm do better than those who receive the standard of care, is it really the best standard of care?

## 2. Overview of clinical trial development

Clinical trials have progressive phases of development, starting with pre-clinical laboratory research, followed by either a pre-clinical phase 0 or phase I trial, and then a succession of phase II, phase III, and usually a phase IV trial. Pre-clinical studies precede human trials, and involve bench research, such as human cell lines, followed by translation into animal models implanted with human xenografts or syngeneic rodent tumors in immune-competent mice for immunological studies.

A phase 0 trial, also known as a micro-dosing exploratory investigational new drug trial (IND), or early phase I trial, is the first translational step into human use, after an investigational agent has been thoroughly studied in animal models. In this phase, only a small amount of drug is used, and the data generated are preliminary without intended indications about safety or effectiveness. A small number of patients with advanced disease and without available treatment options participate, and once the experimental agent is deemed acceptable for human use, a phase I trial is initiated.

Phase I trials are meant to examine the dosing of a new drug, its safety, and pharmacokinetic properties. Classically, the goal is describe the maximum tolerated dose (MTD). Notably, efficacy is not evaluated at this phase [13]. Patients in phase I trials are monitored carefully for side effects. There are approximately 20 enrolled patients, who have advanced disease where no standard treatment exists. Phase I can last for months to a year or more, depending on accruement.

Phase II trials examine the efficacy and pharmacodynamics of the investigational treatment in under 100 patients. Healthy patients are excluded from participation in oncology trials because of the high toxicity associated with cancer treatments. Unfortunately, the efficacy and toxicity of cytotoxic drugs simultaneously increase [14]. In brain tumor patients, efficacy is typically measured by tumor changes, and these are characterized on a set spectrum from complete tumor response to progressive disease, with evaluation performed through radiographic imaging [13]. If a pre-determined level of efficacy is attained, the trial may advance to phase III, otherwise, the clinical trial process is halted. Phase I and II trials may be combined if a drug is already well known for another diagnosis, as there is some existing information on toxicities and dosing.

Phase III trials involve a larger cohort of patients, anywhere from hundreds to thousands of people, and last for years. The intent is to compare the investigational treatment to the standard of care and determine if it confers some advantage over the standard, in terms of efficacy, side effects, or other factors. This phase usually employs both randomization and blinded enrollment, which in combination with larger numbers of participating patients, helps to reduce bias of earlier phase trials. After the completion of phase III, if the study agent possesses benefit over the standard treatment, FDA approval is sought.

Phase IV trials are not always required, and simply serve to answer any lingering questions after the drug has FDA approval, such as side effects that have not been sufficiently explored. Phase IV trials enroll many more patients and may last a long time. Drug companies often sponsor phase IV studies to act as post-marketing surveillance trials (NCI).

The clinical trial process through all of the phases is not easy or rapid. It takes a median of 172 days to open any phase trial, and with three phases this adds up to an extra 1.5 years spent on the administrative process. Many factors play into this slow approval, including inadequate resources for frequent institutional review board (IRB) meetings and unavailability of staff that can be allocated to protocol development. Other barriers, like contracting, or increased litigation and bureaucracy at academic centers, also slow the process. Solutions such as a centralized IRB have been proposed, but not realized. A more efficient administrative path would mean opening trials faster, and consequently patients could obtain the benefits of new treatments sooner; this does not need to come at the expense of ensuring that patient safety and research integrity stay intact [15].

One more streamlined option for drugs entering clinical trials is to apply for accelerated approval (AA). The FDA designed AA so that drugs could be more quickly approved for life-threatening conditions. It is intended for drugs that fill an unmet need in the treatment of a serious condition. Two notable social movements, namely the AIDS and breast cancer movements, helped bring the concept of AA to fruition. Patients who were sick and dying were frustrated by their inability to access promising experimental drugs that still had years before FDA approval [16]. The advent of AA alleviated some of the regulatory sluggishness and hindrances. The results of these activist movements have trickled down to affect treatment of brain tumors; for example, both TMZ and bevacizumab have been granted AA for use in GBM.

AA is faster in part because it relies upon data from surrogate end-points, as opposed to regular approval, which is granted based off of data on real clinical benefit, designated to be either prolonged survival or improved quality of life. Surrogate end-points, such as progression free survival (PFS) or overall radiographic response (ORR), are supposed to reasonably predict an effect on actual clinical measures and give evidence of an acceptable risk-benefit ratio, while

http://dx.doi.org/10.5772/58973

requiring less time to assess. Ideally, the surrogate end-point has been well validated in its relation to clinical benefit, as correlation with the clinical measure does not necessarily mean evidence of clinical improvement will follow suit. A prevalent example is the two drugs encainide and flecainide, which received AA in 1980 for their ability to suppress arrhythmias, a known risk factor in myocardial infarction. After AA, they were prescribed to almost half a million people; physicians even believed that it was unethical for control subjects in a randomized trial not to receive them. However, the completion of a randomized, post-marketing trial found that the drugs actually tripled the risk of death, and they were withdrawn from the market [17]. As shown by this example, simply correlating an end-point with a clinical benefit can be risky. Moreover, although phase II or III trials can provide the data for AA, regular approval is contingent upon the completion of required post-marketing trials that are conducted to demonstrate actual clinical benefit, or the drug may be withdrawn from the market.

Although the importance of post-marketing trials is unquestionable, it is apparent that these are not always conducted in a timely fashion for oncology drugs. The FDA granted AA to 47 new uses for 35 oncology drugs from 1992-2010, but by 2011, 21 had not been given regular approval because the clinical benefit had yet to be proven in a post-marketing trial. Monitoring from the FDA and penalties to companies that do not finish trials in a reasonable time will be necessary to preventing ineffective, or even harmful drugs from staying on the market and being prescribed. Confirming that a post-marketing trial is designed and ready for patient accrual at time that AA is granted would help ensure the drug company's compliance [17, 18].

The FDA and other regulatory agencies are not solely responsible for a challenging clinical trial process. It can also partly be attributed to the complex ethics involved in cancer clinical trials. These ethical issues are important to recognize, and play a part in the physician, patient, and greater regulatory agencies' attitudes towards clinical trial research.

## 3. Ethics of clinical trials

Ethical issues for patients in brain tumor (as well as other oncology and terminal diagnoses) trials can be sorted into a series of fundamental questions. The first question is if terminally ill patients should be considered a vulnerable population? Although the GBM patients who participate in trials are often white, male, and educated, and therefore not classically categorized as vulnerable by society, their status as dying conveys a new vulnerability [19]. A vulnerable group is defined by an inability to protect their own interests or by having cognitive impairments that interfere with decision-making capacity. Physicians and others become concerned when a dying, desperate patient becomes willing to do anything, regardless of proposed risk or benefit, for the chance of an improved outcome. GBM patients undoubtedly suffer from varying degrees of cognitive impairment, and struggle physically and psychologically, so their resulting decision making capacity could very well be reduced. Conversely, these patients arguably make other equally important decisions, such as end-of-life wishes and estate wills.

The debate regarding vulnerability should not produce the conclusion that GBM patients need to be excluded from clinical trials; the very act of exclusion of dying patients can be unjust and harm the progress of medical care [20]. It is presumptive to assume that each patient prefers palliative care to the chance for involvement in research for future treatments, having an avenue to fight their diagnosis, or being valued in the medical research world. The notion that participation in clinical trials by desperate patients is similar to coercion is also incorrect, as being in a situation with inherently limited choices towards the end of life is distinct from coercion [19]. Avoiding the categorization of terminally ill patients participating in trials as exploitation can be achieved by ensuring that the research is essential to the future of the diagnosis, that another population could not replace dying patients, and that risk is minimized [20].

A second ethics issue is the patients understanding of the informed consent process mandatory to entering a trial. Consent is intended to explain the reasons for the trial and what can be expected to happen to a patient as a result of participation. For a phase I trial, the consent process would inform the patient that the study is meant for finding dosing and safety information. Despite this, patients involved in phase I trials often cite their desire for therapeutic benefit as the reason for participation, despite the fact that phase I trials do not anticipate efficacy for patients [14, 21]. A dichotomy between what the researcher, who searches for toxicity and pharmacological details, versus the patient, who wants to get better, hopes to gain is apparent [14]. The fact that patients use phase I trials as a last-ditch effort to fight their disease and to attain a response brings up the natural conclusion that the informed consent process is inadequate. If the consent process were sufficient, the patient would be aware that they very likely would not experience a response in their disease, and that the trial is simply for dosing and safety [21]. However, this gap in understanding is not as simple as inadequate consent. A vital line must be drawn between understanding and appreciation; a patient can comprehend that the chances of receiving a therapeutic benefit are incredibly slim, and that dosing is the end-point, but what they appreciate in this scenario may remain the possibility, however small, of a benefit. Indeed, although only a third of patients report the goal of a phase I trial is for dosing information, a full 92% report it is for safety. Furthermore, it is exceedingly difficult to grasp the psychological state of a person who is dealing with serious illness and fear, and thus inadequate to assume that healthy people fully understand the perspective that gives rise to a terminal patient's decision to participate in a trial with an apparently skewed risk-benefit ratio [19]. Comprehension as a result of the informed consent process needs to be pursued and confirmed along with a realization that patients and researchers may continue to value different end goals. This will avoid exploitation and protect against the formation of false hope in patients.

The third ethics issue is the balance of the risk-benefit ratio, which is exceedingly important in ensuring that a clinical trial should be conducted. The risk-benefit ratio for terminally ill patients has is unique, as they may be more willing to accept risks in order to gain a benefit. For example, it has been historically believed that there has only been an overall response rate of 5%, and a complete response rate of 0.3-0.7%, in phase I anticancer trials. At first glance this seems quite low, and deciding whether or not conducting these trials

http://dx.doi.org/10.5772/58973

is necessary also depends upon the associated risks. However, these numbers do not include newer targeted therapies, and additionally do not contain descriptions of less drastic responses. In fact, more than 60% actually showed at least one objective response (tumor shrinkage of more than 50%). The risk of death by phase I associated toxicities was 0.5% [19]. Horstmann et al. (2005) analyzed 460 oncology trials and found a 10.6% combined complete and partial response rate, and a 34.1% rate of less than partial response or stable disease, which are higher rates than previously recognized (deaths due to toxicity was 0.49%) [22]. It is possible that the benefits of phase I trials have been understated. Horstmann also points out that the retrospective analyses lacked separation by treatment type, which greatly affects toxicity and response. In addition to higher than believed biological response rates, an encouraging result is that psychological value has been discovered in phase I oncology trials. Although a large amount of time and energy must be dedicated by the patient, which is precious at the end of life, it is arguably balanced by the comfort of frequent physician contact and a chance to exert willpower in a powerless situation [19].

Another ethical dilemma in the oncology setting is how the physician-patient relationship is altered by clinical trial participation. This issue is key because physicians are the interface between patients and clinical trial research, and enrollment of patients into trials is heavily dependent upon physician referral. Phase I trials can be frustrating for physicians. A phase I trial is traditionally designed with the 3x3 model of Fibonacci escalation, meaning the first group of patients receives a low dose, the second a higher dose, and the third the highest dose, with dose escalation in each level until a reversible, toxic event occurs. In this design, the majority of patients will receive a sub-therapeutic dose, as disease responses are typically seen at 80-120% of the maximum dose [23]. This means 60-80% of patients in phase I trials receive an ineffective dose, along with any associated toxicities, a low overall response rate, and a historical disease remission rate of just 1%. It becomes understandable why physicians would not be enthusiastic about referring patients to phase I oncology trials. Physicians have no clinical authority over the care of their patient once they are enrolled in a trial, and it is hard to communicate to a patient that even if a benefit were to occur, the chances are not optimized for each patient in a phase I trial because this is fundamentally contrary to the Hippocratic oath [21]. New dosing methods have been suggested to reduce the amount of patients who receive sub-therapeutic doses and to quicken phase I trials. These can take the form of intra-patient escalation, a higher starting dose, fewer patients in each level, and accelerating the dose escalation process [23]. The Fibonacci scheme is no longer widely implemented, which eases some ethical tension for patients and physicians [16]. Changing dosing methods to increase the likelihood of patients benefitting is desirable, but it can blur the lines between research and therapeutics. It implies that phase I trials are for benefit, when they remain to be conducted for research on safety and dosing. With a scheme like intra-patient escalation, physicians may have a greater tendency to think that they are helping their patient, even though the end-point of the phase I trial remains unchanged. Standard medical care and clinical trial research are not one and the same, but physicians and patients alike often fail to see the boundaries [21]. This aside, decreasing the number of patients who are unnecessarily exposed to a drug by employing better dosing schemes is important.

Randomized phase III trials also present issues for the doctor-patient relationship. In order for a physician to send a patient to a clinical trial, they must not believe either arm of the clinical trial is superior; the Hippocratic oath would prevent the physician from accepting randomization in this case. Physicians are inclined to operate under concern for their present patient, not the future generations that will reap the results of a successful clinical trial [24]. However, randomization and blinded enrollment are significant. Trials that do not adequately conceal patient distribution have a greater tendency to find an advantage of the new treatment over the standard. Blinded assessment produces significantly lower and more consistent scores as compared to open assessment [25]. Dealing with ethical issues surrounding randomization is essential. Reluctance of physicians to refer patients to clinical trials is a major obstacle as it begets less effective and less powerful trials due to low patient accrual.

That being said, patient interaction with clinical trials is not wholly dependent upon a relationship with a physician. Patients do seek them out independently or find them as a result of patient advocacy and social movements, as seen with the AIDS and breast cancer activist movements. It would appear that the activist movements gained a victory for terminally ill patients who seek experimental drugs through AA. However, it is feasible that AA is monetarily helpful to pharmacology companies, who can profit once approval is granted, rather than being as advantageous as patients believe it to be. In the AIDS movement, the drugs that were granted AA were extremely expensive, while still being toxic and mediocre [16]. The FDA and congressional regulations are wary of drug companies taking advantage of patients through AA, which is why it is only granted for diseases with extreme need and why, in 1991, the FDA published specific regulations for AA in life-threatening conditions, including a post-marketing trial requirement [26]. The crux of the issue in patients versus approval mechanisms is the ethical argument between the right to take experimental drugs and the need to collect drug data.

In 1980, the United States Supreme Court ruled that patients do not have the right to obtain unapproved drugs (Rutherford vs. U.S.). Gonzales vs. Raich in 2005 resulted in the Supreme Court ruling, "dispensing of new drugs, even when doctors approve their use, must await federal approval" [26]. Recently, the Supreme Court denied the Abigail Alliance's, a non-profit organization founded by a young girl's father hoping to gain access to an experimental drug for his terminally ill daughter, requests to allow drugs to be approved and used after phase I trials, and to let companies financially profit before approval. The possibility of exploitation of sick and desperate patients by drug companies was too conceivable in this case. The facts remain that 66% of oncology drugs entering phase I trials fail to be approved [27]. Thus, accepting the Abigail Alliance's desire for drug approval after phase I trials would be dangerous.

The right to early access to drugs through AA should not compromise further data collection. Once patients have access to a drug through AA, enrolling in the post-marketing trial is not appealing, yet the purpose of the trial is to ultimately understand the risk-benefit ratio, which is critical to patients and should not be undervalued [26]. Although AA is granted with the assumption that the agent will procure clinical benefit, this is not always the case. For example, if a drug receives AA after phase II, the reality is still that 45% of drugs fail phase III testing.

Consequently, AA does need to be granted with caution and the assurance that more data will follow [28]. It is also necessary to understand that rare adverse events may only be illuminated in large randomized trials, and very rare ones may only be discovered after the drug is being taken by large numbers of the population. A possible solution for mitigating the risk of AA would be staggered approval, in which the drug is approved for use in a small subset of a disease, and as more data are collected the drugs' use can be expanded [28]. A second option to reduce the risk associated with AA is expanded access for non-randomized open trials, so that more patients can enroll and receive a drug while data are generated. The National Coalition for Cancer Survivorship and the American Society for Clinical Oncology have advocated for expanded access [26].

The ethics of clinical trials do not have straightforward resolutions; the main point that must be adhered to through any of the ethical debates is protecting patients who have run out of medical options from exploitation or an unacceptably skewed risk-benefit ratio. The fact is that although clinical trials are complex to develop and run, their significance for GBM remains strong even in the midst of ethical and regulatory barriers.

## 4. Challenges in brain tumor clinical trials

Obstacles in brain tumor clinical trials will be discussed in order to illuminate why progress in the field continues to be a struggle. The issues covered will include: challenges to patient selection, trial end-point analyses, and the different trial parameters required for optimal assessment of recently developed targeted, experimental agents.

### 4.1. Patient selection and accrual

Patient accrual and selection in GBM clinical trials can be problematic, because without sufficient patient numbers or stratification, trials become ineffective. GBM is an orphan disease and consequently the number of patients who enter clinical trials is quite low. This problem is exacerbated by physician hesitance to refer patients to trials. As a result of low numbers, statistical power in clinical trials is diminished, which prevents detection of more subtle efficacies. For example, in a randomized clinical trial looking for a 50% increase in survival, 136 patients are needed per arm. To detect a 25% increase in survival, 411 patients must be in each arm. For this reason, in designing a clinical trial for a rare disease, the clinical outcome pre-determined as significant must be carefully considered [29]. By using the same standard for every disease, a drug might be inaccurately deemed ineffective and not worth studying.

Another element in patient selection for brain tumor trials is defining the appropriate control for a treatment comparison. The possibilities include: an untreated baseline from the same patient, an untreated patient in another arm, or historical controls. Historical controls are used to compare efficacy results of many phase I and II trials, but this is not an ideal measure. Historical controls can be derived from possibly flawed literature, and trials may have differed in significant ways, like eligibility criteria, lack of control for corticosteroids, types of imaging analysis, or unaccounted prognostic factors. There is little consistency across trials because of the absence of agreed upon standard care, with the exception of the Stupp protocol after 2005 [30]. With new, targeted therapies, the ideal control for a trial is to procure untreated and treated biological specimens, within the same patient over time. By the patient serving as his/her own control, the amount and function of a target can be easily and thoroughly compared. The issue in this approach lies in the feasibility and cost-effectiveness of multiple surgeries [31].

The GBM patient population is also heterogeneous in regards to individual prognostic factors. Principal prognostic factors described after a recursive partitioning analysis (RPA), performed by the Radiation Therapy Oncology Group, were the patient's age, KPS, neurological function, mental status, and extent of surgery, which is related to survival after 89% of tumor volume resection [4, 32]. Another essential factor for prognosis is tumor location. If patients are not stratified and selected for, with consideration of prognostic factors, it may become impossible to assess whether or not treatment effects are truly due to treatment or individual differences. Understanding of these prognostic factors allows patient to be sorted into four main GBM risk classes, which can be accurately compared amongst one another [32]. Risk groups determined by RPA are important in phase II trials that compare data to historical controls to eliminate patient selection bias [5]. Age is an extremely important as a prognostic factor, followed by performance status for patients older than 50 years, and within that subset, mental status causes a significant split [4, 33].

Highlighting the vitality of prognostic factor description and separation in clinical trials was reported in a retrospective analysis by Perry et al. 1997 of the RTOG database. The group discovered that pre-treatment variables (i.e. prognostic factors) impacted survival more than actual treatment. The variables examined were the duration of symptoms, neurologic abnormalities, tumor grade, age at diagnosis, and post-operative performance status. In their examination of phase II studies, it became apparent that patient selection furnished sufficient explanation of survival differences. It is clear that patient stratification is imperative for accurate treatment analysis, even though it likely increases the required number of patients for trials as subgroups are created [34].

### 4.2. Clinical trial end-points

End point analysis has been a major point of contention and frustration in many GBM clinical trials. There is no single preferred end-point, making comparisons between trials complicated and doubts about a treatment's efficacy hard to resolve. The importance of the end-point cannot be overstated, as an ill-chosen one can make a drug's efficacy seem poorer or better than it actually is, which are both detrimental outcomes. The two main types of end-point analyses for efficacy in brain tumor clinical trials are tumor response (visible tumor effects along with rate and duration of response) and tumor control (PFS or OS). Tumor control is more optimal for targeted therapy effects because it takes into account cytostatic drugs that do not impact tumor burden, as compared to tumor response, which is more sensitive to cytotoxic drugs [34]. Both PFS and tumor response rely upon radiographic imaging analysis, yet this is plagued by unreliability and lack of standardization in brain tumor patients. Radiographic imaging needs meticulous and careful assessment.

*Imaging:* Radiographic imaging is a chief tool for analyzing the results of an interventional agent in clinical trials in all phases. Imaging gives insight into direct and tangible changes in the GBM, but it also comes with many challenges. Treatments may lead to confusing imaging read-outs.

Pseudoprogression is treatment caused changes in edema or contrast enhancement that radiographically mimics increasing tumor burden [35]. Up to 30% of patients have shown psuedoprogression after RT/TMZ, as well as after chemotherapy wafers, immunotoxins delivered with convection enhanced delivery, viral gene therapy, and immunotherapies [36]. A repeat scan must be performed 4-8 weeks later helps to rule out pseudoprogression [37] in order to prevent unnecessary therapy or accidental inclusion of patients in clinical trials for recurrence [35]. Alternatively, pseudoresponse is equally as problematic as it can give rise to the perception that a therapy has caused a response. The corticosteroids used by many patients considerably reduce tumor enhancement on MRI or CT imaging, giving the false appearance of a tumor response [34]. Further, agents that target vascularity alter vessel permeability, and in turn decrease perfusion and enhancement on imaging, without the underlying tumor being affected. One example is the anti-angiogenic agent bevacizumab, which can significantly decrease enhancement within 24 hours on MRI, although the solid tumor is static [38].

There are commonly used methods for assessing imaging in many trials, although no standard is globally applied. Before current methods were proposed, the Levin criteria and the WHO response criteria were used to assess brain tumor imaging. The Levin criteria called for analysis of MRI images to assess the extent of enhancement, edema, and mass effect as compared to a baseline scan. Tumor responses were either categorized as complete, partial, stable disease, or progressive disease [35, 39]. The WHO criteria evaluated contrast-enhanced computed topography (CT) by multiplying the greatest cross-sectional enhancing tumor diameters [35]. The Levin and WHO criteria were subsequently replaced by the Macdonald criteria in 1990 because they did not have adequately defined guidelines, and did not consider artificial enhancement created by factors besides the tumor.

The Macdonald criteria use MRI, contrast-enhancing imaging, which has become the imaging gold-standard method for measuring changes in GBM. There are two different types of MRI assessment. The first is to measure the largest diameter on any single axial section, which can be done using two distinct established criteria, and the second is volumetric measure of tumor size. The first diameter method is the Macdonald Criteria (two dimensional), outlined more than 20 years ago but still widely used, which analyzes the largest enhancing tumor diameter on a single axial gadolinium-enhanced T1-weighted section. This process also considers the greatest perpendicular diameter on that section. The product of the diameters is calculated, and each subsequent imaging study is summed with the previous diameters [40]. These results are then applied to classify the results as complete response (CR), partial response (PR), stable disease (SD), and progressive disease (PD). The Macdonald criteria defines complete response as the disappearance of all enhancing measureable and non-measurable disease for at least 4 weeks, with no new lesions, no corticosteroids, and stable or improved clinical status. A partial response requires greater than 50% decrease in all enhancing perpendicular diameters compared with the baseline, with no new lesions, stable or decreasing corticosteroid use, and stable or improved clinical status. Significant progressive disease is a 25% increase in the sum of the perpendicular diameter products in contrast-enhancing lesion, a new lesion, or clinical deterioration. Stable disease is defined as anything besides complete, partial, or stable response. Clinical status is measured with KPS or Eastern Cooperative Oncology Group (ECOG) performance status (explained below) [34,40]. The criteria take into account corticosteroid use and neurological status changes. Complete and partial responses are combined to comprise what is known as overall radiographic response (ORR), which is the indication of positive treatment efficacy. Radiographic response is used in clinical trials because changes in the size of the tumor are presumably a predictor of symptomatic and survival benefit. ORR can be evaluated in a single arm trial, and it is not convoluted by the history of the disease so it can more accurately predict therapeutic benefit. ORR also has advantage as an end-point because the Macdonald criteria are widely used and relatively objective, so they enable comparison between trials [35]. However, although radiographic response and survival are believed to be related, ORR has not been directly connected to therapeutic benefit, and the significance of a partial versus a complete response is not well characterized [30]. Furthermore, radiographic response is biased against cytostatic agents that produce stable disease as opposed to partial or complete radiographic responses [36].

There are also limitations associated with the Macdonald assessment method. Macdonald criteria do not specify directions for necrotic portions, are restricted in the ability measure irregularly shaped tumors, are subjective to the radiographic reviewer, offer no guidance for multifocal tumors, face challenges in measuring around cysts or surgical cavities, and fail to assess non-enhancing tumor [35, 40, 41]. Ignoring non-enhancing tumor while simply measuring contrast enhancement is insufficient because perfusion of enhancing agents across the BBB can be influenced by many factors, including corticosteroids, inflammation, surgery, ischemia, anti-angiogenic drugs, radiation, radiological methods, seizure, and post-surgical effects [36, 41].

In an effort to rectify these limitations, updates to the Macdonald criteria have been proposed by the Response-Assessment Neurooncology (RANO) working group. The updated criteria consider, without measuring, non-enhancing regions on T2-weighted and FLAIR MRI imaging to visualize response. Any enlargements in these areas are considered as progression, and to be defined as CR, PR, or SD, the non-enhancing regions must be stable or decreased. The definition of stable disease is expanded to be a greater than 25%, but less than 50%, decrease in enhancing disease, along with no new lesions, stable or decreasing corticosteroid use, and stable or increased clinical status. Pseudoprogression is clarified by stating that within the first 12 weeks after radiotherapy, progression can only be determined if all of the enhancement occurs outside the radiation field or is pathologically confirmed [35, 41].

The other diameter measuring method is the one-dimensional RECIST criteria, published in 2000, but not as widely utilized as the Macdonald criteria because it has not been validated in brain tumors [40, 41]. RECIST finds the longest linear enhancing diameter of a lesion in one axial plane, which is repeated on later imaging studies, regardless of changing section or orientation. Non-measurable lesions are less than 10mm, less than 2 times the imaging section thickness, and cannot be cystic foci, necrotic foci, or leptomeningeal lesions. If multiple lesions must be measured, they are done so separately and summed in final analysis [40]. RECIST does not consider steroid use or neurological status, and faces similar challenges as the Macdonald criteria in regards to the difficulty of radiographically measuring a heterogeneous tumor [35]. Macdonald and RECIST have been found to be concordant in other cancers, and recent evidence found that they gave similar responses for tumor response and progression in recurrent GBM treated with irinotecan and bevacizumab [35].

The final MRI method is computer-aided volumetric assessment, in which a computer delineates the border between enhancing and non-enhancing areas over every axial section with enhancement. Border review is conducted by a neuroradiologist to calculate the total enhancing volume. Volumetric measurements can better succeed in controlling measurement variation, and may be more sensitive to early progression and response rates [40]. Nevertheless, defining the borders for measurement is problematic in this heterogeneous tumor [40]. Although there are theoretical advantages, volumetric measurements are not recommended because they are not standardized and the technology is not yet widespread [42].

Newer imaging modalities are a promising solution for imaging confusion. Spectroscopy uses metabolites to better show events in the non-enhancing tumor regions and diffusion imaging uses water diffusion into the tumor to visualize a treatment's efficacy and allow better imaging of the non-enhancing tumor. This helps distinguish between ischemia effects and recurrence. Perfusion imaging is sensitive to blood flow and permeability and therefore an ideal measure for anti-angiogenic therapy. PET scans can help distinguish recurrence versus necrosis post-radiation therapy [30, 36, 41]. T2-weighted or fluid attenuated inversion recovery (FLAIR) MRI imaging can give insight into non-enhancing tumor and the infiltrative tumor burden. These technologies have been used in some studies, although they remain to be standardized [3, 35].

In summary, tumor response on MRI is not infallibly reliable or objective, but PFS is still a common end-point. OS is another often used end-point, and does not rely on radiographic imaging. OS and PFS are explained below.

*Overall survival:* Time from diagnosis or treatment initiation to death, from tumor-related or unrelated causes, is qualified as OS. Because it does not rely upon imaging, OS is a more objective measure. Another advantage over imaging is the ability to compare to historical controls if a comparator trial arm is not present. However, caution is warranted in comparisons to historical controls due to variable start times, eligibility criteria, or less than ideal radiological review [36]. The FDA prefers OS as a gold standard end-point; OS was used in approval for gliadel wafers in recurrent GBM in 1996, gliadel wafers for first line therapy in 2003, TMZ for first line therapy in 2005, and bevacizumab for recurrent GBM in 2009. This is likely a result of the FDA's wariness of imaging subjectivity [43]. However, OS exhibits disadvantages in its inability to account for post-trial life-prolonging therapy, which is far from standardized. End of life care can range widely from antibiotics to aggressive steroid usage [34, 36]. OS also takes significantly longer in trials due to extended follow-up. However, including built in interim analysis such as OS at 12 months can lessen the time needed before analysis. Reduction in time required before measurement is the primary reason PFS is often utilized as an alternative end-point.

*Progression Free Survival:* PFS is the time between tumor stabilization, after surgery or RT/TMZ, and subsequent radiographic tumor progression. Survival and PFS are well correlated, despite inter-patient discrepancies in KPS, age, or prior chemotherapy treatment [29, 30]. PFS is often used as a surrogate end-point for clinical benefit, especially in trials for brain tumors, but it does require special consideration. PFS is optimally assessed through a blinded independent radiology review board, and a control arm has to be included for efficacy comparisons. The FDA is wary of PFS because of its reliance on subjective radiographic imaging. It is unlikely that PFS would provide adequate evidence for AA if a drug were on the market that had already shown significant survival benefit [18]. PFS is free of corruption by life-prolonging treatments [34], and the more frequent occurrence of imaging measurements in comparison to OS. PFS also yields increases in statistical power, facilitating trials involving fewer patients and less time [30]. The standardization of PFS has been improved by setting specified time points for imaging in order to negate time dependent assessment bias [36]. Using 6 month PFS (6moPFS) as the determined end-point is a common choice, as it allows imaging to take place over an adequate amount of time, and this longer time point may be better linked to OS. If 6moPFS were to be substituted for OS as an endpoint in FDA AA decisions, a randomized trial would go from requiring 134 patients and 3.5 years to needing 134 patients and 1.5 years. However, the FDA remains reluctant to accept PFS as a reliable measure.

*1.3.3. Secondary end-points:* There also exist other relevant end-point analyses besides tumor response and tumor control in brain tumor clinical trials. Secondary end-points like quality of life (QOL) or neurocognitive function are significant because radiographic imaging changes do not necessarily give clear insight into the effect of tumor burden or the drug on the patient's everyday life. Survival benefit goes beyond response and survival to encompass improvement of disease-related symptoms and/or QOL. Traditionally, KPS and QOL questions are used to satisfy questions about a treatment's impact on the patient. KPS is frequently used in clinical trials, which measures, on a scale from 0-100, the patient's activity level and medical care requirements. KPS is more related to prognosis and overall physical status than QOL. The ECOG score, also known as the WHO performance score, can also measure performance status. The WHO score is a five-point scale derived from KPS, but it is slightly more simple [44, 45].

The FDA and the North American Brain Tumor Coalition (NABTC) have declared QOL a secondary end-point of interest, but it is notoriously resistant to standardized measurement and therefore it is challenging to validate QOL data to support drug approval [29, 30, 43]. A main problem in measuring QOL is that patients often do not fill out all questionnaires over time, due to symptomatic development, loss of motivation, or doctors and nurses failing to administer or explain questionnaires, so data remain incomplete. There are different questionnaires currently available to measure QOL, but none have become the standard. The MMSE is a questionnaire intended to give insight into QOL, but it is insensitive to mild cognitive impairments and is more appropriate for detecting dementia. QOL questionnaires have been developed by the Functional Assessment of Cancer Therapy (FACT) and the European Organization for the Research and Treatment of Cancer (EORTC) that incorporate information given by the patient and their proxy, although proxies often cannot accurately recapitulate the necessary data and may exaggerate HR-QOL issues while underestimating psychological

http://dx.doi.org/10.5772/58973

problems [34, 46, 47]. The EORTC's QLQ-C30 is a 30 item functional and symptomatic assessment for HR-QOL. A measurement specific for brain cancer developed by this group, the EORTC QLQ-BN20, has 20 items and assesses visual disorder, motor dysfunction, disease symptoms, treatment toxicity, and future uncertainty. The FACT-BR questionnaire is specific to brain cancer and examines physical, social, emotional, and functional measures and is more psychologically, than symptomatically focused [47]. Even if QOL cannot yet be used to support drug approval, it is an important measure in clinical trials of how a patient is coping with treatment, and a worsening QOL needs to be monitored and corrected.

### 4.3. Future of brain tumor clinical trials

The end-points in clinical trials for targeted therapies need to be re-evaluated. Targeted therapies frequently work in a cytostatic fashion, and judging their efficacy on imaging is often inappropriate. Because the biology of GBM is unimaginably complex, it is not likely that a single molecular agent will produce dramatic results on imaging. Instead, taking stock of biological markers before and after treatment will allow a better glimpse at if and how the drug is working. Other cancers have made use of biological markers, but this trend has not yet taken root in brain tumor clinical trials. The relationship between biological molecular changes and tumor response and clinical benefit requires comprehension before markers can be useful. Grasping how molecular markers respond to a treatment will help explain the ideal context for a drug. For example, identifying where it affects a biological pathway can shed light on combination therapy options. Preclinical evaluations in animal models will help define when molecular marker changes are significant in relation to survival or tumor burden. One biological marker in gliomas is phosphorylation of a target receptor in association with tyrosine kinase inhibitor drugs [31]. This measure is direct evaluation of the target, rather than upstream or downstream molecules, which provides a clear picture of the drug's effect on the intended target. However, this does not take into consideration the target as part of a larger biological environment.

An ideal picture of biological events can be gleaned through analysis of surgical tumor samples. The most powerful scenario for efficacy appraisal using biomarkers is to administer the investigational drug before acquiring a tumor sample through biopsy or craniotomy, then give more investigational drug, and finally take another surgical tissue specimen after a specified amount of time has passed. In this model, the changes in biological pathways in direct relation to a drug can be carefully and thoroughly studied, but there are many disadvantages as well. The major obstacle is that not all surgeries are therapeutically necessary. Craniotomies are expensive and risky, while less invasive biopsies are a poor substitute as they may not be representative of the tumor [29, 31].

Moreover, some investigational drugs, namely anti-angiogenic agents, preclude surgery because they interfere with blood clotting, wound healing, and can complicate anesthesia. Immunotherapeutic drugs might also block necessary immune responses in unexpected ways after surgery [31, 34]. When the drug-surgery cycle is feasible, training must be in place for surgeons. In surgery, circumferential dissection yields more viable tissue than inside-out methods, thus standardization of how tissue is acquired is a key control step for clinical trial quality. In anticipation of this issue, surgeons who work with the NABTC have been taught the expected tissue acquisition methods.

Because the drug-surgery model is not always an option for patients, non-invasive marker development will be essential for these cases. Indeed, elucidating appropriate biomarkers and avoiding unnecessary surgery would be preferred in every possible situation. Non-invasive biomarkers were explored in clinical trials on the GBM drug cediranib. The trial utilized non-invasive biomarkers, including circulating progenitor cells (CPCs), circulating endothelial cells (CECs), and amounts of pro-angiogenic proteins in the plasma. These biomarkers were coupled with MRI for perfusion, permeability, and vessel size. Briefly, the study, which will be discussed more below, discovered that the biomarkers were useful to predicting certain tumor behaviors. Furthermore, it was revealed that the drug had a short-lived response, something that may have gone undetected without molecular markers [31]. Fully comprehending the drug's effect is crucial, because subtle windows of efficacy such as this should not be missed or the drug will be mistakenly shelved as ineffective.

Incorporating molecular markers would merit re-vamping of phase 0, I, and II trials, hopefully into a more streamlined process. Trials that use molecular markers would preferably switch from calculating MTD to appropriate biological dose (ABD), instead. As stated previously, MTD works well for cytotoxic agents where a higher the dose equals a higher efficacy. However, ABD can occur well below MTD, and is a function of affecting the target as desired [31].

Phase 0 trials traditionally assess pharmacokinetic and pharmacodynamic properties in a small group of patients, followed by phase I revealing the MTD. An accelerated combined phase 0/I trial of a targeted molecular agent could simultaneously define ABD and gain a preliminary understanding of the drug's action on its target. Actually binding the target with the drug would be a requirement for entering a phase II trial. The phase 0/I design is not meant to replace the dose escalation assessment in phase I or the efficacy analysis in phase II, but it would facilitate an efficient use of time and financial resources by combining dosing with initial target data [29]. Using molecular markers in a phase II trial to show that a molecular agent affects, not just binds the target as intended, would be crucial. Imaging and clinical data would remain helpful as an indirect end-point, especially in combination treatment trials; yet it is vital to keep in mind that a monotherapy clinical trial is unlikely to produce an obvious clinical benefit [31]. Currently, more phase II trials are arising that have surgical arms to facilitate analysis of molecular markers [8]. A phase II trial could go beyond its role for efficacy by identifying a relevant target population. This way, enrolling patients in clinical trials, who are not expected to benefit from it, could be avoided [29].

Comprehending if and how the drug works on the target will produce a knowledgeable foundation for future drug combinations, which is probably the most promising method for GBM treatment [31]. Although a drug may not produce obvious alterations to a clinical or radiographic end-point as monotherapy, its effectiveness could be augmented by adjuvant administration of other carefully selected drugs that simultaneously target relevant connected pathways. Tailoring combinations of targeted molecular agents based on the individual's molecular profile is a future possibility, and trials may come to be designed for patients with different markers [48].

Ahead of many proposed clinical trial design changes, targeted molecular agents have begun to infiltrate clinical trials for GBM, some of which will be explored below. Certain clinical trial changes have taken place, but they are not uniform across the board. In addition to targeted therapies, immunotherapies and other therapies will be discussed, as they are prevalent in the clinical trial landscape and encompass similar trial designs and possible changes, such as use of biomarkers, as targeted molecular agents. The clinical trials discussed are intended to serve as practical examples of the changes, as well as established methods, that are actually taking place in trials, rather than theoretical propositions. Two important points of focus will be end-point analysis and choice of control in the clinical trials. The clinical trials examined below have either been recently completed, or are ongoing. They are organized into categories by the type of interventional agent, namely: anti-angiogenic/receptor tyrosine kinase (RTK) inhibitors, immunotherapies, and other therapy.

## 5. Discussion— Current clinical trials

### 5.1. Receptor tyrosine kinase inhibitor agents

RTK's are an enticing target in GBM because the RTK/ phosphoinositide 3-kinase (PI3K) / protein kinase b (AKT) pathway has mutations in over 80% of tumors [49]. RTKs, such as EGFR, bind and activate PI3Ks, which in turn activate AKT that has many downstream targets and causes apoptosis inhibition while stimulating growth and proliferation [50]. One important downstream target of AKT is hypoxia-inducible factor-1$\alpha$ (HIF-1$\alpha$), a key player in angiogenesis [51]. EGFR is especially ubiquitous with a 40% alteration rate through mutation, rearrangement, or amplification [49, 52]. PI3K is not the only mediator in functional RTK signaling; in fact *in vivo* activation of various RTKs prohibits GBM from being dependent on any single RTK for important downstream signaling [52]. GBMs are so variable that they can be comprised of cells with different driver genes of RTKs, such as EGFR and PDGF, exhibiting various activation statuses from cell to cell. Therapeutically, a silver lining is that these coexisting subpopulations have shared early genetic mutations, suggesting the existence of a possibly targetable precursor cell [53]. RTK therapy has given sub-par evidence of efficacy in trials thus far. Clinical trial results may improve if targeted molecular therapy addresses the presence of the target and the circuitry in which it occurs, the appropriate type of trial evaluation, that GBMs are complex networks with cross-talk and feedback loops, and the tendency of cancer cells to rapidly mutate due to genomic instability. Each of these elements is likely to impact the effectiveness of any targeted therapy. A lesson should be learned from the failure of HIV monotherapy and success of combination therapy as an example of the approach needed in quickly mutating diseases [54]. This begs the question of why RTKs are evaluated as monotherapy in clinical trials and expected to produce clinical benefit when the efficacy of a single agent is highly unlikely due to ubiquitous presence of different activated RTKs in GBM.

Erraticism in RTK profiles from patient to patient and even within one tumor is precisely why combination therapy for RTK inhibitors would be necessary to demonstrate therapeutic success. Combinations might even be optimized if they are based on the individual's specific RTK activation profile [52]. This will not be an easy undertaking, as the experience with some drugs' efficacy, namely cediranib, not correlating with the target expression indicates. Targets are not biologically isolated, and their expression does not guarantee a targeted treatment will have results. Combination therapy comes with its own issues in teasing out toxicities and efficacy of different agents.

Ensuring that the RTK inhibitors, especially anti-angiogenic therapies, actually impact the tumor is paramount to understanding their influence on efficacy. Imaging issues have already been discussed; anti-angiogenic drugs can cause convoluted imaging read-outs with transient improvement in edema and mass effect. As such, biomarkers will be vital in clinical trials, as well as other imaging options, such as T2 and FLAIR MRI or PET with amino acid tracers [36, 37]. Finally, the side effects of RTKs are not negligible, and may affect future treatments, such as surgery due to inhibited wound healing [29]. Selecting the patient population that is most likely to benefit is essential for reducing unnecessary exposures to these drugs.

#### *5.1.1. Bevacizumab*

Bevacizumab is a humanized, monoclonal antibody that inhibits vascular endothelial growth factor (VEGFA), the ligand of the VEGF receptor, a receptor tyrosine kinase associated with angiogenesis. Angiogenesis is vital to embryogenesis in order to develop the vascular system from endothelial cells. When a tumor becomes too large (greater than 1-2mm) to rely on the host vasculature, it may transition from avascular to vascular prompted by hypoxia-induced activation of pro-angiogenic factors such as VEGF and transforming growth factor beta (TGF-β). VEGF is an important inducer of angiogenesis, and is over-expressed in GBM, as well as many other cancers [55]. Bevacizumab was granted FDA accelerated approved for the treatment of recurrent GBM on May 5$^{th}$, 2009, based on the evidence for objective tumor response provided by two phase II studies. The process of bevacizumab through clinical trials is discussed.

#### *5.1.2. AVF3708*

This phase II trial was designed to study GBM in its first or second recurrence and give evidence for AA. The trial had two arms: bevacizumab as monotherapy and bevacizumab with Irinotecan, and was historically controlled. To be eligible, patients may have had prior surgery or biopsy, prior RT/TMZ, demonstrable radiographic evidence of progression after therapy, stable or decreasing corticosteroid use 5 days before the baseline MRI, and a KPS ≥ 70. The median age of the bevacizumab arm was 54 years, and KPS was stratified in groups of 70-80 and 90-100. There were 85 patients in the bevacizumab monotherapy arm; the irinotecan and bevacizumab arm were not analyzed for approval because the FDA stated that the efficacy of bevacizumab and irinotecan were inseparable. 6moPFS was the designated primary trial end-point. However, the primary end-point per the FDA was objective response rate, as 6moPFS needs a comparative control to show results. An independent review committee determined the objective response rate according to Macdonald response criteria, and the MRI readings were confirmed 4 weeks later. Secondary end-points were the duration of response and safety. Historical control data was from an analysis by Wong et al [56] of eight phase II trials at the M.D. Anderson Cancer Center, which included 225 GBM patients. In these studies, both CT and MRI imaging were used, scans were performed every 2 months, and criteria similar to Macdonald were used. In the AVF3708 trial, MRI imaging was conducted every six weeks with Macdonald criteria. The historical control objective response rates were assumed to be 5% for the bevacizumab monotherapy arm, and 15% for the 6moPFS. A significant 28.2% objective response rate with 1 CR and 23 PR, and a duration of 5.6 months was reported. The FDA reported a 25.9% response rate with 4.5 months duration. The discordance rate for objective response rate assessments between two assigned, independent review radiologists was 47.1% and a third radiologist failed to agree with the first two 14.3% of the time. The high frequency of disagreement highlights exactly why the FDA is hesitant about MRI usage in clinical trials, especially with anti-angiogenic therapies that are known to change MRI readings, as stated previously [38]. The 6moPFS reported by the trial sponsor (Genentech) was significant at 43.6%, the 6moPFS reported by the FDA was significant at 36%, and as reported by the investigator was significant at 42.6%. The discrepancy was purportedly due to the fact that Genentech used a 5.52 month cut-off, while the FDA adhered to 6 months. Although historical controls are not ideal due to possible population differences, tumor assessment frequency and criteria, along with type of follow-up, Genentech proposed that such a large change in 6moPFS is a reasonable predictor of clinical benefit.

AVF3708 suffered from lack of clarity over the end-point of choice, since the FDA disagreed with Genentech. The study also relied upon historical controls, which are never optimal, and due to poor planning was unable to use data from the bevacizumab and irinotecan arm. Finally, although the study used Macdonald criteria, the objective response rate was obviously a point of contention with disagreement between reviewers. Despite these issues, this data was used to support AA.

#### *5.1.3. NCI 06-C-0064E*

A second phase II trial examined the efficacy of bevacizumab in recurrent GBM, as compared to historical controls. It used the same tumor assessment criteria (Macdonald) with an independent review process, but collected MRI every 4 instead of 6 weeks. The median age of the patients (n=56) was 54 years, and KPS was stratified with a group scoring 70-80 and a group scoring 90-100. Patients had previously undergone surgery, radiation, and systemic chemo-therapy. Once again, PFS was the determined end-point, but it was agreed that the data on objective response rate and the duration of the response would be used to support bevacizu-mab approval. A 19.6% response rate with a median duration of 3.9 months was reported. These data supported AA along with AVF3708.

#### *5.1.4. Post-marketing trials*

After AA was granted based on these phase II trials, two post-marketing phase III clinical trials, as required by the FDA after AA, were initiated. They were intended to confirm the efficacy of bevacizumab, but this time in the primary tumor setting, and the trials have recently have reported results. The first trial, AVF4396g, was sponsored by the drug company Hoffman-La Roche and was a randomized, double-blind, placebo-controlled study of bevacizumab in combination with RT/TMZ for 921 newly diagnosed GBM patients. The median age in the treatment group was 57 years and in the placebo group it was 56 years. KPS was stratified with 32.6% and 30.3% having a score of 50-80 in the treatment and placebo groups, respectively, and 67.4% and 69.7% having a score of 90-100 in the treatment and placebo groups, respectively. Patients were also organized into RPA classes, with the majority being in class IV. The primary end-points were designated as OS and PFS, although the FDA declared OS as the principal regulatory end-point. Updated Macdonald criteria were used for imaging assessment. Patients were randomized with recursive partitioning analysis to receive RT/TMZ with or without bevacizumab (FDA 2009). The median PFS was significantly higher at 10.6 months in the bevacizumab arm versus 6.2 months in the placebo arm. OS was not significantly different in the experimental versus placebo groups, 72.4% and 66.3% at 1 year, and 33.9% and 30.1% at two years, respectively. No change was observed in QOL or neurocognitive function [57].

The second phase III trial was sponsored by the National Cancer Institute, and enrolled 978 patients, 637 of whom were eligible to undergo randomization to receive RT/TMZ with bevacizumab or a placebo. The median age was 58 years in the randomized group. There was a KPS of 60-80 in 40% and 39% of the treatment and placebo groups, respectively, and a KPS of 90-100 in 60% and 61% of the treatment and control groups, respectively. The majority of patients had total resection, although roughly a third had partial resection. RPA class stratification was used, with most patients being in class IV. There was no significant effect on OS, 15.7 months in the bevacizumab group and 16.1 months in the placebo arm. OS was similar to the AVF4396g study, but PFS differed, possibly due to a statistical difference in the pre-specified alpha level for progression ($p<0.01$). PFS was improved at 10.7 versus 7.3 months. This study reported that over time patients experienced worsened quality of life, a greater symptom burden, and a decline in neurocognitive function [58].

The phase III trials failed to show a direct clinical benefit for survival, which jeopardizes the continued usage of bevacizumab in GBM, at least in the upfront setting. Disturbingly, these two trials presented contrasting data on the impact on the quality of life for GBM patients. This was puzzling as both studies used the EORTC's QLQ-30 and BN20 questionnaires for quality of life assessment. AVF4396g used updated Macdonald imaging criteria that took into account non-enhancing tumor, so the possibility of missing a progression in disease was reduced, which could have affected QOL [57]. The lessening of edema and subsequent reduced need for corticosteroids is the purported benefit to QOL seen in AVF4396g. Differences in statistics and imaging criteria between the post-marketing trials are not negligible, and point to the challenge of which results are to be most convincing.

Bevacizumab is a germane example of a drug that received AA, only to disappoint in confirmatory trials. If bevacizumab is indeed harmful to the quality of life, as suggested by the NCI's phase III trial, its presence on the market is concerning, although the differences in primary vs recurrent setting may clarify that. It could be speculated that early studies and AA were flawed in their reliance on imaging dependent end-points as their initial primary considerations. Objective response and 6moPFS may not accurately predict clinical benefit. The issues with imaging in the trial are substantiated by the almost 50% frequency of disagreement in AVF3708 between radiological reviewers according to the FDA. AA is also based on much smaller trials, whereas the phase III trials combined looked at almost 2,000 patients, so statistical power is greatly improved. It remains to be seen how bevacizumab will be prescribed in the future, now that it is has a debatable effect on survival. It has not been removed from the market, and continues to be evaluated in clinical trials.

### 5.1.5. *Cediranib*

A receptor tyrosine kinase inhibitor that recently went through clinical trials is Cediranib (AZD2171), a pan-VEGFR inhibitor with some activity against related structures c-Kit and-which acts against platelet-derived growth factor receptors (PDGFRA and B). A phase II trial involving 31 recurrent GBM patients receiving cediranib monotherapy, with the primary end-point being APF6, was conducted. The median age was 53 years and median KPS was 90 and patients were not stratified. Secondary end-points were radiographic response, median OS, and toxicity. Various imaging modalities were employed (assessment was changed to include 2D and volumetric measurements) and analysis of plasma and urinary biomarkers was undertaken. In summary, the median OS was 227 days and the APF6 was 25.8%. A radiographic partial response was detected in 17/30 (56.7%) patients with volumetric measurements, and with 8/30 (27%) using Macdonald criteria instead of volumetric analysis. This is a significant example of the differences that can arise between different imaging assessment methods. As compared to historical controls (Wong et al. analysis 1999), the results were deemed encouraging [59]. The baseline levels of different biomarkers were unable to be correlated with PFS or OS, but were postulated to be helpful for pharmacodynamics. However, some biomarkers did exhibit significant change, independent of PFS or OS, after treatment. A significant correlation was stated between some dynamic biomarkers and radiographic response and survival. This study demonstrated that the majority of patients reduced or stopped their corticosteroid dosages, but this was contingent upon continued treatment with cediranib. The study results were overall positive, and the vitality of combined therapy was re-iterated due to the belief that cediranib normalizes vessels to make other treatments more effective [60].

A phase III randomized, placebo controlled, partially blinded study was initiated after the promising phase II results. Phase III was a 3 arm study of 325 recurrent GBM patients investigating cediranib monotherapy, cediranib with lomustine (nitrosourea approved for use in GBM), and lomustine monotherapy. This phase took the important step of moving to combination therapy. The median age in each arm was 54 years. The patients were stratified according to KPS with 50%, 48%, and 36.2% having a score of 70-80 in each arm, respectively and 50, 51.2, and 62.5% having a KPS of 90-100 in the respective arms. Patients had previously been treated with RT/TMZ. The primary end-point was PFS, assessed by centralized, independent, blinded radiographic review, which used updated Macdonald criteria for T1, T2 and FLAIR MRI imaging. It should be noted that this evolved from the phase II trials that used volumetrics for imaging analysis and APF6. The soluble biomarkers VEGF, VEGFR2, and bFGF from plasma were measured in relation to baseline levels, but they were determined to be unrelated to predicting outcome in the trial. Biomarkers did not prove helpful in this trial, which was disappointing. The trial did not meet its PFS goal of significance, and did not impact OS. Since 136 patients received salvage therapy of bevacizumab monotherapy or combination therapy, survival could have been biased, yet salvage therapy was established to be similar in the different arms. Perhaps the disappointing results can be partially attributed to changes in imaging analysis methods over the course of the trial phases. There were secondary benefits of lengthened time to neurologic deterioration and reduced steroid dependence. The combination of cediranib and lomustine was not ideal, as cediranib heightened lomustine associated toxicities, although these were manageable. The idea that cediranib might be better in combination with RT, according to pre-clinical results, was proposed. Two phase II studies on cediranib and radiation are ongoing [2].

### 5.2. Immunotherapy

Immunotherapy has been gaining momentum as the next attractive treatment option for GBM. It promises fewer side effects, and greater efficacy because it uses the host's own immune defense mechanisms to fight cancer while sparing normal tissue. Important immune cells to be activated are naïve and memory T cells, natural killer cells (NK), and natural killer T cells (NKT). Immunotherapies seem to show good evidence of impacting survival in clinical trials with relatively minimal toxicities [61].

Although immunotherapy is promising, there are inherent challenges and limitations. The BBB is often discussed in immunotherapy, but its role is a subject of debate. However, the BBB may not be as impenetrable as formerly proposed. Antigens from the CNS do end up in cervical and nasal lymph nodes. Also, lymphocytes are capable of crossing the BBB. In fact, activated T cells express certain molecules that enable them to penetrate the BBB [62]. Inflammatory chemokines stimulate lymphocyte arrest and binding of cell adhesion molecules to integrins, which is fundamental to immune cells entering the brain. Furthermore, lower numbers of immune molecules and cells, like CD4 and human leukocyte antigen (HLA) class I, have been correlated to worse prognosis and survival, which would not be expected if the brain was exclusive to the immune system [63].

In addition to the BBB, antigen identification is also challenging. While other cancers express tumor-specific antigens for obvious targeting, GBM has very few cancer specific antigens [63]. Even epidermal growth factor variant III (EGFRvIII), which is found solely on GBM cells, is expressed in just 20-30% of tumors. Also, because an antigen is tumor specific does not mean that it is immunogenic [64]. GBM cells do not adequately present antigens, limiting the activation of T cells [62]. A third formidable obstacle to immunotherapy is the profound immunosuppression of GBM patients, both in the tumor microenvironment and systemically. Immune suppression is typically profound and cannot be completely overcome, which is a disadvantage for immunotherapy efficacy but an advantage in avoiding a different risk of immunotherapy, that of accidentally inducing autoimmunity. The occurrence of an autoimmune reaction is a risk because tumor cells are technically host cells, so they have inherent tolerance systems put in place to avoid autoimmunity, and expression patterns similar to host cells [63].

Therapies that are effective despite immunosuppression issues can run into a major obstacle, which is tumoral immune editing. If a therapy effectively targets certain antigens, the tumor may subsequently change its reliance on these antigens [65]. This was illustrated by the loss of EGFRvIII expression in many recurrent tumors after administration of an EGFRvIII targeted vaccine, rindopepimut. Vaccines using whole tumor lysates or combination therapy are a possible solution to immune editing.

In addition to immune system obstacles, immunotherapy faces the same problems as other therapies with clinical trial design, imaging limitations, and end-point selection. Reliance on pre-clinical animal models is not optimal because the models have limits as surrogates, and translating the therapy's effects into humans is complex. Moreover, obtaining an immune response does not necessarily bestow improved survival or longer time to progression [65]. Finally, immunotherapy trials are very expensive. The simplest phase III immunotherapy cancer trial with approximately 300 patients, easy immunotherapy manufacturing, and efficient clinical readouts, surgery, and imaging might cost about 20 million dollars. A larger trial that has personalized therapy and is more technology reliant could cost in the hundreds of millions [64].

### *5.2.1. Rindopepimut*

Another popular and prevalent vaccine for GBM is Rindopepimut (CDX-110), an EGFRvIII specific 14-mer peptide. EGFRvIII is unique in that it is solely expressed on GBM cells. An in-frame deletion causes fusion of two parts of the molecule, ultimately leading to constitutive activation that is implicated in tumorigenicity, tumor cell migration, and resistance to chemotherapy and radiation [62].

A phase II clinical trial (ACT III) with intradermally administered rindopepimut plus GM-CSF and maintenance TMZ in 65 newly diagnosed EGFRvIII positive GBM patients reported a PFS of 12.3 months (compared to 6.3 historically) and an OS of 24.6 months (compared to 15.0 historically). Patients had to have undergone gross total resection and traditional TMZ/RT without progression. The median age was 56 years and the median KPS was 90 [62]. The historical control cohort consisted of 17 patients treated at the center at the same time and the populations were matched for positive EGFRvIII status, gross total resection, treatment with RT/TMZ, and no progression for 3 months post treatment [66]. The primary end-point was considered PFS. Methylation of MGMT resulted in a significantly increased PFS. After these positive results, new clinical trials were initiated.

The current investigations of rindopepimut are a phase III trial (ACT IV) for newly diagnosed GBM patients and a phase II trial (ReACT) of recurrent GBM patients. ACT IV aims to include 700 EGFRvIII positive patients who have had gross total and incomplete resection, in an effort to reduce bias towards grossly resected patients, and who have completed standard chemoradiation. Completion is expected in 2016 [62]. The trial is a 2 arm, randomized study, comparing rindopepimut to a TMZ control, with OS as the primary measure, and PFS and safety and tolerability as secondary measures. Results have not yet been released (Clinicaltrials.gov, NCT01480479). ReACT is studying the efficacy of rindopepimut in combination with bevacizumab for patients with relapsed EGFRvIII positive GBM. Patients are sorted into two groups: those who have received and are refractory to bevacizumab, and those who have not previously received bevacizumab. Within those two groups, patients will be randomly assigned to receive rindopepimut/GM-CSF or a placebo (KLH) while continuing, re-starting, or starting bevacizumab therapy. Group 1 is bevacizumb naïve and receives bevacizumab plus rindopepimut/GM-CSF. Group 2 is bevacizumab naïve and receives bevacizumab plus a KLH placebo. Group 2C is bevacizumab refractory and receives bevacizumab plus rindopepimut/GM-CSF. The primary end-point for Groups 1 and 2 is 6moPFS, and the secondary end-points are safety and tolerability, antitumor activity, and EGFRvIII specific immune responses. OS is notably absent as an end-point. The primary end-point in group 2C will be ORR. Imaging analyses are performed using RANO criteria. Patients must have had prior surgery and chemoradiation, be EGFRvIII positive, and be in their first or second relapse of primary GBM or first relapse of secondary GBM. Completion is anticipated for 2014 with 168 patients. Preliminary results were released in November 2013. The OS for Group 1 was 12.0 months versus 7.9 months in Group 2. The PFS was 3.7 months in group 1 as compared to 2.0 months in group 2. Interestingly, the occurrence of tumor response (>50% shrinkage) for group 1 was 37% per investigator review and was 32% per expert panel review. For group 2 it was 19% per investigator review and 25% per expert panel review. Once again, this demonstrates the objective nature of imaging analyses. The results also indicate that patients who are EGFRvIII positive do have a poorer prognosis. In Group 2C the OS was 5.6 months and the PFS was 1.9 months. In preliminary ReACT data it was suggested that the anti-EGFRvIII titer is predictive of patient outcome. The results for ReACT are continuing to be assessed, but show a trend towards efficacy (Clinicaltrials.gov, NCT01498328).

There are limitations in the analysis and use of rindopepimut. An obvious problem with rindopepimut is that only 20-30% of GBMs express EGFRvIII. Furthermore, upon recurrence it has been documented that between 82-91% of tumors lose EGFRvIII expression after recurrence [62, 67]. Importantly, EGFRvIII expression has not been significantly related to survival. Furthermore, trial design was not ideal in rindopepimut testing. The ACT III trial did not take into account certain prognostic factors, like mutation of isocitrate dehydrogenase one/two (IDH1/2), which is known to positively affect survival; patients in the trial also had various salvage therapies that may have influenced survival. The historical control population was also much smaller than the experimental group (n=17 vs. n=65). Despite matched eligibility criteria, discrepancies between the rindopepimut study population and the historical population used for comparison in ACT III are possible and would be problematic. Bias in the clinical trials of rindopepimut could also have arisen from the fact that KPS scores were quite high; in ACT III the median KPS was 90. KPS is a key prognostic factor and may indicate that patients in these trials had a better prognosis overall. Moreover, patients in these trials underwent gross total resection, which is not realistic to the greater GBM patient population, but ACTIV and ReAct do attempt to address this by including patients with less than gross total resection [62].

### 5.3. Other therapies

An intriguing non-drug option for GBM patients is the Novo-TTF system, approved by the FDA in 2011. NovoTTF is a portable device that is worn almost continuously, with the exception of short daily breaks for personal needs. It emits low intensity, intermediate frequency, alternating electronic fields that are non-invasive. Electronic fields disturb cell division by triggering microtubule misalignment necessary for the metaphase to anaphase transition. The fields also cause movement of intracellular macromolecules and organelles in telophase. Ultimately, the cytokinetic division of the cell is impossible after failed segregation and distribution of chromosomes, organelles, and microtubules, and cell death occurs [59]. Dividing cells have unique shapes and electric features, making rapidly multiplying cancer cells sensitive to electric field treatment.

NovoTTF was tested in 237 recurrent GBM patients in a phase III trial comparing NovoTTF monotherapy to any active chemotherapy, as determined by the physician's judgment. The median age of patients was 54 years and the median KPS was 80. The primary end-point was OS and the secondary end-points were PFS, PFS6, radiological response, 1 year survival, QOL, and safety. A central review board did imaging analysis using the MacDonald criteria. Selected patients must have had radiation, with or without TMZ, and 80% had failed 2 or more chemotherapies and had more than one recurrence. The primary end-point of OS was not significant at 14% versus 9.6% in the active control arm. PFS6 was improved at 21% compared to 15%. The failure to produce improved survival might have been unavoidable in a patient population with more than one recurrence and failure of other treatments; other trials involving recurrent patients often enroll patients on their first recurrence. Despite not reaching survival significance, NovoTTF was approved. An important result contributing to approval was NovoTTF's effect on QOL, assessed via QLQ-30 [59]. Enhanced QOL is attributable to the absence of serious chemotherapy related toxicities, such as nausea, anemia, fatigue, and serious infections, although, some patients treated with NovoTTF did have worsened neurologic events, including headaches and convulsion.

The FDA approval of NovoTTF was surprising in light of the FDA's hesitance on relying unstandardized QOL measures. However, the decision to approve NovoTTF is understood through its contingency upon the dearth of treatments for recurrent GBM. Re-resection and re-irradiation are feasible in only a handful of recurrent patients, and chemotherapy has an extremely low response rate of less than 10%. Approval for an intervention that does not improve survival would is far more feasible in a disease like GBM that has such a poor prognosis. The vote for approval was very close (7 to 6) and can be classified as a "non-inferiority" approval, meaning NovoTTF is not better nor worse than other therapies, and it may improve QOL [59]. Here the risk-benefit ratio was tantamount to the drug succeeding in clinical trials. It is an example of how skewed the ratio is in a severe diagnosis such as GBM. The benefit did not have to be great because other approved agents have very low benefits in comparison to significant side effects.

## 6. Conclusion

The ideal design of clinical trials for GBM patients remains elusive. The conflict between OS, PFS, and ORR as primary end-points continues, with the FDA staying with OS. Radiographic imaging assessment remains an obstacle for PFS and ORR, which is evidenced by disagreement between radiographic reviewers (as seen in studies with bevacizumab). Although imaging criteria are being updated, the most likely progress will be through different imaging methods, like T2 MRI and FLAIR. Alternatively, biomarkers are becoming more important. They are already being used in trials, but there is still a gap in comprehension of how and when they are most useful. In RTK inhibitor clinical trials biomarkers were assessed, yet they did not always have predictive value or an expected relationship to an end-point. However, this does not mean that biomarkers are useless. Connecting tumoral and survival end-points to biomarkers will require further study, and they are indeed continuing to be analyzed in clinical trials.

Many investigational agents discussed above undergo changes to their end-points as the drug advances from phase to phase in the clinical trial. Rindopepimut is an example of the myriad end-points that may be used for assessing any one agent. Furthermore, as each investigational agent seems to use a different control cohort, there is especially variability in the historical cohorts chosen for comparative analyses, which are drawn from several literature sources. Lack of consistency across trials or even phases is detrimental because it creates confusion and complexity in analyzing investigational agents. Also, many drugs in clinical trials end up being disappointing despite promising early phase results. This phenomenon could be attributed to limitations in early phase clinical trials, such as small sample size, absence of a comparator arm, or bias in patient selection. Protecting drugs in early phases who have not demonstrated clear efficacy and safety from entering the market will continue to be an ethical and sometimes legal battle; collecting data is absolutely vital to the welfare of current and future patients and it cannot be compromised.

Another major issue is the tendency to focus on monotherapy (or monotherapy plus RT/TMZ). Monotherapy is helpful in determining how a drug works, but beyond this the therapeutic effects would be greatly augmented by creating relevant combination therapies. GBM evolves too quickly and frequently for any monotherapy to become a "cure". Moreover, combination therapy in the form of novel drugs, in comparison to a new drug added to the RT/TMZ regimen, is not common and needs more focus. Combining novel drugs is admittedly tricky, yet it holds promise.

Clinical trials are the avenue for progress in GBM. The obstacles that inhibit the success of clinical trials are formidable, but not unsolvable. Greater patient participation, better standardization across and within clinical trials, and innovative end-points and combination therapy are the way forward.

## Acknowledgements

The authors would like to thank the University of Colorado Department of Neurosurgery, The University of Colorado Cancer Center, the Cancer League of Colorado, and the National Institutes of Health RO1 # 11066485 for support.

## Author details

Helen Madsen, Justin E. Hellwinkel and Michael W. Graner*

*Address all correspondence to: michael.graner@ucdenver.edu

Department of Neurosurgery, University of Colorado School of Medicine, USA

## References

[1] Stupp R, Mason WP, van den Bent MJ, Weller M, Fisher B, Taphoorn MJ, et al. Radiotherapy plus concomitant and adjuvant temozolomide for glioblastoma. N Engl J Med. 2005;352(10):987-96.

[2] Batchelor TT, Mulholland P, Neyns B, Nabors LB, Campone M, Wick A, et al. Phase III randomized trial comparing the efficacy of cediranib as monotherapy, and in combination with lomustine, versus lomustine alone in patients with recurrent glioblastoma. J Clin Oncol. 2013;31(26):3212-8.

[3] Zuniga RM, Torcuator R, Jain R, Anderson J, Doyle T, Ellika S, et al. Efficacy, safety and patterns of response and recurrence in patients with recurrent high-grade gliomas treated with bevacizumab plus irinotecan. J Neurooncol. 2009;91(3):329-36.

[4] Lacroix M, Abi-Said D, Fourney DR, Gokaslan ZL, Shi W, DeMonte F, et al. A multivariate analysis of 416 patients with glioblastoma multiforme: prognosis, extent of resection, and survival. J Neurosurg. 2001;95(2):190-8.

[5] Lamborn KR, Chang SM, Prados MD. Prognostic factors for survival of patients with glioblastoma: recursive partitioning analysis. Neuro Oncol. 2004;6(3):227-35.

[6] Krex D, Klink B, Hartmann C, von Deimling A, Pietsch T, Simon M, et al. Long-term survival with glioblastoma multiforme. Brain : a journal of neurology. 2007;130(Pt 10):2596-606.

[7] Bleeker FE, Molenaar RJ, Leenstra S. Recent advances in the molecular understanding of glioblastoma. J Neurooncol. 2012;108(1):11-27.

[8] Omuro AM, Faivre S, Raymond E. Lessons learned in the development of targeted therapy for malignant gliomas. Mol Cancer Ther. 2007;6(7):1909-19.

[9] Friedman HS. State-of-the-art Therapy for Glioblastoma Multiforme. US Oncological Disease, 2007. 2007;1(2):103-4.

[10] Carlson B. Therapeutic vaccine for brain cancer succeeds using a unique approach. Biotechnology healthcare. 2011;8(3):31-2.

[11] Shahar T, Nossek E, Steinberg DM, Rozovski U, Blumenthal DT, Bokstein F, et al. The impact of enrollment in clinical trials on survival of patients with glioblastoma. J Clin Neurosci. 2012;19(11):1530-4.

[12] Field KM, Drummond KJ, Yilmaz M, Tacey M, Compston D, Gibbs P, et al. Clinical trial participation and outcome for patients with glioblastoma: multivariate analysis from a comprehensive dataset. J Clin Neurosci. 2013;20(6):783-9.

[13] Markman M. The needs of science vs the needs of patients: ethical concerns in cancer clinical trials. Cleveland Clinic journal of medicine. 2003;70(12):1008-9, 13-4, 16.

[14] Kodish E, Stocking C, Ratain MJ, Kohrman A, Siegler M. Ethical issues in phase I oncology research: a comparison of investigators and institutional review board chairpersons. J Clin Oncol. 1992;10(11):1810-6.

[15] Dilts DM, Sandler AB. Invisible barriers to clinical trials: the impact of structural, infrastructural, and procedural barriers to opening oncology clinical trials. J Clin Oncol. 2006;24(28):4545-52.

[16] Zohar S, O'Quigley J. Re: Dose escalation methods in phase I cancer clinical trials. J Natl Cancer Inst. 2009;101(24):1732-3; author reply 3-5.

[17] Fleming TR. Surrogate endpoints and FDA's accelerated approval process. Health affairs. 2005;24(1):67-78.

[18] Johnson JR, Ning YM, Farrell A, Justice R, Keegan P, Pazdur R. Accelerated approval of oncology products: the food and drug administration experience. J Natl Cancer Inst. 2011;103(8):636-44.

[19] Agrawal M, Emanuel EJ. Ethics of phase 1 oncology studies: reexamining the arguments and data. JAMA. 2003;290(8):1075-82.

[20] Henry B, Scales DC. Ethical challenges in conducting research on dying patients and those at high risk of dying. Accountability in research. 2012;19(1):1-12.

[21] Miller M. Phase I cancer trials. A collusion of misunderstanding. The Hastings Center report. 2000;30(4):34-43.

[22] Horstmann E, McCabe MS, Grochow L, Yamamoto S, Rubinstein L, Budd T, et al. Risks and benefits of phase 1 oncology trials, 1991 through 2002. N Engl J Med. 2005;352(9):895-904.

[23] Eisenhauer EA, O'Dwyer PJ, Christian M, Humphrey JS. Phase I clinical trial design in cancer drug development. J Clin Oncol. 2000;18(3):684-92.

[24] Taylor KM, Feldstein ML, Skeel RT, Pandya KJ, Ng P, Carbone PP. Fundamental dilemmas of the randomized clinical trial process: results of a survey of the 1,737 Eastern Cooperative Oncology Group investigators. J Clin Oncol. 1994;12(9):1796-805.

[25] Jadad AR, Moore RA, Carroll D, Jenkinson C, Reynolds DJ, Gavaghan DJ, et al. Assessing the quality of reports of randomized clinical trials: is blinding necessary? Controlled clinical trials. 1996;17(1):1-12.

[26] Okie S. Access before approval--a right to take experimental drugs? N Engl J Med. 2006;355(5):437-40.

[27] Falit BP, Gross CP. Access to experimental drugs for terminally ill patients. JAMA. 2008;300(23):2793-5.

[28] Eichler HG, Pignatti F, Flamion B, Leufkens H, Breckenridge A. Balancing early market access to new drugs with the need for benefit/risk data: a mounting dilemma. Nat Rev Drug Discov. 2008;7(10):818-26.

[29] Chang SM, Lamborn KR, Kuhn JG, Yung WK, Gilbert MR, Wen PY, et al. Neurooncology clinical trial design for targeted therapies: lessons learned from the North American Brain Tumor Consortium. Neuro Oncol. 2008;10(4):631-42.

[30] Nelson R. Brain-tumour clinical-trial endpoints: FDA public workshop. Lancet Oncol. 2006;7(3):205-6.

[31] Lang FF, Gilbert MR, Puduvalli VK, Weinberg J, Levin VA, Yung WK, et al. Toward better early-phase brain tumor clinical trials: a reappraisal of current methods and proposals for future strategies. Neuro Oncol. 2002;4(4):268-77.

[32] Gorlia T, van den Bent MJ, Hegi ME, Mirimanoff RO, Weller M, Cairncross JG, et al. Nomograms for predicting survival of patients with newly diagnosed glioblastoma: prognostic factor analysis of EORTC and NCIC trial 26981-22981/CE.3. Lancet Oncol. 2008;9(1):29-38.

[33] Curran WJ, Jr., Scott CB, Horton J, Nelson JS, Weinstein AS, Fischbach AJ, et al. Recursive partitioning analysis of prognostic factors in three Radiation Therapy Oncology Group malignant glioma trials. J Natl Cancer Inst. 1993;85(9):704-10.

[34] Perry JR, DeAngelis LM, Schold SC, Jr., Burger PC, Brem H, Brown MT, et al. Challenges in the design and conduct of phase III brain tumor therapy trials. Neurology. 1997;49(4):912-7.

[35] Chinot OL, Macdonald DR, Abrey LE, Zahlmann G, Kerloeguen Y, Cloughesy TF. Response assessment criteria for glioblastoma: practical adaptation and implementation in clinical trials of antiangiogenic therapy. Curr Neurol Neurosci Rep. 2013;13(5):347.

[36] Reardon DA, Galanis E, DeGroot JF, Cloughesy TF, Wefel JS, Lamborn KR, et al. Clinical trial end points for high-grade glioma: the evolving landscape. Neuro Oncol. 2011;13(3):353-61.

[37] Stupp R, Tonn JC, Brada M, Pentheroudakis G, Group EGW. High-grade malignant glioma: ESMO Clinical Practice Guidelines for diagnosis, treatment and follow-up. Ann Oncol. 2010;21 Suppl 5:v190-3.

[38] Cohen MH, Shen YL, Keegan P, Pazdur R. FDA drug approval summary: bevacizumab (Avastin) as treatment of recurrent glioblastoma multiforme. Oncologist. 2009;14(11):1131-8.

[39] Kreisl TN, Kim L, Moore K, Duic P, Royce C, Stroud I, et al. Phase II trial of single-agent bevacizumab followed by bevacizumab plus irinotecan at tumor progression in recurrent glioblastoma. J Clin Oncol. 2009;27(5):740-5.

[40] Henson JW, Ulmer S, Harris GJ. Brain tumor imaging in clinical trials. AJNR Am J Neuroradiol. 2008;29(3):419-24.

[41] Wen PY, Macdonald DR, Reardon DA, Cloughesy TF, Sorensen AG, Galanis E, et al. Updated response assessment criteria for high-grade gliomas: response assessment in neuro-oncology working group. J Clin Oncol. 2010;28(11):1963-72.

[42] Eisenhauer EA, Therasse P, Bogaerts J, Schwartz LH, Sargent D, Ford R, et al. New response evaluation criteria in solid tumours: revised RECIST guideline (version 1.1). Eur J Cancer. 2009;45(2):228-47.

[43] FDA. FDA Briefing Document Oncology Drug Advisory Committee Meeting BLA STN 125085/169 Avastin® (bevacizumab) In: Administration UFaD, editor. Available from: http://www.fda.gov/ohrms/dockets/ac/09/briefing/2009-4427b1-01-FDA.pdfMarch 31, 2009.

[44] Yates JW, Chalmer B, McKegney FP. Evaluation of patients with advanced cancer using the Karnofsky performance status. Cancer. 1980;45(8):2220-4.

[45] Peus D, Newcomb N, Hofer S. Appraisal of the Karnofsky Performance Status and proposal of a simple algorithmic system for its evaluation. BMC medical informatics and decision making. 2013;13:72.

[46] Meyers CA, Hess KR. Multifaceted end points in brain tumor clinical trials: cognitive deterioration precedes MRI progression. Neuro Oncol. 2003;5(2):89-95.

[47] Taphoorn MJ, Sizoo EM, Bottomley A. Review on quality of life issues in patients with primary brain tumors. Oncologist. 2010;15(6):618-26.

[48] Sargent DJ, Conley BA, Allegra C, Collette L. Clinical trial designs for predictive marker validation in cancer treatment trials. J Clin Oncol. 2005;23(9):2020-7.

[49] Joshi AD, Loilome W, Siu IM, Tyler B, Gallia GL, Riggins GJ. Evaluation of tyrosine kinase inhibitor combinations for glioblastoma therapy. PLoS One. 2012;7(10):e44372.

[50] Fan QW, Weiss WA. Targeting the RTK-PI3K-mTOR axis in malignant glioma: overcoming resistance. Curr Top Microbiol Immunol. 2010;347:279-96.

[51] Kaur B, Khwaja FW, Severson EA, Matheny SL, Brat DJ, Van Meir EG. Hypoxia and the hypoxia-inducible-factor pathway in glioma growth and angiogenesis. Neuro Oncol. 2005;7(2):134-53.

[52] Stommel JM, Kimmelman AC, Ying H, Nabioullin R, Ponugoti AH, Wiedemeyer R, et al. Coactivation of receptor tyrosine kinases affects the response of tumor cells to targeted therapies. Science. 2007;318(5848):287-90.

[53] Snuderl M, Fazlollahi L, Le LP, Nitta M, Zhelyazkova BH, Davidson CJ, et al. Mosaic amplification of multiple receptor tyrosine kinase genes in glioblastoma. Cancer Cell. 2011;20(6):810-7.

[54] Huang TT, Sarkaria SM, Cloughesy TF, Mischel PS. Targeted therapy for malignant glioma patients: lessons learned and the road ahead. Neurotherapeutics. 2009;6(3): 500-12.

[55] Gerber HP, Ferrara N. Pharmacology and pharmacodynamics of bevacizumab as monotherapy or in combination with cytotoxic therapy in preclinical studies. Cancer Res. 2005;65(3):671-80.

[56] Wong ET, Hess KR, Gleason MJ, Jaeckle KA, Kyritsis AP, Prados MD, et al. Outcomes and prognostic factors in recurrent glioma patients enrolled onto phase II clinical trials. J Clin Oncol. 1999;17(8):2572-8.

[57] Chinot OL, Wick W, Mason W, Henriksson R, Saran F, Nishikawa R, et al. Bevacizumab plus radiotherapy-temozolomide for newly diagnosed glioblastoma. N Engl J Med. 2014;370(8):709-22.

[58] Gilbert MR, Dignam JJ, Armstrong TS, Wefel JS, Blumenthal DT, Vogelbaum MA, et al. A randomized trial of bevacizumab for newly diagnosed glioblastoma. N Engl J Med. 2014;370(8):699-708.

[59] Stupp R, Wong ET, Kanner AA, Steinberg D, Engelhard H, Heidecke V, et al. NovoTTF-100A versus physician's choice chemotherapy in recurrent glioblastoma: a randomised phase III trial of a novel treatment modality. Eur J Cancer. 2012;48(14): 2192-202.

[60] Batchelor TT, Duda DG, di Tomaso E, Ancukiewicz M, Plotkin SR, Gerstner E, et al. Phase II study of cediranib, an oral pan-vascular endothelial growth factor receptor tyrosine kinase inhibitor, in patients with recurrent glioblastoma. J Clin Oncol. 2010;28(17):2817-23.

[61] Gustafson MP, Knutson KL, Dietz AB. Therapeutic vaccines for malignant brain tumors. Biologics : targets & therapy. 2008;2(4):753-61.

[62] Babu R, Adamson DC. Rindopepimut: an evidence-based review of its therapeutic potential in the treatment of EGFRvIII-positive glioblastoma. Core evidence. 2012;7:93-103.

[63] Jackson CM, Lim M, Drake CG. Immunotherapy for Brain Cancer: Recent Progress and Future Promise. Clin Cancer Res. 2014;20(14):3651-9.

[64] Goldman B, DeFrancesco L. The cancer vaccine roller coaster. Nat Biotechnol. 2009;27(2):129-39.

[65] Rolle CE, Sengupta S, Lesniak MS. Challenges in clinical design of immunotherapy trials for malignant glioma. Neurosurg Clin N Am. 2010;21(1):201-14.

[66] Weller M, Kaulich K, Hentschel B, Felsberg J, Gramatzki D, Pietsch T, et al. Assessment and prognostic significance of the epidermal growth factor receptor vIII mutation in glioblastoma patients treated with concurrent and adjuvant temozolomide radiochemotherapy. Int J Cancer. 2014;134(10):2437-47.

[67] Jackson SE, Chester JD. Personalised cancer medicine. Int J Cancer. 2014.

Chapter 14

# Clinical Presentation of Brain Tumors

Christie Adams, Joan Sullivan and Todd W. Vitaz

Additional information is available at the end of the chapter

http://dx.doi.org/10.5772/59046

## 1. Introduction

Understanding the clinical picture and the signs and symptoms produced by brain tumors is complicated by the extreme heterogeneity amongst these patients. This is secondary to the variability in size, location, pathology and rate of growth of the tumor. In general symptoms can be broadly divided into two categories generalized or focal. Most generalized symptoms are caused by the mass effect and resulting increased intracranial pressure or global cerebral dysfunction caused by the lesion [1]. These typically are clues that a neurological abnormality exists, but are not usually helpful in determining lesion localization.

## 2. Generalized symptoms

The most common generalized symptoms are shown in table 1. Headache is the most frequent symptom and occurs in approximately 48-56% of brain tumor patients [2,3]. Headache patterns and location vary greatly depending on mechanism and pathophysiology and this is described in a subsequent section. In general, headaches can be either localized or global in nature and the intensity and rate of progression may provide insight into the rate of growth of the lesion. Lesions with a long history of slowly worsening symptoms over years tend to be more slow growing and benign whereas acute onset headaches with a rapid crescendo pattern are worrisome for a more ominous course. The classic brain tumor headache is one of a global headache often radiating to the vertex or periorbital region which is associated with nausea and vomiting and worse in the am (secondary to $CO_2$ retention and subsequent vasodilation during sleep).

| | |
|---|---|
| Headache | 52% |
| Memory loss/cognitive dysfunction | 35% |
| Seizures | 32% |
| Personality Changes | 23% |
| Nausea and Vomiting | 13% |

**Table 1.** The common generalized symptoms of brain tumor patients [3].

Cognitive changes are not only a common presenting symptom of brain tumors, but also tend to persist even after treatment of the tumor and can affect the patient's overall quality of life and survival [4]. These neurocognitive deficits encompass memory problems, personality changes, and mood disturbances. In some instances, these changes are drastic enough to cause alarm for the patient or family member and lead directly to the diagnosis. These scenarios often include sudden changes, such as the loss of skills related to executive functioning such as paying bills, following directions, job performance or driving and automobile (figure 1).

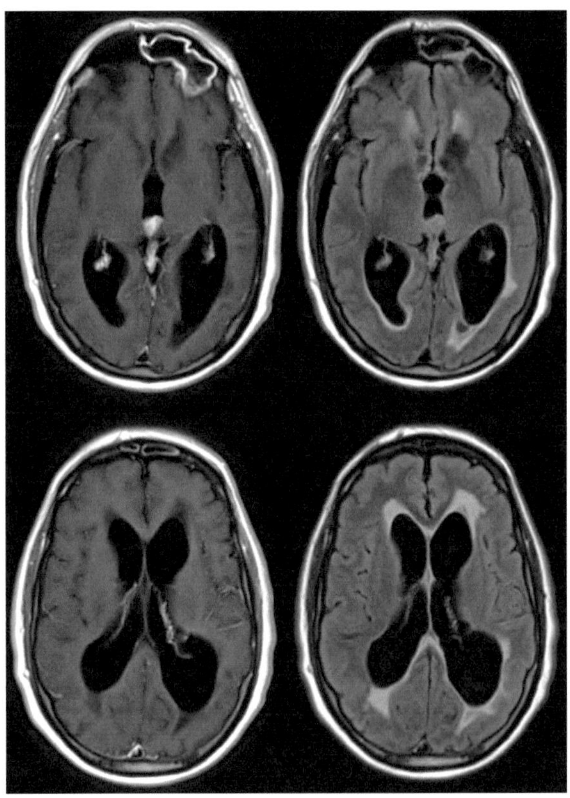

**Figure 1.** MRI scan from an elderly patient with a pineal mass and associated hydrocephalus who presented with acute confusion consisting of difficulty driving and paying bills.

http://dx.doi.org/10.5772/59046

However, in other cases, these changes are slow and insidious and may often be overlooked or attributed to other causes such as aging or stress. In some instances these issues present only following a visit from a distant family member or friend who has not seen or interacted with the patient recently. It is also not uncommon for these issues to remain completely unrecognized and discovered only after specific questioning and inquiry by a physician or as the result of specialized neuropsychological testing. In fact when formal neuropsychological testing is performed on this population of patients almost all of them show at least mild to moderate dysfunction in at least one cognitive domain [4]. It has only been over the past decade that the magnitude and impact that these cognitive deficits have on such patients has been truly recognized.

A majority of cognitive processes, including planning, motivation, personality, judgment, and abstraction, are controlled by the frontal lobe. However, a significant amount of these processes require input from various other regions of the brain including the parietal and temporal lobes. Therefore, neurocognitive changes are seen with tumors in multiple locations. The tools for evaluation of cognitive deficits will be discussed in a separate section.

Like cognitive deficits, seizures are another symptom of brain tumors that may be present on presentation, or may develop later during the disease process. Tumor-related seizures include both general and focal seizures. The seizure semiology (pattern and symptoms) may provide insight into lesion localization especially in cases with focal seizures. There is a distinction that can be made in the incidence of seizures for various types of brain tumors. Patients with primary brain tumors are more likely to present with seizures or subsequently develop them as compared to patients with brain metastases [5]. In addition, patients with low grade gliomas have seizures more commonly than those with high grade gliomas. One study showed as much as a 85% rate of seizures in those with low grade gliomas as compared to 49% in those with glioblastoma multiforme [5].

Seizures occur secondary to irritation of the cerebral cortex either from the brain tumor itself or the surrounding peritumoral edema. Seizures can result from lesions in any area of the cerebral cortex but are more frequently seen in patients with lesions in the frontal or temporal lobes. Lesions in the brainstem and cerebellum almost never cause seizure activity. Seizures in essence occur as a result of this cortical irritation which causes a "short circuit" within the brain where depolarization rapidly spreads to surrounding areas. Seizure types are broken down into several categories based on the symptoms at the time of seizure onset and whether or not the seizure activity remains focused or spreads throughout the brain. Generalized seizures are those where a large portion of the brain is affected at the onset and as a result of this the patient becomes unresponsive at the onset. Secondary generalized seizures such as the classic partial complex seizure are very common and frequently occur with lesions located in the medial temporal lobe. In these cases symptoms typically start with rhythmic movement on the side contralateral to the lesion but then eventually progress to generalized seizure activity resulting in a loss of alertness and tonic and/or clonic movements on both sides of the body. Patients with generalized or secondary generalized seizures almost always lose consciousness during the event and typically have a period of post-ictal confusion that can last for minutes to hours following such events. However, a less common type of generalized seizure commonly referred to as absence seizures presents with brief starring spells without motor movements. These episodes can occur hundreds of times per day and are not usually associated with post-ictal confusion. Finally, focal seizures occur when the abnormal electrical depolarization remains contained to a small area of the brain. Symptoms with this type of seizure depend on the area involved but usually results in either episodic periods of uncontrolled motor movement and twitching or sensory complaints. The classic Jacksonian March Seizure is commonly seen with lesions in or around the primary motor cortex. These patients exhibit episodes of tonic-clonic activity that typically starts in one area of the contralateral extremity such as the distal leg and the involved activity spreads ("marches") to include a progressively larger area of the body (entire leg and then arm) as the seizure progresses. Patients with focal seizures almost always retain consciousness and awareness during their episodes [1].

Unlike patients with other causes of epilepsy, patients with lesional epilepsy secondary to a brain tumor often progress in frequency, intensity and severity if they remain untreated. It is not uncommon to see a patient with a low-grade glioma who had "a spell" several years ago which was never investigated or brought to the attention of a physician until the patient suffers either repeated or more intense attacks at a later date. The treatment of epilepsy in brain tumor patients varies on a case to case basis. We do not generally recommend prophylactic antiepileptics on these patients for many reasons. Most importantly class I data shows that the routine use of such medications doesn't prevent these patients from having seizures, but does significantly raise the incidence of drug related side effects [6]. In addition, many of these drugs are metabolized through the cytochrome P450 pathway in the liver and can affect the bioavailability of many chemotherapeutic agents and can thus affect the efficacy and side effect profile of these other medications [6]. We typically reserve the use of antiepileptics for patients who present with a seizure or develop one during treatment or for rare instances of "high-risk" patients with temporal lobe lesions who require awake mapping procedures. In these unusual cases we may treat the patient only in the perioperative period. For patients requiring treatment we commonly use leviteracitam unless the use of this is contraindicated. This medication is typically well tolerated by the majority of these patients however in rare instances it can cause or exacerbate headaches or cognitive dysfunction in this patient population. The duration of treatment for patients who present with seizure activity and then do not have any further events remains controversial. In many instances the surgical removal of the epileptogenic trigger may be enough to provide long-term control; however, we recommend continuing antiepileptic medications for at least 6 months or longer and routinely perform EEG prior to considering discontinuation of any antiepileptic medications. If EEG is normal or shows only diffuse changes than medications can usually be stopped safely; however if it shows significant sharp waves or other electrical evidence of cortical irritation than we will routinely advise patients to continue treatment for at least one to two years.

Nausea and vomiting associated with brain tumors is typically a result of the increasing ICP from the space-occupying lesion. However, when occurring in the absence of other symptoms it is often difficult to make the diagnosis which is typically made only after extensive workup for other causes such as gastrointestinal issues have been ruled out. In rare instances lesions

http://dx.doi.org/10.5772/59046

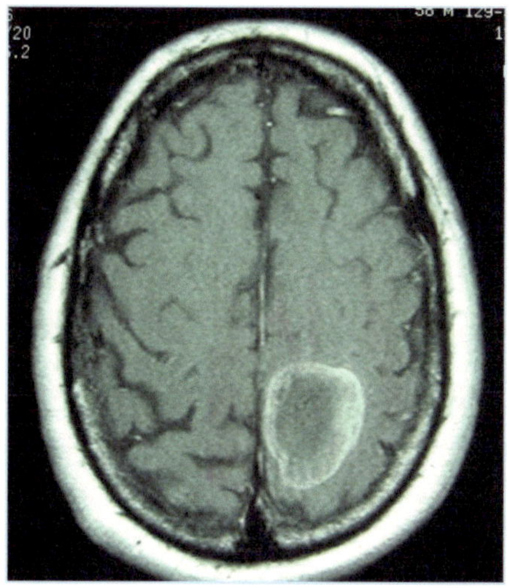

**Figure 2.** MRI showing lesion in motor cortex in a patient who presented with right sided weakness.

in the brainstem or other parts of the posterior fossa can lead to pure nausea and or vomiting without other complaints.

## 3. Focal symptoms

Compared to the generalized symptoms described above, focal symptoms of brain tumors can commonly offer clues as to the location of the lesion. This stems from the fact that focal deficits are created from the tumor or resulting edema compressing a specific portion of the brain parenchyma or cranial nerves. Therefore, from the knowledge of the structure and function of the brain, we are able to use the focal deficits found on a patient's exam to predict the location of the tumor.

| | |
|---|---|
| Motor deficits | 33% |
| Language deficits or aphasia | 32% |
| Visual deficits | 22% |
| Sensory deficits | 13% |
| Dizziness, balance problems or ataxia | 9% |

**Table 2.** The common focal symptoms of brain tumor patients [3].

Motor deficits from brain tumors can range from specific weakness in certain extremities to generalized weakness throughout the body. Focal motor deficits occur from a lesion situated in or around the precentral cortex (figure 2).

Lesions in the prefrontal area, caudate or basal ganglia can also cause motor deficits but this is typically more of a coordination or fine motor control issue as opposed to hemiplegia. Deficits can also occur when the lesion affects the descending fibers associated with a specific area of the motor cortex. These types of focal deficits are commonly very noticeable to patients and often lead to them seeking medical attention sooner. In some cases, the tumor itself may not be in a specific motor cortex region, but edema from the tumor extends to that region. In those cases, weakness is typically very responsive to treatment with steroids.

Like focal motor deficits, sensory deficits are also seen when the tumor or associated edema are lying in a region controlling sensory function such as the post-central gyrus or other areas of the parietal lobe. Some of the common sensory deficits that are seen include: graphesthesia abnormalities, stereoagnosis abnormalities, loss of proprioception, and abnormalities in pain and touch sensation. Graphesthesia is the ability to determine a number or letter that is written on the palm of the hand without watching as it is drawn. Stereoagnosis refers to the ability to determine what an object is that is placed in the hand when the eyes are closed. Proprioception refers to the ability to sense where in space a part of the body is. All of these abilities, along with the ability to sense touch, pain, and temperature can be diminished when a brain tumor is affecting the sensory areas of the parietal lobe [1].

When tumors occur in the regions of the brain controlling or contributing to speech and language, specific forms of aphasia and language deficits can be seen. Statistics show that language deficits of some sort occur in 30-53% of brain tumor patients [7,8]. Like all symptoms, language function will be affected differently in brain tumor patients, but most commonly tumors in the fronto-temporal region are responsible for causing aphasia [7].

Two regions of the brain, known as Broca's and Wernicke's area, are the most documented regions for language control. In greater than 85% of people, these areas are located in the left hemisphere, in the temporal region adjacent to the Sylvian fissure. Broca's area is located in the frontal operculum and typifies the expressive language control center, controlling a person's ability to facilitate speech. The location of Wernicke's area is much more variable; however, in most patients it is located in the posterior aspect of the superior or middle temporal gyrus. It is associated with the control of receptive language, a person's ability to understand both written and spoken language.

The four most common types of aphasia include: Broca's aphasia, Wernicke's aphasia, global aphasia and anomic aphasia. A brain tumor causing Broca's aphasia would limit a patient's ability to express their thoughts. These patients understand what they want to say, but the ability to form fluent, sensical words and phrases has been lost. On the other hand, a lesion causing Wernicke's aphasia would cause a patient to create non-sensical, non-meaningful speech. They can speak fluently, but their words and phrases have no meaning. These patients typically are not aware of the meaningless of their speech (figure 3).

When both Broca's and Wernicke's area have been affected, global aphasia results. These patients can neither express nor understand speech and language. This includes spoken language in addition to reading and writing. This can occur with large lesions affecting both the dominant frontal and temporal lobes or from smaller lesions which affect the angular gyrus on the

http://dx.doi.org/10.5772/59046

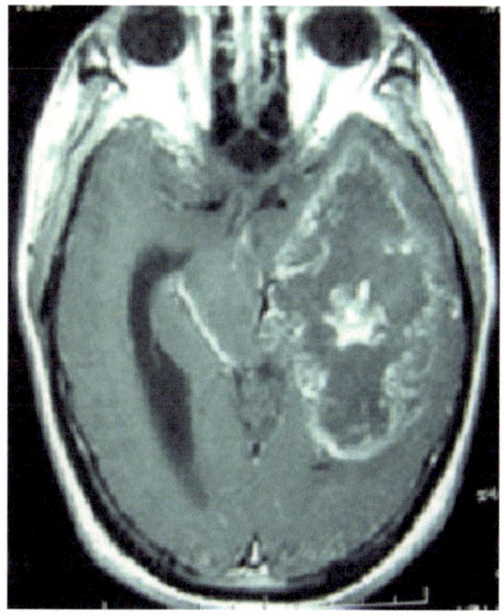

**Figure 3.** MRI scan of patient presenting with Wernicke's type aphasia.

dominant side. Finally anomic aphasia occurs when a lesion damages the left temporal region in addition to other lesions in the language pathways. This is best illustrated in a patient who has primarily word finding and naming difficulties. Speech will be fluent to start a sentence, but the patient will then lose the ability to produce the next word. Anomic aphasia is the most common form of language deficit in brain tumor patients [7].

The visual pathway is not specific to one hemisphere or lobe of the brain. Rather it encompasses both hemispheres, multiple cranial nerves, and travels from the retina posteriorly to the occipital lobe. Therefore, there are multiple locations in which visual deficits can be created from a brain tumor. Even compression on the optic nerve creates variability in visual deficits depending on the location along the cranial nerve. When compression occurs at the optic chiasm, bitemporal hemianopsia occurs, meaning that a patient is unable to see temporal peripheral fields out of both eyes. This type of visual loss is very common in patients with tumors in the pituitary region, particularly with non-functioning adenomas that extend into the suprasellar space and cause compression of the optic chiasm [9] (figure 4).

However, if compression from the lesion is only on one side of the optic nerve, than visual impairment is only experienced on the affected side. Patients can also complain of changes related to decreased visual acuity. This can occur with lesions anywhere along the optic system. In addition, it is a frequent complaint among patients with hydrocephalus or increased intracranial pressure in which case it is likely secondary to papilledema. Lesions in the occipital lobe cause a homonymous hemianopsia in which the patient loses vision in the contralateral portion of both eyes (figure 5). The onset of visual deficits is typically very gradual, and may not cause the patient to seek medical attention until the deficits are very severe. In fact in patients with benign slow growing lesions symptoms may not become evident until the patient experiences and accident from running into an object that they didn't visualize secondary to an enlarged blind spot.

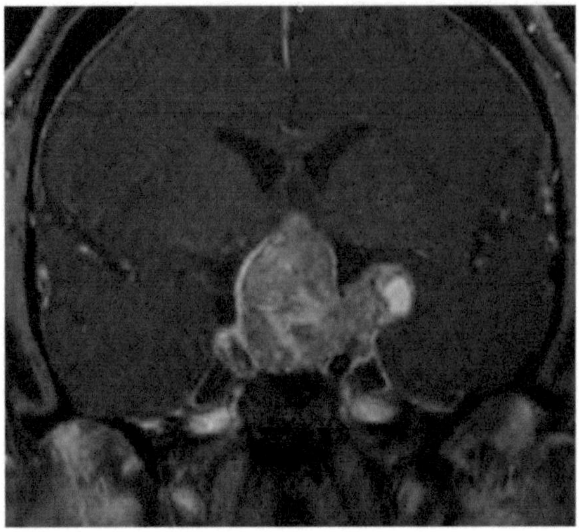

**Figure 4.** Coronal MRI of a patient with a large pituitary mass compressing the optic chiasm causing bitemporal hemianopsia.

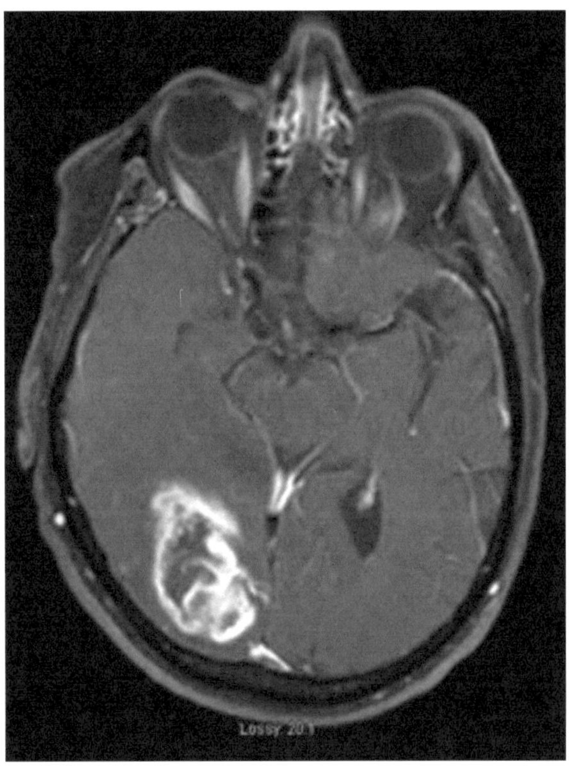

**Figure 5.** MRI scan of patient presenting with a left homonymous hemianopsia from a right occipital lesion.

http://dx.doi.org/10.5772/59046

Cranial nerve dysfunction is much less common than the other above symptoms. These typically occur with lesions affecting the skull base and in many instances multiple cranial nerves may be involved. In general the cranial nerves with pure motor functions (i.e. Facial nerve) are much more resistant to compressive forces than sensory nerves (i.e. Acoustic and vestibular nerves) (figure 6). In patients with metastatic disease the occurrence of multiple cranial neuropathies is an ominous sign and usually signifies the presence of leptomeningeal disease.

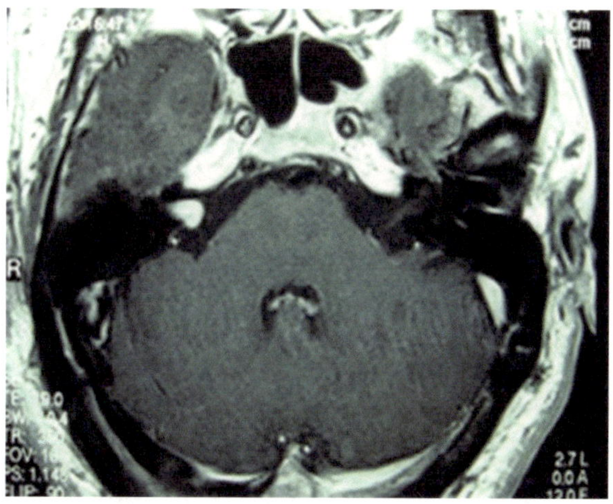

**Figure 6.** Axial post contrast MRI of patient with a small right acoustic neuroma who presented with hearing loss.

## 4. Headaches

Headaches are probably the most common complaint among brain tumor patients. Headaches can arise from many different pathological reasons. In some instances the headaches are unrelated to the imaging abnormalities and thus may not improve with treatment whereas in others the headaches are directly related to the pathological abnormalities.

In many instances the headaches are the result of increased intracranial pressure. This headache pattern is often associated with either large tumors or those lesions that have significant surrounding peritumoral edema (figure 7). The skull is a fixed rigid space with a limited volume. Therefore any changes in that volume directly affect the pressure within the skull. During early stages or with slowly growing lesions the CNS has the ability to autoregulate and compensate for these changes in tumor or edema volume by decreasing spinal fluid or changes in venous engorgement. However, sudden rapid changes in tumor size or edema can cause changes that cannot be overcome by these typical compensatory mechanisms and thus cause a dramatic change in intracranial pressure (ICP). This relationship of pressure and volume in the skull is referred to as the Monroe-Kelli Doctrine [1].

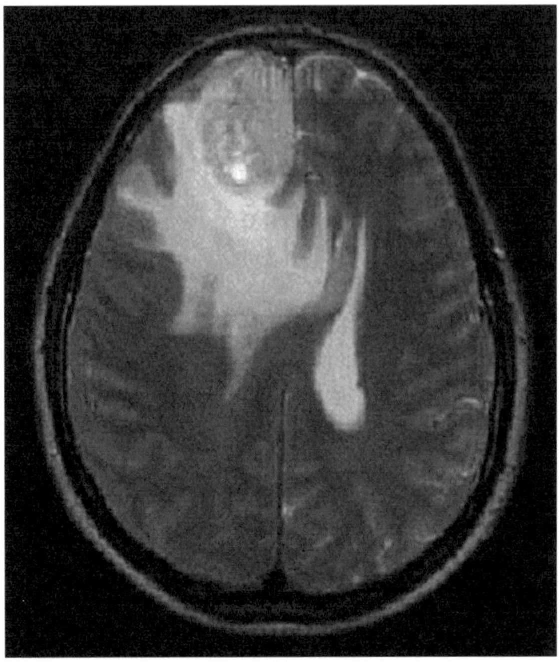

(a)

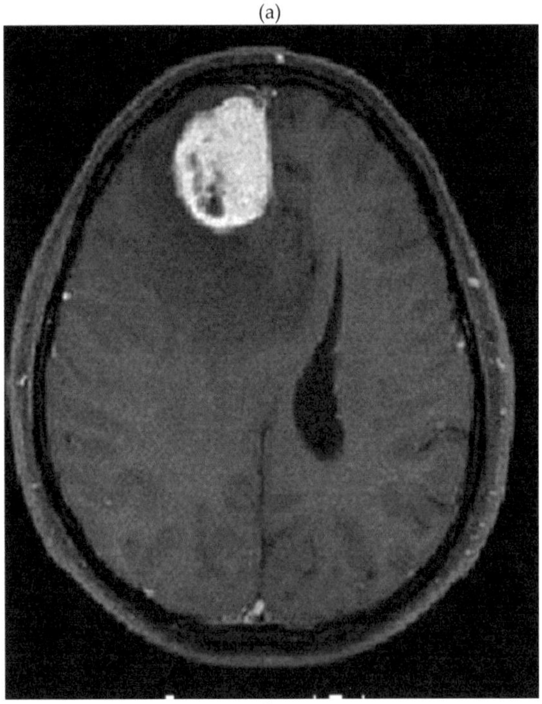

(b)

**Figure 7.** Axial T2-weighted and post contrast T1-weighted MRI scan showing significant edema and midline shift secondary to a tumor and surrounding edemawhich resulted in headache secondary to increased ICP

http://dx.doi.org/10.5772/59046

Typically headaches associated with this type of pathology are reported as global or frequently refer pain to the convexity or bifrontal/periorbital region. These headaches are usually progressive with time and are crescendo in nature. The speed at which they worsen varies depending on the rate of change in ICP. These headaches are usually worse in the morning and often associated with nausea and or vomiting. Vague visual complaints, likely the result of increased pressure in the optic nerve sheath, are often common.

Some lesions result in obstructive hydrocephalus (figure 1). The pattern and disease progression are often similar to headaches from more general increased ICP. These patients often have cognitive deficits as a result of involvement of the lateral ventricles and frontal horns. In severe cases alterations in mental status can occur and at times rapidly progress to death if emergent interventions are not instituted.

Headaches as the result of dural inflammation or irritation tend to me more focal. This can be the result of focal involvement of the dura by lesions such as meningiomas or metastasis or from stretching of the dura from tumor growth. A majority of the dura in innervated by the trigeminal nerve. As a result pain can at times be referred to the face, preauricular or periorbital region.

However, in most cases the headaches are located unilaterally ipsilateral to the pathology and in some instances directly correlated with lesion location. In my experience headaches that are directly correlated with the location of imaging abnormalities almost always improve with surgical resection.

Tumors in the sellar region can commonly cause stretching of the diaphragm sella (figure 8). These headaches commonly radiate to the periorbital or bifrontal region. The intensity and frequency of these types of headaches commonly fluctuate and can be sporadic in nature likely do to transient changes in local inflammation or pressure in the lesion itself.

Tumors that invade or compress the trigeminal nerve typically cause a very classic headache syndrome. Many of these patients experience facial pain syndromes similar to classic trigeminal neuralgia. This can often be dysesthetic in nature and frequently can become very severe and debilitating. The pain is always on the side of the lesion unless there is involvement of the brainstem. Unlike classic trigeminal neuralgia patients pain related to these lesions typically does not respond to medical management (gabapentin, pregabalin or carbamazepine) (figure 9).

In rare instances tumors can be large enough to compress or stretch the large arteries in the brain. Headaches from this cause are infrequent and vary in nature and symptomatology. On the other hand headaches as the result of tumor bleeding tend to be very classic. These headaches are often thunderclap or sudden onset in nature and occur instantaneously with a high intensity. Mental status changes and nausea and vomiting may accompany this type of headache depending on the volume and degree of hemorrhage (figure 10). Table three shows the most common histologies for brain metastasis which result in hemorrhage.

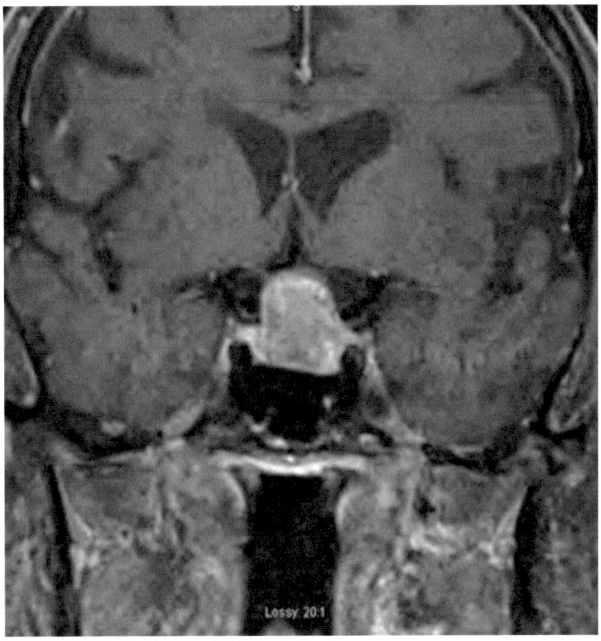


**Figure 8.** Coronal MRI of a patient with a small pituitary macroadenoma who presented with headache likely the result of stretching of the diaphragm sella.

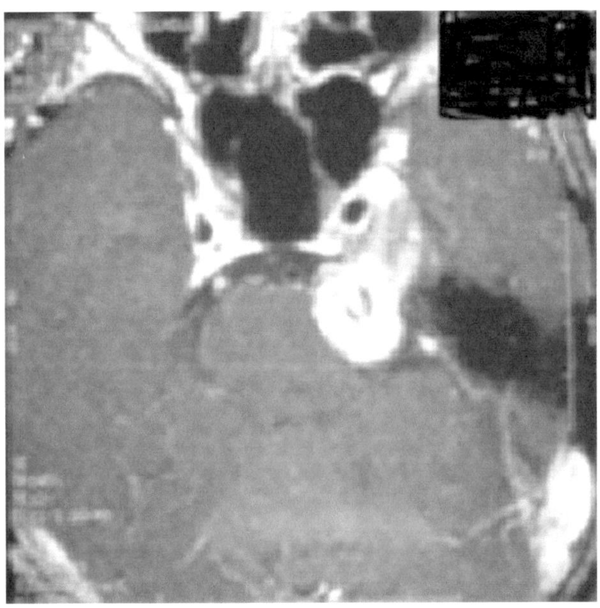

**Figure 9.** Axial post contrast MRI of patient with left sided facial pain who was found to have a small trigeminal neuroma compressing the trigeminal nerve.

http://dx.doi.org/10.5772/59046

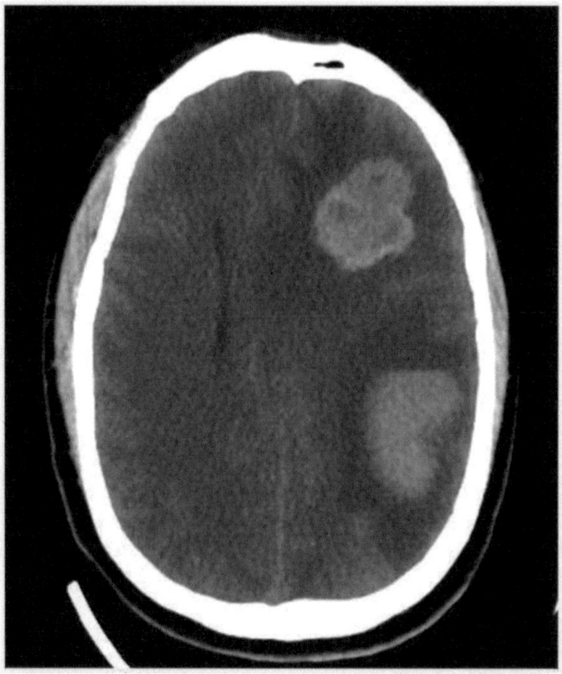

**Figure 10.** CT scan from a patient with remote history of melanoma who presented with thunderclap headache.

| |
|---|
| **Lung adenocarcinoma** |
| **Melanoma** |
| **Renal cell Carcinoma** |
| **Choriocarcinoma** |
| **Papillary Thyroid** |

**Table 3.** Most common histologies for brain metastasis that result in hemorrhage

Lesions located in the posterior fossa can cause headaches that refer pain to the vertex especially if there is associated hydrocephalus. In addition, pain may also be referred to the auricular and post auricular region secondary to innervation of the petrous dura and tentorium. These patients may also complain of pain in the suboccipital region. In rare instances of tonsilar herniation either from posterior fossa lesions or hydrocephalus patients may complain of severe neck pain at the base of the skull which worsens with extension.

The determination of which headache patient to image is always a difficult decision for the primary care or emergency room doctor as there are many more patients who complain of headaches who don't have intracranial pathology that those who do. My recommendations have always been that for adult patients who previously have not had significant headaches but then start having gradually progressive headaches that imaging should be strongly considered. Patients with rapidly deteriorating headaches or those with thunderclap onset deserve more urgent evaluation. A strong index of suspicion should also be entertained when new headaches occur with nausea and vomiting and persist despite routine headache management. Headaches associated with any other neurological finding or seizure activity also demand urgent imaging. In most instances MRI with and without contrast is the gold standard as CT scanning even when performed with contrast can have significant false negative rates. CT scanning may be adequate when intracranial hemorrhage or hydrocephalus are of concern based on clinical suspicion.

## 5. Cognitive evaluation for brain tumor patients

A majority of patients harboring brain tumors experience changes in cognitive or high level executive functioning [10-14]. Many patients may complain of subjective deficits which often are difficult to characterize, while others can slowly develop large abnormalities and be unaware of the slowly progressive changes (figure 11).

Unless patients are exhibiting major confusion and disorientation these complaints often go unassessed and unaddressed for these patients. In addition, most will exhibit at least partial improvement if a cognitive rehabilitation program is instituted before symptoms become too devastating [15].

Objective screening tests are limited and vary in efficacy in this patient population. Extensive neuropsychological batteries are time consumptive and require a trained neuropsychologist which is not available at most major brain tumor centers or smaller community treatment facilities. In addition, these deficits can change with time and are affected by all treatment modalities: surgery, radiation and chemotherapy. Therefore any reliable screening tool must also take into account the effect of "learning" from prior administrations.

Not until the past decade has the importance of assessing cognitive function and evaluating the impact of treatment on such function come into the forefront, despite the known association with cognitive functioning on quality of life and overall survival [16-18]. Only recently have prospective studies incorporated some aspect of cognitive evaluation in their study design. The mini-mental status evaluation (MMSE) is the most frequently used tool in clinical practice as well as for many large research studies. This test has numerous drawbacks including extremely low sensitivity and specificity in this patient population. In addition a "ceiling effect" exists [4]. Many patients score normal results on this test despite having significant cognitive impairments.

For the past five years I have been using the Montreal Cognitive Assessment Tool (MoCA) with my tumor patients. This is a free screening tool (available at www.mocatest.org) can be administered by office staff or physicians with minimal training and excellent inter-observer reliability. This tool assesses several aspects of cognitive function including: executive function, visuo-spatial function, naming, memory, attention, abstraction, language, orienta-

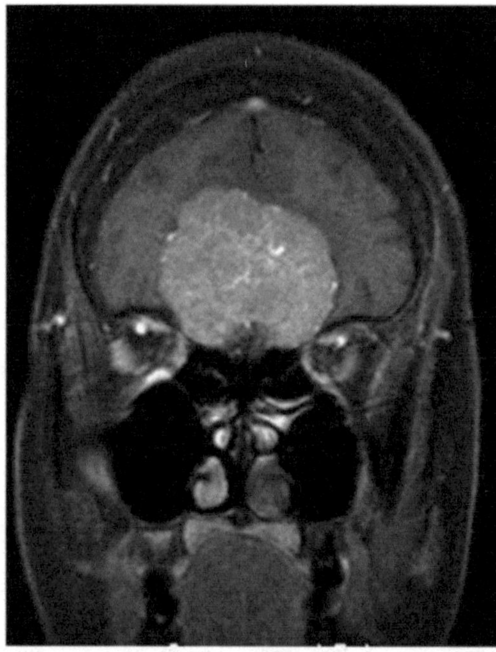

(a)

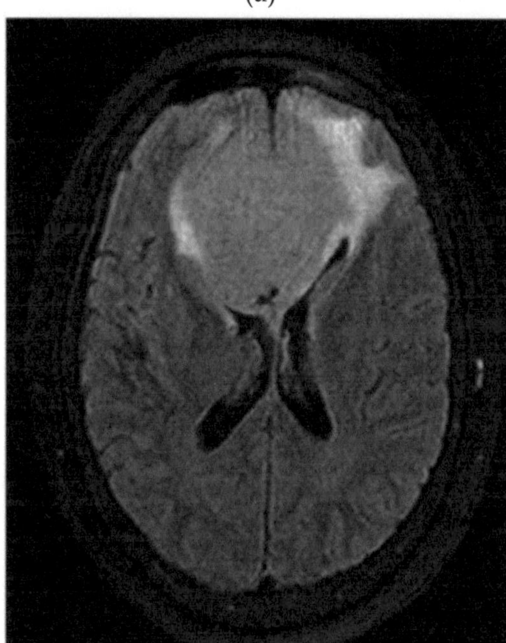

(b)

**Figure 11.** Axial post-contrast T1-weighted and FLAIR MRI in patient with a large olfactory groove meningioma who presented with cognitive dysfunction.

tion; and has been used extensively as a screening tool and for serial examinations for numerous different pathological conditions from dementia to heart failure.

The MoCA is more sensitive than the MMSE for detecting mild cognitive impairment (MCI) [19-21]. Olson compared the efficacy of MoCA vs MMSE in a group of patients with brain metastasis by administering both tests to patients at a similar time point after diagnosis of their brain metastasis. Ninety-eight percent of patients completed the test in less than 15 minutes, and 88% of patients took less than 10 minutes. Based on the results of the study (using normal cutoff scores for both tests) 80% of patients were classified as having at least mild cognitive impairment on the MoCA (score <26) vs. 30% using the MMSE (score <26) [22].

In 2011 the same group reported the results of 58 brain metastasis patients who were studied prospectively [4]. Once again both groups were administered MoCA and MMSE tests, 67% of the patients also underwent formal neuropsychological assessment (NPA) which consisted of a battery of tests taking 3-4 hours to complete. This formal testing was performed within 2 weeks of administration of the screening tests. Study analysis showed that only 7% of patients scored normal on the NPA and an additional 38% had borderline results, the remainder of the patients had cognitive impairment in greater than two domains. MMSE results showed abnormal cognitive function in only 12.8% and MoCA showed impairment in 53.8%. Thus it is clearly illustrated based on the poor sensitivity that the MMSE is a poor screening tool for determining cognitive impairment in these patients and has limited value. The MoCA was more sensitive in determining mild cognitive impairment but still failed to illustrate all cases [4]. Finally, in yet another study they were able to show that the results of the MoCA were highly correlated with overall survival in patients undergoing treatment for brain metastasis but failed to show a relationship of survival to MMSE results [22].

## Author details

Christie Adams, Joan Sullivan and Todd W. Vitaz*

*Address all correspondence to: todd.vitaz@spectrumhealth.org

Department of Clinical Neurosciences Spectrum Health Medical Group, and College of Human Medicine, Michigan State University, Grand Rapids, Michigan, USA

## References

[1] Ellenbogen R, Abdulrauf S, Sekhar L. Principles of Neurological Surgery. 2012.

[2] Forsyth P, Posner J. Headaches in patients with brain tumors: a study of 111 patients. Neurology. 1993;43(9):1678.

[3] Chandana S, Movva S, Arora M, Singh T. Primary Brain Tumors in Adults. Am Fam Physician. 2008 May 15;77(10):1423-1430

[4] Olson R, Iverson G, Carolan H, Parkinson M, Brooks B, McKenzie M. Prospective comparison of two cognitive screening tests: diagnostic accuracy and correlation with community integration and quality of life. Journal of Neurooncology 2011; 105: 337-344

[5] Lote K, Stenwig AE, Skullerud K, Hirschberg H. Prevalence and prognostic significance of epilepsy in patients with gliomas. Eur J Cancer. 1998;34(1):98.

[6] Glantz et al Neurology 2000.

[7] Davie G, Hutcheson K, Barringer D, Weinberg J, Lewin J. Aphasia in patients after brain tumour resection. Aphasiology 2009;23(9):1-11.

[8] Recht L, McCarthy K, O'Donnell B, Cohen R, Drachman D. Tumour-associated aphasia in left hemisphere primary brain tumours: The importance of age and tumor grade.

[9] Snyder PJ. Gonadotroph adenomas. In: The Pituitary, 2nd, Melmed S (Ed), Blackwell Science Inc., Malden, MA 2002. p.575.

[10] Chang E, Wefel J, Maor m, Hassenbush S, Mahajan A, Lang F et al. A pilot study of neurocognitive function in patients with one to three new brain metastases initially treated with stereotactic radiosurgery alone. Neurosurgery 2007;60(2): 277-284.

[11] Herman M, Tremont-Lukats I, Meyers C, Trask D, Froseth C, Renschler et al. Neurocognitive and functional assessment of patient with brain metasteses: a pilot study. American Journal of Clinical Oncology 2003;26(3): 273-279.

[12] Mehta M, Shapiro W, Glantz M, Patchell R, Weitzner M, Meyers C, et al. Lead-in phase to randomized trial of motexafin gadolinium and whole-brain radiation for patients with brain metastases: centralized assessment of magnetic resonance imaging, neurocognitive, and neurologic end points. Journal of Clincal Oncology 2002;20(16): 3445-3453.

[13] Murray K, Scott C, Zachariah B, Michalski J, Demas W, VoraN, et al. Importance of the mini-mental status examination in the treatment of patients with brain metastases: a report from the radiation oncology group protocol. International Journal of Radiation Oncology Biology and Physics 2000;48(1): 59-64.

[14] Taphorn M, Klein M. Cognitive deficits in adult patients with brain tumours. Lancet Neurology 2004;3(3): 159-68.

[15] Olson R, Chhanabhai T, McKenzie M. Feasibility study of the Montreal Cognitive Assessment (MoCA) in patients with brain metastases. Supportive Care Cancer 2008;16: 1273-1278

[16] Meyers C, Hess K, Yung W, Levin V. Cognitive function as a predictor of survival in patients with recurrent malignant glioma. Journal of clinical Oncology 2000;18: 646-650.

[17] Meyers C, Smith J, Bezjak A, Mehta M, Liebmann J, Illidge T, et al. Neurocognitive function and progression in patients with brain metastases treated with whole-brain radiation and metoxafin gadolinium: results of a randomized phase III trial. Journal of Clinical Oncology 2004;22: 157-165.

[18] Sherman A, Jaeckle K, Meyers C. Pretreatment cognitive performance predicts survival in patients with leptomeningeal disease. Cancer 2002;95: 1311-1316.

[19] Guthier S, Reisberg B, Zaudig M, Petersen R, Ritchie K, Broich K, et al. Mild cognitive impairment. Lancet 2006;367(9518): 1262-1270.

[20] Nasreddine Z, Phillips N, Bedirian V, Charbonneau S, Whitehead V, Collin I, et al. The montreal cognitive assessment, MoCA: a brief screening tool for mild cognitive impairment. Journal of American Geriatric Society 2005;53(4): 695-699.

[21] Smith T, Gildeh N, Holmes C. The montreal cognitive assessment: validity and utility in a memory clinic setting. Canadian Journal of Psychiatry 2007;52(5): 329-332.

[22] Olson R, Tyldesley S, Carolan H, Parkinson M, Chhanabhai T, McKenzie M. Prospective comparison of the prognostic utility of the mini mental state examination and the montreal cognitive Assessment in patients with brain metastases. Supportive Care Cancer 2011;19: 1849-1855

Section 3

# Immunotherapy for Brain Tumors

Chapter 15

# Immune Modulation by Tumor-Derived Extracellular Vesicles in Glioblastoma

Justin E. Hellwinkel, Helen Madsen and Michael Graner

Additional information is available at the end of the chapter

http://dx.doi.org/10.5772/59037

## 1. Introduction

Glioblastoma multiforme (GBM) is a highly aggressive and malignant brain tumor that is largely resistant to surgical, radiological, and chemotherapeutic intervention. It is characterized as a WHO Grade IV astrocytoma with high infiltrative capacity into brain parenchyma, resulting in debilitating cognitive deficits. Features such as diffuse tumor margins, high vascularity, and necrosis are cardinal indications for GBM diagnosis [1]. Current treatment regimens include a combination of surgery and radiotherapy, along with adjuvant temozolomide. This line of therapy has been successful in extending patient survival to 15 months [2]. However, the significant emotional and financial cost incurred by patients and their families during this process can be devastating. All three approaches employ a shotgun approach with nonspecific effects leading to reduced quality of life and increased burden of disease. Despite advances in the management of many other tumor types, glioblastoma has not experienced the same success and median survival still remains 15 months. An alarming 8% average survival at 3 years stresses the urgent need for more effective treatments [3]. Emerging novel therapeutics aim to manipulate the immune system for selective destruction of cancerous tissue, while leaving healthy brain tissue undisturbed. These approaches offer promise for a selective approach of tumor elimination with reduced side effects and improved quality of life. However, immunotherapeutic success has also been limited, due to lack of understanding of the influence of cancer cells on the immune system. Better understanding of the glioma and immune interface will allow for more effective immune manipulations in order to generate anti-tumor responses. Recent studies have identified intercellular signaling modalities as critical components for tumor growth. Extracellular vesicles released from GBM cells have been revealed to be potent modulators of the local environment to facilitate malignancy and mitigate destruction of the tumor by immune cells. Specific mechanisms of vesicle-induced changes are becoming more evident and offer novel targets for future therapies. Elucidating intracellular changes and signaling cascades that lead to phenotypic deviation of naïve immune cells will reveal points of regulation to manipulate for tumor destruction. This chapter aims to examine the multifaceted roles of GBM-derived extracellular vesicles on immune cells. We will discuss the current state of knowledge about the mechanisms by which extracellular vesicles alter the tumor microenvironment, along with new findings relating to transformation of T cells by extracellular vesicles. Phenotypic changes, functional pathways, and protein profiles of immune cells will be discussed to gain an understanding of the means of transformation. These changes will also be assessed over time to highlight potential early markers of tumor influence that may be used for diagnostic or prognostic application. Finally, we will discuss considerations for new immunotherapies relating to immune cell transformation induced by extracellular vesicles.

## 2. Tenacity of brain tumors

### 2.1. Failure of current therapies

#### *2.1.1. Traditional therapies*

Despite recent advancements in approaches to cancer treatment, GBM remains a complex and problematic cancer to target. Diffuse borders of GBM tumors invade sensitive brain tissue and make complete surgical resection particularly difficult. Incidentally, cancerous cells are left behind, which allows the tumor to repopulate the resection cavity and enables recurrent tumor growth. Radiation therapy is commonly utilized to eliminate portions of tumor remaining after surgery and in recurrent settings. Although radiation has shown to provide survival benefit, innocent bystander damage to nearby brain structures still remains a major obstacle in this field. Newer technologies, including gamma knife surgery, allow for a more targeted approach to access remaining tumor and reduce the risk of complications from a second surgery [4]. Despite this, damage to healthy tissue still occurs and the inability to target every cancerous cell constituting the tumor remains problematic. The addition of the alkylating agent temozolomide to GBM treatment has extended overall survival and progression-free survival for patients receiving surgical resection and radiation [5]. A multimodal approach in the treatment of GBM offers the most promising outcome for patients. However, prognosis remains dismal and quality of life is poor because these treatment options do not specifically target glioma cells. In recent years, alternative approaches have been explored that more specifically isolate cancerous cells and remove support from surrounding structures. Gliadel wafers implanted into the surgical resection bed provide survival benefit by releasing anti-tumor agent, carmustine, locally to target areas of infiltrating tumor. Since most GBM tumors will recur in a 2 cm margin surrounding the resection cavity, carmustine impregnated wafers are able to focus on this area, while sparing other sensitive structures. The ease of implantation and regional release of drug makes this method attractive, yet overall survival and quality of life is equal to temozolomide alone, and wafers offer no benefit in recurrent settings [6]. Electric field devices offer a novel approach to GBM destruction by emitting alternating electric fields to slow and prevent tumor progression. However, incomplete understanding of the mechanism by which electric fields can slow tumor growth has hindered success of this therapy. The noninvasive nature of electric field technology offers promise for enhanced quality of life and ease of treatment delivery integrated into patient's daily lives. Unfortunately, these devices have shown to confer minimal benefit in survival over chemotherapy [7].

### 2.1.2. *Monoclonal antibodies*

Utilization of natural defense mechanisms offers the most potential to support the failing triad of traditional therapies in GBM. One element of immunotherapy that has gained momentum in recent years has been the use of monoclonal antibodies. Monoclonal antibodies offer antigenic specificity and have been successful in controlling a variety of other cancers in different stages including breast, lung, and melanoma [8]. The strength behind antibody treatment lies in their ability to circulate to identify distant metastasis and specifically target tumor-specific antigens. The first major obstacle for antibody therapy in GBM is delivery across a selective blood-brain barrier and maintenance of the antibody binding pocket once penetration is complete. Since GBM almost never metastasizes outside the cranial cavity, antibodies must be able to access the tumor *in situ* by crossing over the blood-brain barrier easily. The second major barrier for antibody therapy is the existence of few tumor-specific antigens on the surface of GBM cells. Although some antigens have been identified to date, tumors have been shown to adapt quickly to change expression of surface molecules in the face of antigen-specific attack. Thus, even if these antigens have roles in aiding tumor progression, they are not ideal targets because they are not necessary for tumor survival. In addition, the vast heterogeneity of GBM tumors precludes a single target approach. Therefore, soluble factors constituting the tumor microenvironment have been targeted. GBM tumors are highly vascularized and release abundant amounts of vascular endothelial growth factor (VEGF) into the external environment to induce local angiogenesis. Their high metabolic needs require sustained nutrient delivery directly to the tumor site, so much that the cores of GBM tumors contain areas of necrosis. Bevacizumab is a monoclonal antibody that binds and neutralizes VEGFA in the brain tumor environment to reduce vascularization and limit nutrient delivery. It is currently the only monoclonal antibody approved for use in recurrent GBM and is implemented during various disease states in clinical trials [9]. Bevacizumab remains a passive treatment option that has been successful in restricting tumor growth, but does not actively kill cancerous cells. Some studies have suggested bevacizumab promotes development of structurally competent blood vessels around the tumor, rather than the compromised leaky vessels that typically grow in tumor sites [10]. This modification may help ameliorate symptoms caused by cerebral edema, but does not slow nutrient delivery to GBM tumors. To date, bevacizumab has conferred minimal overall survival benefit, although time to recurrence and quality of life are reportedly improved [11]. Currently available treatment options offer a variety of approaches that demonstrate clinical benefit, but none substantially extend survival or decrease burden of disease for patients.

### 2.1.3. *Tumor-specific immunotherapy*

The heterogeneity and adaptability of GBM tumors needs to be met with a dynamic and adaptable treatment strategy in order to maintain remission or eliminate the tumor altogether. Manipulation of the adaptive immune system against GBM is the goal of future immunotherapies as a means to specifically identify cancerous cells for destruction. Vast molecular differences between patients and within individual patient tumors have prevented identification of common components to target. New approaches employ *ex vivo* stimulation of patient's adaptive immune cells with their own tumor followed by injection of the activated cells back into circulation. The goal of this approach is to initiate a level of immune stimulation that will specifically target tumor antigens typically hidden *in vivo*, while protecting the patient from autoimmune complications. The promise for initiation of an adaptive response stems from identification of lymphocytes within GBM tissue during autopsies and the later understanding of tumor specificity of these cells [12]. Although unable to eliminate the tumor, it became clear that lymphocytes play a role in antitumor immunity. Activated lymphocytes have a unique ability to migrate into brain parenchyma, thus *ex vivo* activation of the adaptive immune response has been explored as a means of eliciting antitumor responses [13]. Variations in type of tumor material, incubation conditions, adaptive cell types, and course of treatment have been under rigorous investigation to optimize tumor destruction [12,14,15]. Tumor-specific antigens continue to be ideal targets, but tumors rarely rely on a single antigen, and targeting overexpressed molecules could critically disrupt healthy cells that need those antigens for survival. Molecular targets including EphA2, IL-13R2a, EGFRvIII and survivin have been implicated in GBM progression and offer potential pathways and signaling modalities for cellular immunotherapies to target [16–19]. Other potential sources of tumor antigens include protein complexes, chaperones, RNA, and whole cell lysate [20]. These approaches offer the benefit of stimulating a varied approach of tumor destruction because of the immune cells' innate ability to distinguish harmful from harmless. The potential for response against multiple tumor antigens is greater with unbiased access to native tumor material (antigens), thus the immune response has a better chance to elicit a multidimensional attack against the heterogeneous GBM. The two primary approaches employing these strategies include autologous T cell transfer and dendritic cell vaccines.

Autologous T cell transfer has been referred to as passive immunotherapy because the T cells are stimulated *ex vivo* and reintroduced to the patient as antigen specific, activated cells. Dendritic cell vaccines are an active type of therapy, in which dendritic cells are isolated from the patient and pulsed with tumor antigen before reintroduction to the patient. The dendritic cell then has the opportunity to present antigen in secondary lymphoid tissue to lymphocytes in the ideal environment for activation. Both approaches continue to be studied in order to identify the optimal approach to adaptive immune activation. Sipuleucel-T was the first FDA-approved dendritic cell vaccine to exhibit survival benefit for any type of cancer and created a new realm of potential for personal immunotherapy [21]. Utilization of this treatment strategy for GBM is much more difficult, primarily because Sipuleucel-T relies on the presence of a tumor antigen found on the subset of cells that respond well to treatment. Dendritic cell vaccines for GBM currently under investigation in clinical trials employ differential antigenic approaches in hope of producing an ideal cocktail [22–24]. However, passive and active immunotherapies have not yet transformed the landscape of GBM due to complexity of the disease. In fact, very few patients have exhibited tumor regression for any substantial period of time [25]. A major obstacle that must be overcome when developing these immunogenic responses is the immunosuppressive environment induced by GBM. Once the burden of immunosuppression is alleviated, immunotherapeutic strategies and their effectors will have a better chance to infiltrate, identify, and kill cancerous cells.

### 2.2. Immune manipulation by gliomas

Malignant brain tumors are known to correspond with multiple mechanisms of immune suppression. Although phenotypic changes have been well documented, specific mechanisms inducing the alterations are less well understood. Presence of modified immune cells transformed by the tumor environment presents obstacles investigators need to consider when developing new therapeutics utilizing the immune system. GBM cells can modulate their external environment through release of soluble factors and expression of discrete molecules on the cell surface. One soluble factor released from GBM that appears to have a major role in tumor progression is transforming growth factor beta (TGFβ) [26]. TGFβ has a wide range of effects capable of suppressing immune responses including inhibition of IL-2 receptor on T cells, down regulation of MHC molecules on antigen presenting cells, and even neutralization of activated lymphocytes entering the tumor environment ([26,27]. Inhibitors of TGFβ and neutralizing antibodies have shown promise in mitigation of glioma growth and immune suppression [28]. To further enhance immune suppression in the local environment, GBM recruits and converts naïve cells. Transformation of monocytes to immunosuppressive macrophages is one of the most significant changes GBM produces in the microenvironment. Tumor associated macrophages (TAMs) can comprise of classically activated M1 macrophages or alternatively actived M2. TAMs are predominantly of the M2 phenotype and are the most common immune infiltrate in glioma [29]. Evidence has shown TAMs can comprise up to 40% of the tumor mass in GBM, thus the suppressive roles are highly apparent [30]. Unlike M1 macrophages, M2 TAMs do not release proinflammatory and chemoattractive factors, but instead aid in tumor progression and attenuate activity of infiltrating lymphocytes. TAMs can arise from both circulating monocytes and resident microglia near the tumor site [31]. Gliomas ability to tip the balance towards the M2 phenotype is important for tumor survival and progression because of the protection conferred to evade immune destruction. TAMs isolated from glioma express very little MHCII or costimulatory molecules CD80/86 and this phenotype can be transferred to naïve monocytes introduced to the same cell culture media [29,32]. Impaired release of TNF$\alpha$ from glioma macrophages can also be transferred to naïve monocytes in cell culture, providing a regionally dependent inhibitory modulation of monocytes in the GBM environment. In addition to reductions in TNF$\alpha$ release, TAMs actively suppress the extracellular space by constitutively expressing immunosuppressive cytokines IL-10 and TGFβ [33]. This active inhibition is supported by impaired cytotoxic capabilities of TAMs, which generates a highly immunocompromised environment for GBM to grow [34]. Converted TAMs further propagate the glioma environment through release of matrix metalloproteases and growth factors for endothelial cells and tumor cells alike [35]. In order to remove the inhibition caused by glioma TAMs, it will be necessary to tip the balance back towards the classically activated M1 phenotype without causing autoimmunity or inflammatory consequences.

Glioma patients exhibit varying degrees of lymphopenia, but often a great proportion of remaining cells are regulatory T cells. This phenomenon has been observed in many types of cancer and is thought to act as a driving force to maintain immunosuppression and propagate tumor cells. It is unclear whether regulatory T cell production is driven primarily by MDSC, tumor-released proteins, alternative signaling pathways, or carefully selected from the natural T cell population. Anti-CD25 treatment options have shown benefit in the glioma setting, which could help tilt the balance back towards an immunostimulatory environment [36]. Although the presence of a high concentration of regulatory T cells persists, some T cells have the capability to become active and access the tumor bed. Tumor-infiltrating lymphocytes (TILs) are antigen-specific lymphocytes capable of penetrating the blood-brain barrier in an effort to confer immunity against a growing tumor. The presence of TILs in gliomas indicates patients are not entirely tolerant to the tumor and attempt to mount a response against it, thus yielding a more favorable prognosis for patients. However, the TILs do not respond to mitogenic stimulation and proliferate very poorly in the face of a challenge [37]. The exact origin and capabilities of TILs are not clear, but their ineffectiveness in tumor destruction generates an opportunity to learn about transformation. Similar activation abilities have been reported with B cells isolated from peripheral circulation of GBM patients, whereas immunoglobulin production is hindered when cells were stimulated [38].

# 3. Extracellular vesicles

## 3.1. Genesis

Extracellular vesicles (EVs) arise primarily from two distinct biogenesis pathways during healthy and pathological conditions. Release of vesicles can occur by direct shedding of plasma membrane (microvesicles) or though invagination of an endosome to form a multi-vesicular body, which later fuses with the plasma membrane (exosomes) [39]. Distinction of origin is controversial, since components of the plasma membrane and intracytosolic proteins are found in both. Overlapping similarities in size, density, membrane proteins and morphology suggests differential nomenclature is not necessary, but the specific difference between the types of extracellular vesicles is not fully understood [40]. Shuttling of contents into EVs occurs through random capture during vesicle formation and through selection based on mechanisms remaining to be elucidated [41]. EVs are released by many cell types in normal and pathological states, including lymphocytes, dendritic cells, neurons, reticulocytes, and tumors [42–46]). These vesicles contain distinct cargo that resemble the cell from which they were released and can be identified in circulating fluids such as urine, breast milk, plasma, saliva, cerebrospinal fluid, and amniotic fluid [47]. EVs vary in size from 30-2,000 nm in diameter, which ultimately dictates the amount of cargo they can carry. Enhanced release of extracellular vesicles from cancer cells is an indicator that they may have a role in aiding in tumor progression [48]. Release is further heightened in cancer cells exposed to radiation or hypoxic conditions [49,50]. Due to their presence in these fluids and the specific signature they contain, EVs are ideal vehicles for transfer of large amounts of information to modulate the external environment and signal immune complexes.

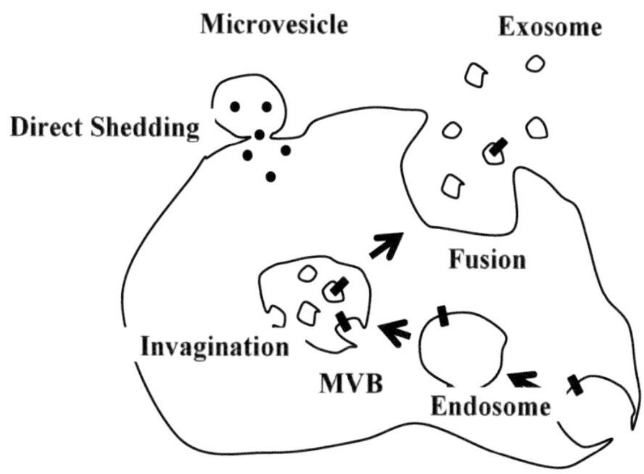


Abbreviations used in this figure. MVB: Multivesicular body

**Figure 1.** Release pathways for microvesicles and exosomes. Microvesicles are directly shed from the cellular membrane and capture contents by inclusion of nearby particles. Exosomes are formed through endosomal invaginations, which form multivesicular bodies and fuse with the plasma membrane. Shuttling of exosomal contents is more selective due to machinery available

### 3.2. Waste receptacles

EVs are responsible for a multitude of roles in intercellular communication. Enrichment of discrete molecules suggests well-organized machinery dictates packaging of internal contents before release. These small packets of information can be transferred long distances with specificity for a recipient cell. However, their pleiotropic roles in a healthy setting are still not fully understood. They were originally thought to be waste receptacles for cells lacking lysosome machinery, since release was first identified during reticulocyte maturation [45]. Other studies have confirmed packaging of waste products into extracellular vesicles, along with cytotoxic substances, including chemotherapeutic agents [51]. This evidence provides a novel mechanism of drug resistance in cancerous cells and a potential target to induce sensitivity to toxic drugs as well. Controlling drug transport can allow for delivery of chemotherapeutic drugs at a lower concentration and provide increased efficacy. This is particularly important in GBM in order to preserve healthy brain tissue typically damaged by toxic drugs during treatment.

### 3.3. Immune response

In addition to waste disposal, EVs are now known to be important factors in antigen presentation [42]. Immunostimulatory properties of EVs were first recognized by Raposo et al. when they found MHC class II molecule enrichment on the surface of extracellular vesicles released from EBV-transformed B cells. These EVs were sufficient to elicit an antigen-specific T cell response. These data present a mechanism for rapid amplification of specific immune response via presentation of peptides bound to MHC II molecules. Later studies confirmed presence of co-stimulatory molecules on the surface of vesicles and amplification of CD4+ and CD8+ responses through horizontal transfer of MHC II loaded EVs from activated dendritic cells to maturing dendritic cells [52]. Further mechanisms of immune activation by EVs include activation of NK cells and monocytes [53,54]. Extracellular vesicles represent an ideal booster for immune responses, but also contain a kill switch to dampen response and tightly regulate clearance of pathogens. Activated lymphocytes release EVs containing Fas ligand and APO2 ligand, which are both capable of inducing cell death [55]. It is postulated that release of cytotoxic components from activated cells ensures moderation of excessive immune responses and reduces autoimmunity. The expression and composition of EVs in a normal immune response is highly controlled and deliberate to ensure modulation at appropriate times.

### 3.4. Horizontal transfer of information

Intercellular communication via EVs allows for transfer of large amounts of information to maintain homeostasis and normal physiological function. Some functions that have been identified to date include tissue repair, stem cell regeneration, synaptic plasticity, neuronal communication, and viral transmission [56–59]. EVs contain many components that resemble the host cell, but also contain discrete pieces of information that may be useful for identification of specific signaling capabilities. Valadi et al. first described packaging and transfer of messenger RNA (mRNA) and microRNA (miRNA) in extracellular vesicles in 2007 [60]. EVs from healthy mast cells were harvested and analyzed based on genetic content. Interestingly, no DNA was found within EVs, which suggests they signal exclusively through epigenetic changes and signaling mechanisms in the recipient cell. mRNA found in EVs released from mast cells exhibited functionality and was found to be unique from the donor cell. This discovery revealed a new complexity to intercellular communication by means of modifying protein expression and gene regulation through horizontal transfer of packets of information. Later studies have been able to identify distinct miRNA signatures in pathological conditions not found in normal cells. These signatures have been well documented in ovarian cancers, lung cancer, and GBM [61–63]. mRNA contained within GBM extracellular vesicles control a variety of cellular functions to promote tumorigensis, including enhancement of angiogenic, proliferative, and migratory pathways. Identification of cargo released from cancerous cells offers critical information about components that are deliberately shuttled out of the cell, possible influence on the local environment, and the potential to act as a peripheral biomarker for diagnostic or prognostic applications. Genetic signatures are particularly valuable in the brain tumor arena because of their ease of collection and sensitivity to identify of tumor progression.

## 4. Tumor-derived EVs

### 4.1. EVs and tumor microenvironment

The Taylor group first identified release of tumor-derived EVs in 1979 [46]. Their seminal study was met with antagonism because it was not believed that small particles like these could have any substantial effect on tumor propagation. Later studies confirmed these small cellular surrogates could act locally and peripherally and their bioactive cargo had significance in the cancer setting [64,65]. EV cargo varies between cells and disease states and the significance of inclusion of certain cargo is just beginning to be understood. EVs are capable of carrying proteins, lipids, carbohydrates and nucleic acids in endless combinations. The restrictive size of the EV compartments dictates the amount of material that can be packaged, thus tumor cells must selectively package opportunistic cargo to facilitate tumor progression. Tumor specific antigens MART1 and HER2/Neu have been identified in EVs released from cells with respective mutations, implicating a role for EVs in horizontal transfer of cancer promoting agents [48]. Much like transfer of viral peptides, EVs offer a mechanism to exponentially facilitate cancer progression through delivery of disease-specific antigens. In the brain tumor setting, EVs have been shown to carry and transfer the truncated EGFRvIII from GBM cells containing the mutation, to GBM cells without the mutation [66]. EGFR mutant variant III may be associated with over 50% of GBM tumors and indicates a negative prognosis for patients [67]. Rapid onset and growth of this subset of GBM relies on the presence of EGFRvIII on the plasma membrane surface. EV delivery of the mutated receptor to neighboring cells presents a partial explanation for the relentless aggressiveness of these tumors. Besides tumor antigens, EVs also carry factors to modify the extracellular environment to ensure tumor survival. Active matrix metalloprotease (MMP) and other matrix remodeling enzymes have been identified as EV cargo and are capable of compromising the rigidity of the extracellular matrix [68]. GBM tumors are notoriously invasive around the borders of the tumor margin and it is likely that EVs play a role in promoting invasion. Other factors carried by GBM EVs include angiogenic proteins VEGF and IL-6, which aid in recruiting new blood vessels to the tumor site. Many other pieces of cargo have been identified to date, but the functional consequences of their presence is not clear. Identification of a tumor signature from tumor-derived EVs offers promise for noninvasive biopsy type analysis and could aid in treatment before large changes can be seen from imaging.

GBM EVs have been shown to participate in modulation of the external environment through a variety of pathways, although specific molecules responsible for the changes are not known. Exogenous brain tumor EVs are capable of enhancing proliferation of GBM cells in a dose-dependent manner, which generate a positive feedback loop *in vivo* [69]. Thus, EVs are partially or largely responsible for rapid propagation of tumor cells. GBM cells often induce their own proliferation through autocrine growth factor signaling, but for cells that have not yet acquired the correct mutations, EVs offer a mechanism to promote proliferation. In addition to proliferation, glioma EVs promote migration of tumor cells as well [70]. Effectively, GBM tumors generate their own chemoattractive gradient away from the core of the tumor towards the external environment. This process is further exacerbated by radiation treatment, as the GBM cells release greater amounts of EVs and exhibit enhanced migration towards their EVs [49]. Extensive proteomic studies have begun to identify material responsible for some of these changes. Profiling all the material contained within tumor-derived EVs and understanding the correct balance of information will help to better characterize targets in the future.

### 4.2. Tumor-derived EVs and immune response

#### *4.2.1. Cellular decoys*

Extracellular vesicles are optimal vehicles for transfer of large amounts of information to amplify signaling without cell-to-cell contact. While this elegant ability can amplify an immune response against pathogens extremely rapidly, it can also be used as a mechanism of immune manipulation by brain tumor cells. The pleiotropic roles of tumor-derived EVs on immune modulation are not fully understood and it is likely the effects in the brain tumor environment may be unique compared to other tumor types. Many of the studies conducted on tumor-derived EVs have occurred *in vitro* or using murine models, but offer great insight about the modulatory capacities and potency of EVs. The immense immunosuppressive roles of tumor-derived EVs reveal the importance of these signaling modalities in the cancer setting. Modulation of both innate and adaptive immune responses undermines the immune system's redundancy against harmful stimuli. Tumor EVs have been shown to inhibit cytotoxic capabilities of natural killer (NK) cells that typically patrol cellular surface antigens for danger signals [71] and presence of MHC. One of the mechanisms by which this occurs is through expression of danger signal MICA on the surface of EVs released into the extracellular space. Binding of MICA on the surface of EVs by NK cells prevents them from identifying the problematic cells and leads to inactivation of NK cells through down regulation of MICA binding protein, NKG2D [72]. This process creates difficulty for future attempts to activate this subset of NK cells in the presence of real tumor and the continued release of tumor EVs as cellular decoys perpetuates inhibition. Similarly, tumor EVs have shown to attenuate humoral immunity by binding antigen-specific antibodies and misguiding antibody-dependent cellular cytotoxicity away from the tumor [73]. Expression of cell surface antigens on the surface of EVs introduces a unique obstacle for treatments targeting surface molecules. Immune cells and pharmacological agents in development will have to circumnavigate the decoy EVs to specifically access tumor cells.

#### *4.2.2. Monocyte transformation*

Another worrisome consequence of tumor EVs is their ability to restrict peripheral blood monocytes from fully maturing to dendritic cells [74]. As a central hub bridging innate and adaptive immunity, dendritic cells are critical for developing a specific and adaptable anti-tumor response. The potential of immunotherapy relies heavily on the premise of selective destruction by adaptive cells that have been fully educated by dendritic cells about tumor antigens to target. Further evidence has revealed EVs can not only inhibit, but also promote a transformation of monocytes towards a myeloid-derived suppressor cell (MDSC) phenotype. MDSCs are critically important for facilitation of glioma growth, as discussed above, and can comprise a large portion of glioma mass [29]. Tumor-derived EVs induce release of immunosuppressive factors from MDSC including TGFβ and PGE2 and also down regulate expression of MHCII on monocyte cell surfaces, limiting activation potential [75,76].

### 4.2.3. Migratory capacity

The phenotypic changes of naïve immune cells exposed to tumor-derived EVs dictates the functionality of the immune response to perpetuate tumor growth. One of the most important functional consequences of tumor-derived EVs is the ability to alter migratory capacity of PBMCs. Preliminary data from our group has demonstrated attenuation of migration of mitogen-activated PBMCs moving towards glioma EVs (Figure 2). Migration is a necessary component of activated PBMCs in order to properly activate and then destroy cells of interest. When brain tumor EVs are present, this process is disrupted, which can prevent even the best tumor-specific cells from reaching their targets. Interestingly, studies have demonstrated brain tumor EVs can enhance tumor cell migration as discussed above. If glioma EVs truly facilitate glioma migration while diminishing immune cell migration, it is possible similar pathways are altered in both cell types. Better understanding of the exact mechanisms and pathways involved will lead to pharmacologic targets that could reverse migratory effects. Because EVs are packets of complex information, identification of a switch to reverse both processes simultaneously will be challenging. However, immune cells can still enter the tumor site to promote tumor growth, thus tumor-derived EVs do not entirely eliminate PBMC entry into brain parenchyma. They may, however, select for immune cells that will only aid in tumor progression, such as MDSCs, and limit migration of anti-tumor cells. This selective entry could help explain why resident immune cells at the tumor site do not destroy the tumor and presents a reason for the limited success of immunotherapies that do not address EV presence. Alternatively, brain tumor EVs in peripheral circulation may prevent movement of activated dendritic cells to secondary lymphoid tissue, severely compromising their ability to activate an adaptive immune response.

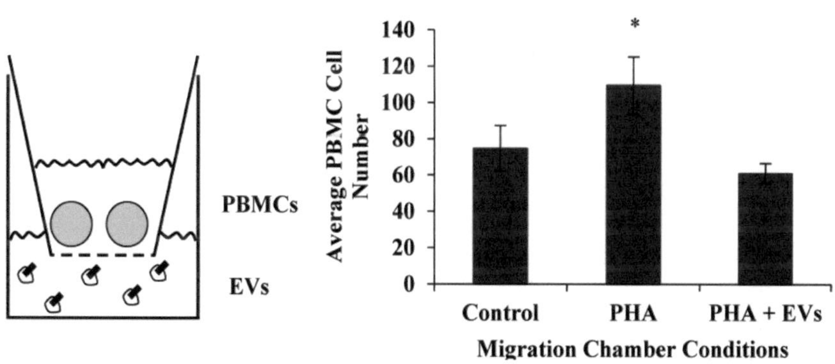


Abbreviations used in this figure. PHA: Phytohemagglutinin; EVs: Extracellular Vesicles; PBMC: Peripheral Blood Mononuclear Cell

**Figure 2.** Average migration of naïve PBMCs in the presence of mitogenic stimuli with or without extracellular vesicles. PBMCs were placed in the top of a migration chamber with PHA and the bottom chamber contained EVs or media. The number of PBMCs that migrated to the bottom chamber was quantified after 24 hours. *=$p < 0.01$.

### 4.3. Altered function of T cells

Aberrations of T cell phenotypes and functional capacities in the cancer setting have been described, but specific mechanisms of alteration are not well understood. T cell deficits induced by tumor EVs are among the most important transformations necessary to protect tumors from immune destruction. T cells cultured with tumor EVs exhibit reduced capacity for interleukin-2 (IL-2) production, thus limiting the proliferative potential for activated T cells [77]. In addition, tumor EVs can direct apoptosis of activated T cells though Fas/Fas-L binding [78]. Expression of the Fas death signal on the surface of activated cells typically is used as a shut off switch to prevent development of autoimmunity during normal pathogenic clearance. Cancer cells are able to take advantage of the molecule expression by releasing EVs containing Fas-L on their surface to kill threatening T cells from afar. Tumor EVs have also proven to be capable of suppressing mitogenic activation abilities of naïve T cells in the ovarian cancer setting, exacerbating the attenuation of immunogenic responses [79]. Although little work has been conducted analyzing the transformation of T cells exposed to glioma exosomes, evidence exists that brain tumor EVs decrease quantities of cytotoxic CD8 cells and inhibit interferon gamma release from remaining cells [80]. Our studies analyzing intracellular signaling cascades within naïve T cells exposed to glioma EVs reveal aberrations of many signaling pathways seen in other cancer types, including T cell receptor signaling (Figure 3). Analysis of just a few members of the signaling cascade can predict the overall activation status of this pathway and isolate particular proteins of interest to better understand how inhibition is occurring. Inhibition of the T cell receptor cascade by EVs is of particular importance for immunotherapies, which rely on generation of antigen-specific anti-tumor cells. Although many other factors in the tumor microenvironment can alter T cell signaling, EVs appear to play a substantial role in creating this change. Much like the effects of tumor EVs on monocytes, T cells can be inhibited and converted to a suppressive phenotype [81]. Induction of regulatory T cells by tumor EVs cultivates immunosuppressive factors in the tumor microenvironment to further prevent activation of cells that may threaten tumor survival. Elevated levels of regulatory T cells are common across many types of cancer and soluble factors pushing naïve cells towards a regulatory phenotype have been characterized from gliomas [36]. Tumor EVs by themselves are capable of inducing this transformation and may be an important factor to target in order to prevent transformation.

### 4.4. Transformation of T cells over time

To date, no studies have analyzed the transformation of T cells in GBM over time or over the course of treatment. Understanding the process of cellular transformation can offer information about response to treatment or act as a prognostic predictor before changes can be seen on radiological imaging. Other research in the brain tumor EV field has been able to correlate EV contents to the constitution of tumor cells, which will allow EVs to act as a liquid biopsy to track treatment. Perhaps as important are the downstream consequences of changing EV contents released from GBM and the amount of time needed to produce

http://dx.doi.org/10.5772/59037

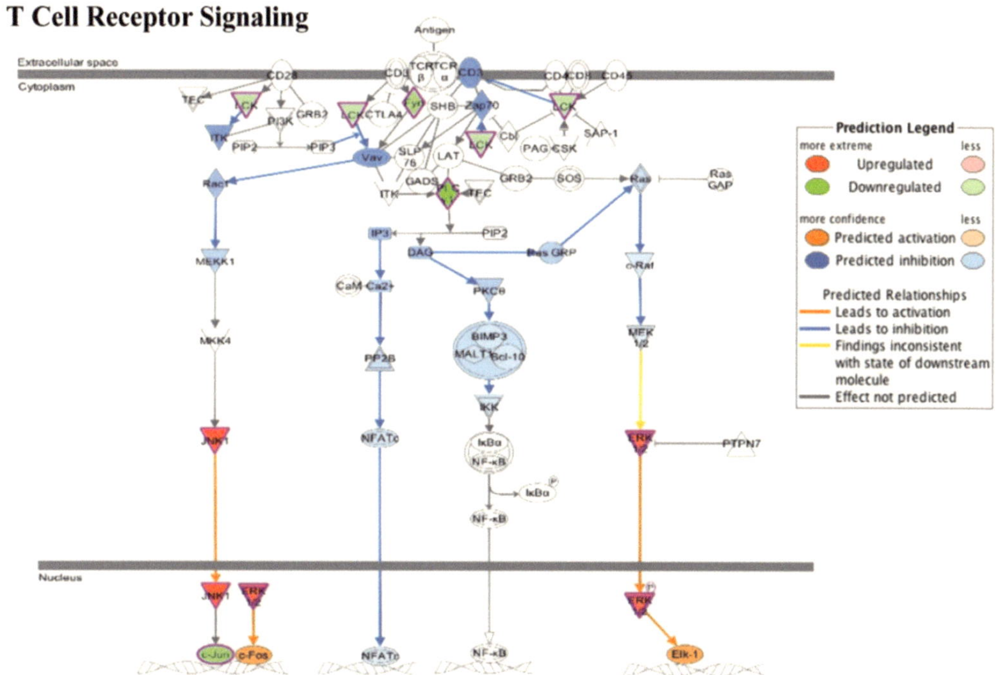


**Figure 3.** PBMCs were incubated with PHA and EVs for 72 hours and intracellular signaling molecules were quantified using protein arrays. Output from Ingenuity Pathway Analysis revealed pathways predicted to change based on EV exposure.

functional immune consequences. Better understanding of pathways affected earliest could offer insight about which functions the tumors consider a priority to eliminate. Transformation of stimulated T cells after exposure to brain tumor-derived EVs occurs quickly and we have been able to characterize some of the important changes that occur in the first 72 hours of glioma EV presence (Table 1). By analyzing protein expression profiles, we observed the transformation of intracellular signaling pathways within naïve T-cells exposed to tumor-derived extracellular vesicles at 72 hours compared to 2 hours. Apoptotic and developmental cascades were affected in the early stages, whereas migratory pathways become increasingly dysregulated during later time points. These data parallel previous studies in other tumor types, but here we are able to identify early activation of apoptotic pathways that do not persist for a prolonged period of time in GBM. Instead, the EVs continue to transform T cells without killing them, with a focus on modification of migratory capacity and cytotoxicity of cells. Modification of invasive capacity of T cells within tumor is an important functional deficit induced by glioma EVs. Lymphocyte entry into brain parenchyma is loosely restricted by the blood-brain barrier and EVs may offer another obstacle preventing activated T cells from accessing tumor cells.

| Function | Predicted Activation State | Z-Score |
|---|---|---|
| Binding of blood cells | Decreased | -2.000 |
| Proliferation of T lymphocytes | Decreased | -2.028 |
| Formation of cytoskeleton | Decreased | -2.043 |
| Chemotaxis of cells | Decreased | -2.227 |
| Adhesion of immune cells | Decreased | -2.323 |
| Cytotoxicity of leukocytes | Decreased | -2.414 |
| Migration of cells | Decreased | -3.469 |

**Table 1.** PBMCs were incubated with PHA and EVs for 2 or 72 hours, and then purified for T cells and analyzed for intracellular signaling changes. Output from Ingenuity Pathway Analysis revealed functions predicted to change based on protein expression. Z-score represents confidence of associated functions change.

# 5. Manipulation of EVs in the tumor setting

## 5.1. T cell rescue

GBM EVs utilize a variety of mechanisms to enhance tumor malignancy as discussed above. However, the functional impact they have on naïve immune cells is still under investigation. Disruption of function of naive T cells in the circulation of GBM patients may reveal a significant barrier in production of anti-tumor responses in immunotherapy. Our data reveal EVs alter migration pathways in T cells that have not seen tumor before, and EVs can functionally inhibit and convert naïve T-cells. However, GBM patients are not significantly globally immune compromised and are able to mount healthy responses against communicable diseases as well as grafted organs. This suggests specific immune tolerance to cancerous cells, but it is not known whether cells that have been transformed by extracellular vesicles can be rescued when challenged with a pathogen or if this is the job of truly naïve T cells. Determining activation abilities of GBM tolerant T cells will be necessary in order to understand how to develop new therapies to compensate for vesicle-induced modulation and to reactivate or ablate affected cells.

## 5.2. EV release

Because of the known roles of EVs in propagating tumor survival, disruption of EV genesis, release, or fusion may all offer viable solutions to lessen negative consequences of EV exposure. In recent years, better understanding of packaging and release mechanisms have been discovered. Some studies have been able to effectively inhibit release of EVs by inhibition of neutral sphingomyelinases, which are necessary for EV formation [82]. Other inhibitors of vesicle release have exhibited reduction in tumor growth *in vivo*, which further underlines the importance of tumor EVs in the microenvironment [83]. Many other targets aimed to reduce EV release are under investigation, but an obstacle in this approach is the removal of healthy EVs as well. EVs are known to maintain homeostasis by communicating with every cell in the body and generating an effective immune response in a noncancerous setting. The consequences of nonselective EV removal are not understood, thus the safest inhibitor will need to access the tumor site and selectively prevent EV release in a controlled manner. As more evidence emerges concerning packaging and release of EVs, better targets will become available to prevent the negative effects of tumor EV on supporting cells.

### 5.3. Therapeutic EVs

Engineered EVs represent a new mechanism for drug delivery and therapeutic potential in the GBM setting. They maintain stability in circulation, protect cargo from metabolism and can penetrate the blood-brain barrier to deliver cargo to a specific cell [41]. Their potential has not been fully realized due to the complexity of specific binding, but it is possible in the future that EVs will be engineered with high affinity for cellular targets. This delivery method would provide a wide variety of benefits over antibody delivery, which has been the predominant method of specific targeting in recent years. However, even the best targeted EV will not have the dynamic capabilities of the natural immune system, thus EVs are under investigation as a means to enhance the immune response against tumors. Because tumor-derived EVs contain tumor antigen, EVs have been explored as an antigen delivery mechanism from dendritic cells in order to prime an adaptive antitumor response. One approach that has been explored is loading of tumor antigens onto MHC molecules on EV surfaces by pulsing dendritic cells with tumor antigen [43]. EVs released from dendritic cells in a nontumor setting are potent immunostimulatory agents because of their ability to express antigen, costimulatory molecules, and adhesion molecules. Artificial activation of dendritic cells must be sufficient to produce mature cells, which express these molecules on their cell surface, in order to be incorporated on to EV surface [84]. Full maturation of dendritic cells prior to antigen pulsing is necessary to generate optimal antitumor responses. Once cells are loaded with antigen, EVs can be isolated and reintroduced to the patient, or the activated dendritic cells can be injected directly into the patient to elicit a response *in vivo* [69]. Studies are still under investigation to determine the best method of transfer and optimal conditions for incubation of stimulated cells to produce effective antitumor responses. Another approach to utilize tumor antigens within EVs is by direct vaccination of tumor exosomes to generate specific immunity. Interestingly, GBM EVs are not immunosuppressive in a tumor naïve setting. Prophylactic glioma EV injection before tumor implantation in mice leads to rejection of tumor [85]. These mice exhibit no evidence of tumor growth over time and when challenged with a second tumor implantation, mice successfully rejected the graft again. However, EV delivered after tumor implantation has no effect on tumor rejection. This evidence reveals potential immunostimulatory capacity of GBM EVs in the correct setting. However, the tremendous obstacle in utilizing EVs is that treatment for tumors must come after the tumor is established. Understanding and mimicking the optimal environment in patients may allow for self-vaccination against their own tumor.

### 5.4. Gene therapy

Gene therapy is gaining recognition as a possible avenue for future GBM treatment because of its ability to recruit the immune system for a targeted therapy approach. It has many forms, ranging from virotherapy with a conditionally replicating virus to genetic immunotherapy. By altering the genetics of target (or attack) cells, gene therapy is efficient while minimizing detrimental systemic effects. Gene therapy employs a vector, either viral or non-viral, to deliver genes to the cancer cells. Viral vectors are the most frequently used [86], and are being explored in multiple glioblastoma clinical trials. An example is using a retroviral vector that codes for an artificial molecule against a tumor-specific antigen to genetically modify T cells. The artificial molecules are chimeric antigen receptors (CARs). Fusing an extracellular variable domain from a high affinity monoclonal antibody specific for a tumor-associated antigen with an intercellular signaling domain from CD3ξ of an antigen specific T cell receptor creates a CAR. When the target antigen activates the extracellular domain, downstream signaling is initiated to activate the T cell [87]. The survivability of viral vectors has been an issue, and there are safety concerns with ensuring viruses are rendered non-replicative. To minimize risk of this therapy, non-viral vectors, including EVs, are currently being explored. EVs have been shown to be inherently capable of transferring genetic material, so using them for targeted gene therapy is logical. Their small size, bi-lipid membrane for protecting cargo, natural, non-viral state, capacity to be taken up by target cells, and stability during laboratory work are all advantages [88]. It is also possible that EVs could reduce non-specific delivery and immunogenicity issues. One group has been able to deliver short interfering RNA (siRNA) to disrupt gene expression in the brain using EVs as a vehicle in order to achieve targeted gene knockdown. In this study, dendritic cells altered to express an EV membrane protein, Lamp2b, were fused to neuron-specific rabies virus glycoprotein peptide 3 (RVG peptide-3). The EVs isolated from the culture media of these cells were loaded with siRNA via electroporation, and they were targeted to neurons with RVG-p3. Although administered systemically, the EVs were able to specifically deliver siRNA to neurons, microglia, and oligodendrocytes in the brain and produce gene knockdown. Moreover, the mRNA and protein levels of the gene were strongly knocked down (approximately 60%) [89]. Recently, a group studied a non-toxic peptide-based carrier loaded with VEGF-siRNA and BCNU, an approved chemotherapy for GBM treatment, to target GBM cells [90]. The VEGF-siRNA and BCNU were both efficiently delivered to cultured GBM cells, and VEGF expression was successfully reduced. The combination of gene therapy and drugs is an exciting possibility and EVs offer an ideal mechanism of transfer as newer therapies become available. Gene therapy is promising because it offers the opportunity deliver novel therapies directly and efficiently into the brain. It also holds the potential for combination therapy, such as gene therapy/engineered drug delivery with immunotherapy, which is the most probable method for successful treatment in this complicated and unpredictable disease.

## 6. Conclusion

The GBM microenvironment is a complex and heterogeneous conglomeration of many factors working in concert to ensure survival of the tumor. Extracellular vesicles represent a component that has not been well studied and may offer a way for GBM to exhibit dynamic adaptation. Current clinical trials investigate neutralization or blockage of individual molecules, but a single driver does not define the heterogeneous nature of GBM. The complexity of the tumor is likely to parallel the complexity of its signaling modalities. Extracellular vesicles provide transfer of discrete packets of information as a means of influencing countless pathways in facilitation of tumor progression. Here we discuss paracrine, autocrine, and immune modulatory effects of GBM-derived extracellular vesicles. Environmental modulation is necessary for GBM progression and extracellular vesicles influence many of the necessary changes needed for tumor survival. The adaptability of GBM to tolerate toxic insults is characteristic of the tumor's vigor. We are just now beginning to understand the complexity of extracellular vesicle packaging to produce a tumorigenic environment. As we understand more about the role of each signaling moiety contained within the vesicles, more information dictating treatment can be generated based on their overall composition. Appropriate treatment regimens will then be catered to each patient to more efficiently target GBM cells for destruction.

## Acknowledgements

The authors would like to thank the University of Colorado Department of Neurosurgery, The University of Colorado Cancer Center, the Cancer League of Colorado, and the National Institutes of Health RO1 # 11066485 for support.

## Author details

Justin E. Hellwinkel, Helen Madsen and Michael Graner*

*Address all correspondence to: michael.graner@ucdenver.edu

Department of Neurosurgery, University of Colorado School of Medicine, USA

## References

[1] Louis DN, Ohgaki H, Wiestler OD, Cavenee WK, Burger PC, Jouvet A, et al. The 2007 WHO classification of tumours of the central nervous system. Acta Neuropathol. 2007;114:97–109.

[2] Stupp BR, Dietrich P, Kraljevic SO, Pica A, Maillard I, Maeder P, et al. Promising survival for patients with newly diagnosed glioblastoma multiforme treated with concomitant radiation plus temozolomide followed by adjuvant temozolomide. J. Clin. Oncol. 2002;20(5):1375–1382.

[3] Smoll NR, Schaller K, Gautschi OP. Long-term survival of patients with glioblastoma multiforme (GBM). J. Clin. Neurosci. [Internet]. 2013 May [cited 2014 Aug 5];20(5): 670–5. Available from: http://www.ncbi.nlm.nih.gov/pubmed/23352352

[4] Skeie BS, Enger PØ, Brøgger J, Ganz JC, Thorsen F, Heggdal JI, et al. Γ Knife Surgery Versus Reoperation for Recurrent Glioblastoma Multiforme. World Neurosurg. [Internet]. 2012 Dec [cited 2014 Jul 21];78(6):658–69. Available from: http://www.ncbi.nlm.nih.gov/pubmed/22484078

[5] Stupp BR, Dietrich P, Kraljevic SO, Pica A, Maillard I, Maeder P, et al. Promising survival for patients with newly diagnosed glioblastoma multiforme treated with concomitant radiation plus temozolomide followed by adjuvant temozolomide. J. Clin. Oncol. 2002;20(5):1375–1382.

[6] Hart M, Grant R, Garside R. Chemotherapy wafers for high grade glioma. Cochrane Database Syst. Rev. [Internet]. 2011 [cited 2014 Aug 5];(3). Available from: http://onlinelibrary.wiley.com/doi/10.1002/14651858.CD007294.pub2/pdf/standard

[7] Stupp R, Wong ET, Kanner A a, Steinberg D, Engelhard H, Heidecke V, et al. NovoTTF-100A versus physician's choice chemotherapy in recurrent glioblastoma: a randomised phase III trial of a novel treatment modality. Eur. J. Cancer [Internet]. 2012 Sep [cited 2014 Jul 16];48(14):2192–202. Available from: http://www.ncbi.nlm.nih.gov/pubmed/22608262

[8] Jackson SE, Chester JD. Personalised cancer medicine. Int. J. Cancer [Internet]. 2014 May;00. Available from: http://www.ncbi.nlm.nih.gov/pubmed/24789362

[9] Cohen MH, Shen YL, Keegan P, Pazdur R. FDA drug approval summary: bevacizumab (Avastin) as treatment of recurrent glioblastoma multiforme. Oncologist [Internet]. 2009 Nov [cited 2014 Jul 23];14(11):1131–8. Available from: http://www.ncbi.nlm.nih.gov/pubmed/19897538

[10] Norden AD, Drappatz J, Wen PY. Novel anti-angiogenic therapies for malignant gliomas. Lancet Neurol. [Internet]. 2008 Dec [cited 2014 Aug 5];7(12):1152–60. Available from: http://www.ncbi.nlm.nih.gov/pubmed/19007739

[11] Dixit S. Immunotherapy for high-grade glioma. Futur. Oncol. 2014;10(6):911–915.

[12] Steinbok P, Thomas JP, Dolman CL. Intratumoral autologous mononuclear cells in the treatment of recurrent glioblastoma multiforme. A phase 1 (toxicity) study. J. Neurooncol. 1984;2(2):147–151.

[13] Ransohoff RM, Kivisäkk P, Kidd G. Three or more routes for leukocyte migration into the central nervous system. Nat. Rev. Immunol. [Internet]. 2003 Jul [cited 2014 Jul 15];3(7):569–81. Available from: http://www.ncbi.nlm.nih.gov/pubmed/12876559

[14] Komata T, Kanzawa T, Kondo Y, Kondo S. Telomerase as a therapeutic target for malignant gliomas. Oncogene [Internet]. 2002 [cited 2014 Aug 5];21(4):656–663. Available from: http://europepmc.org/abstract/MED/11850793

[15] Tsuda N, Shichijo S, Harada M, Kamura T, Shigemori M. Recognition of ADP-ribosylation factor 4-like by HLA-A2-restricted and tumor-reactive cytotoxic T lymphocytes from patients with brain tumors. 2002;(2):319–327.

[16] Liu F, Park PJ, Lai W, Maher E, Chakravarti A, Durso L, et al. A Genome-Wide Screen Reveals Functional Gene Clusters in the Cancer Genome and Identifies EphA2 as a Mitogen in Glioblastoma. Cancer Res. [Internet]. 2006 Nov 15 [cited 2014 Aug 5];66(22):10815–10823. Available from: http://cancerres.aacrjournals.org/cgi/doi/10.1158/0008-5472.CAN-06-1408

[17] Kahlon KS, Brown C, Cooper LJN, Raubitschek A, Forman SJ, Jensen MC. Specific Recognition and Killing of Glioblastoma Multiforme by Interleukin 13-Zetakine Redirected Cytolytic T Cells Specific Recognition and Killing of Glioblastoma Multiforme by Interleukin 13-Zetakine Redirected Cytolytic T Cells. Cancer Res. 2004;64(24):9160–9166.

[18] Heimberger AB, Iressa ZD, Learn CA, Archer GE, Mclendon RE, Chewning TA, et al. Brain Tumors in Mice Are Susceptible to Blockade of Epidermal Growth Factor Receptor (EGFR) with the Oral, Brain Tumors in Mice Are Susceptible to Blockade of Epidermal Growth Factor Receptor (EGFR) with the Oral, Specific,. Clin. Cancer Res. 2002;8(11):3496–3502.

[19] Guvenc H, Pavlyukov MS, Joshi K, Kurt H, Banasavadi-Siddegowda YK, Mao P, et al. Impairment of glioma stem cell survival and growth by a novel inhibitor for Survivin-Ran protein complex. Clin. Cancer Res. [Internet]. 2013 Feb 1 [cited 2014 Aug 5];19(3):631–42. Available from: http://www.ncbi.nlm.nih.gov/pubmed/23251006

[20] Ballestrero A, Boy D, Moran E, Cirmena G, Brossart P, Nencioni A. Immunotherapy with dendritic cells for cancer. Adv. Drug Deliv. Rev. [Internet]. 2008 Jan;60(2):173–183. Available from: http://www.ncbi.nlm.nih.gov/pubmed/17977615

[21] Kantoff P, Higano C, Shore N, Berger R, Small E, Penson D, et al. Sipuleucel-T immunotherapy for castration-resistant prostate cancer. N. Engl. J. Med. [Internet]. 1970 [cited 2014 Aug 5];363(5):411–422. Available from: http://scholar.google.com/scholar?hl=en&btnG=Search&q=intitle:new+england+journal#2

[22] Yamanaka R, Abe T, Yajima N, Tsuchiya N, Homma J, Kobayashi T, et al. Vaccination of recurrent glioma patients with tumour lysate-pulsed dendritic cells elicits immune responses: results of a clinical phase I/II trial. Br. J. Cancer [Internet]. 2003 Oct 6 [cited 2014 Aug 5];89(7):1172–9. Available from: http://www.pubmedcentral.nih.gov/articlerender.fcgi?artid=2394324&tool=pmcentrez&rendertype=abstract

[23] Kikuchi T, Akasaki Y, Abe T, Fukuda T, Saotome H, Ryan JL, et al. Vaccination of glioma patients with fusions of dendritic and glioma cells and recombinant human interleukin 12. J. Immunother. 2004;27(6):452–459.

[24] Rutkowski S, De Vleeschouwer S, Kaempgen E, Wolff JE a, Kühl J, Demaerel P, et al. Surgery and adjuvant dendritic cell-based tumour vaccination for patients with re-

lapsed malignant glioma, a feasibility study. Br. J. Cancer [Internet]. 2004 Nov 1 [cited 2014 Aug 5];91(9):1656–62. Available from: http://www.pubmedcentral.nih.gov/articlerender.fcgi?artid=2409960&tool=pmcentrez&rendertype=abstract

[25] Rosenberg S a, Yang JC, Restifo NP. Cancer immunotherapy: moving beyond current vaccines. Nat. Med. [Internet]. 2004 Sep;10(9):909–915. Available from: http://www.pubmedcentral.nih.gov/articlerender.fcgi?artid=1435696&tool=pmcentrez&rendertype=abstract

[26] Bodmer S, Strommer K, Frei K, Siepl C, de Tribolet N, Heid I, et al. Immunosuppression and transforming growth factor-beta in glioblastoma. Preferential production of transforming growth factor-beta 2. J. Immunol. [Internet]. 1989 Nov;143(10):3222–3229. Available from: http://www.ncbi.nlm.nih.gov/pubmed/2809198

[27] Kehrl J, Wakefield L. Production of transforming growth factor beta by human T lymphocytes and its potential role in the regulation of T cell growth. J. Exp. Med. [Internet]. 1986 [cited 2014 Aug 5];163(5):1037–1050. Available from: http://jem.rupress.org/content/163/5/1037.abstract

[28] Vega E a, Graner MW, Sampson JH. Combating immunosuppression in glioma. Future Oncol. [Internet]. 2008 Jun;4(3):433–442. Available from: http://www.pubmedcentral.nih.gov/articlerender.fcgi?artid=3425388&tool=pmcentrez&rendertype=abstract

[29] Badie B, Schartner J. Role of microglia in glioma biology. Microsc. Res. Tech. [Internet]. 2001 Jul 15;54(2):106–13. Available from: http://www.ncbi.nlm.nih.gov/pubmed/11455617

[30] Kennedy BC, Maier LM, D'Amico R, Mandigo CE, Fontana EJ, Waziri A, et al. Dynamics of central and peripheral immunomodulation in a murine glioma model. BMC Immunol. [Internet]. 2009 Jan;10:11. Available from: http://www.pubmedcentral.nih.gov/articlerender.fcgi?artid=2654428&tool=pmcentrez&rendertype=abstract

[31] Morioka T, Baba T, Black KL, Streit WJ. Immunophenotypic analysis of infiltrating leukocytes and microglia in an experimental rat glioma. Acta Neuropathol. [Internet]. 1992 Jan;83(6):590–597. Available from: http://www.ncbi.nlm.nih.gov/pubmed/1636377

[32] Kostianovsky a. M, Maier LM, Anderson RC, Bruce JN, Anderson DE. Astrocytic Regulation of Human Monocytic/Microglial Activation. J. Immunol. [Internet]. 2008 Oct;181(8):5425–5432. Available from: http://www.jimmunol.org/cgi/doi/10.4049/jimmunol.181.8.5425

[33] Rodrigues JC, Gonzalez GC, Zhang L, Ibrahim G, Kelly JJ, Gustafson MP, et al. Normal human monocytes exposed to glioma cells acquire myeloid-derived suppressor cell-like properties. Neuro. Oncol. [Internet]. 2010 Apr;12(4):351–65. Available from: http://www.pubmedcentral.nih.gov/articlerender.fcgi?artid=2940603&tool=pmcentrez&rendertype=abstract

[34] Hussain SF, Yang D, Suki D, Grimm E, Heimberger AB. Innate immune functions of microglia isolated from human glioma patients. J. Transl. Med. [Internet]. 2006 Jan; 4:15. Available from: http://www.pubmedcentral.nih.gov/articlerender.fcgi?artid=1501057&tool=pmcentrez&rendertype=abstract

[35] Kamoshida G, Ogawa T, Oyanagi J, Sato H, Komiya E, Higashi S, et al. Modulation of matrix metalloproteinase-9 secretion from tumor-associated macrophage-like cells by proteolytically processed laminin-332 (laminin-5). Clin. Exp. Metastasis [Internet]. 2014 Mar [cited 2014 Aug 5];31(3):285–91. Available from: http://www.ncbi.nlm.nih.gov/pubmed/24292405

[36] Fecci PE, Sweeney AE, Grossi PM, Nair SK, Learn C a, Mitchell D a, et al. Systemic anti-CD25 monoclonal antibody administration safely enhances immunity in murine glioma without eliminating regulatory T cells. Clin. Cancer Res. [Internet]. 2006 Jul; 12(14 Pt 1):4294–4305. Available from: http://www.ncbi.nlm.nih.gov/pubmed/16857805

[37] Miescher S, Whiteside TL, de Tribolet N, von Fliedner V. In situ characterization, clonogenic potential, and antitumor cytolytic activity of T lymphocytes infiltrating human brain cancers. J. Neurosurg. [Internet]. 1988 Mar;68(3):438–48. Available from: http://www.ncbi.nlm.nih.gov/pubmed/3257792

[38] Bielamowicz K, Khawja S, Ahmed N. Adoptive cell therapies for glioblastoma. Front. Oncol. [Internet]. 2013 Jan [cited 2014 Jul 28];3(November):275. Available from: http://www.pubmedcentral.nih.gov/articlerender.fcgi?artid=3823029&tool=pmcentrez&rendertype=abstract

[39] Denzer K, Kleijmeer MJ, Heijnen HF, Stoorvogel W, Geuze HJ. Exosome: from internal vesicle of the multivesicular body to intercellular signaling device. J. Cell Sci. [Internet]. 2000 Oct;113 Pt 19:3365–74. Available from: http://www.ncbi.nlm.nih.gov/pubmed/10984428

[40] Kesimer M, Scull M, Brighton B, DeMaria G, Burns K, O'Neal W, et al. Characterization of exosome-like vesicles released from human tracheobronchial ciliated epithelium: a possible role in innate defense. FASEB J. [Internet]. 2009 Jun [cited 2014 Aug 4]; 23(6):1858–68. Available from: http://www.pubmedcentral.nih.gov/articlerender.fcgi?artid=2698655&tool=pmcentrez&rendertype=abstract

[41] EL Andaloussi S, Mäger I, Breakefield XO, Wood MJ a. Extracellular vesicles: biology and emerging therapeutic opportunities. Nat. Rev. Drug Discov. [Internet]. 2013 May;12(5):347–357. Available from: http://www.ncbi.nlm.nih.gov/pubmed/23584393

[42] Raposo G, Nijman HW. B lymphocytes secrete antigen-presenting vesicles. J. Exp. Med. [Internet]. 1996;183(March):1161–1172. Available from: http://jem.rupress.org/content/183/3/1161.abstract

[43] Zitvogel L, Regnault A, Lozier A, Wolfers J. Eradication of Established Murine Tumor Using a Novel Cell-Free Vaccine: Dendritic Cell-Derived Exosomes. Nat. Med.

[Internet]. 1998;(March). Available from: http://www.nature.com/nm/journal/v4/n5/abs/nm0598-594.html

[44] Fauré J, Lachenal G, Court M, Hirrlinger J, Chatellard-Causse C, Blot B, et al. Exosomes are released by cultured cortical neurones. Mol. Cell. Neurosci. [Internet]. 2006 Apr [cited 2014 Jul 14];31(4):642–8. Available from: http://www.ncbi.nlm.nih.gov/pubmed/16446100

[45] Johnstone RM, Adam M, Hammonds JR, Turbide C. Vesicle Formation during Reticulocyte Maturation. J. Biol. Chem. 1987;262(1):9412–9420.

[46] Taylor D, Doellgast G. Quantitation of Peroxidase-Antibody Using Column Binding to Membrane Chromatography Fragments. Anal. Biochem. 1979;59(1):53–59.

[47] Simpson R, Lim J, Moritz R, Mathivanan S. Exosomes: Proteomic Insights and Diagnostic Potential. Expert Rev. Proteomics. 2009;6(3):267–83.

[48] Andre F, Schartz N, Movassagh M. Malignant effusions and immunogenic tumour-derived exosomes. Lancet [Internet]. 2002 [cited 2014 Aug 5];360:295–305. Available from: http://www.sciencedirect.com/science/article/pii/S0140673602095521

[49] Arscott WT, Tandle AT, Zhao S, Shabason JE, Gordon IK, Schlaff CD, et al. Ionizing Radiation and Glioblastoma Exosomes: Implications in Tumor Biology and Cell Migration. Transl. Oncol. [Internet]. 2013 Dec;6(6):638–IN6. Available from: http://linkinghub.elsevier.com/retrieve/pii/S1936523313800034

[50] King HW, Michael MZ, Gleadle JM. Hypoxic enhancement of exosome release by breast cancer cells. BMC Cancer [Internet]. 2012 Jan [cited 2014 Aug 5];12(1):421. Available from: http://www.pubmedcentral.nih.gov/articlerender.fcgi?artid=3488584&tool=pmcentrez&rendertype=abstract

[51] Safaei R, Larson BJ, Cheng TC, Gibson M a, Otani S, Naerdemann W, et al. Abnormal lysosomal trafficking and enhanced exosomal export of cisplatin in drug-resistant human ovarian carcinoma cells. Mol. Cancer Ther. [Internet]. 2005 Oct [cited 2014 Jul 25];4(10):1595–604. Available from: http://www.ncbi.nlm.nih.gov/pubmed/16227410

[52] Théry C, Duban L, Segura E, Véron P, Lantz O, Amigorena S. Indirect activation of naïve CD4+T cells by dendritic cell-derived exosomes. Nat. Immunol. [Internet]. 2002 Dec [cited 2014 Jul 21];3(12):1156–62. Available from: http://www.ncbi.nlm.nih.gov/pubmed/12426563

[53] Simhadri VR, Reiners KS, Hansen HP, Topolar D, Simhadri VL, Nohroudi K, et al. Dendritic cells release HLA-B-associated transcript-3 positive exosomes to regulate natural killer function. PLoS One [Internet]. 2008 Jan [cited 2014 Aug 5];3(10):e3377. Available from: http://www.pubmedcentral.nih.gov/articlerender.fcgi?artid=2566590&tool=pmcentrez&rendertype=abstract

[54] Baj-Krzyworzeka M, Szatanek R, Weglarczyk K, Baran J, Zembala M. Tumour-derived microvesicles modulate biological activity of human monocytes. Immunol.

Lett. [Internet]. 2007 Nov 15 [cited 2014 Aug 5];113(2):76–82. Available from: http://www.ncbi.nlm.nih.gov/pubmed/17825925

[55] Martínez-Lorenzo MJ, Anel a, Gamen S, Monle n I, Lasierra P, Larrad L, et al. Activated human T cells release bioactive Fas ligand and APO2 ligand in microvesicles. J. Immunol. [Internet]. 1999 Aug;163(3):1274–1281. Available from: http://www.ncbi.nlm.nih.gov/pubmed/10415024

[56] Gatti S, Bruno S, Deregibus MC, Sordi A, Cantaluppi V, Tetta C, et al. Microvesicles derived from human adult mesenchymal stem cells protect against ischaemia-reperfusion-induced acute and chronic kidney injury. Nephrol. Dial. Transplant [Internet]. 2011 May [cited 2014 Jul 19];26(5):1474–83. Available from: http://www.ncbi.nlm.nih.gov/pubmed/21324974

[57] Ratajczak MZ, Kucia M, Jadczyk T, Greco NJ, Wojakowski W, Tendera M, et al. Pivotal role of paracrine effects in stem cell therapies in regenerative medicine: can we translate stem cell-secreted paracrine factors and microvesicles into better therapeutic strategies? Leukemia [Internet]. 2012 Jun;26(6):1166–1173. Available from: http://www.ncbi.nlm.nih.gov/pubmed/22182853

[58] Chivet M, Hemming F, Pernet-Gallay K, Fraboulet S, Sadoul R. Emerging role of neuronal exosomes in the central nervous system. Front. Physiol. [Internet]. 2012 Jan [cited 2014 Jul 14];3(May):145. Available from: http://www.pubmedcentral.nih.gov/articlerender.fcgi?artid=3361079&tool=pmcentrez&rendertype=abstract

[59] Pelchen-Matthews A, Raposo G, Marsh M. Endosomes, exosomes and Trojan viruses. Trends Microbiol. [Internet]. 2004 Jul;12(7):310–316. Available from: http://www.ncbi.nlm.nih.gov/pubmed/15223058

[60] Valadi H, Ekström K, Bossios A, Sjöstrand M, Lee JJ, Lötvall JO. Exosome-mediated transfer of mRNAs and microRNAs is a novel mechanism of genetic exchange between cells. Nat. Cell Biol. [Internet]. 2007 Jun [cited 2014 Jul 11];9(6):654–9. Available from: http://www.ncbi.nlm.nih.gov/pubmed/17486113

[61] Taylor DD, Gercel-Taylor C. MicroRNA signatures of tumor-derived exosomes as diagnostic biomarkers of ovarian cancer. Gynecol. Oncol. [Internet]. 2008 Jul [cited 2014 Jul 10];110(1):13–21. Available from: http://www.ncbi.nlm.nih.gov/pubmed/18589210

[62] Rabinowits G, Gerçel-Taylor C, Day JM, Taylor DD, Kloecker GH. Exosomal microRNA: a diagnostic marker for lung cancer. Clin. Lung Cancer [Internet]. 2009 Jan [cited 2014 Jul 15];10(1):42–6. Available from: http://www.ncbi.nlm.nih.gov/pubmed/19289371

[63] Skog J, Würdinger T, Rijn S Van. Glioblastoma microvesicles transport RNA and protein that promote tumor growth and provide diagnostic biomarkers. Nat. cell … [Internet]. 2008;10(12):1470–1476. Available from: http://www.nature.com/ncb/journal/v10/n12/abs/ncb1800.html

[64] Lee TH, D'Asti E, Magnus N, Al-Nedawi K, Meehan B, Rak J. Microvesicles as mediators of intercellular communication in cancer--the emerging science of cellular "debris". Semin. Immunopathol. [Internet]. 2011 Sep;33(5):455–467. Available from: http://www.ncbi.nlm.nih.gov/pubmed/21318413

[65] Rak J. Microparticles in cancer. Semin. Thromb. Hemost. [Internet]. 2010 [cited 2014 Aug 5];1(212):888–906. Available from: https://www.thieme-connect.com/products/ejournals/abstract/10.1055/s-0030-1267043

[66] Al-Nedawi K, Meehan B, Micallef J, Lhotak V, May L, Guha A, et al. Intercellular transfer of the oncogenic receptor EGFRvIII by microvesicles derived from tumour cells. Nat. Cell Biol. [Internet]. 2008 May;10(5):619–624. Available from: http://www.ncbi.nlm.nih.gov/pubmed/18425114

[67] Pedersen M, Meltorn M. The type III epidermal growth factor receptor mutation Biological significance and potential target for anti-cancer therapy. Ann. ... [Internet]. 2001 [cited 2014 Aug 5];:745–760. Available from: http://annonc.oxfordjournals.org/content/12/6/745.short

[68] Dolo V, Ginestra a, Cassará D, Ghersi G, Nagase H, Vittorelli ML. Shed membrane vesicles and selective localization of gelatinases and MMP-9/TIMP-1 complexes. Ann. N. Y. Acad. Sci. [Internet]. 1999 Jun;878(Iv):497–499. Available from: http://www.ncbi.nlm.nih.gov/pubmed/10415753

[69] Graner M. Brain tumor exosomes and microvesicles: pleiotropic effects from tiny cellular surrogates. Mol. Targets CNS Tumors [Internet]. 2011 [cited 2014 Aug 5];Available from: http://www.intechopen.com/source/pdfs/19928/InTech-Brain_tumor_exosomes_and_microvesicles_pleiotropic_effects_from_tiny_cellular_surrogates.pdf

[70] Epple LM, Griffiths SG, Dechkovskaia AM, Dusto NL, White J, Ouellette RJ, et al. Medulloblastoma exosome proteomics yield functional roles for extracellular vesicles. PLoS One [Internet]. 2012 Jan;7(7):e42064. Available from: http://www.pubmedcentral.nih.gov/articlerender.fcgi?artid=3407172&tool=pmcentrez&rendertype=abstract

[71] Liu C, Yu S, Zinn K, Wang J, Zhang L, Jia Y, et al. Murine Mammary Carcinoma Exosomes Promote Tumor Growth by Suppression of NK Cell Function. J. Immunol. [Internet]. 2006 Jan;176(3):1375–1385. Available from: http://www.jimmunol.org/cgi/doi/10.4049/jimmunol.176.3.1375

[72] Ashiru O, Boutet P, Fernández-Messina L, Agüera-González S, Skepper JN, Valés-Gómez M, et al. Natural killer cell cytotoxicity is suppressed by exposure to the human NKG2D ligand MICA*008 that is shed by tumor cells in exosomes. Cancer Res. [Internet]. 2010 Jan 15 [cited 2014 Aug 5];70(2):481–9. Available from: http://www.pubmedcentral.nih.gov/articlerender.fcgi?artid=2817492&tool=pmcentrez&rendertype=abstract

[73] Battke C, Ruiss R, Welsch U, Wimberger P, Lang S, Jochum S, et al. Tumour exosomes inhibit binding of tumour-reactive antibodies to tumour cells and reduce ADCC. Cancer Immunol. Immunother. [Internet]. 2011 May;60(5):639–648. Available from: http://www.ncbi.nlm.nih.gov/pubmed/21293856

[74] Wieckowski E, Whiteside TL. Human tumor-derived vs dendritic cell-derived exosomes have distinct biologic roles and molecular profiles. Immunol. Res. [Internet]. 2006 Jan;36(1-3):247–54. Available from: http://www.ncbi.nlm.nih.gov/pubmed/17337785

[75] Xiang X, Poliakov A, Liu C. Induction of myeloid-derived suppressor cells by tumor exosomes. ... J. Cancer [Internet]. 2009 [cited 2014 Aug 5];2633(December 2008):2621–2633. Available from: http://onlinelibrary.wiley.com/doi/10.1002/ijc.24249/full

[76] Poutsiaka D, Schroder E. Membrane vesicles shed by murine melanoma cells selectively inhibit the expression of Ia antigen by macrophages. J. ... [Internet]. 1985 [cited 2014 Aug 5];2(I):138–144. Available from: http://www.jimmunol.org/content/134/1/138.short

[77] Clayton A, Mitchell JP, Court J, Mason MD, Tabi Z. Human tumor-derived exosomes selectively impair lymphocyte responses to interleukin-2. Cancer Res. [Internet]. 2007 Aug 1 [cited 2014 Jul 17];67(15):7458–66. Available from: http://www.ncbi.nlm.nih.gov/pubmed/17671216

[78] Taylor DD, Gerçel-Taylor C. Tumour-derived exosomes and their role in cancer-associated T-cell signalling defects. Br. J. Cancer [Internet]. 2005 Jan;92(2):305–311. Available from: http://www.pubmedcentral.nih.gov/articlerender.fcgi?artid=2361848&tool=pmcentrez&rendertype=abstract

[79] Poutsiaka DD, Taylor DD, Levy EM, Black PH. Inhibition of recombinant interferon-gamma-induced Ia antigen expression by shed B16 F10 melanoma cell membrane vesicles. J. Immunol. [Internet]. 1985 Jan;134(1):145–50. Available from: http://www.ncbi.nlm.nih.gov/pubmed/3917273

[80] Liu Z-M, Wang Y-B, Yuan X-H. Exosomes from murine-derived GL26 cells promote glioblastoma tumor growth by reducing number and function of CD8+T cells. Asian Pac. J. Cancer Prev. [Internet]. 2013 Jan [cited 2014 Aug 5];14(1):309–14. Available from: http://www.ncbi.nlm.nih.gov/pubmed/23534743

[81] Szajnik M, Czystowska M, Szczepanski MJ, Mandapathil M, Whiteside TL. Tumor-derived microvesicles induce, expand and up-regulate biological activities of human regulatory T cells (Treg). PLoS One [Internet]. 2010 Jan;5(7):e11469. Available from: http://www.pubmedcentral.nih.gov/articlerender.fcgi?artid=2908536&tool=pmcentrez&rendertype=abstract

[82] Trajkovic K, Hsu C, Chiantia S, Rajendran L, Wenzel D, Wieland F, et al. Ceramide triggers budding of exosome vesicles into multivesicular endosomes. Science [Inter-

net]. 2008 Feb 29 [cited 2014 Aug 4];319(5867):1244–7. Available from: http://www.ncbi.nlm.nih.gov/pubmed/18309083

[83] Chalmin F, Ladoire S.-associated Hsp72 from tumor-derived exosomes mediates STAT3-dependent immunosuppressive function of mouse and human myeloid-derived suppressor. J. ... [Internet]. 2010 [cited 2014 Aug 5];120(2):457–471. Available from: http://www.jci.org/articles/view/40483

[84] Segura E, Nicco C, Lombard B. ICAM-1 on exosomes from mature dendritic cells is critical for efficient naive T-cell priming. ... [Internet]. 2005;106(1):216–223. Available from: http://bloodjournal.hematologylibrary.org/content/106/1/216.short

[85] Graner MW, Alzate O, Dechkovskaia AM, Keene JD, Sampson JH, Mitchell D a, et al. Proteomic and immunologic analyses of brain tumor exosomes. FASEB J. [Internet]. 2009 May [cited 2014 Jul 14];23(5):1541–57. Available from: http://www.pubmedcentral.nih.gov/articlerender.fcgi?artid=2669426&tool=pmcentrez&rendertype=abstract

[86] Castro MG, Cowen R, Williamson IK, David a, Jimenez-Dalmaroni MJ, Yuan X, et al. Current and future strategies for the treatment of malignant brain tumors. Pharmacol. Ther. [Internet]. 2003 Apr;98(1):71–108. Available from: http://linkinghub.elsevier.com/retrieve/pii/S0163725803000147

[87] Hegde M, Bielamowicz K, Ahmed N. Novel Approaches and Mechanisms of Immunotherapy for Glioblastoma. Discov. Med. 2014;(93):145–54.

[88] Lee Y, El Andaloussi S, Wood MJ a. Exosomes and microvesicles: extracellular vesicles for genetic information transfer and gene therapy. Hum. Mol. Genet. [Internet]. 2012 Oct 15 [cited 2014 Jul 14];21(R1):R125–34. Available from: http://www.ncbi.nlm.nih.gov/pubmed/22872698

[89] Vlassov A V, Magdaleno S, Setterquist R, Conrad R. Exosomes: current knowledge of their composition, biological functions, and diagnostic and therapeutic potentials. Biochim. Biophys. Acta [Internet]. 2012 Jul;1820(7):940–948. Available from: http://www.ncbi.nlm.nih.gov/pubmed/22503788

[90] Yi N, Oh B, Kim HA, Lee M. Combined delivery of BCNU and VEGF siRNA using amphiphilic peptides for glioblastoma. J. Drug Target. [Internet]. 2014 Feb [cited 2014 Aug 5];22(2):156–64. Available from: http://www.ncbi.nlm.nih.gov/pubmed/24219243

Chapter 16

# Immunology and Immunotherapy in Brain Tumors — Immune Failure and Potential Counteractions

Soliman Oushy and Michael W. Graner

Additional information is available at the end of the chapter

http://dx.doi.org/10.5772/59044

## 1. Introduction

The status of the immune system plays a major role tumor progression. Lewis Thomas proposed the association between immune surveillance and tumor progression as early as the 1950's. He suggested that the adaptive immune system has evolved to detect changes in the body's own cell surfaces due to damage or mutation. T cells, which specialize in monitoring cell surfaces, usually in the context of MHC molecular presentation, carry out this role; if a cell is deemed to be abnormal, it is destroyed before a mutant clone has time to proliferate and progress. Thus, the development of cancer could be seen as a failure of the immune system.

This chapter will discuss the ongoing interaction between the tumor development and the immune system, a process that has been called immunoediting. We will focus on tumors involving the central nervous system in both adult and pediatric settings—high grade gliomas (WHO grades III and IV tumors). We will review of the normal mechanisms employed by the immune system in combating tumor cells including cytotoxic T cells, Th1/Th2 cells, Natural Killer (NK) cells, B cells, macrophages, and the complement system.

Furthermore, we will explore the topic of tumor-associated antigens (TAA) in brain tumors, where we will start the review of alternative tactics of brain tumor treatments using immunotherapy. Although there have been relatively few successes in the field of immunotherapy, we will review the recent developments in brain tumor immunotherapy research and the different on-going clinical trials.

## 2. The immune system

### 2.1. General defense mechanisms

The immune system is the backbone of the body's defense against foreign invaders including bacteria, fungi, parasites, and viruses. The ability of humans to resist infections is composed of multiple systems working together, the first of which are the physical barriers of innate immunity lining the human body and entry points—skin and mucous membranes. Those physical barriers possess special properties that help fend off unwanted microorganisms including the ability to regenerate and secretion of antibiotics—defensin and cathelicidin families. However, under certain circumstances the physical barriers fail, allowing foreign intruders to venture deep inside the body requiring the activation of the immune system.

The immune system is comprised of two major divisions: the innate and adaptive immune systems. The innate system is not specific to a single pathogen, but is dependent on specific group of proteins and cells to recognize conserved features of pathogens. The main components of the innate system include 1) physical epithelial barriers discussed above, 2) phagocytic leukocytes, 3) dendritic cells, 4) natural killer (NK) cells, and 5) circulating plasma proteins. Using toll-like receptors (TLRs), the innate system is able to recognize pathogen-associated molecular patterns (PAMPs) and damage-associated molecular patterns (DAMPs) and respond within minutes. The adaptive immune system, on the other hand, is capable of recognizing new antigens and forming memory cells. The adaptive immune is activated when pathogens overcome the defenses of the innate system. Adaptive responses, however, are slow to respond at initial exposure to a new pathogen since specific clones of B and T cells are not yet activated. There are two types of adaptive immunity: humoral and cell-mediated immunity. Humoral immunity is mediated via antibodies secreted by B-lymphocytes whereas cell-mediated immunity is carried out by T-lymphocytes.

### 2.2. Induction of immune responses to antigens

Consider a scenario where a pathogen bypasses the physical barriers of the innate immune system. The pathogen is then recognized as foreign, taken up by professional antigen-presenting cells (APCs) and delivered to the nearest lymph node via the lymphatic system where T lymphocytes are activated. Alternatively, antigens can reach the lymph node by passive drainage where they are taken up by macrophages and dendritic cells (DCs). The antigens are then processed and presented to T-lymphocytes in association with MHC molecules. The simultaneous binding of T-cell receptor (TCR) to major histocompatibility complex (MHC) molecules and stimulation via APC's co-stimulatory molecules initiates T-cell activation. The T-lymphocyte may be a "helper T cell" that is now capable of aiding in activating "killer T cells" (cytotoxic T-lymphocytes, CTLs) and B-lymphocytes.

### 2.3. Immune surveillance

Immune surveillance is the theory that the immune system evolved not only to protect the body against foreign pathogens but also host cells that become tumorigenic. This idea,

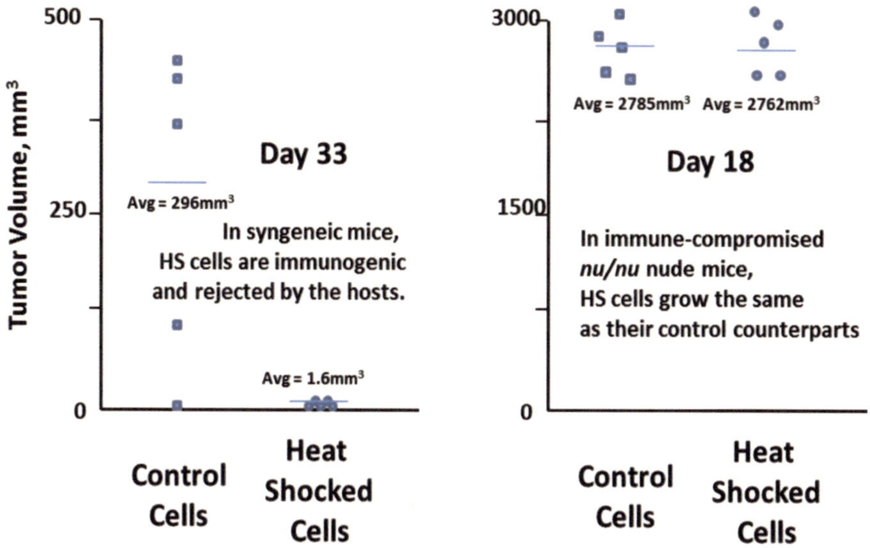


**Figure 1.** Immune mechanisms in tumor growth control: Tumor cells rendered immunogenic (by heat shock) are rejected by immune competent hosts, but grow unrestricted in immune-compromised mice. In this experiment, heat-shocked murine brain tumor cells became immunogenic (possibly due to the release of stress proteins) compared to non-heat shocked cells and were rejected following injection into syngeneic, immune-competent hosts. However, in immune-compromised mice (athymic nude mice, in this case, lacking T lymphocytes), heat shocked tumor cells grew equally large tumors as the non-heat shocked cells, indicating that the heat stress did not compromise cell viability, and that an intact immune system is required for rejection of the implanted tumors. Note differences in day of tumor measurements and the differences in the tumor volume axes.

proposed in the 1950's, was quite prescient given that self monitoring done by T-cells was not discovered until 20 years later [1]. There is some evidence for this attractive notion: 1) Patients with T-cell immunodeficiencies have a higher incidence of tumors, e.g. AIDS patients have a higher incidence Burkitt's lymphoma and Kaposi's sarcoma; 2) Organ transplant patients treated with immunosuppressive drugs had 25 to 100 fold increase in tumor incidence relative to healthy controls; 3) Tumor-Infiltrating Lymphocytes (TILs) have been identified that are capable of recognizing tumor-associated antigens. The most persuasive evidence, however, comes from the chemically-induced sarcomas in RAG2$^{-/-}$mice. RAG2 knockout mice fail to produce mature B and T cells due to lack of recombinase enzymes that are necessary to generate mature and functional antibodies and T-cell receptors [2]. Tumor cells induced in this knockout strain could be transplanted to new knockout hosts with 100% take rate, whereas wild-type mice of the same strain rejected 60% of the tumor challenges [3]. These experiments suggested that the immune system plays an active role in defending the body against cancerous cells. Additionally, this suggests that certain types of tumors or cells within a tumor may be strongly immunogenic inciting an immune response, while other cells may be weakly immunogenic. For instance, cells that are driven (eg, by heat stress) to be immunogenic are rejected by immune-competent syngeneic hosts, but those cells will grow at the same rates as control (unstressed) cells in immune-compromised (*nu/nu*) mice (Figure 1). We can then conclude that the immune system of mice plays a role in determining the pro-or anti-immune phenotypes of tumors that arise in mice, and possibly humans, a process termed immunoediting.

### 2.4. Immunoediting

The interaction between the immune system and tumor development has been termed immunoediting. One can think of the role of the immune system in immunoediting as the selective force on tumors, a process analogous to Darwinian selection. The process of immune editing can result into 3 outcomes: 1) the tumor cells are successfully eliminated as seen in the WT mice (Figure 1); 2) The tumor cells and lymphocytes exist in equilibrium; 3) Tumor cells initiate several responses that result in the suppression of the immune system or avoidance of immune effectors.

#### *2.4.1. Tumor cell elimination*

Compared to normal cells, tumor cells display a variety of metabolic abnormalities leading to the expression of damage associated molecular patterns (DAMPs) [4], as well as the stress expression of NK ligands such as MICA/B and ULBP families [5]. The expression of DAMPs and other stress molecules leads to the activation of the innate immune system, which in turn activates the adaptive immune system via APCs and cytokine release. The adaptive response yields stimulated effector lymphocytes. The end result is macrophage and lymphocyte infiltration of the tumor. If the abnormal clone is successfully eliminated, the process of immunoediting ends here. If the abnormal clone persists, however, then it can exists in equilibrium or grow beyond the control of the immune system [6].

#### *2.4.2. Equilibrium*

Another outcome to the infiltration of tumors by lymphocytes is incomplete eradication of the tumor. In this scenario, the abnormal clone and lymphocytes exist in equilibrium where the lymphocytes keep the tumor in check, but fail to entirely eradicate it, aided by regulatory T cells (Tregs, a subset of lymphocytes with immune suppressive properties) [7]. This may result in tumor dormancy (sometimes called "occult" cancers), but the mechanisms of this are poorly understood [8, 9].

#### *2.4.3. Escape*

The third phase of the immunoediting paradigm is escape of the tumor from immune attacks. This is often regarded as an "immune sculpting" phenomenon [10] that leads to immune pressure selection and outgrowth of unrecognized tumor clones. In combination with the aforementioned Tregs, the tumor may reach sufficient size that it can generate its own immune suppressive microenvironment, leading to growth and metastases in the face of an ineffectual immune response. In light of tumor selection and tumor-induced immune suppression, what factors lead to immune recognition of tumors?

## 3. Detection of neoplastic tissue

The immune system is generally very successful in eliminating viral infections and certain virus-induced tumors due to the vast difference in structure between viral and self-antigens. So, how are tumors lacking a viral etiology recognized and eliminated?

### 3.1. Tumor associated antigens

TAAs are antigens that are expressed by tumor cells and not readily found on corresponding normal cells. TAA can be found on normal cells, but are usually overexpressed or abnormally expressed on tumor cells. There are several types of TAAs: 1) viral gene products; 2) mutant gene products; 3) normal gene products. Viral antigens are expressed in tumors caused by viral infections: e.g. HTLV-1 and HTLV-2 viruses causing mycosis fungoides, human papilloma virus (HPV) in cervical cancer, Epstein-Barr virus (EBV) in Burkitt's lymphoma, and hepatitis B and C viruses (HBV, HCV) in hepatocellular carcinomas [11]. Mutant gene products are often found in transformed cells that may be part of the transformation process, or caused by physical and chemical carcinogens resulting in mutated proteins. Mutant gene products vary from one patient to the other and represent tumor-specific antigens (TSA). It has been estimated that tumors may have scores to hundreds of mutations that lead to recognizable epitopes [12].

Normal gene products are found on corresponding normal cells, but may overexpressed by tumors, such as epidermal growth factor family members (eg, HER2/Neu [13]). Others may be inappropriately expressed outside developmental or differential stages, such as oncofetal antigens and differentiation antigens. Differentiation antigens are lineage specific antigens that are usually overexpressed e.g. prostate-specific antigen (PSA) or the melanoma antigens MART1, TRP1, and tyrosinase. Oncofetal antigens are normally expressed in fetal tissue but not adult tissue. Perhaps the most familiar oncofetal antigen is the carcinoembryonic antigen (CEA) found in patients with colon carcinoma, amongst others. A review describing a comprehensive database for tumor antigens may be found here [14].

### 3.2. Effectors of the immune system

How does the immune system manage to eliminate tumors once an abnormal clone is recognized? Perhaps the most important cell in the topic of anti-tumor resistance is the CD8+cytotoxic T-lymphocyte (CTL).

CTLs are capable of recognizing TAAs presented on MHC class I molecules, which are present on the surface of most cells in humans. Following activation, CD8+CTLs undergo clonal expansion and migrate towards the tumor. CTLs then eliminate abnormal clones by inducing apoptosis through perforin or Fas-mediated pathways. Additionally, CTLs secrete IFN $\gamma$ upon engagement of their TCR, attracting macrophages. CTLs, however, can be inactivated upon arrival to tumor site as identified in melanoma patients [15, 16]. As a component of normal regulatory mechanisms, CTLs carry a surface marker, PD-1, that when engaged inactivates the

CTL. Many tumor types, however, up regulate PD-1 ligand (PD-L1 or PD-L2) in order to suppress and evade CTL activity.

Another notable cell belongs to a subset of CD4+T-lymphocytes, the type 1 T-helper cell (Th1). Th1 cells play a major role in recognition of antigens, production of lymphokines, activation of CD8+CTLs, and attracting M1 macrophages. Th1 cells then could play an important role in development of cancer vaccines [17].

Natural Killer (NK) cells are part of the immune system and are also known as large granular lymphocytes (LGLs). Being part of the immune system, NK cells can recognize a range of tumors and stress related markers without prior exposure to antigen (eg, via immunization). NK cells play a role in cancer immunity attacking cells that down regulate MHC class I molecules. Certain types of cancer cells down-regulate MHC class I molecules as an attempt to evade CTLs; the abnormal clone, however, risks detection and elimination by NK cells for reduced expression of surface MHC molecules [18].

Macrophages play a major role in cancer, exhibiting both anti-and pro-cancer behavior. Macrophages are part of the innate immune system and can be divided into the opposing M1 and M2 type macrophages. M1 activity inhibits cell proliferation and causes tissue damage. M2 activity promotes proliferation and repair. Tumors are capable of promoting M2 macrophage phenotypes which then aid in tumor angiogenesis, immune suppression, and tumor progression [19].

Dendritic cells (DC) are professional antigen-presenting cells and are a transitional link between the innate and adaptive immune system, inducing and maintaining T-cell immunity. DCs are outfitted with antigen-processing machinery (APM) allowing them to uptake and process TAAs. Processed TAAs are then loaded on MHC class I and II and presented to the appropriate T-cells. Thus, activated DCs are responsible for antigen specific immune responses by promoting activation and proliferation of T-cells. DCs can be divided into 2 major groups: plasmacytoid and classical DC. Plasmacytoid DCs play a role in antiviral immune response. Classical DCs can be further classified based on surface marker and function e.g. Langerhans cell in human epidermis. DCs are potential vectors for immune priming as vaccines against cancer antigens [20].

Antibodies play an interesting role in cancer immunity. Tumor-reactive serum antibodies from patients have long been viewed as resources for antigen detection, both in terms of vaccine potential and as exploitable biomarkers [21]. In other cases, antibodies isolated from cancer patients were tested for reactivity against cancer cell lines in vitro and in vivo. The antibodies showing specificity for tumors were all germ-line encoded and most belonged to the IgM class, binding to surface carbohydrates on malignant cells [22]. The utility of endogenous anti-tumor antibodies has not been clearly exploited, but may play a role in vaccine scenarios [23].

### 3.3. The immune response

Immune system activation is classically initiated when foreign antigens are taken up by professional APCs such as DCs, which migrate to the nearest draining lymph node. Figure 2 shows a highly diagrammatic and simplified version of this phenomenon. Protein antigens are processed during transit and beyond so that peptides may be loaded onto MHC Class I and Class II molecules for surface display by the APC. Once in the lymph node, the APC presents the antigen to the corresponding naïve T-cell to activate it. Activation of the T-cell requires two signals: 1) presentation/display of the processed peptide to the T-cell; and 2) co-stimulation of the T-cell by direct contact with APC surface molecules and by the secretion of activating cytokines (interferons, IL-12, IL-15, granulocyte macrophage-colony stimulating factor [GM-CSF], etc) by the APC. For Signal 1, the peptide displayed must fit into the peptide binding cleft of the host's MHC molecules and bind with sufficient affinity that the peptide-MHC is stably presented at the APC surface. The "T-cell of destiny" will be one whose T-cell receptor (TCR) recognizes the displayed peptide in the context of the MHC molecule. Thus, the T-cell must be antigen-specific. For Signal 2, the APC must be sufficiently stimulated upon and following antigen uptake that it produces co-stimulatory molecules such as CD80 and CD86, whose receptor, CD28, awaits on the T-cells. The APC will also produce the aforementioned stimulatory cytokines, as well, contributing to the activation of T-cells. This cell-cell interaction, with the various presentation of antigens and ligands to receptors requires close contact between the cells, and has been termed "the immunological synapse" [24]; for further review, see [25].

### 3.3.1. *Tumor evasion*

Given the descriptions of the immune system cited earlier, one would think that attempts by the immune system to eradicate tumors are a rare phenomenon. In fact, TAAs are found in the sera of some cancer patients. Still, however, the development of many human cancers is not blocked by the immune system. A likely explanation considers the antigenic properties of abnormal clones; certain cancers utilize the tolerance of the immune system to self-antigens by only expressing proteins that fly under the immunologic radar. Another possibility is immunoevasion—strategies employed by antigenic tumors after initial insult by the immune system.

### 3.3.2. *Immunoevasion*

The strategies of immunoevasion enable tumor cells to grow and create clinically relevant tumors. The immune system acts as a selective force on the initial tumor, allowing abnormal clones to escape elimination. Perhaps the most obvious evasive maneuver employed by tumor cells is to hide their identity by ceasing to display specific TAA and TSA. By doing so, abnormal clones evade elimination by cytotoxic T-lymphocytes. Consider a melanoma patient who was vaccinated with tyrosinase protein expressed by his melanoma cells. Initially, his melanoma regressed as a result of the immune response. Soon, however, tyrosinase-negative clones emerge while the tyrosinase-positive clones continue to regress. The tyrosinase-negative clones continue to proliferate rapidly until his death, a process called "immune escape". A possible explanation to the rise of the tyrosinase-negative melanoma cells is the diverse population of abnormal clones created by faulty DNA replication in cancerous cells. The tyrosinase-negative clone was then selected for by the immune system. This scenario is evident

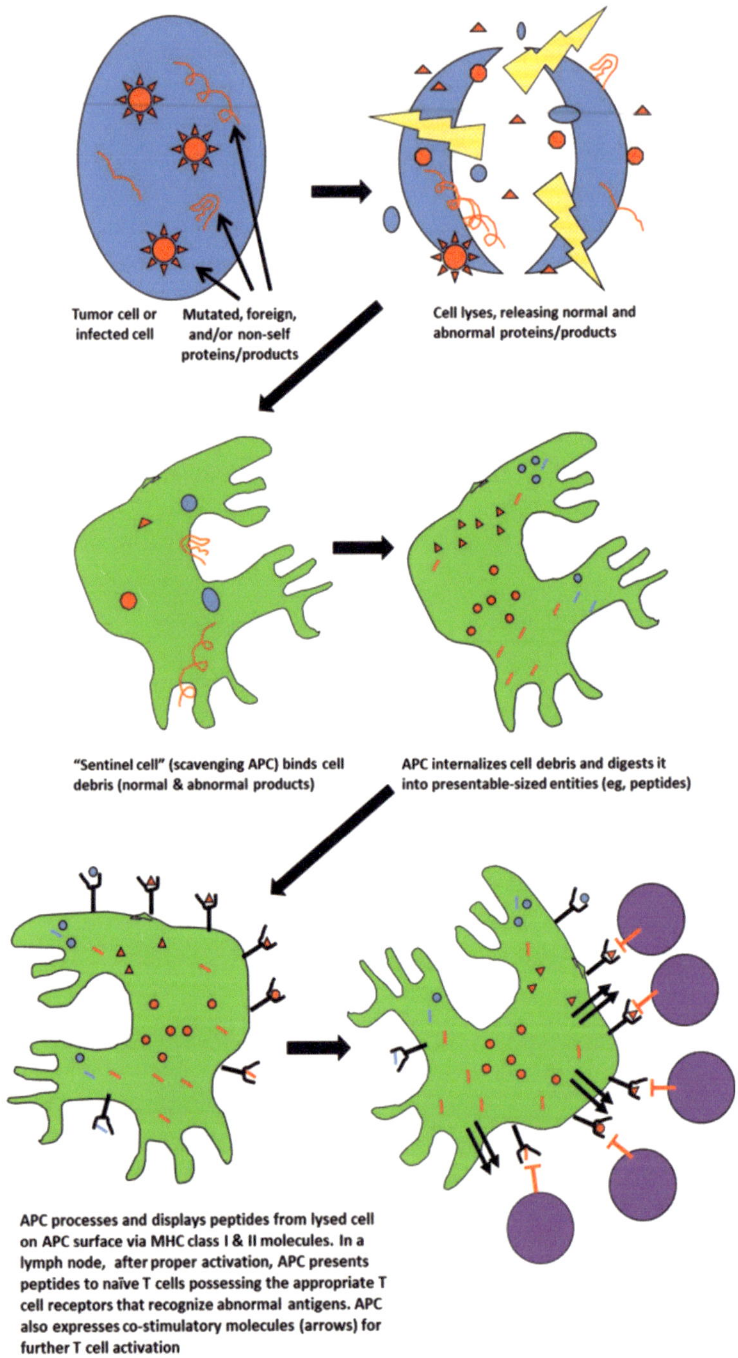


**Figure 2.** Antigen uptake, processing, and presentation. Pathogenic cells may lyse for a number of reasons, releasing normal and abnormal (viral, mutated, mis-expressed) proteins or other products. Scavenging Antigen Presenting Cells (APCs) may encounter the debris, internalize, and process it into peptides that are loaded onto MHC molecules and presented with co-stimulation to T cells in the lymph node, activating the T cell.

both in murine [26] and human studies [27], and is a concern where a particular antigen may be inconsequential to tumor physiology.

Some antigens, however, are essential for the function of tumor cells and neoplastic growth. In cancer cells that cannot down regulate TAAs, an alternative immunoevasive strategy is employed—downregulation of MHC class I molecules by repressing MHC gene transcription, instability of MHC at the cell surface by reduction of $\beta 2$ microglobulin, or with proteasomal or transporter associated with antigen processing (TAP) deficiencies leading to poor peptide processing/loading [27]. Such strategy can be seen in various forms of human cancers (e.g. lung, breast, colon, head & neck squamous cell carcinoma). Such downregulation or loss of MHC class I expression in human cancer represents a poor prognosis. Nevertheless, downregulation of cell surface MHC class I molecules attracts the attention of Natural Killer (NK) cells. NK cells patrol the body looking for cells that have reduced their cell surface display of MHC molecules. Decreased level of MHC class I molecules or total loss prompts destruction of cells by NK cells. This phenomenon explains why certain cancers block a minute fraction of surface MHC class I molecules. Perhaps this small fraction of surface MHC molecules prevents NK cell attack, but strategies to upregulate MHC I expression would be a consideration [28].

Another way by which abnormal clones evade NK cells is by repressing NKG2D ligands—stress-signaling proteins displayed by cells in stressful situations such as viral infections and neoplastic transformations. NK cells display a receptor on its surface (NKG2D) capable of recognizing various stress signals such as MICA and MICB. Binding of the NKG2D receptor to stress signals results in activation of NK cell's cytotoxic response and rapid killing of cells expressing the stress signals. Abnormal clones then can repress expression of NKG2D ligands in various ways, such as by secretory release or shedding of NKG2DLs [29] or regulation of expression at several levels [30]. The shedding strategy employed by human melanoma cells allows for continued expression of stress signals such as MICA, but as decoy ligands—the stress signals are released in surrounding medium instead of being displayed on cell surface. This diverts the attention of NK cells and CTLs from the ligands displayed on the cells surface.

Macrophages also play a role in tumor elimination responding to several signals on the surface of tumor cells. One protein expressed on the surface of various normal cells throughout the body, CD47, is used to protect the cells from random attacks by macrophages. Consider the downregulation of CD47 in erythrocytes as they progress through their life cycle. Such downregulation ensures that older cells are discarded by macrophages. Circulating malignant mammary cells have used CD47 to their advantage; by over-expressing CD47, they are able to evade the innate immune system acting via macrophages [31].

Not only can tumor cells evade the attacks of the immune system, but also they can launch counterattacks on lymphocytes. Cytotoxic lymphocytes utilize the Fas Ligand (FasL) molecule on its surface to bind and activate Fas receptors on target cells. Activation of Fas receptors leads to activation of the extrinsic apoptotic pathway. Cancer cells acquire resistance to the FasL through mechanisms that are not well understood. This leads to abnormal clones that are resistant to destruction by cytotoxic T-lymphocytes. Additionally, they also acquire the ability to synthesize and secrete soluble forms of FasL. The secretion of FasL does not affect the already resistant strain; however, some studies have shown that they do affect some lymphocytes leading to activation of extrinsic apoptotic pathway and lymphocyte death. This strategy ensures a safe microenvironment for the growing neoplasm [32].

In addition to FasL, some human cancers have been shown to secrete TGF- $\beta$ or Interleukin-10 (IL-10). Both IL-10 and TGF- $\beta$ are immunosuppressive agents secreted by normal cells of the immune system with TGF- $\beta$ being is the most potent immunosuppressive cytokine. TGF- $\beta$ has many biological effects including the inhibition of 1) APC antigen presentation; 2) APC maturation; 3) T-cell activation and differentiation. Studies have shown that TGF- $\beta$ is upregulated in glioma clones that are resistant to CTLs [33]. IL-10 on the other hand is capable of downregulating the expression of MHC class II antigens and Type 1 T-Helper (Th1) cytokines. The expression of IL-10 in glioma tissue has been correlated with tumor grade [34, 35].

In addition to CTLs and macrophages, tumor cells have been shown to recruit regulatory T-lymphocytes (Treg) to essentially fend off attacks by other lymphocytes. Treg cells are capable of suppressing T-helper lymphocytes and CTLs. These may be immature T cells committed to the regulatory lineage, or antigen-driven induced Tregs [36]. Research has shown that the percentage of Treg cells increases by 3-5 fold in cancer patients especially in tumor infiltrating lymphocytes (TILs). Furthermore, the degree of Treg infiltration correlates with tumor grade [37]. The ability of tumor cells to attract Treg cells depends on the secretion of chemokine CCL22. CCL22 acts on CCR4, a receptor on the surface of Treg cells to attract Treg cells towards the tumor [38, 39]. While present in the tumor, Treg cells are capable of indirectly suppressing both the humoral and cellular branch of the immune system through inactivation of T-helper cells. The existence of Treg cells in the tumor mass questions the association between the total number of TILs and tumor prognosis. TILs were assumed to be cytotoxic T-cells, but if a substantial fraction of TILs are Treg cells then this notion casts a shadow of doubt over the significance of TILs in tumors [40].

Myeloid-derived suppressor cells (MDSCs) are another cell type recruited by tumors to evade host immune defenses. MDSCs comprise a heterogeneous group of immature myeloid cells that play a major role in the immune suppressive tumor microenvironment (TME) [41]. As a part of their normal physiologic role, immature myeloid cells play a role in replenishing DCs and macrophages in early phases of trauma and stress and avoiding immune pathology in later stages [42]. The TME, however, influences local myeloid cells to become immunosuppressive [43]. Additionally, tumors initiate myelopoiesis, thus recruiting more immature myeloid cells [44]. MDSCs play a role in tumor progression by inhibiting T-cell response and their elimination has been shown to improve anti-tumor immunity [45]. Although treatment aimed at MDSCs could potentially be effective, efforts at characterizing MDSCs have been fruitless providing inadequate information to understand their phenotypical and functional heterogeneity.

### 3.4. Immunology of the CNS

The ability to restrict collateral damage caused by the immune response is essential, especially in the CNS. As a result, a status of immunological privilege is maintained in the brain limiting the magnitude of the immune response and inflammation.

Due to the delicate nature of the cells composing the central nervous system (CNS), the blood brain barrier (BBB) tightly controls molecular passage and cellular migration in and out of the CNS. The BBB is composed of both capillary and post capillary vessels. The ability of the BBB to tightly regulate passive diffusion of hydrophilic molecules results from the selectivity of the tight junctions (TJ) between endothelial cells in the CNS vasculature [46]. Consequently, the BBB has been implicated in the regulating the immune response in the CNS by restricting molecular access to cerebral interstitial fluid (CIF).

As discussed above, the activation of the immune response is maintained throughout the body: APCs uptake antigen, migrate to lymphatics, appropriate T-helper cells and CTLs are activated. However, professional antigen presenting cells (APCs) such as dendritic cells in the systemic circulation have not been described in CNS parenchyma, but DCs are present in vascular-rich regions of the CNS [47]. Instead, microglia are the primary resident APCs in the CNS [48]. Microglia express MHC class II antigens and T-cell co-stimulatory molecules giving them the ability to present antigens to T-helper cells. Once antigens are taken up by APCs in the CNS, presentation of the antigen seems to take place in the cervical lymph nodes (Dunn et al., 2007). T-cells are not normally found in the brain unless activated [49], but T-cells and antibodies do have access to the brain [50].

Migration of leukocytes towards the CNS starts with the interaction between leukocytes attracted to chemokines and adhesion molecules on endothelial cells. The chemokines secreted by the site of inflammation activate G protein-signaling, thus activating the leukocyte and upregulating integrins. Through a tight interaction involving adhesion molecules on lymphocytes and endothelial cells (VCAMs, ICAMs, and LFAs), the cells transmigrate into the parenchyma [51].

# 4. Neoplasia in the CNS

## 4.1. Glioblastoma multiforme (GBM)

Brain tumors exist as two distinct types, malignant and benign. This chapter will focus malignant tumors originating in the brain, primarily glioblastoma multiforme (GBM). Tumors originating from astrocytes/glial cells are named gliomas with (GBM) being the most common and aggressive primary adult brain tumor. GBM is a grade IV astrocytoma arising from astrocytes and is characterized by central areas of necrosis surrounded by anaplastic cells. Median survival time is less than 15 month and significantly less for patients with recurrent tumors [52]. GBM can present as primary or secondary tumor. Primary GBM is generally seen in older patients as a result of EGFR overexpression, PTEN mutations, and mdm2 gene amplification [53]. Primary GBM is thought to be a single step transformation with no clinical background. Secondary GBM is seen in younger patients as a slow multi-step transformation process. Secondary GBM results from p53 inactivation or overexpression of PDGF ligand, receptor, or both [54].

### 4.2. Glioma immunity vs immune suppression

A number of potential TSA and TAA have been identified in gliomas (a listing may be found here [55]) including a number of antigens previously found in melanoma (eg, gp100, MAGE-1 and-3, MART-1, NY-ESO-1, tyrosinase and related proteins 1 and 2). Others include tenascin-C, IL13R$\alpha$2, EphA2, and EGFRvIII. Whole proteins or peptides derived from these antigens could be used in vaccine scenarios with a goal of providing antigen to APCs (presumably DCs), usually in the context of an adjuvant or immune stimulant to promote antigen uptake and activation of the DCs. Alternatively, the DCs may be harvested as progenitors from patients, differentiated and bulk-proliferated ex vivo, supplied with antigen, and then returned to the patient as a cellular vaccine. In other scenarios, lysates or particular proteins that may "sample" the antigenic peptide repertoire of the tumor (eg, heat shock proteins or chaperone proteins) [56, 57] may be employed to provide "blanket" immunogenicity by theoretically supplying all antigens rather than selected ones.

Unfortunately, gliomas are capable of employing some or all of the immunoevasive strategies discussed above. Patients with malignant gliomas often have weak adaptive immune systems due to the increased percentage of Tregs [58, 59]. In addition, malignant gliomas have been shown to secrete TGF-$\beta$ and VEGF capable of direct immune suppression as well as inducing myeloid-derived suppressor cells [60]. VEGF has been shown to inhibit NF-$\kappa$B signaling in hematopoietic progenitor cells, thus inhibiting dendritic cell maturation.

### 4.3. Current therapies

Available therapies for GBM and other brain tumors include chemotherapy, fractionated radiotherapy, and image-guided tumor resection. Current chemotherapeutic options for glioblastoma include Gliadel wafers (carmustine/BCNU), cisplatin, and temozolomide (the drug that is part of the standard of care regimen concurrent with radiation, and then in the adjuvant setting [52].

Carmustine is an alkylating agent and was the first drug approved for the treatment of GBM. Carmustine inhibits cancer growth via alkylation of O6-guanine position on DNA and thus crosslinking the helix. Carmustine has shown modest improvement in patient survival in early trials (reviewed here [61]) and has been the cornerstone of GBM adjuvant therapy. Although carmustine can cross the blood brain barrier (BBB), delivery to target site is difficult. Additionally, carmustine effectiveness hindered by its short half-life, systemic toxicity and tendency for chemo-resistance.

For better delivery of carmustine to action site, Gliadel wafers are used. Gliadel wafers are made of carmustine-loaded biodegradable polymers placed in the resection cavity formerly occupied by the tumor post-surgical excision. As the polymer is degraded, carmustine is slowly released. A study conducted by Westphal et al. in 2003 [62] showed that Gliadel-treated patients had a median survival rate of 13.9 month compared to 11.6 month in placebo controls. The complications of Gliadel wafers are serious and life threatening--seizures, edema, and hydrocephalus [63, 64].

The current standard of care for GBMs is maximal surgical resection followed by concurrent fractionated radiation and temozolomide (TMZ), with TMZ then given in the adjuvant setting

[52]. There are variations on this theme, including the addition of the anti-VEGFA antibody bevacizumab (as a form of anti-angiogenesis), but surgery, radiation, and TMZ are the staples [65]. TMZ is an oral DNA alkylating agent capable of crossing the BBB and inducing apoptosis [66, 67]. Attempts at combination treatments using TMZ and other chemotherapy drugs have shown little or no benefit when compared to TMZ alone [68]. TMZ efficacy varies, however, in patients depending on the action of the enzyme repairing the lesion produced by the drug, O6 methyl guanine DNA methyl transferase (MGMT) [69].

Cisplatin is a cis platinum complex containing 2 chloride and 2 amine groups. Once in the body, cisplatin triggers apoptosis by crosslinking DNA. Cisplatin's efficacy on brain tumors has shown few benefits. A phase 3 trial showed no significant outcome improvement in patients administered carmustine and radiation therapy versus cisplatin, carmustine, and radiation therapy [70].

#### *4.3.1. Understanding Glioma-Associated Antigens (GAAs)*

Considering the low median survival time, current therapies are inadequate and there is a strong need for novel therapies with superior safety and efficacy. In order to develop new therapies, it's important to be familiar with potential glioma-specific molecular targets. In light of the potential utility of immunotherapy as a novel therapeutic strategy for patients with GBM, this section will discuss Glioma-Associated Antigens (GAA), some of which were briefly mentioned above.

**IL13R$\alpha$2**

IL13R$\alpha$2 is a glycoprotein overexpressed on the surface of many glioma cells. The only other normal tissue where IL13R$\alpha$2 can be found is in the testes; therefore it represents a great potential target for glioma therapy [71].

**EphA2**

A receptor tyrosine kinase overexpressed on the plasma membrane of gliomas and tumor-associated vasculature. EphA2 is thought to play a role in developmental processes and carcinogenesis. EphA2 has been shown to provoke a response from cytotoxic T-lymphocytes against glioma clones [72].

**EGFRvIII**

Type III variant mutation of EGFR (EGFRvIII) is seen with patients with primary and recurrent GBM and is currently the most prevalent TSA found on glioma. EGFRvIII promotes and enhances carcinogenesis [73]; EGFRvIII encodes a constitutively active tyrosine kinase that does not need to dimerize nor bind ligand for activity [74, 75].

**Survivin**

Although not specific for gliomas, survivin belongs to the inhibitor-of-apoptosis protein family that is overexpressed in the majority of human cancers [76]. It is considered a marker of poorer prognosis in patients with GBM [77].

### WT1

Wilm's Tumor 1 (WT1) is a transcription factor that is important in the developmental biology of many organs; its mis-expression may drive epithelial-to-mesenchymal transitions prevalent in many cancers [78]. WT1 is overexpressed in solid tumors, leukemias, and gliomas [79]. WT1 has both oncogenic and tumor suppressor capacities depending on mutational status, over-expression, and tissue source [80]. It is considered to be a viable tumor antigen with multiple applications [81].

### SOX

Sry-related high mobility group box (SOX) is a family of transcription factors involved in directing the development of various tumors and cell types [82]. SOX2, SOX5, SOX6, and SOX11 are preferentially overexpressed in tumors of the CNS [83] and in glioma stem cell lines [84].

## 5. Immunotherapy

Understanding how cancer escapes the immune system provides clues for researchers and clinicians to intervene at critical points and empower the immune system. Although the field of cancer immunotherapy has much to prove, it has the potential to treat various forms of cancer with high specificity and relatively low toxicities. The superior therapeutic specificity in particular makes immunotherapy an attractive, tolerable alternative or possible adjuvant to chemotherapy for patients. Available cancer immunotherapeutic options include vaccines, monoclonal antibodies, adoptive cell therapy (ACT), and cytokine therapy, and the so-called "checkpoint blockades".

### 5.1. Glioma vaccines

Vaccines harness the immune system and allow it to target glioma-associated antigens via the processes of antigen provision/uptake to APCs, followed by the stimulation of specific lymphocytes by the APCs. The field of antitumor vaccines is one of the most studied and established modalities of immunotherapy. There are 3 general types of glioma vaccines: whole cell/tumor lysate vaccines, peptide-based vaccines, and dendritic cell vaccines. These vaccines may be used with various adjuvants or immune stimulants; they may be used amidst the standard of care; they may involve additional immune stimulation or regulatory suppression strategies.

Whole cell glioma vaccines involve administration of irradiated allogeneic or autologous glioma cells providing multiple GAA for the immune system to target. Obviously, autologous whole cell vaccines would provide the most personalized treatment using GAAs specific to each patient. On the other hand, such tumor cells may also provide tumor suppressive entities [85]. Manufacturing whole cell vaccines, however, is a very demanding task especially when handling large-scale glioma cell cultures, and when time is of the essence for patients with short times to progression [86]. Additionally, this approach puts patients at a theoretical risk

http://dx.doi.org/10.5772/59044

for autoimmune encephalomyelitis [87]. However, several autologous cell vaccine trials by Schneider et al among others have reported no major adverse effects [88].

An alternative to whole cell glioma vaccine and their associated autoimmunity risks are peptide-based vaccines. Peptide-based vaccines use synthetic peptides based on shared GAA epitopes. Unlike whole cell glioma vaccines, peptide-based vaccines target one or few GAAs specific to each patient's tumor. This may be beneficial in generating higher levels of specific responses to a particular antigen; it may also provide an easier outlet for immune escape by antigen loss. However, this strategy does present a lower risk for development of autoimmunity, and peptide manufacturing is relatively simple compared to handling large-scale glioma cell cultures. Peptide-based vaccines targeting EGFRvIII have been shown to be safe and potentially beneficial in the ACTIVATE (A Complementary Trial of an Immuno-therapy Vaccine Against Tumor-Specific EGFRvIII) series of trials (including ACT II, ACT III, ACT IV, ReACT [89, 90]). The ACTIVATE phase II trial recruited 18 patients with EGFRvIII expressing tumors that received CDX-110 (14-amino acid EGFRvIII epitope conjugated to a keyhole limpet hemocyanin as a hapten carrier with GM-CSF as an adjuvant) along with standard radio-and chemotherapy. The median time to progression was 14.2 month and median survival was 26 month; no adverse events were recorded. ACT IV is a phase III trial comparing vaccine/GM-CSF+TMZ vs TMZ and placebo alone (see Table 1).

A somewhat different version of peptide-based therapy is that of chaperone protein or "heat shock protein" (HSP)-based vaccines [56, 57]. The concept here is that chaperone/HSPs bind intracellular peptides as part of their chaperone duties. Thus, purification of particular chaperone/HSPs from tumor cells results in a population of peptides that are specific to that particular tumor, even though the chaperone/HSPs may appear identical. Upon vaccination, this would provide APCs with a "peptide fingerprint" of the tumor, making the vaccine tumor—and patient—specific, even if the chaperone proteins were ubiquitous in different cell types (see Figure 3). The current chaperone protein vaccine in use for GBMs is variously called Prophage, Oncophase, and HSPPC-96; the protein purified from tumors for vaccine generation is glucose-regulated protein (GRP) 94, also called glycoprotein (gp) 96.

A key common feature of most peptide-based vaccines is the inclusion of immune stimulatory factors as adjuvants (eg, DNA constructs such as polyICLC [91], GM-CSF [92], Freund's adjuvant [93], TLR agonists [94], and cytokines [95]). This is necessary because the lack of APC stimulation will result in poor activation of T cells, with possible conversion to an anergic state. The chaperone/HSP vaccines utilize the "danger signal" effects of extracellular HSPs as innate immune stimulators to essentially provide their own adjuvanticity [96]. An advantage of peptide antigens of known sequence is that provides investigators with a means of immune monitoring by measuring and tracking the immune response, by T cell readouts [97] and sometimes by antibody responses [23]. One question that remains is whether results from immune monitoring yield true prognostic information, as often there is a positive correlation with immune measures of vaccination, but these do not necessarily appear related to clinical benefit [98].

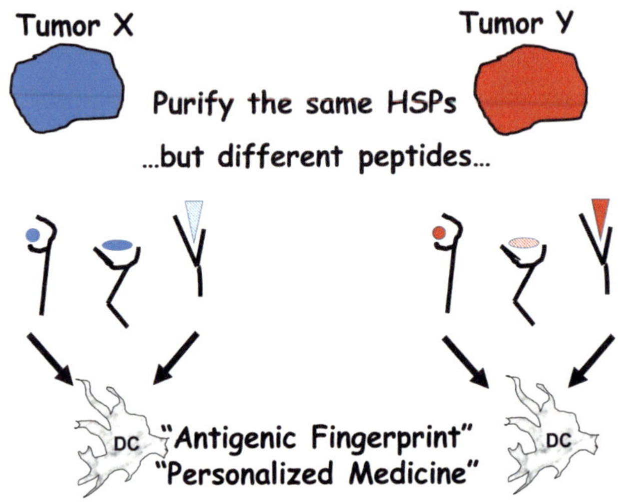


**Figure 3.** Chaperone/Heat Shock Protein (HSP) vaccines from tumors. Various HSPs have been shown to be immunogenic when purified from tumors. However, purification of the same HSPs from different tumors does not generate cross-protection (eg, if HSPs are purified from Tumor X and used as a vaccine, but the host is challenged with Tumor Y, there will be no anti-tumor protection, because the antigenic peptide repertoire differs between the two tumors, even if the HSPs appear the same).

| Trial Name | Phase | n | Therapy | Primary Outcome | Trial Identifier |
|---|---|---|---|---|---|
| Vaccine therapy + sargramostim | I | 9 | ISA-51/survivin peptide vaccine + sargramostim | Safety | NCT01250470 |
| HSPPC-96 vaccine + Temozolamide | II | 55 | HSPPC-96 + Temozolamide | Safety | NCT00905060 |
| ACT III | II | 82 | CDX-110 1 TMZ 1 RT | Progression-free survival | NCT00458601 |
| ACT IV | III | 440 | CDX-110 1 TMZ | Overall survival | NCT01480479 |

**Table 1.** Summary of ongoing peptide-based vaccine trials for malignant glioma. Data obtained from National Institutes of Health. Information is available by Trial Identifier at http://www.clinicaltrials.gov.

## 5.2. Antibodies

Antibodies are utilized in cancer immunotherapy usually as human, humanized, or mouse-human chimeric monoclonal antibodies (mAb) that target tumor-associated antigens (TAA) and tumor-specific antigens (TSA), generally on the surfaces of cancer cells, or targeted against secretory molecules. There are 2 categories of mAbs most frequently used: naked and conjugated antibodies. Naked antibodies work independently without an attached radiolabel or toxin. Once bound to the target cell, naked antibodies mark cells to be eliminated by the immune system, usually neutrophils and macrophage. If such mAbs target surface receptors, they may interfere with ligand binding or downstream function. Conjugated or "armed" antibodies, on the other hand, are mAbs joined to a toxin, chemotherapy drug or a radioactive particle. Conjugated antibodies are essentially vehicles specific for targeting abnormal clones, sparing normal cells from toxic therapy. Regardless of the type, it is crucial that the mAb bind with high affinity and specificity to target [99]. Monoclonal antibody therapy has been successful in treating lymphomas (rituximab), breast cancer (trastuzumab), and more recently, recurrent glioblastoma (bevacizumab). Malignant gliomas are vascular tumors producing vascular endothelial growth factor (VEGF), which promotes angiogenesis and tumor progression. Bevacizumab is a humanized monoclonal antibody against VEGFA administered in combination with chemotherapy [100]. Inhibition of VEGF via bevacizumab followed by cytotoxic chemotherapy and radiation therapy has generated encouraging results in several studies [100].

The use of mAbs to treat GBM has been investigated in preclinical systems. Y10, anti-EGFRvIII naked murine IgG2a, significantly increased survival time in mice bearing EGFRvIII expressing tumors by an average of 286% [101]. Additionally, Y10 was shown to inhibit cell proliferation and DNA synthesis in vitro by complement activation and antibody dependent cell-mediated cytotoxicity (ADCC). Another type of anti-EGFRvIII (or "delta 2-7") is mAb 806, which has also shown pre-clinical efficacy against EGFR-amplified tumors [102] and has shown good targeting capability and pharmacokinetics in a phase I study [103]. Anti-EGFRvIII mAbs such as L8A4 (murine IgG1) have also been radiolabeled and utilized in pre-clinical testing [104], including boronation [105].

Given the role of EGFR in the progression of malignant glioma, efforts to inhibit EGFR have culminated in phase I study conducted by Faillot et al which demonstrated the ability of murine anti-EGFR mAb EMD55900 to bind the tumor in vivo and is well tolerated in patients [106]. Repeated infusions only resulted in one patient developing human anti-mouse antibodies (HAMA response). Despite the substantial binding of EMD55900 to targets, phase I/II clinical trials using EMD55900 administered intravenously showed no significant tumor regression [107]. The use of another anti-EGFR antibody (chimeric humanized), cetuximab, showed good tolerability but limited efficacy in patients with recurrent GBMs [108]. A recently-developed chimeric humanized anti-EGFR antibody, nimotuzumab, is in clinical trials for malignant gliomas, but the studies are not mature enough to provide much information [109].

### 5.3. DC Immunotherapy

The superior antigen presenting ability of DCs has been harnessed in novel cancer vaccination strategies. DC vaccines take advantage of the antigen presenting machinery of these cells to activate CD4+ and CD8+ T cells that are specific for TAAs/TSAs. DCs are generated using autologous peripheral blood leukocytes that are incubated with specific cytokines to induce differentiation of monocytes into DCs; the type of cytokine used dictates the quality of DCs generated e.g. GM-CSF and IFN$\alpha$ generate DCs highly potent in T-cell activation. DCs are then pulsed with 1) synthetic tumor antigens (TAAs) or 2) autologous tumor lysate, or 3) tumor RNAs to promote activation and antigen presentation, and are injected back into the patient [110].

Phase I trials assessing safety have been carried out by Yu et al. in 7 patients (+2 with anaplastic astrocytomas) who received injections of autologous glioma peptide pulsed-DCs; these peptides were acid-eluted from tumor cell surfaces (presumably from MHC molecules). Four out of 7 patients developed tumor specific T cell cytotoxicity, and others had T cell infiltrates into their tumors at reoperation [111]. The Cedar Sinai experience in DC vaccine clinical trials is discussed here [112]. In another phase I trial done by Liau et al., 12 patients were administered DCs also pulsed with autologous glioma-eluted peptides from surface of resected tumors. Fifty percent of the patients showed increased systemic and intracranial immunologic responses while reporting no adverse effects from vaccination [113]. More recent studies by that group have utilized autologous tumor lysate as the antigen source due to its availability from surgical resection, whereas the use of specific GAAs requires patients to express suitable MHC molecules able to present the GAA [114]. Prins et al have also conducted a phase I trial using TLR7 agonists (imiquimod or polyICLC) combined with autologous tumor lysate-pulsed DC vaccination. Twenty-three GBM patients were enrolled showing a mean overall survival of 31 months and 47% 3-year survival [115]. The use of DC vaccines pulsed with tumor-derived RNAs (total polyA+RNAs or specific mRNAs) was demonstrated almost 20 years ago [116], and this strategy has made it to clinical trials for patients with GBMs [117]. An advantage of RNA as a source of antigen is that it can be prepared by standard conditions, or synthesized cheaply.

DC-based vaccine trials have been prevalent in neuro-oncology, and many of those are reviewed here [110], along with a listing of current DC vaccine trials in glioma (Table 2).

| Trial Name | Phase | n | Therapy | Primary Outcome | Identifier |
|---|---|---|---|---|---|
| ATTAC | I | 16 | CMV pp65-LAMP mRNA-loaded DCs | Safety | NCT00639639 |
| NY-ESO-1 intranodal vaccine | I | 30 | DEC-205-NY-ESO-1 fusion protein + sirolimus | Safety | NCT01522820 |
| Vaccine therapy for recurrent GBM | I | 50 | BTSC mRNA-loaded DCs | Safety | NCT00890032 |
| Phase I study of DC vaccine | I | 40 | Allogenic stem cell lysate | Safety | NCT02010606 |
| DC vaccine for patients with brain tumors | II | 60 | Autologous tumor lysate + adjuvant | Most effective combination of DC vaccine components | NCT01204684 |
| ICT-107 | IIb | 200 | TAA | Overall survival | NCT01280552 |
| DCVax-L | III | 300 | Autologous tumor cell lysate | Progression-free survival | NCT0045968 |

**Table 2.** Summary of ongoing DC vaccine clinical trials for malignant glioma. Data obtained from National Institutes of Health. Available at http://www.clinicaltrials.gov.

### 5.4. Adoptive Cell Therapy (ACT)

ACT is the manipulation of autologous cells ex vivo to be infused back into the patient. ACT aims to amplify cell lines that best fight cancer including 1) TILs 2) peripheral blood mononuclear cells (PBMCs) 3) lymphokine-activated killer cells (LAKs) and 4) antigen specific CTLs.

ACT originated as a way to restore viral immunity in patients undergoing hematopoietic stem cell transplant and to prevent cytomegalovirus (CMV) reactivation in transplant patients. Early use of adoptive cell transfer to treat non-viral malignancies was seen in attempts to treat hematologic malignancies and melanoma. Steinbok et al. was the first to demonstrate the possibility of ACT in treatment of gliomas in 1984 [118]. Steinbok collected autologous PBMCs to be re-infused into the cavity created post tumor excision. The study, however, showed no significant beneficial outcomes. Newer technologies and a better understanding of the cells involved have made ACT an attractive approach. However, the ex vivo generation of large quantities of specifically reacting cells is cumbersome, expensive, and not necessarily available everywhere.

#### *5.4.1. Cytotoxic T-Lymphocytes*

Based on the findings that CTLs can bypass the BBB and migrate into brain parenchyma (reviewed here [119]. GAA-reactive CTLs isolated from peripheral blood and glioma tissue might mount a favorable antitumor response in glioma patients. Glioma tissues are infiltrated with GAA-specific CTLs that could be expanded ex-vivo using IL-2 and subsequently selected for antigen specificity [120]. Once GAA-specific CTLs have been isolated, ex-vivo manipulations include cloning high affinity TCRs, expression of chimeric antigen receptors (CARs), and T-cell subtype selection. Cloning high affinity TCRs is done by isolating CD8+T cells with high GAA affinity for particular antigens and cloning TCR $\alpha$ and $\beta$genes to be exogenously induced in bulk CD8+cells. ACT using high affinity TCR T-cells has resulted in regression of metastatic melanoma [121], suggesting the potential of applying this method to glioma therapy. ACT of various types using CTLs has a history in glioma trial therapy, but none have shown consistent benefit [122].

Chimeric Antigen Receptors (CARs) are chimeric molecules composed of epitope-binding domain of mAb fused to CD3 signal transduction domain (Gross et al., 1989). CAR is an alternative to transgenic high-affinity TCRs and don't require the expression of MHC molecules. CAR-T cells have just reached clinical trial stage in GBMs (NCT02209376 at ClinicalTrials.gov) targeting EGFRvIII. Other targets include IL13R$\alpha$2 [123], HER2/Neu (EGFR2) [124], and 3$^{rd}$ generation anti-EGFRvIII cells [125].

#### *5.4.2. LAK cells*

Lymphokine-Activated Killer (LAK) cells are activated prior to exposure to IL-2 in vitro. LAK cells possess cytotoxic machinery capable of lysing abnormal clones (allogeneic and autologous) sparing normal cells. As a result of the toxic systemic effect of IL-2 administration, *in vivo* human trials using LAK cells are limited and researchers have resorted to ex vivo LAK trials, with an occasional long-term survivor [126]. Administration of LAK cells into post excision cavity combined with IL-2 therapy has shown to increase median survival from 26 weeks to 53 weeks in patients with recurrent GBM [127]. LAK cells, however, have limited specificity to tumors in vivo and their tumor recognition mechanisms are not well understood.

### *5.4.3. Lymphodepletion*

Lymphodepletion is the process killing white blood cells to enhance adoptive transfer therapy possibly in vaccination scenarios. Lymphodepletion induces homeostatic proliferation, a situation where lymphocytes proliferate in an enriched cytokine environment and with lowered thresholds of stimulation and decreased numbers of Tregs [128]. Lymphodepletion has a long history in the ACT therapies in melanoma, where there have been objective response rates of greater than 50% [129]. There is also a suggestion that the lymphopenia induced by TMZ chemotherapy may actually benefit anti-tumor vaccination by driving homeostatic proliferation [130], and this may aid in Treg depletion by mAb blockade [131]. Dose-dense TMZ regimens may induce more myelotoxicity, however [132].

## 6. Virotherapy

Oncolytic virotherapy is the use of genetically engineered viruses for the treatment of malignancies. Oncolytic viruses are engineered to specifically infect malignant cells, thus sparing the normal tissue surrounding the tumor [133]. The intracellular replication of the oncolytic virus then results in cancer cell lysis and release of viral progeny that infects additional cancerous cells [134]. The use of oncolytic viruses for GBM treatment has been tested in clinical trials for the last 15 years with multiple phase I trials completed and some ongoing, proving to be a safe option. Two treatment strategies exist in virotherapy 1) replication-incompetent viruses and 2) replication-competent viruses. Replication-incompetent viruses exert their therapeutic effect through the delivery of transgenes that exert their effect through multiple mechanisms, one of which is discussed below [133]. Replication-competent viruses exert their therapeutic effect via replication and lysis of target tumor cells [133].

Concerns about uncontrolled viral infection in hosts led researchers to use replication-incompetent viruses for initial attempts in oncolytic virus therapies. Replication-incompetent adenoviruses and retroviruses are then engineered with the herpes simplex virus thymidine kinase gene (HSV-TK), which produces a cytotoxic metabolite from the drug ganciclovir [135]. Ram et al. used a replication-incompetent retrovirus engineered with HSV-TK for the first phase I clinical trial [136]. Fifteen patients received viral injections to the tumor site and oral gancyclovir with no adverse effects. Median survival time was 8.1 month; however, the lack of statistical significance in phase III trials [137] led researchers to study replication-competent oncolytic viruses (OVs).

OVs are attenuated viruses capable of lysing target tumor cells and activation of the local immune response to tumor antigen release [138]. There currently exist 4 different OVs used in published clinical trials. Herpes Simplex Virus G207 is among the OVs used in clinical trials. G207 is unable to replicate in normal cells because it lacks ribonucleotide reductase. In the first

http://dx.doi.org/10.5772/59044

of 2 separate phase I clinical trials, of the 21 patients injected with G207, 8 patients demonstrated reduction in tumor size shown on MRI scans [139]. In the second trial, investigators demonstrated successful replication of the virus in the tumor [140]. Although safe, OVs tested to date have proven less efficacious than expected. However, there are efforts to create new viruses equipped with cytotoxic agents and other viruses specifically targeting the stem cell population of GBM [141, 142]. There are also studies showing safety testing of a polio virus-rhino virus chimera that shows high targeting capacities for tumors (due to overexpression of the poliovirus receptor NECL5) and replication within tumor cells due to putative biochemical abnormalities [143, 144]. There is a newly-opened trial based on this virus (NCT01491893 at ClinicalTrials.gov). Other clinical trials involving viral therapy are listed in Table 3.

| Trial Name | Phase | Viral Modifications | n | Primary Outcome | Identifier |
|---|---|---|---|---|---|
| **MV-CEA for recurrent glioblastoma** | I | Carcinoembryonic antigen-expressing | 40 | Safety, MTD, viral propagation and expression | NCT00390299 |
| **NDV-HUJ in glioblastoma** | I/II | HUJ strain | 30 | Progression-free survival | NCT01174537 |
| **DNX2401 and TMZ in recurrent glioblastoma** | I | Mutation in E1A and RGD-related integrin expression | 31 | No. of patients with adverse events | NCT01956734 |

**Table 3.** Selected ongoing oncolytic viral clinical trials for malignant glioma. Data obtained from National Institute of Health. Available at http://www.clinicaltrials.gov.

## 7. Immune checkpoint blockade

As mentioned above, certain molecules expressed on T cells, with ligands or counter receptors expressed on tumors or Tregs, may provide an avenue of control over maintenance of an activated T cell status or denial of a suppressive effect. One such T cell surface molecule is cytotoxic T lymphocyte antigen 4 (CTLA4), which is a receptor that downregulates T cell activity by binding to CD80 and/or CD86 on other T cells, particularly Tregs. Ipilimumab is an antibody that binds to CTLA4 and prevents its binding to CD80/86, thus maintaining the activated state of the T cell (and running some risk for autoimmunity) [145]. This antibody is approved for the treatment of therapy-resistant metastatic melanoma [146], and has been in clinical trials for patients with brain metastases [146]. There is currently a clinical trial open for patients with recurrent GBM utilizing this drug (NCT02017717, at ClinicalTrials.gov) as well as the anti-PD-1 antibody nivolumab (below).

PD-1 and PD-1L/PD-2L are another pair of T cell inhibitory receptors/ligands. The ligands PD-1L or PD-2L are often upregulated on cancer cells, where engagement with PD1 on T cells leads to T cell apoptosis [147]. Nivolumab is an antibody directed against PD-1 that prevents interaction with surface ligands on other cells, thus preventing the immune suppression induced by the tumor [147]. As mentioned, this antibody is used along with ipilimumab as checkpoint blockades in a clinical trial for patients with recurrent gliomas.

## 8. Conclusion

Glioblastoma Multiforme (GBM) remains the most common CNS malignancy with abysmal prognosis. Our current GBM therapies are clearly inadequate stressing the need for new treatment modalities. Immunotherapy is an emerging cancer treatment, potentially utilized alongside surgery, radiation, and chemotherapy. The dynamic interactions within the tumor microenvironment dictate the balance between tumor elimination and escape. Additionally, high-grade gliomas employ a multitude of strategies to evade the immune system. Early trials, however, using anti-tumor vaccines and adoptive cell therapy have demonstrated the potential anti-tumor efficacy and feasibility of such approaches. Moreover, several promising phase III trials are underway, and continual research provides more information and more data that indicate immunotherapy is a viable option for the treatment of patients with these devastating diseases.

## Author details

Soliman Oushy* and Michael W. Graner

Department of Neurosurgery,University of Colorado School of Medicine, Anschutz Medical Campus, Aurora, USA

## References

[1] Thomas L. On immunosurveillance in human cancer. The Yale journal of biology and medicine. 1982;55(3-4):329-33.

[2] Shinkai Y, Rathbun G, Lam KP, Oltz EM, Stewart V, Mendelsohn M, et al. RAG-2-deficient mice lack mature lymphocytes owing to inability to initiate V(D)J rearrangement. Cell. 1992;68(5):855-67.

[3] Shankaran V, Ikeda H, Bruce AT, White JM, Swanson PE, Old LJ, et al. IFNgamma and lymphocytes prevent primary tumour development and shape tumour immunogenicity. Nature. 2001;410(6832):1107-11.

[4] Hou W, Zhang Q, Yan Z, Chen R, Zeh Iii HJ, Kang R, et al. Strange attractors: DAMPs and autophagy link tumor cell death and immunity. Cell Death Dis. 2013;4:e966.

[5] Huergo-Zapico L, Acebes-Huerta A, Lopez-Soto A, Villa-Alvarez M, Gonzalez-Rodriguez AP, Gonzalez S. Molecular Bases for the Regulation of NKG2D Ligands in Cancer. Frontiers in immunology. 2014;5:106.

[6] Pardoll D. Does the immune system see tumors as foreign or self? Annu Rev Immunol. 2003;21:807-39.

[7] Quezada SA, Peggs KS, Simpson TR, Allison JP. Shifting the equilibrium in cancer immunoediting: from tumor tolerance to eradication. Immunol Rev. 2011;241(1): 104-18.

[8] Quesnel B. Tumor dormancy and immunoescape. APMIS : acta pathologica, microbiologica, et immunologica Scandinavica. 2008;116(7-8):685-94.

[9] Udagawa T. Tumor dormancy of primary and secondary cancers. APMIS : acta pathologica, microbiologica, et immunologica Scandinavica. 2008;116(7-8):615-28.

[10] Mittal D, Gubin MM, Schreiber RD, Smyth MJ. New insights into cancer immunoediting and its three component phases--elimination, equilibrium and escape. Curr Opin Immunol. 2014;27:16-25.

[11] White MK, Pagano JS, Khalili K. Viruses and Human Cancers: a Long Road of Discovery of Molecular Paradigms. Clin Microbiol Rev. 2014;27(3):463-81.

[12] Srivastava N, Srivastava PK. Modeling the repertoire of true tumor-specific MHC I epitopes in a human tumor. PLoS One. 2009;4(7):e6094.

[13] Milani A, Sangiolo D, Montemurro F, Aglietta M, Valabrega G. Active immunotherapy in HER2 overexpressing breast cancer: current status and future perspectives. Ann Oncol. 2013;24(7):1740-8.

[14] Vigneron N, Stroobant V, Van den Eynde BJ, van der Bruggen P. Database of T cell-defined human tumor antigens: the 2013 update. Cancer Immun. 2013;13:15.

[15] Lee PP, Yee C, Savage PA, Fong L, Brockstedt D, Weber JS, et al. Characterization of circulating T cells specific for tumor-associated antigens in melanoma patients. Nat Med. 1999;5(6):677-85.

[16] Boon T, Coulie PG, Van den Eynde BJ, van der Bruggen P. Human T cell responses against melanoma. Annu Rev Immunol. 2006;24:175-208.

[17] Kennedy R, Celis E. Multiple roles for CD4+T cells in anti-tumor immune responses. Immunol Rev. 2008;222:129-44.

[18] Yokoyama WM, Kim S, French AR. The dynamic life of natural killer cells. Annu Rev Immunol. 2004;22:405-29.

[19] Komohara Y, Jinushi M, Takeya M. Clinical significance of macrophage heterogeneity in human malignant tumors. Cancer Sci. 2014;105(1):1-8.

[20] Ueno H, Klechevsky E, Morita R, Aspord C, Cao T, Matsui T, et al. Dendritic cell subsets in health and disease. Immunol Rev. 2007;219:118-42.

[21] Tan HT, Low J, Lim SG, Chung MC. Serum autoantibodies as biomarkers for early cancer detection. FEBS J. 2009;276(23):6880-904.

[22] Brandlein S, Pohle T, Ruoff N, Wozniak E, Muller-Hermelink HK, Vollmers HP. Natural IgM antibodies and immunosurveillance mechanisms against epithelial cancer cells in humans. Cancer Res. 2003;63(22):7995-8005.

[23] Schmittling RJ, Archer GE, Mitchell DA, Heimberger A, Pegram C, Herndon JE, 2nd, et al. Detection of humoral response in patients with glioblastoma receiving EGFRvIII-KLH vaccines. J Immunol Methods. 2008;339(1):74-81.

[24] Dustin ML, Chakraborty AK, Shaw AS. Understanding the structure and function of the immunological synapse. Cold Spring Harbor perspectives in biology. 2010;2(10):a002311.

[25] CA J, P T, M W, M S. Immunobiology 5: The Immune System in Health and Disease. 5 ed. New York: Garland Publishers; 2001.

[26] Sanchez-Perez L, Kottke T, Diaz RM, Ahmed A, Thompson J, Chong H, et al. Potent selection of antigen loss variants of B16 melanoma following inflammatory killing of melanocytes in vivo. Cancer Res. 2005;65(5):2009-17.

[27] Slingluff CL, Jr., Chianese-Bullock KA, Bullock TN, Grosh WW, Mullins DW, Nichols L, et al. Immunity to melanoma antigens: from self-tolerance to immunotherapy. Adv Immunol. 2006;90:243-95.

[28] Bubenik J. MHC class I down-regulation: tumour escape from immune surveillance? (review). Int J Oncol. 2004;25(2):487-91.

[29] Baragano Raneros A, Suarez-Alvarez B, Lopez-Larrea C. Secretory pathways generating immunosuppressive NKG2D ligands: New targets for therapeutic intervention. Oncoimmunology. 2014;3:e28497.

[30] Ullrich E, Koch J, Cerwenka A, Steinle A. New prospects on the NKG2D/NKG2DL system for oncology. Oncoimmunology. 2013;2(10):e26097.

[31] Steinert G, Scholch S, Niemietz T, Iwata N, Garcia SA, Behrens B, et al. Immune escape and survival mechanisms in circulating tumor cells of colorectal cancer. Cancer Res. 2014;74(6):1694-704.

[32] Ramaswamy M, Cleland SY, Cruz AC, Siegel RM. Many checkpoints on the road to cell death: regulation of Fas-FasL interactions and Fas signaling in peripheral immune responses. Results and problems in cell differentiation. 2009;49:17-47.

[33] Hau P, Jachimczak P, Schlaier J, Bogdahn U. TGF-beta2 signaling in high-grade gliomas. Curr Pharm Biotechnol. 2011;12(12):2150-7.

[34] Huettner C, Czub S, Kerkau S, Roggendorf W, Tonn JC. Interleukin 10 is expressed in human gliomas in vivo and increases glioma cell proliferation and motility in vitro. Anticancer Res. 1997;17(5A):3217-24.

[35] Nitta T, Hishii M, Sato K, Okumura K. Selective expression of interleukin-10 gene within glioblastoma multiforme. Brain Res. 1994;649(1-2):122-8.

[36] Sakaguchi S, Powrie F. Emerging challenges in regulatory T cell function and biology. Science. 2007;317(5838):627-9.

[37] Heimberger AB, Abou-Ghazal M, Reina-Ortiz C, Yang DS, Sun W, Qiao W, et al. Incidence and prognostic impact of FoxP3+regulatory T cells in human gliomas. Clin Cancer Res. 2008;14(16):5166-72.

[38] Gobert M, Treilleux I, Bendriss-Vermare N, Bachelot T, Goddard-Leon S, Arfi V, et al. Regulatory T cells recruited through CCL22/CCR4 are selectively activated in lymphoid infiltrates surrounding primary breast tumors and lead to an adverse clinical outcome. Cancer Res. 2009;69(5):2000-9.

[39] Olkhanud PB, Baatar D, Bodogai M, Hakim F, Gress R, Anderson RL, et al. Breast cancer lung metastasis requires expression of chemokine receptor CCR4 and regulatory T cells. Cancer Res. 2009;69(14):5996-6004.

[40] Bacic D, Uravic M, Bacic R, Sutic I, Petrosic N. Augmentation of regulatory T cells (CD4+CD25+Foxp3+) correlates with tumor stage in patients with colorectal cancer. Collegium antropologicum. 2011;35 Suppl 2:65-8.

[41] Lindau D, Gielen P, Kroesen M, Wesseling P, Adema GJ. The immunosuppressive tumour network: myeloid-derived suppressor cells, regulatory T cells and natural killer T cells. Immunology. 2013;138(2):105-15.

[42] Gabrilovich DI, Nagaraj S. Myeloid-derived suppressor cells as regulators of the immune system. Nat Rev Immunol. 2009;9(3):162-74.

[43] Biswas SK, Mantovani A. Macrophage plasticity and interaction with lymphocyte subsets: cancer as a paradigm. Nat Immunol. 2010;11(10):889-96.

[44] Youn JI, Kumar V, Collazo M, Nefedova Y, Condamine T, Cheng P, et al. Epigenetic silencing of retinoblastoma gene regulates pathologic differentiation of myeloid cells in cancer. Nat Immunol. 2013;14(3):211-20.

[45] Khaled YS, Ammori BJ, Elkord E. Myeloid-derived suppressor cells in cancer: recent progress and prospects. Immunol Cell Biol. 2013;91(8):493-502.

[46] Abbott NJ, Ronnback L, Hansson E. Astrocyte-endothelial interactions at the blood-brain barrier. Nat Rev Neurosci. 2006;7(1):41-53.

[47] McMahon EJ, Bailey SL, Miller SD. CNS dendritic cells: critical participants in CNS inflammation? Neurochem Int. 2006;49(2):195-203.

[48] Aloisi F. Immune function of microglia. Glia. 2001;36(2):165-79.

[49] Hickey WF, Hsu BL, Kimura H. T-lymphocyte entry into the central nervous system. J Neurosci Res. 1991;28(2):254-60.

[50] Bullard DE, Bigner DD. Applications of monoclonal antibodies in the diagnosis and treatment of primary brain tumors. J Neurosurg. 1985;63(1):2-16.

[51] Engelhardt B. Immune cell entry into the central nervous system: involvement of adhesion molecules and chemokines. J Neurol Sci. 2008;274(1-2):23-6.

[52] Stupp R, Mason WP, van den Bent MJ, Weller M, Fisher B, Taphoorn MJ, et al. Radiotherapy plus concomitant and adjuvant temozolomide for glioblastoma. N Engl J Med. 2005;352(10):987-96.

[53] Verhaak RG, Hoadley KA, Purdom E, Wang V, Qi Y, Wilkerson MD, et al. Integrated genomic analysis identifies clinically relevant subtypes of glioblastoma characterized by abnormalities in PDGFRA, IDH1, EGFR, and NF1. Cancer Cell. 2010;17(1):98-110.

[54] Ohgaki H, Kleihues P. Genetic pathways to primary and secondary glioblastoma. Am J Pathol. 2007;170(5):1445-53.

[55] Reardon DA, Wucherpfennig KW, Freeman G, Wu CJ, Chiocca EA, Wen PY, et al. An update on vaccine therapy and other immunotherapeutic approaches for glioblastoma. Expert Rev Vaccines. 2013;12(6):597-615.

[56] Graner MW, Bigner DD. Chaperone proteins and brain tumors: potential targets and possible therapeutics. Neuro Oncol. 2005;7(3):260-78.

[57] Yang I, Fang S, Parsa AT. Heat shock proteins in glioblastomas. Neurosurg Clin N Am. 2010;21(1):111-23.

[58] Fecci PE, Mitchell DA, Whitesides JF, Xie W, Friedman AH, Archer GE, et al. Increased regulatory T-cell fraction amidst a diminished CD4 compartment explains cellular immune defects in patients with malignant glioma. Cancer Res. 2006;66(6): 3294-302.

[59] Humphries W, Wei J, Sampson JH, Heimberger AB. The role of tregs in glioma-mediated immunosuppression: potential target for intervention. Neurosurg Clin N Am. 2010;21(1):125-37.

[60] Waziri A. Glioblastoma-derived mechanisms of systemic immunosuppression. Neurosurg Clin N Am. 2010;21(1):31-42.

[61] Jones A. Cerebral astrocytomata--trends in radiotherapy and chemotherapy: a review. Journal of the Royal Society of Medicine. 1978;71(9):669-74.

[62] Westphal M, Hilt DC, Bortey E, Delavault P, Olivares R, Warnke PC, et al. A phase 3 trial of local chemotherapy with biodegradable carmustine (BCNU) wafers (Gliadel wafers) in patients with primary malignant glioma. Neuro Oncol. 2003;5(2):79-88.

[63] Weber EL, Goebel EA. Cerebral edema associated with Gliadel wafers: two case studies. Neuro Oncol. 2005;7(1):84-9.

[64] Gallego JM, Barcia JA, Barcia-Marino C. Fatal outcome related to carmustine implants in glioblastoma multiforme. Acta neurochirurgica. 2007;149(3):261-5; discussion 5.

[65] Weller M, Cloughesy T, Perry JR, Wick W. Standards of care for treatment of recurrent glioblastoma--are we there yet? Neuro Oncol. 2013;15(1):4-27.

[66] Roos WP, Batista LF, Naumann SC, Wick W, Weller M, Menck CF, et al. Apoptosis in malignant glioma cells triggered by the temozolomide-induced DNA lesion O6-methylguanine. Oncogene. 2007;26(2):186-97.

[67] Villano JL, Seery TE, Bressler LR. Temozolomide in malignant gliomas: current use and future targets. Cancer Chemother Pharmacol. 2009;64(4):647-55.

[68] Koukourakis GV, Kouloulias V, Zacharias G, Papadimitriou C, Pantelakos P, Maravelis G, et al. Temozolomide with radiation therapy in high grade brain gliomas: pharmaceuticals considerations and efficacy; a review article. Molecules. 2009;14(4): 1561-77.

[69] Sarkaria JN, Kitange GJ, James CD, Plummer R, Calvert H, Weller M, et al. Mechanisms of chemoresistance to alkylating agents in malignant glioma. Clin Cancer Res. 2008;14(10):2900-8.

[70] Buckner JC, Ballman KV, Michalak JC, Burton GV, Cascino TL, Schomberg PJ, et al. Phase III trial of carmustine and cisplatin compared with carmustine alone and standard radiation therapy or accelerated radiation therapy in patients with glioblastoma multiforme: North Central Cancer Treatment Group 93-72-52 and Southwest Oncology Group 9503 Trials. J Clin Oncol. 2006;24(24):3871-9.

[71] Debinski W. An immune regulatory cytokine receptor and glioblastoma multiforme: an unexpected link. Crit Rev Oncog. 1998;9(3-4):255-68.

[72] Hatano M, Eguchi J, Tatsumi T, Kuwashima N, Dusak JE, Kinch MS, et al. EphA2 as a glioma-associated antigen: a novel target for glioma vaccines. Neoplasia. 2005;7(8): 717-22.

[73] Batra SK, Castelino-Prabhu S, Wikstrand CJ, Zhu X, Humphrey PA, Friedman HS, et al. Epidermal growth factor ligand-independent, unregulated, cell-transforming potential of a naturally occurring human mutant EGFRvIII gene. Cell Growth Differ. 1995;6(10):1251-9.

[74] Chu CT, Everiss KD, Wikstrand CJ, Batra SK, Kung HJ, Bigner DD. Receptor dimerization is not a factor in the signalling activity of a transforming variant epidermal growth factor receptor (EGFRvIII). Biochem J. 1997;324 (Pt 3):855-61.

[75] Wikstrand CJ, Reist CJ, Archer GE, Zalutsky MR, Bigner DD. The class III variant of the epidermal growth factor receptor (EGFRvIII): characterization and utilization as an immunotherapeutic target. J Neurovirol. 1998;4(2):148-58.

[76] Cheung CH, Huang CC, Tsai FY, Lee JY, Cheng SM, Chang YC, et al. Survivin-biology and potential as a therapeutic target in oncology. OncoTargets and therapy. 2013;6:1453-62.

[77] Lv S, Dai C, Liu Y, Shi R, Tang Z, Han M, et al. The Impact of Survivin on Prognosis and Clinicopathology of Glioma Patients: A Systematic Meta-Analysis. Mol Neurobiol. 2014.

[78] Miller-Hodges E, Hohenstein P. WT1 in disease: shifting the epithelial-mesenchymal balance. J Pathol. 2012;226(2):229-40.

[79] Rushing EJ, Sandberg GD, Horkayne-Szakaly I. High-grade astrocytomas show increased Nestin and Wilms's tumor gene (WT1) protein expression. International journal of surgical pathology. 2010;18(4):255-9.

[80] Yang L, Han Y, Suarez Saiz F, Minden MD. A tumor suppressor and oncogene: the WT1 story. Leukemia. 2007;21(5):868-76.

[81] Oka Y, Tsuboi A, Elisseeva OA, Udaka K, Sugiyama H. WT1 as a novel target antigen for cancer immunotherapy. Curr Cancer Drug Targets. 2002;2(1):45-54.

[82] Castillo SD, Sanchez-Cespedes M. The SOX family of genes in cancer development: biological relevance and opportunities for therapy. Expert Opin Ther Targets. 2012;16(9):903-19.

[83] de la Rocha AM, Sampron N, Alonso MM, Matheu A. Role of SOX family of transcription factors in central nervous system tumors. American journal of cancer research. 2014;4(4):312-24.

[84] Ikushima H, Todo T, Ino Y, Takahashi M, Saito N, Miyazawa K, et al. Glioma-initiating cells retain their tumorigenicity through integration of the Sox axis and Oct4 protein. J Biol Chem. 2011;286(48):41434-41.

[85] Webster WS, Thompson RH, Harris KJ, Frigola X, Kuntz S, Inman BA, et al. Targeting molecular and cellular inhibitory mechanisms for improvement of antitumor memory responses reactivated by tumor cell vaccine. J Immunol. 2007;179(5):2860-9.

[86] Okada H, Lieberman FS, Walter KA, Lunsford LD, Kondziolka DS, Bejjani GK, et al. Autologous glioma cell vaccine admixed with interleukin-4 gene transfected fibroblasts in the treatment of patients with malignant gliomas. J Transl Med. 2007;5:67.

[87] Wikstrand CJ, Bigner DD. Immunobiologic aspects of the brain and human gliomas. A review. Am J Pathol. 1980;98(2):517-68.

[88] Schneider T, Gerhards R, Kirches E, Firsching R. Preliminary results of active specific immunization with modified tumor cell vaccine in glioblastoma multiforme. J Neurooncol. 2001;53(1):39-46.

[89] Xu LW, Chow KK, Lim M, Li G. Current vaccine trials in glioblastoma: a review. Journal of immunology research. 2014;2014:796856.

[90] Sampson JH, Heimberger AB, Archer GE, Aldape KD, Friedman AH, Friedman HS, et al. Immunologic escape after prolonged progression-free survival with epidermal growth factor receptor variant III peptide vaccination in patients with newly diagnosed glioblastoma. J Clin Oncol. 2010;28(31):4722-9.

[91] Okada H, Kalinski P, Ueda R, Hoji A, Kohanbash G, Donegan TE, et al. Induction of CD8+T-cell responses against novel glioma-associated antigen peptides and clinical activity by vaccinations with {alpha}-type 1 polarized dendritic cells and polyinosinic-polycytidylic acid stabilized by lysine and carboxymethylcellulose in patients with recurrent malignant glioma. J Clin Oncol. 2011;29(3):330-6.

[92] Sampson JH, Archer GE, Mitchell DA, Heimberger AB, Herndon JE, 2nd, Lally-Goss D, et al. An epidermal growth factor receptor variant III-targeted vaccine is safe and immunogenic in patients with glioblastoma multiforme. Mol Cancer Ther. 2009;8(10): 2773-9.

[93] Hailemichael Y, Overwijk WW. Peptide-based anticancer vaccines: The making and unmaking of a T-cell graveyard. Oncoimmunology. 2013;2(7):e24743.

[94] Baxevanis CN, Voutsas IF, Tsitsilonis OE. Toll-like receptor agonists: current status and future perspective on their utility as adjuvants in improving anticancer vaccination strategies. Immunotherapy. 2013;5(5):497-511.

[95] Decker WK, Safdar A. Cytokine adjuvants for vaccine therapy of neoplastic and infectious disease. Cytokine Growth Factor Rev. 2011;22(4):177-87.

[96] Graner MW, Bigner DD. Therapeutic aspects of chaperones/heat-shock proteins in neuro-oncology. Expert Rev Anticancer Ther. 2006;6(5):679-95.

[97] Zaritskaya L, Shurin MR, Sayers TJ, Malyguine AM. New flow cytometric assays for monitoring cell-mediated cytotoxicity. Expert Rev Vaccines. 2010;9(6):601-16.

[98] Ogi C, Aruga A. Immunological monitoring of anticancer vaccines in clinical trials. Oncoimmunology. 2013;2(8):e26012.

[99] Glassman PM, Balthasar JP. Mechanistic considerations for the use of monoclonal antibodies for cancer therapy. Cancer biology & medicine. 2014;11(1):20-33.

[100] Norden AD, Drappatz J, Wen PY. Novel anti-angiogenic therapies for malignant gliomas. Lancet neurology. 2008;7(12):1152-60.

[101] Sampson JH, Crotty LE, Lee S, Archer GE, Ashley DM, Wikstrand CJ, et al. Unarmed, tumor-specific monoclonal antibody effectively treats brain tumors. Proc Natl Acad Sci U S A. 2000;97(13):7503-8.

[102] Luwor RB, Johns TG, Murone C, Huang HJ, Cavenee WK, Ritter G, et al. Monoclonal antibody 806 inhibits the growth of tumor xenografts expressing either the de2-7 or amplified epidermal growth factor receptor (EGFR) but not wild-type EGFR. Cancer Res. 2001;61(14):5355-61.

[103] Scott AM, Lee FT, Tebbutt N, Herbertson R, Gill SS, Liu Z, et al. A phase I clinical trial with monoclonal antibody ch806 targeting transitional state and mutant epidermal growth factor receptors. Proc Natl Acad Sci U S A. 2007;104(10):4071-6.

[104] Reist CJ, Archer GE, Kurpad SN, Wikstrand CJ, Vaidyanathan G, Willingham MC, et al. Tumor-specific anti-epidermal growth factor receptor variant III monoclonal antibodies: use of the tyramine-cellobiose radioiodination method enhances cellular retention and uptake in tumor xenografts. Cancer Res. 1995;55(19):4375-82.

[105] Yang W, Wu G, Barth RF, Swindall MR, Bandyopadhyaya AK, Tjarks W, et al. Molecular targeting and treatment of composite EGFR and EGFRvIII-positive gliomas using boronated monoclonal antibodies. Clin Cancer Res. 2008;14(3):883-91.

[106] Faillot T, Magdelenat H, Mady E, Stasiecki P, Fohanno D, Gropp P, et al. A phase I study of an anti-epidermal growth factor receptor monoclonal antibody for the treatment of malignant gliomas. Neurosurgery. 1996;39(3):478-83.

[107] Stragliotto G, Vega F, Stasiecki P, Gropp P, Poisson M, Delattre JY. Multiple infusions of anti-epidermal growth factor receptor (EGFR) monoclonal antibody (EMD 55,900) in patients with recurrent malignant gliomas. Eur J Cancer. 1996;32A(4):636-40.

[108] Neyns B, Sadones J, Joosens E, Bouttens F, Verbeke L, Baurain JF, et al. Stratified phase II trial of cetuximab in patients with recurrent high-grade glioma. Ann Oncol. 2009;20(9):1596-603.

[109] Bode U, Massimino M, Bach F, Zimmermann M, Khuhlaeva E, Westphal M, et al. Nimotuzumab treatment of malignant gliomas. Expert Opin Biol Ther. 2012;12(12): 1649-59.

[110] Anguille S, Smits EL, Lion E, van Tendeloo VF, Berneman ZN. Clinical use of dendritic cells for cancer therapy. Lancet Oncol. 2014;15(7):e257-67.

[111] Yu JS, Wheeler CJ, Zeltzer PM, Ying H, Finger DN, Lee PK, et al. Vaccination of malignant glioma patients with peptide-pulsed dendritic cells elicits systemic cytotoxicity and intracranial T-cell infiltration. Cancer Res. 2001;61(3):842-7.

[112] Akasaki Y, Black KL, Yu JS. T cell immunity in patients with malignant glioma: recent progress in dendritic cell-based immunotherapeutic approaches. Front Biosci. 2005;10:2908-21.

[113] Liau LM, Prins RM, Kiertscher SM, Odesa SK, Kremen TJ, Giovannone AJ, et al. Dendritic cell vaccination in glioblastoma patients induces systemic and intracranial T-cell responses modulated by the local central nervous system tumor microenvironment. Clin Cancer Res. 2005;11(15):5515-25.

[114] Prins RM, Wang X, Soto H, Young E, Lisiero DN, Fong B, et al. Comparison of glioma-associated antigen peptide-loaded versus autologous tumor lysate-loaded dendritic cell vaccination in malignant glioma patients. J Immunother. 2013;36(2):152-7.

[115] Prins RM, Soto H, Konkankit V, Odesa SK, Eskin A, Yong WH, et al. Gene expression profile correlates with T-cell infiltration and relative survival in glioblastoma patients vaccinated with dendritic cell immunotherapy. Clin Cancer Res. 2011;17(6):1603-15.

[116] Boczkowski D, Nair SK, Snyder D, Gilboa E. Dendritic cells pulsed with RNA are potent antigen-presenting cells in vitro and in vivo. J Exp Med. 1996;184(2):465-72.

[117] Vik-Mo EO, Nyakas M, Mikkelsen BV, Moe MC, Due-Tonnesen P, Suso EM, et al. Therapeutic vaccination against autologous cancer stem cells with mRNA-transfected dendritic cells in patients with glioblastoma. Cancer Immunol Immunother. 2013;62(9):1499-509.

[118] Steinbok P, Thomas JP, Grossman L, Dolman CL. Intratumoral autologous mononuclear cells in the treatment of recurrent glioblastoma multiforme. A phase 1 (toxicity) study. J Neurooncol. 1984;2(2):147-51.

[119] Ransohoff RM, Kivisakk P, Kidd G. Three or more routes for leukocyte migration into the central nervous system. Nat Rev Immunol. 2003;3(7):569-81.

[120] Rosenberg SA, Restifo NP, Yang JC, Morgan RA, Dudley ME. Adoptive cell transfer: a clinical path to effective cancer immunotherapy. Nat Rev Cancer. 2008;8(4):299-308.

[121] Morgan RA, Dudley ME, Wunderlich JR, Hughes MS, Yang JC, Sherry RM, et al. Cancer regression in patients after transfer of genetically engineered lymphocytes. Science. 2006;314(5796):126-9.

[122] Ishikawa E, Takano S, Ohno T, Tsuboi K. Adoptive cell transfer therapy for malignant gliomas. Adv Exp Med Biol. 2012;746:109-20.

[123] Kong S, Sengupta S, Tyler B, Bais AJ, Ma Q, Doucette S, et al. Suppression of human glioma xenografts with second-generation IL13R-specific chimeric antigen receptor-modified T cells. Clin Cancer Res. 2012;18(21):5949-60.

[124] Ahmed N, Salsman VS, Kew Y, Shaffer D, Powell S, Zhang YJ, et al. HER2-specific T cells target primary glioblastoma stem cells and induce regression of autologous experimental tumors. Clin Cancer Res. 2010;16(2):474-85.

[125] Sampson JH, Choi BD, Sanchez-Perez L, Suryadevara CM, Snyder DJ, Flores CT, et al. EGFRvIII mCAR-modified T-cell therapy cures mice with established intracere-

bral glioma and generates host immunity against tumor-antigen loss. Clin Cancer Res. 2014;20(4):972-84.

[126] Lillehei KO, Mitchell DH, Johnson SD, McCleary EL, Kruse CA. Long-term follow-up of patients with recurrent malignant gliomas treated with adjuvant adoptive immunotherapy. Neurosurgery. 1991;28(1):16-23.

[127] Hayes RL, Koslow M, Hiesiger EM, Hymes KB, Hochster HS, Moore EJ, et al. Improved long term survival after intracavitary interleukin-2 and lymphokine-activated killer cells for adults with recurrent malignant glioma. Cancer. 1995;76(5):840-52.

[128] Boyman O, Letourneau S, Krieg C, Sprent J. Homeostatic proliferation and survival of naive and memory T cells. Eur J Immunol. 2009;39(8):2088-94.

[129] Hershkovitz L, Schachter J, Treves AJ, Besser MJ. Focus on adoptive T cell transfer trials in melanoma. Clin Dev Immunol. 2010;2010:260267.

[130] Sampson JH, Aldape KD, Archer GE, Coan A, Desjardins A, Friedman AH, et al. Greater chemotherapy-induced lymphopenia enhances tumor-specific immune responses that eliminate EGFRvIII-expressing tumor cells in patients with glioblastoma. Neuro Oncol. 2011;13(3):324-33.

[131] Mitchell DA, Cui X, Schmittling RJ, Sanchez-Perez L, Snyder DJ, Congdon KL, et al. Monoclonal antibody blockade of IL-2 receptor alpha during lymphopenia selectively depletes regulatory T cells in mice and humans. Blood. 2011;118(11):3003-12.

[132] Neyns B, Tosoni A, Hwu WJ, Reardon DA. Dose-dense temozolomide regimens: antitumor activity, toxicity, and immunomodulatory effects. Cancer. 2010;116(12): 2868-77.

[133] Mohyeldin A, Chiocca EA. Gene and viral therapy for glioblastoma: a review of clinical trials and future directions. Cancer J. 2012;18(1):82-8.

[134] Sze DY, Reid TR, Rose SC. Oncolytic virotherapy. Journal of vascular and interventional radiology : JVIR. 2013;24(8):1115-22.

[135] Moolten FL, Wells JM. Curability of tumors bearing herpes thymidine kinase genes transferred by retroviral vectors. J Natl Cancer Inst. 1990;82(4):297-300.

[136] Ram Z, Culver KW, Oshiro EM, Viola JJ, DeVroom HL, Otto E, et al. Therapy of malignant brain tumors by intratumoral implantation of retroviral vector-producing cells. Nat Med. 1997;3(12):1354-61.

[137] Rainov NG. A phase III clinical evaluation of herpes simplex virus type 1 thymidine kinase and ganciclovir gene therapy as an adjuvant to surgical resection and radiation in adults with previously untreated glioblastoma multiforme. Hum Gene Ther. 2000;11(17):2389-401.

[138] Price RL, Chiocca EA. Evolution of malignant glioma treatment: from chemotherapy to vaccines to viruses. Neurosurgery. 2014;61 Suppl 1:74-83.

[139] Markert JM, Medlock MD, Rabkin SD, Gillespie GY, Todo T, Hunter WD, et al. Conditionally replicating herpes simplex virus mutant, G207 for the treatment of malignant glioma: results of a phase I trial. Gene Ther. 2000;7(10):867-74.

[140] Markert JM, Liechty PG, Wang W, Gaston S, Braz E, Karrasch M, et al. Phase Ib trial of mutant herpes simplex virus G207 inoculated pre-and post-tumor resection for recurrent GBM. Mol Ther. 2009;17(1):199-207.

[141] Grandi P, Peruzzi P, Reinhart B, Cohen JB, Chiocca EA, Glorioso JC. Design and application of oncolytic HSV vectors for glioblastoma therapy. Expert Rev Neurother. 2009;9(4):505-17.

[142] Dey M, Ulasov IV, Lesniak MS. Virotherapy against malignant glioma stem cells. Cancer Lett. 2010;289(1):1-10.

[143] Dobrikova EY, Goetz C, Walters RW, Lawson SK, Peggins JO, Muszynski K, et al. Attenuation of neurovirulence, biodistribution, and shedding of a poliovirus:rhinovirus chimera after intrathalamic inoculation in Macaca fascicularis. J Virol. 2012;86(5): 2750-9.

[144] Goetz C, Gromeier M. Preparing an oncolytic poliovirus recombinant for clinical application against glioblastoma multiforme. Cytokine Growth Factor Rev. 2010;21(2-3):197-203.

[145] Patel SP, Woodman SE. Profile of ipilimumab and its role in the treatment of metastatic melanoma. Drug design, development and therapy. 2011;5:489-95.

[146] Queirolo P, Spagnolo F, Ascierto PA, Simeone E, Marchetti P, Scoppola A, et al. Efficacy and safety of ipilimumab in patients with advanced melanoma and brain metastases. J Neurooncol. 2014;118(1):109-16.

[147] Mamalis A, Garcha M, Jagdeo J. Targeting the PD-1 pathway: a promising future for the treatment of melanoma. Archives of dermatological research. 2014;306(6):511-9.

Section 4

# Herbal Medicine Treatments for Brain Tumors

Chapter 17

# Clinical Effects of Saireito for Patients with Advanced Stage Glioblastoma

Yasushi Shibata

Additional information is available at the end of the chapter

http://dx.doi.org/10.5772/58979

## 1. Introduction

Glioblastoma is the one of the most malignant brain tumors. The average survival of patients with glioblastoma is approximately one year, despite aggressive therapeutic efforts. Glioblastoma is associated with peritumoral brain edema. This brain edema is caused by tumor infiltration into the normal brain and breakdown of the blood brain barrier. Osmotic diuretics, like glycerol and mannitol, are frequently used to reduce brain edema. The effective duration of these osmotic diuretics is a few hours, so frequent intravenous infusions are required to control brain edema in these patients. Steroids are effective for repairing the damaged blood brain barrier. Therefore, the patients with advanced glioblastoma need to be administered long-term osmotic diuretics and steroids. Both of these types of agents have various side effects. Saireito is a commercially available Chinese herbal medicine that combines Syousaikotou and Goreisan, both of them are also commercially available Chinese herbal medicine. Syousaikotou has steroid-like effects and Goreisan has a diuretic effect. There have been some clinical reports of a beneficial effect of Saireito or Goreisan for chronic subdural hematoma and other conditions. However, there have been no reports about the clinical effects of Saireito in patients with malignant brain tumors. We evaluated the clinical effects of Saireito for patients with advanced stage glioblastoma.

## 2. Patients and methods

Saireito was administered to eight patients diagnosed with advanced stage glioblastoma. The tumor locations were cerebral in seven cases and in the pons in one case. There were four males and four females. The age of the patients ranged from 38 to 86 years old. Seven patients underwent tumor resection and were pathologically diagnosed with glioblastoma. One patient did not receive surgery because of the high age, so glioblastoma was diagnosed clinically. The seven patients who received surgery were treated with postoperative radiation and chemotherapy. Five patients underwent repeat surgery and additional radiation therapy for recurrence. All patients received temozolomide chemotherapy and interferon immunotherapy wherever possible. Saireito (2.7 g) was given three times a day for all patients with advanced stage disease. Saireito was given through a nasogastric tube for the patients who could not take the medication orally.

## 3. Representative case report

A 74-year-old male presenting with memory disturbance and right hemiparesis was diagnosed to have a left frontal brain tumor using brain magnetic resonance imaging (MRI). The tumor was surgically removed, and the pathological diagnosis was glioblastoma. He received postsurgical radiation therapy and concomitant oral chemotherapy with temozolomide. After these initial therapies, maintenance chemotherapy with temozolomide and intravenous infusion of interferon were continued. His consciousness deteriorated one year after the initial therapy. He could not take medication orally, so we started parenteral nutrition using a nasogastric tube. Brain MRI showed an increase in bilateral frontal edema (Fig. 1). Therefore, we first administered intravenous glyceol; however, we considered permanent intravenous administration of glyceol to be difficult. Therefore, we started parenteral Saireito administration and terminated the intravenous glyceol treatment. The patient's condition remained unchanged, so he discharged, and the nasogastric parenteral nutrition and Saireito administration were continued at his home. He underwent repeat short-term hospitalization for scheduled chemotherapy and intravenous infusion of interferon (Fig. 2)

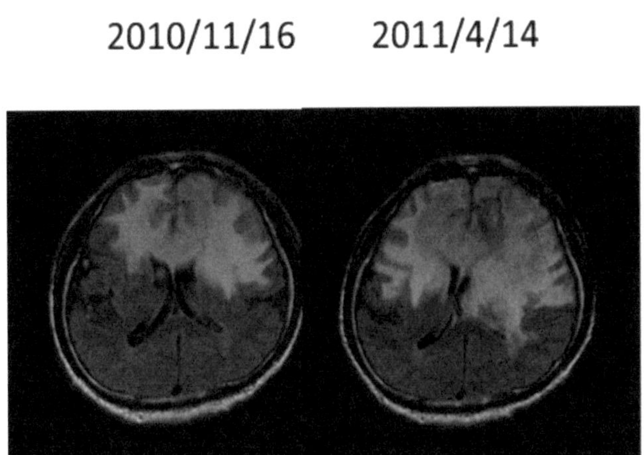


**Figure 1.** Fluid attenuated inversion recovery (FLAIR) MRI image

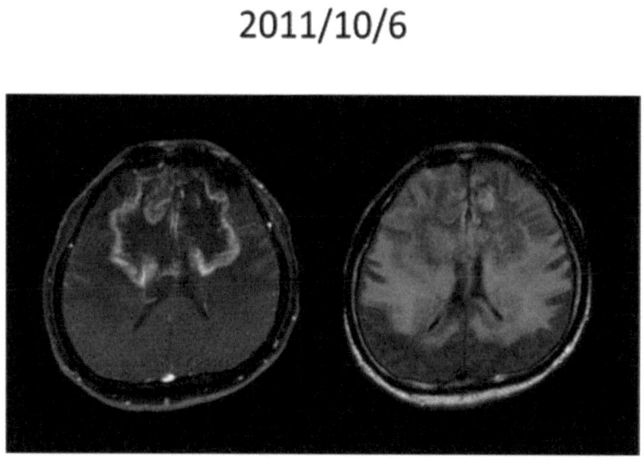


**Figure 2.** Gadolinium-DTPA enhanced T1 weighted image and FLAIR image

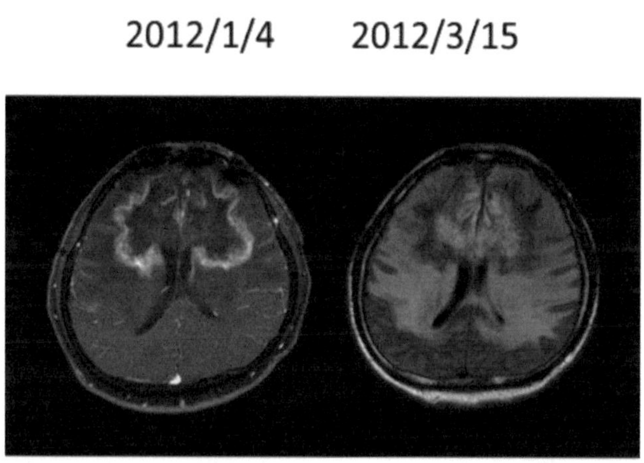


**Figure 3.** Gadolinium-DTPA enhanced T1 weighted image and FLAIR image

About one year after the initiation of Saireito, he developed intestinal bleeding and pleural effusion. Chest and abdominal computed tomography showed multiple tumors. The parenteral nutrition and medication were terminated. He died because of intestinal bleeding two years after the initial diagnosis of the brain tumor. The final brain MRI showed a stable brain tumor and perifocal edema (Fig. 3). The tumor diameter on fluid attenuated inversion recovery (FLAIR) and gadolinium-diethylene triamine pentaacetic acid (DTPA)-enhanced T1-weighted MRI (GdT1) was plotted in Figure 4. Before the administration of Saireito, the tumor diameter in FLAIR was continuously increasing. After the initiation of Saireito administration, the tumor diameter in FLAIR became stable, although the tumor diameter in GdT1 continuously increased. Because of his poor renal function, GdT1 MRI was not performed during the early stage of follow-up.

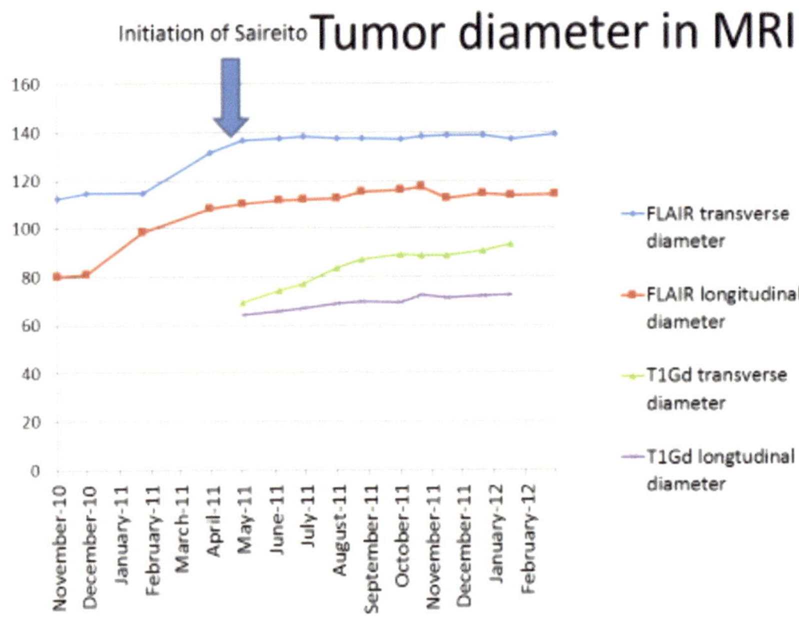


**Figure 4.** Temporal change of Tumor diameter in MRI

## 4. Results

All eight patients died. The survival time of the patients ranged from four to 35 months, with a mean of 18.4 months, and a median of 22 months. Saireito was given to all of the patients until almost the end of the life. The direct causes of death were tumor growth in four patients, central nervous system failure without tumor growth in one patient, and another malignancy, pneumonia and a hyperglycemic coma in one patient each. The continuous glycerol infusion was stopped after Saireito administration in all patients. The steroid administration was stopped for two patients and reduced for two patients after Saireito administration. The interval from the initiation of Saireito to death ranged from one to 12 months, with a mean of 5.9 months and a median of three months. The Karnofsky performance status (KPS) was used to assess the patient's general condition [1]. The KPS of all patients who received Saireito was less than 50 at the time of initiation. The radiation therapy oncology group recursive partitioning analysis (RTOG RPA) was used as an index of the prognosis [2]. The RTOG RPA of all patients who received Saireito was Stage VI. The mean prognosis of RTOG RPA Stage VI is

http://dx.doi.org/10.5772/58979

five months. Therefore, a prolongation of survival was observed for four of the eight patients. For the patients who took Saireito for less than four months, no prolongation of survival was observed. On the other hand, prolonged survival was observed in the patients who took Saireito for more than six months. No significant side effects of Saireito were observed. The administration of Saireito is covered by the Japanese health insurance system, and the cost of Saireito is less than 400 Japanese yen per day.

| Age | Sex | onset to death | Saireito Intake | Intake to death | Cause of death |
|---|---|---|---|---|---|
| 75 | M | 24 | 12 | 13 | Intestinal bleeding |
| 68 | F | 35 | 4 | 4 | neural without tumor |
| 86 | M | 4 | 2 | 2 | hyperglycemic coma |
| 62 | F | 4 | 1 | 1 | Brain Tumor |
| 59 | M | 20 | 2 | 2 | Brain Tumor |
| 58 | M | 31 | 8 | 8 | Pneumonia |
| 38 | F | 11 | 11 | 11 | Brain Tumor |
| 38 | F | 20 | 7 | 8 | Brain Tumor |
| Mean | | 19.7 | 5.9 | 6.1 | |
| Median | | 22 | 3 | 3 | |

**Table 1.** Summary of the patients

## 5. Discussion

Saireito is a mixture of Syousaikotou and Goreisan. Syousaikotou has mild steroid-like effects. In animal studies, Syousaikotou increased the secretion of corticotrophin-releasing hormone and adrenocorticotropic hormone (ACTH), resulting in an increased cortisol concentration [3] [4]. Cortisol is effective for decreasing inflammation and brain edema. Long-term administration of Saireito does not have the typical side effects of conventional steroids. Saireito and Goreisan have diuretic effects by controlling the aquaporin function at the cell membrane [5]. Long-term glycerol infusion is associated with some side effects, such as electrolyte imbalance. However, these side effects have been reported to be rare for Saireito.

There have been some clinical reports about the effective applications of Saireito and Goreisan for cerebral edema, chronic subdural hematoma and edema at the extremities [6, 7]. However, the clinical application of Saireito for malignant brain tumors has not been reported previously. The clinical effects should be confirmed by a randomized controlled study. However, the low cost and apparently rare side effects appear to be major advantages of this Chinese herbal medicine.

## 6. Conclusion

Saireito was found to be both safe and effective for patients with advanced stage glioblastoma. Some patients could stop taking glycerol and steroids. Among the eight patients evaluated in the study, death due to tumor growth was observed in four patients. A prolongation of survival was observed in four of the eight patients. This Chinese herbal medicine appears to be effective, and is associated with both a low cost and rare side effects, thereby warranting further studies in a larger number of patients.

## Acknowledgements

I appreciate my mentors, collaborators and the patients.

## Author details

Yasushi Shibata*

Department of Neurosurgery, Mito Medical Center, University of Tsukuba/ Mito Kyodo General Hospital, Mito, Ibaraki, Japan

## References

[1] Mackworth N, Fobair P, Prados MD. Quality of life self-reports from 200 brain tumor patients: comparisons with Karnofsky performance scores. J Neurooncol 1992;14:243-253.

[2] Curran WJ, Jr., Scott CB, Horton J, Nelson JS, Weinstein AS, Fischbach AJ, Chang CH, Rotman M, Asbell SO, Krisch RE, et al. Recursive partitioning analysis of prognostic factors in three Radiation Therapy Oncology Group malignant glioma trials. J Natl Cancer Inst 1993;85:704-710.

[3] Nakano Y, et. a. The effect of Saireito on the Human hypothalamic-pituitary-adrenal axis.. Hormone and clinic (In Japanese) 1993;41:97-99.

[4] Nakano Y, Suda T, Tozawa F, Dobashi I, Sato Y, Ohmori N, Sumitomo T, Demura H. Saireito (a Chinese herbal drug)-stimulated secretion and synthesis of pituitary ACTH are mediated by hypothalamic corticotropin-releasing factor. Neurosci Lett 1993;160:93-95.

[5] Isohama Y. Diuretic effect of chinese herbal medicine and aquaporin (In Japanese). Pharmacia 2011;47:1117-1120.

http://dx.doi.org/10.5772/58979

[6] Hayashi A. Effectiveness of Gorei-San for eliminating brain edema due to intracranial malignant brain tumors (In Japanese). Kampo and recent therapy (In Japanese) 2008;17:226-231.

[7] Kitahara M. Clinical effect of Saireito for chronic subdural hematoma (In Japanese). Science of Kampo Medicine 2010;34.

Chapter 18

# Cannabidiol and Cancer — An Overview of the Preclinical Data

Marta Solinas, Valentina Cinquina and
Daniela Parolaro

Additional information is available at the end of the chapter

http://dx.doi.org/10.5772/59193

## 1. Introduction

In this chapter the state of art of the pre-clinical evidences of cannabidiol (CBD) anti-tumour effects on different kinds of cancer will be discussed. As you will see in the following paragraphs, CBD is a phytocannabinoid devoid of any psychotropic activity which exerts some of its effects through modulation of different components of the endocannabinoid system. For a more clear comprehension, a brief introduction on the endocannabinoid system itself is here provided.

## 2. The endocannabinoid system: A brief overview

The endocannabinoid system (eCB) is a signalling system that consist of the cannabinoid $CB_1$ and $CB_2$ receptors, their intrinsic lipid ligands, named endocannabinoids (eCBs), such as the N-arachidonoylethanolamide (anandamide, AEA) and the 2-arachidonoylglycerol (2AG), and the associated enzymatic machinery, comprising transporters, biosynthetic and degradative enzymes. It has been recently discovered and was thoroughly explored by scientists in the past 15 years.

The cannabinoid $CB_1$ and $CB_2$ receptors are G protein coupled receptors. $CB_1$ receptors are mainly present in the central nervous system (CNS) with low to moderate expression in periphery; on the contrary, $CB_2$ receptors are highly localized in the immune system with much lower and more restricted distribution in the CNS [1,2].

Soon after the characterization of the cannabinoid receptors came the discovery of their endogenous ligands. The two major known endogenous ligands are anandamide (AEA) and 2-arachidonoylglycerol (2AG) [3-6]. Both derive from arachidonic acid and are produced postsynaptically from phospholipid precursors through activity-dependent activation of specific phospholipase enzymes [7]. Later on, a number of other eCB ligands have been discovered including N-arachidonoyldopamine (NADA), N-arachidonoylglycerolether and O-arachidonoylethanolamine [8].

AEA and 2AG are characterized by different biosynthetic and metabolic pathways, showing distinct mechanisms of regulation. AEA can be synthesized through different pathways from the phospholipid precursors N-arachidonoyl-phosphatidylethanolamine, the most important of which is a direct conversion catalysed by an N-acyl-phosphatidylethanolamine selective phosphodiesterase. 2AG principal way of synthesis is through activation of phospholipase C and subsequent production of diacylglycerol, which is rapidly converted to 2AG by diacylglycerol lipase. After its re-uptake, AEA is hydrolysed by the enzyme fatty acid amide hydrolase (FAAH), producing arachidonic acid and ethanolamine, while 2AG is primarily metabolized by monoacylglycerol lipase (MAG lipase), leading to the formation of arachidonic acid and glycerol [9]. eCBs may bind not only to the well known $CB_1$ and $CB_2$ receptors, but also to other receptors. For instance, AEA may activate the potential vanilloid receptor type 1 (TRPV1) intracellularly [10]. Moreover, 'orphan' G protein coupled receptor, GPR55, has been recently proposed as putative cannabinoid receptor [11], as has been the peroxisome proliferator activated receptor, PPAR [12,13]. $CB_1$ and $CB_2$ receptors still remain the best known targets for AEA and 2AG, though interacting with different affinity: AEA has the highest affinity to both receptors, whereas 2AG has the highest efficacy on both receptors [14].

eCB synthesis can be induced by physiological or pathological stimuli and results in their immediate release, with subsequent activation of cannabinoid receptors. Therefore eCBs are synthesized and released "on demand" by post-synaptic cells, involving the cleavage of membrane phospholipid precursors. Each member of the endocannabinoid machinery tightly controls the synthesis, release and degradation of the eCBs, finely tuning the signalling system.

The eCB system has been found altered in several diseases, as multiple sclerosis and spinal cord injury, neuropathic pain, cancer, atherosclerosis, stroke, myocardial infarction, hypertension, glaucoma, obesity/metabolic syndrome and osteoporosis, thus paving the way for new therapeutic strategies aimed at restoring normal eCB system functionality [15].

Currently, the term 'cannabinoid' refers more than 100 terpenophenols derived from *Cannabis sativa* [16], as well as to synthetic compounds that directly or indirectly interact with cannabinoid receptors. The most psychoactive component of the plant *Cannabis sativa* is $\Delta^9$-tetrahydrocannabinol ($\Delta^9$-THC): its biological actions as well as the ones of synthetic cannabinoid compounds (synthetic compounds active on cannabinoid receptors) are primarily mediated by $CB_1$ and $CB_2$ receptors. Cannabinoids classification comprises phytocannabinoids (subclassified in different categories according to their chemical structures, such as $\Delta^9$-THC, $\Delta^8$-THC, cannabinol, CBD and cannabicyclol), synthetic compounds active on cannabinoid receptors (i.e., JWH133, WIN55212-2, SR141716) and endocannabinoids (i.e., AEA and 2AG) which are produced endogenously (Figure 1).

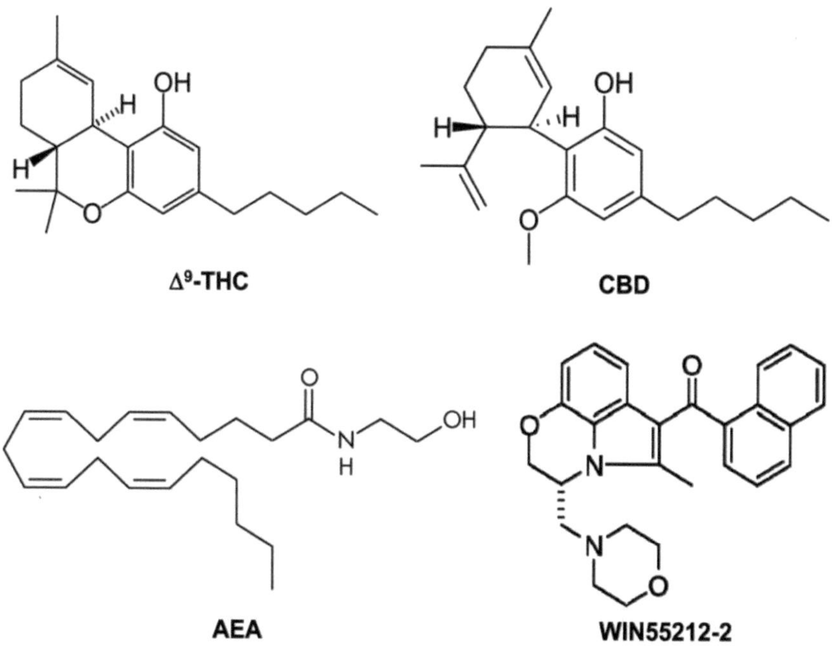


**Figure 1.** Chemical structures of Δ$^9$-tetrahydrocannabinol (Δ$^9$-THC), cannabidiol (CBD), anandamide (AEA) and WIN55212-2

## 3. Cannabinoids and cancer

Till now, most of cannabinoids applications in clinical practice of cancer patients comprised palliate wasting, emesis and pain that often accompany cancer. The discovery of a potential utility of these compounds for targeting and killing cancer cells led to a significant advancement in cannabinoid use in cancer treatment. In 1975 Munson et al. [17] demonstrated that the administration of Δ$^9$-THC, Δ$^8$-THC and cannabinol inhibited the growth of Lewis lung adenocarcinoma cells *in vitro* as well as *in vivo* after oral administration in mice. From then on, the interest in anti-carcinogenic properties of cannabinoids substantially decreased, until the discovery of the eCB system and the cloning of the specific cannabinoid receptors, $CB_1$ and $CB_2$. In the past decades, more and more evidences have contributed to assess and define the anti-tumourigenic effect of several cannabinoid compounds, including Δ$^9$-THC, cannabidiol (CBD), synthetic agonists, endocannabinoids and endocannabinoid transport or degradation inhibitors. These molecules have proved valuable against tumour cell proliferation and angiogenesis, and induce apoptosis in various cancer types, *i.e.* lung, glioma, thyroid, lymphoma, skin, pancreas, uterus, breast, prostate and colorectal carcinoma, both *in vitro* and *in vivo* [18-26]. Moreover, other mechanisms adopted by cannabinoids to counteract tumourigenesis are currently emerging and comprise interference with tumour neovascularization, cancer cell migration, adhesion, invasion and metastasisation [27].

Notwithstanding these promising anti-tumour effects, the clinical application of $\Delta^9$-THC and other cannabinoid agonists is often limited by their unwanted psychoactive side effects. In line with this fact, in recent years increasing interest has been focused on non-psychoactive cannabinoid compounds with structural affinity for $\Delta^9$-THC, such as cannabidiol (CBD). Interestingly, although its very low affinity for both $CB_1$ and $CB_2$ receptors, CBD has been recently reported to act with unexpectedly high potency *in vitro* as antagonist of $CB_1$ receptors in the mouse vas deferens [28] and brain [29] tissues, and to behave as inverse agonist at human $CB_2$ receptors [29]. Moreover, other putative CBD's molecular targets are TRPV, 5-$HT_{1A}$, GPR55 and PPAR$\gamma$ receptors (Figure 2).

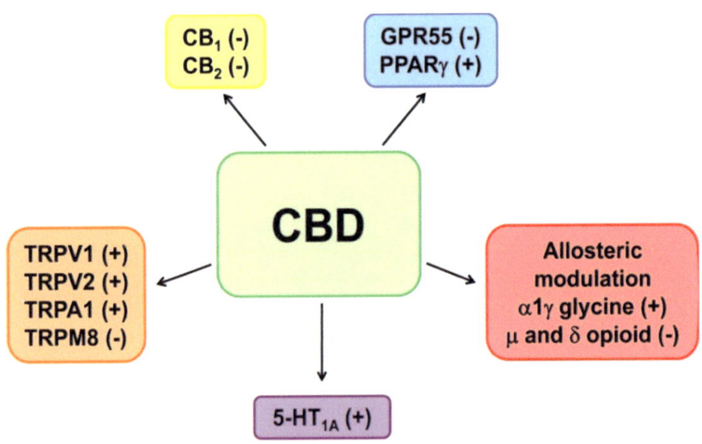


**Figure 2.** Some of the potential biological targets of CBD (with the permission of the authors [30])

Several studies reported the beneficial effects of CBD in the treatment of pain and spasticity and other CNS pathologies, as multiple sclerosis, Huntington disease, Parkinson etc. Moreover, many reports demonstrated its anti-tumour effects: it is characterized by a pro-apoptotic anti-metastatic activity and inhibits cancer cell migration, adhesion and invasion.

The aim of this chapter is to report the state of art on the efficacy of CBD in the modulation of the different steps of tumourigenesis in several types of cancer. The results here presented highlight the importance of future further exploration of CBD and/or of CBD analogues as alternative agents for tumour therapy, at least for breast cancer, glioma, lung tumour and leukaemia. The data available so far are summarized in Table 1 and are discussed in detail in the following paragraphs.

## 4. CBD and breast cancer

In 2006 Ligresti et al. [31] first demonstrated that CBD potently and selectively inhibits the proliferation of human breast cancer cells. This compound was able to strongly inhibit the growth of different breast tumour cell lines (MCF7, MDA-MB-231) *in vitro*, with an $IC_{50}$ of

| Cancer | *In vitro effect* | Receptor involvement | ROS production | Molecular cell signalling | Autophagy | Apoptosis | *In vivo effect* | Reference |
|---|---|---|---|---|---|---|---|---|
| Breast | ↓ proliferation | $CB_2$; TRPV1 | ↑ | NC | NC | + | ↓ xenografts growth ↓ lung metastases | [26] |
| | ↓ viability | non-$CB_1$; non-$CB_2$; non-TRPV1 | ↑ | ↓ pAkt; ↑ cytochrome C Bid translocation | + | + | NC | [29] |
| | ↓ invasion | NC | ↑ | ↓ Id-1; ↑ pERK | NC | NC | ↓ tumour growth ↓ size and number of metastases | [27,28] |
| Glioma | ↓ proliferation | non-$CB_1$; partial-$CB_2$; non-TRPV1 | ↑ | ↓ pERK; ↓ pAkt; ↓ HIF-1$\alpha$ ↑ cytochrome C caspase activation | NC | + | ↓ tumour growth | [33,34,37,38] |
| | ↓ proliferation and invasiveness | NC | NC | NC | NC | NC | NC | [35] |
| | ↓ migration | non-$CB_1$; non-$CB_2$; non-TRPV1 | NC | Ptx insensitive | NC | NC | NC | [39] |
| | ↓ invasiveness | NC | NC | ↓ Id-1 | NC | NC | NC | [46] |
| Leukaemia | ↓ viability | NC | NC | caspase-3 activation | NC | + | NC | [40] |
| | ↓ viability | $CB_2$ | ↑ | ↓ p-p38 caspase activation; ↓ Bid ↑ cytochrome C | NC | + | ↓ tumour burden ↑ tumour cell apoptosis | [41] |
| Lung | ↓ invasion | $CB_1$; $CB_2$; TRPV1 | NC | ↑ p-p38; ↑ p-ERK; ↑ TIMP-1 ↓ PAI-1 | NC | NC | ↓ lung metastases ↓ PAI-1 in xenografts | [49,50] |
| Thyroid | cytostatic effect | NC | NC | NC | NC | + | NC | [26] |
| Thymoma | ↓ viability | NC | ↑ | NC | NC | + | NC | [53] |
| Colon | ↓ proliferation | $CB_1$; TRPV1; PPAR$\gamma$ | NC | ↓ Akt; ↑ 2AG ↑ caspase-3; ↑ COX-2 | NC | + | ↓ ACF, polyps and tumours | [55] |

NC=not checked ↑ increase; ↓ decrease

**Table 1.** Effects of CBD on different types of cancer

about 6 μM. Worth to note, its effect on non cancer cells resulted far less potent. Further on, by the use of xenografts obtained by *s.c.* injection into athymic mice of human MDA-MB-231 breast carcinoma, the authors demonstrated that CBD and CBD-rich extracts (containing approximately 70% CBD together with lesser amounts of other cannabinoids) not only inhibited tumour growth *in vivo*, but also reduced lung metastases deriving from intrapaw injection of MDA-MB-231 cells. The possible cellular and molecular mechanisms underlying these effects may include induction of a combination of mechanisms by CBD, involving direct TRPV1 activation and/or $CB_2$ indirect activation (via FAAH), as well as induction of oxidative stress.

Subsequent work form McAllister and coworkers [32] demonstrated that CBD not only affected breast cancer cell proliferation, but it also interfered with invasion and metastasis, two other crucial final and fatal steps of breast cancer cell progression. Analysis on three different groups of cannabinoid compounds (phytocannabinoids with affinity for $CB_1$ and $CB_2$ receptors; phytocannabinoids with no appreciable affinity for $CB_1$ and $CB_2$ receptors; synthetic compounds with affinity for $CB_1$ and $CB_2$ receptors) revealed that CBD was shown to be one of the most effective inhibitors of human breast cancer cell proliferation, being as potent as $\Delta^9$-THC and CP55940 in inhibiting MDA-MB-231 and MDA-MB-436 cell growth respectively, and resulting as the most potent inhibitor of the MDA-MB-231 cell migration. By the use of Boyden chamber the authors also investigated the effect of several cannabinoids on the ability of MDA-MB-231-the most aggressive breast cancer cell line-to migrate and invade a reconstituted basement membrane: CBD demonstrated once more to be the most potent inhibitor of cell invasion. Further investigation concerned the identification of the cellular mechanism underlying CBD effect on cell growth and invasion. CBD was predicted to act through the regulation of key genes involved in the control of cell proliferation and invasion. In particular, attention was focused on Id-1 protein, an inhibitor of basic helix-loop helix transcription factors, which overexpression in breast cancer cells stimulates proliferation, migration and invasion. In fact, CBD exerted inhibition of Id-1 expression at the same concentrations already proved to be effective against proliferation and invasion (0.1, 1 and 1.5 μM). It is worth noting that CBD has no effect on invasiveness in cells that ectopically expressed Id-1. CBD therefore revealed a non toxic exogenous agent able to significantly decrease Id-1 expression in breast cancer cells and, at the same time, effective at reducing tumour aggressiveness.

Later work from the same group elucidated the cellular pathways involved in the down-regulation of Id-1 expression by CBD and leading to inhibition of human breast cancer proliferation and invasiveness [33]. First of all, they demonstrated that CBD-induced up-regulation of the extracellular signal-regulated kinase phosphorylation (p-ERK) was responsible for inhibition of Id-1 expression and subsequent human breast cancer cell proliferation and invasion. Indeed, the ERK inhibitor, U0126, partially reverted the ability of CBD to inhibit proliferation and invasion and attenuated its effect on Id-1 expression. Besides ERK up-regulation, also the production of reactive oxygen species (ROS) seems to play a role in CBD inhibitory effect on Id-1. In fact, CBD ability to inhibit proliferation, invasion and Id-1 expression was reversed by the use of tocopherol, a ROS scavenger. In addition to Id-1, CBD also modulates the pro-differentiation factor Id-2, inducing its up-regulation. Consistent with the work from Ligresti [31], CBD also demonstrated *in vivo* efficacy: it reduced primary tumour mass as well as the size and number of metastatic foci in two models of metastasis.

The most recent contribute to the elucidation of the cellular mechanism elicited by CBD to induce cell death in breast cancer cells comes from an excellent paper of Shrivastava et al. [34]. According to the experiments that they performed on both estrogen receptor positive and estrogen receptor negative breast cancer cells, CBD (0.1-10 μM for 24 h) induced a concentration-dependent cell death. Worth to note, the effective concentrations of CBD in tumour cells have little effect on MCF-10A cells, a line of non tumourigenic, mammary cells. This effect resulted to be independent of $CB_1$, $CB_2$ and TRPV1 receptor activation. Cell morphology assessed through electron microscopy revealed to be consistent with the coexistence of autophagy and apoptosis. These events were promoted by the induction of endoplasmic reticulum (ER) stress and the inhibition of Akt/mTOR/4EBP1 signalling. Also ROS production induced by CBD seems to play a role, since ROS inhibition through tocopherol blocked the induction of apoptosis and autophagy. Further investigation of the cellular mechanisms involved in CBD-induced programmed cell death (PCD) demonstrated that this compound reduced mitochondrial membrane potential, triggered the translocation of the Beclin2 Interacting Protein (Bid) to the mitochondria and the release of cytochrome C to the cytosol and, ultimately, the activation of the intrinsic apoptotic pathway. The relationship between CBD-induced apoptosis and autophagic cell death was also explored through blockade of each form of the PCD with specific caspase and autophagy inhibitors. In the first case, caspase inhibition reduced CBD pro-apoptotic effect and corresponded to lower levels of protein markers in breast cancer cells. On the other hand, the inhibition of autophagy enhanced the level of CBD-induced apoptosis and determined an increase in protein marker expression. As suggested by these data, blockade of CBD-induced autophagy likely results in a compensatory increase of apoptosis as an alternative means of PCD. CBD-induced PCD thus depends on a precise balance between apoptosis and autophagy which could be mediated by Beclin1. Though its mechanism of action is not clearly elucidated, Beclin1 is considered a key signalling molecule in the autophagic process. It has been recently suggested that Beclin1 is cleaved by caspases and that such cleaved form is incapable of inducing autophagy [31,32]. CBD treatment (5 to 10 μM) resulted in the cleavage of Beclin1. This is consistent with induction of caspases activity and suggests that Beclin1 may likely have a role in CBD-mediated cell death. The consequent cleavage product translocates to the mitochondria, where it induces apoptosis by enhancing the release of cytochrome C [35,36]. The cleavage and consequent translocation of cleaved Beclin1 to the mitochondria induced by CBD treatment may thus be crucial among the mechanisms elicited by CBD to modulate the balance between autophagy and apoptosis in breast cancer cells.

As a whole this work highlights the presence of a complex mutual regulation of autophagy and mitochondria-mediated apoptosis in CBD-induced breast cancer cell death. The very promising data here reported support the idea that this non toxic compound could likely represent either a new therapeutic opportunity for breast cancer treatment or the starting point for a second generation compound to be tested in clinic.

In Figure 3 it is depicted a schematic representation of the signalling pathways associated with CBD effect in breast cancer cell proliferation and invasion.

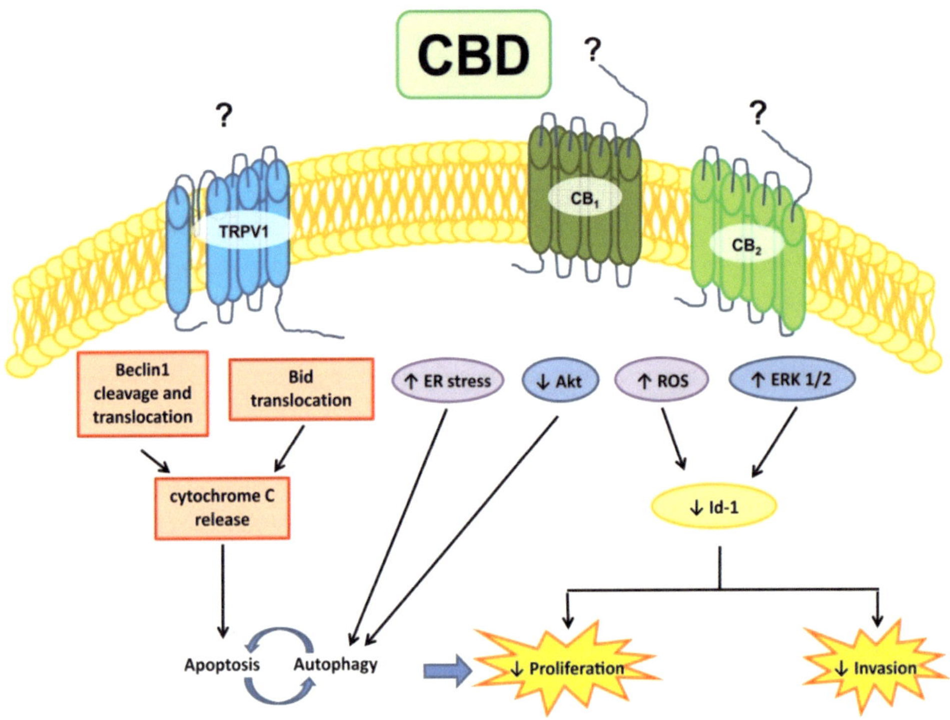


**Figure 3.** Schematic representation of the signalling pathways associated with CBD effects on breast cancer (with the permission of the authors [30])

## 5. CBD and glioma

Moreover, CBD also exhibited anti-tumoural properties in gliomas, a class of brain tumours of glial origin characterized by a high morphological and genetic heterogeneity accounting for over 30% of all primary brain tumours. Gliomas are characterized by a high proliferative rate, aggressive invasiveness and insensitivity to radio-and chemotherapy, and are considered among the most rapidly growing and devastating solid tumours.

In a seminal paper Jacobsson et al. [37] first demonstrated that CBD displayed a serum-dependent effect on C6 murine glioma cell proliferation. Massi et al. [38] afterwards reported

http://dx.doi.org/10.5772/58965

http://dx.doi.org/10.5772/58965

http://dx.doi.org/10.5772/58962

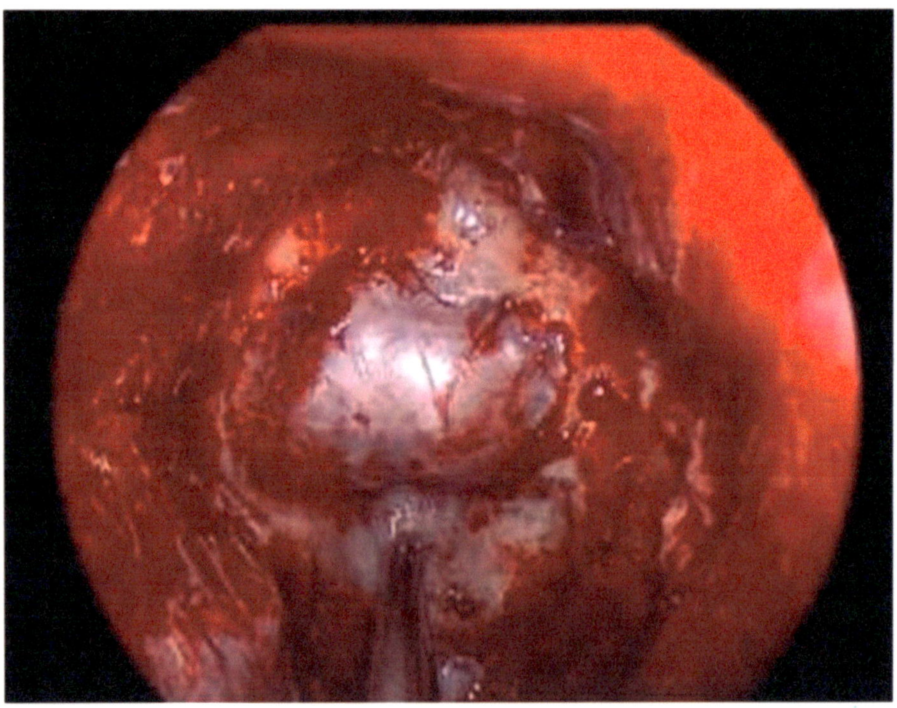

http://dx.doi.org/10.5772/59051

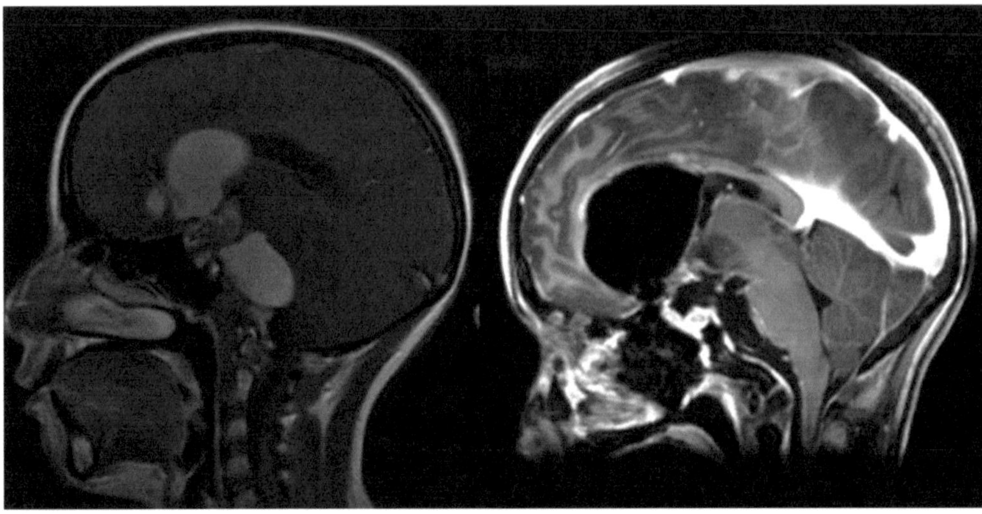

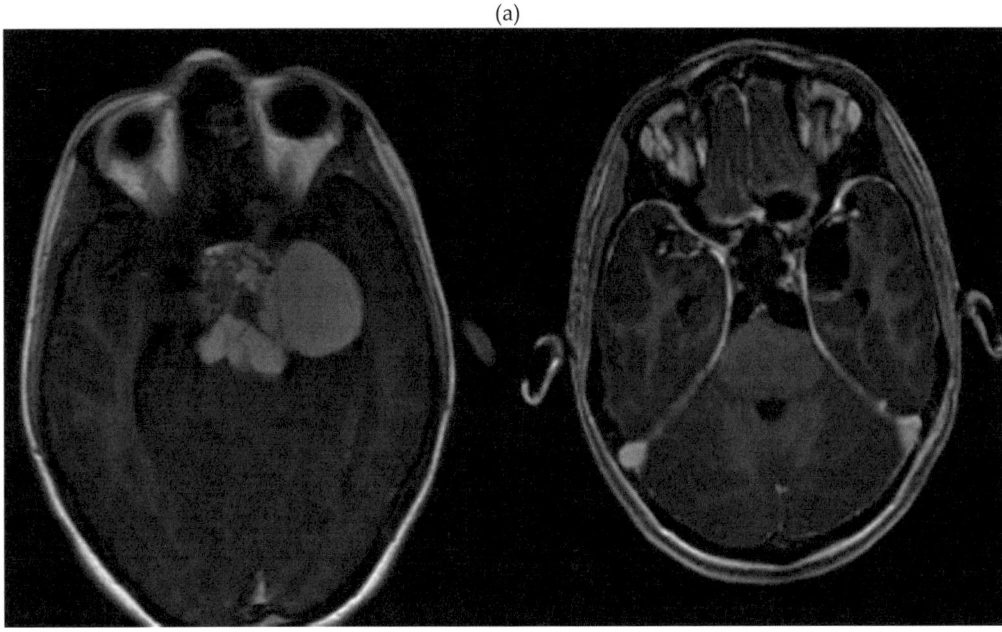

http://dx.doi.org/10.5772/58961

http://dx.doi.org/10.5772/59981

http://dx.doi.org/10.5772/58973

http://dx.doi.org/10.5772/58973

http://dx.doi.org/10.5772/59046

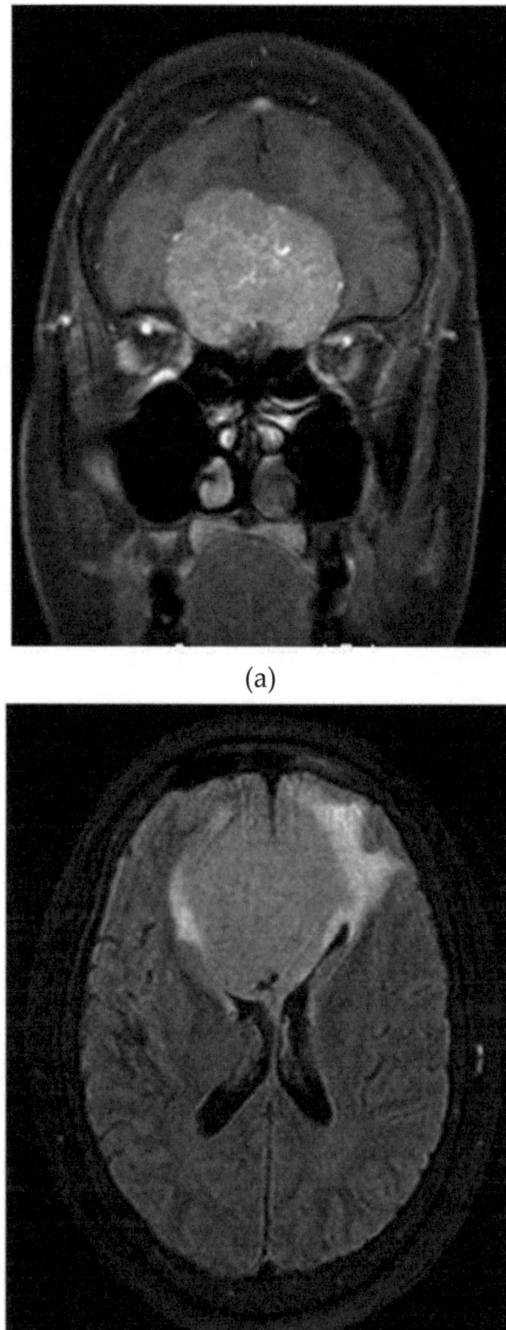

http://dx.doi.org/10.5772/59037

http://dx.doi.org/10.5772/59044

http://dx.doi.org/10.5772/59044

http://dx.doi.org/10.5772/59044

http://dx.doi.org/10.5772/59193

in 2004 an effective inhibition of U87-MG and U373 human glioma cell proliferation *in vitro* following CBD treatment, associated with the induction of apoptosis. Exposure of both cell lines to CBD for 24 h induced a concentration-and time-dependent inhibition of the mitochondrial oxidative metabolism, with an $IC_{50}$ value of 25 μM. The authors then evaluated the effect of intratumoural *in vivo* treatment with CBD, in tumour xenografts generated by subcutaneous injection of glioma cells in the flank region of immune-deficient mice. The treatment caused a significant reduction (60% mean) of the tumour growth over a 23-day period of observation [38]. Data from flow-cytometric analysis and ssDNA detection assay indicated that this reduction was correlated to CBD ability to induce a PCD. Of note, subsequent investigation demonstrated that CBD as no effect on the viability of non transformed primary glial cells [39].

Analysis of the cellular mechanisms responsible for CBD anti-proliferative effect demonstrated the lack of significant stimulation of cannabinoid and vanilloid receptors [38]. The sole $CB_2$ receptor antagonist SR144528 only weakly and transiently reverted CBD effect, a partial antagonism being present only over a 24 h-period and restricted to just one glioma cell lineage. Further data from the same work demonstrated for the first time that CBD anti-tumour effect depend on its ability to induce an oxidative stress state in the tumour cells: indeed this molecule induced an elevated and early production of ROS, a corresponding depletion of intracellular glutathione and an increase of activity of the GSH-associated enzymes. Consistent with these evidences, the anti-proliferative effect of the drug was reversed by the anti-oxidant, tocopherol. It is worth noting that CBD did not affect ROS production in non transformed primary glial cells [39]. Subsequent investigation of the cellular events implicated in glioma cell death demonstrated that CBD induces a time-dependent release of cytochrome C and activation of caspase-8, caspase-9 and caspase-3: both the intrinsic and the extrinsic pathways of apoptosis result therefore involved in CBD effect [39].

Further support to the efficacy of CBD in inhibiting the growth of different glioblastoma cell lines (SF126, U251 and U87-MG) comes from a work from Marcu et al. [40]. In their paper the authors demonstrated not only that CBD appears more potent that $\Delta^9$-THC, but also that combination treatment of $\Delta^9$-THC with CBD determined an enhancement of $\Delta^9$-THC inhibitory effect on glioblastoma cell growth, but not on invasiveness [40]. Accordingly, Torres et al. [41] recently confirmed that association of CBD with $\Delta^9$-THC treatment greatly reduced the viability of several human glioma cells and determined an enhancement of both autophagy and apoptosis, with corresponding triggering of caspase-3 activation. Exposure of xenografts generated from U87-MG cells in nude mice to submaximal concentrations of CBD in combination with $\Delta^9$-THC inhibited tumour growth at a higher extent than the treatment with the individual compounds: these data suggest a potential use of the combinatory therapy as a strategy to allow reduction of the amount of the psychoactive $\Delta^9$-THC in potential cancer treatment.

The cellular mechanism involved in the synergistic action of the combined therapy were investigated by Marcu et al. [40]: double treatment with CBD and $\Delta^9$-THC *in vitro* induced cell cycle arrest, stimulation of ROS production and sustained activation of caspases-3,-7 and-9, with consequent induction of apoptosis, together with specific modulation of the extracellular signal-regulated kinase, ERK. Exposure to each individual compound was unable to induce these specific effects, suggesting that the signal transduction pathways affected by the combination treatment were unique. Recent results form Parolaro's group [42] apparently disagree with Marcu's data, as in their hands CBD *per se* strongly down-regulates ERK, as well as another signalling molecule playing a crucial role in tumour cell proliferation, such as PI3K/Akt, both in U87-MG cells and in cannabinoid-resistant T98G human glioma cell lines. Moreover, CBD also profoundly down-regulated the hypoxia-inducible transcription factor HIF-1$\alpha$, one of the most critical stimuli for cell survival, motility and tumour angiogenesis. These evidences suggest that HIF-1$\alpha$, together with ERK and Akt, represent three of the multiple molecular targets through which the CBD exerts its anti-neoplastic activity [42].

Talking about the mechanisms elicited by CBD to prevent glioma growth, further *ex vivo* investigations, performed on glioma tumour tissues excised from nude mice treated *in vivo* with CBD, showed its ability to modulate the lipoxygenases (LOX) pathway and the endocannabinoid system [43]. Biochemical analysis indicated a significant decrease of 5-LOX activity and content and of its end-product leukotriene B4, as well as a marked stimulation of the fatty acid amide hydrolase (FAAH), and a decrease of AEA content. In contrast, cyclooxygenase (COX)-2 activity and content were not affected by CBD.

CBD ability to reduce tumour growth is not only restricted to cell proliferation, but several data also support its effects on glioma cell migration and invasiveness. As a matter of fact, CBD inhibited U87-MG glioma cells migration in a concentration-dependent way, at concentrations lower than those required to inhibit cell proliferation [44]. Treatment with the selective cannabinoid receptor antagonists SR141716 ($CB_1$), SR144528 ($CB_2$) or by pretreatment with pertussis toxin were not able to antagonize CBD anti-migratory effect, thus indicating no involvement of classical cannabinoid receptors and/or $G_{i/o}$ protein coupled receptors. Cell invasiveness, evaluated through a reconstituted basement membrane in a Boyden chamber test, was reduced after CBD treatment in U251 glioma lineage [40].

Worth to note, an activation of TRPV2 receptor by CBD have recently [45] demonstrated to inhibit human glioma cell proliferation and overcome carmustine resistance of glioma cells. This mechanisms seems to involve increase in $Ca^{2+}$influx and consequent drug uptake, synergizing with cytotoxic agents to induce apoptosis of glioma cells. Interestingly this effect was limited to tumour cells, whereas it is absent in normal human astrocytes.

At last, Soroceanu and coworkers [46] recently investigated the role of the transcriptional regulator Id-1 in modulating the invasiveness of glioma cells. As previously reported for breast cancer, Id-1 expression levels positively correlate with glioma cell invasiveness in culture and with histopathological grades in patient biopsies. The authors showed that CBD significantly down-regulates Id-1 gene expression and associated glioma cell invasiveness and self-renewal, and glioma progression *in vivo*, thus suggesting that Id-1 may be an additional target for CBD.

As a whole, CBD seems to counteract glioma cell proliferation and invasion through multiple mechanisms. Most of them are summarized in Figure 4.

http://dx.doi.org/10.5772/59193

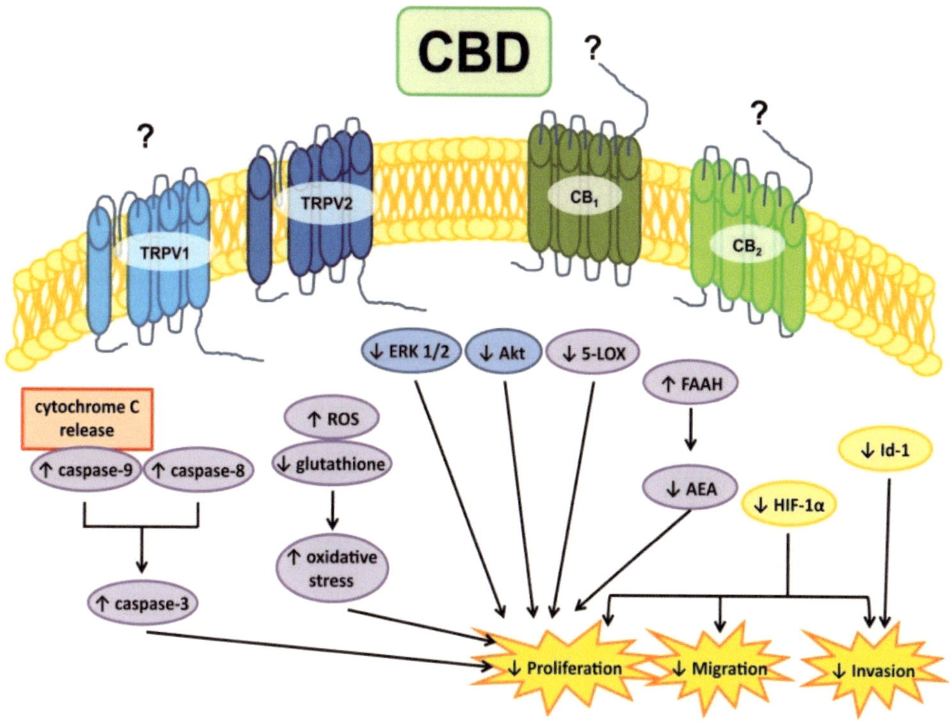


**Figure 4.** Schematic representation of the signalling pathways associated with CBD effects on glioma

## 6. CBD and leukaemia/lymphoma

Gallily et al. [47] first evidenced the possible role of CBD in the treatment of lymphoblastic diseases. They demonstrated that 24 h-treatment with CBD induced apoptosis in human acute myeloid leukaemia HL-60 cell line: the effect was dose-dependent and involved caspase-3 activation. On the contrary, CBD treatment had no effect on human monocytes from normal individuals.

By far the most important work in this field was from McKallip et al. [48]. They exposed the murine EL-4 lymphoma cell line and the human Jurkat and Molt-4 leukaemia cell lines to CBD (1-10 μM) and demonstrated that this compound is able to reduce the number of viable cells and to induce apoptosis, both *in vitro* and *in vivo*, in a $CB_2$ receptor dependent way. In particular, treatment with CBD *in vivo* led to a significant reduction in tumour burden and determined a higher level of apoptotic tumours in EL-4-bearing mice [48].

As far as the cellular mechanisms are concerned, CBD effect on Jurkat cells *in vitro* involved the activation of caspase-8, caspase-9, and caspase-3, caused the cleavage of poly(ADPribose) polymerase, and corresponded to a decrease in full-length Bid: these concerted events support a possible cross-talk between the intrinsic and extrinsic apoptotic pathways. CBD exposure caused a loss of mitochondrial membrane potential and the subsequent release of cytochrome C, thus further confirming the crucial role of mitochondria in PCD regulation by CBD. Moreover, as previously observed in other tumour cells, CBD treatment corresponded to an increase of ROS production as well as in the expression of the NAD(P)H oxidases Nox4 and $p22^{phox}$. Treatment with the ROS scavengers or the NAD(P)H oxidase inhibitors prevented both CBD-mediated induction of apoptosis and ROS increase. Finally, CBD down-regulated phosphorylation and consequent activation of p38 mitogen-activated protein kinase, but did not affect p-ERK and p-JNK levels. Exposure to a $CB_2$-selective antagonist or to a ROS scavenger reverted this effect, thus suggesting that CBD may involve $CB_2$ receptors and regulation of Nox4 and $p22^{phox}$ expression in its action [48].

As a whole, CBD may represent a novel and highly selective candidate for leukaemia treatment. It is worth noting that previous evidences indicated that human leukaemias and lymphomas expressed significantly higher levels of $CB_2$ receptors compared to other tumour cell lines. For this reason the observation that CBD mediates apoptosis through $CB_2$ receptors is particularly relevant, suggesting the possibility that tumours of immune origin may be highly sensitive to the $CB_2$-mediated effects of CBD [49].

## 7. CBD and lung cancer

Lung cancer is characterized by a particularly aggressive biological nature and is, at present, poorly responsive to available therapy. For this reason, a series of targets and therapeutic strategies for its treatment are currently being investigated [50-53].

Ramer's research group is one of the most active interested in preclinical lung cancer research. They recently [54-56] evaluated CBD effects on A549 cells, a line of human lung carcinoma cells expressing both $CB_1$ and $CB_2$, as well as TRPV1 receptors, with particular focus on invasiveness. By the use of Matrigel invasion assay, they demonstrated that CBD induces an impaired invasion of A549 cells; this impairment was reversed by antagonists to both $CB_1$ and $CB_2$ receptors as well as to TRPV1. Moreover, they observed that invasion decrease determined by CBD treatment corresponded to an upregulation of tissue inhibitor of matrix metalloproteinases-1 (TIMP-1); on the other hand, knocking down of TIMP-1 expression through a siRNA approach was able to reverse the CBD-elicited decrease in tumour cell invasiveness. These evidences suggest that there may be a causal link between the TIMP-1 up-regulation and CBD anti-invasive action. CBD was also shown to induce phosphorylation of two mitogen-activated protein kinases, p38 and p42/44: these have been identified as upstream mechanisms leading to TIMP-1 induction and subsequent decrease of invasiveness. Interestingly, these events are all prevented by exposure to cannabinoids or TRPV1 receptor antagonists.

The authors also performed *in vivo* studies in thymic aplastic nude mice [54]: in such model, intravenous injection of CBD at a dose of 5 mg/kg in animals caused a significant inhibition of A549 lung metastasis, further supporting the possible therapeutic benefit of CBD adoption. Together with the strong inhibition of A549 cell invasion, CBD treatment induced a corresponding down-regulation of the plasminogen activator inhibitor PAI-1 expression and secretion, another factor playing an important role in the regulation of cell spreading [55].

CBD-driven decrease in PAI-1 secretion and cell invasion were suppressed by exposure to $CB_1$ and $CB_2$ receptors as well as to TRPV1 receptor antagonists. Recombinant human PAI-1 led to a concentration-dependent up-regulation of invasiveness, while PAI-1 siRNA caused down-regulation, suggesting a crucial role of PAI-1 in A549 invasiveness. The same experiments were also performed in two other human lung cancer cell lines, H460 and H358, and key data were confirmed.

PAI-1 also revealed crucial *in vivo*: CBD treatment (5 mg/kg) of A549 xenografts of rats determined its significant down-regulation [55].

One of the most important aspects in these works resides in the dose-range at which CBD effectively inhibits invasion. In fact, treating human lung cancer cells for 72 h with CBD the authors observed a significant effect at a concentration as low as 0.01 μM, corresponding to a 33% inhibition when compared to control vehicle. At the same conditions [56] an equimolar concentration of $\Delta^9$-THC caused a 68% inhibition of cell invasion. Nonetheless, it is worth noting that CBD anti-invasive effect occurred in a range of therapeutically relevant concentrations: as a matter of fact, as reported from a clinical study on healthy volunteers, CBD reached peak plasma concentrations between 0.01 μM and 0.05 μM following administration of SativexTM (1:1 ratio of $\Delta^9$-THC and CBD) at the buccal dose of 10 mg or at the self-titrated doses during chronic therapy [57].

In their most recent work, Ramer et al. [58] demonstrated that CBD reduces cell viability in lung cancer cell lines (A549, H460) and primary cells from a patient with lung cancer, this effect being associated with apoptosis. The cellular mechanisms induced by CBD involve an initial up-regulation of COX-2 and PPAR-γ, both *in vitro*, in A549 and H460 cell lines, and *in vivo*, in A549-xenografted nude mice, and a subsequent nuclear translocation of PPAR- by COX-2-dependent prostaglandins.

As a whole, these evidences contribute to elucidate the mechanisms underlying CBD anti-invasive action on human lung cancer cells and strongly support its possible use as a therapeutic option for the treatment of highly invasive types of cancers.

## 8. CBD and endocrine tumours

Among the endocrine malignancies, the most common one is thyroid cancer. This kind of tumour is characterized by overactivation of Ras, that may depend on activating mutations in the ras gene or on overactivation of receptor tyrosine kinase receptors. According to these observations, new strategies for the treatment of thyroid cancer should reasonably point at Ras as crucial molecular target.

Ligresti et al. [31] first exposed KiMol cells – rat thyroid cells transformed with the v-K-ras oncogene – to CBD treatment: this phytocannabinoid caused anti-proliferative effects in association with a cell cycle block at the G1/S phase transition, which was accompanied by a pro-apoptotic action.

Further studies from Lee et al. [59] demonstrated a marked CBD pro-apoptotic effect in both murine thymocytes and EL-4 thymoma cells: this effect was time-and concentration-related. In particular, according to time-course analyses, CBD-mediated apoptosis occurred earlier in EL-4 cells than in thymocytes. The cellular events triggered by CBD were similar in both T cells: ROS generation played a pivotal role, although the basal level of ROS in thymocytes was lower than that in EL-4 cells. Exposure to the glutathione precursor N-acetyl-L-cysteine (NAC) markedly attenuated CBD-driven induction of apoptosis, and reverted the decrease of cellular thiols levels.

In conclusion, unlike monocytes, T cells, both primary and immortalized, are all sensitive and similarly responding to CBD, as demonstrated by the fact that CBD induced oxidative stress in thymocytes, EL-4 cells and splenocytes [60]. ROS generation proved to play a central role in this response.

## 9. CBD and colon cancer

Colon cancer is one of the principal causes of morbidity and mortality in Western countries. Its aetiology seems to reside in a series of histopathological and molecular changes that transform normal colonic epithelial cells, give rise to Aberrant Crypt Foci (ACF) and polyps as intermediate steps, and at last develops a colorectal carcinoma.

First investigation about CBD effect on SW480 colon and LNCaP prostate carcinoma cells comes from Sreevalsan et al. [61]. They demonstrated that CBD inhibits cell growth in both cell lines. This anti-proliferative effect corresponds to an induction of apoptosis. Moreover, CBD induced mRNA expression of several dual specificity phosphatases and protein tyrosine phosphatases. This is particularly relevant given that the anti-tumoural effects of many cannabinoids include modulation of intracellular kinase. The pro-apoptotic activity of CBD was phosphatase-dependent in both cell lines, on the other hand, cannabinoid receptors mediated its effects only in prostate cancer cells, whereas their role in colon carcinoma is controversial.

Izzo and coworkers recently [62] investigated the effect of CBD in a preclinical animal model of colon cancer based on azoxymethane (AOM) administration in mice. AOM causes in exposed cells occurrence of ACF (preneoplastic lesions), polyps, and tumour formation, as well as up-regulation of p-Akt, iNOS and COX-2 and the down-regulation of caspase-3. The authors demonstrated that CBD possesses effective chemopreventive properties: it reduced ACF, polyps and tumours and counteracted AOM-induced p-Akt and caspase-3 changes. Moreover, *in vitro* studies performed in colorectal carcinoma cell lines evidenced that CBD protected DNA from oxidative damage, increased endocannabinoid levels and reduced cell proliferation in a $CB_1$-, TRPV1-and PPAR-$\gamma$-antagonists sensitive manner.

Based on these promising data and on its safety records, it is likely to consider CBD a worthy candidate for clinical consideration in colon cancer prevention.

## 10. CBD and angiogenesis

More and more evidences indicate that a new promising therapeutic target for cancer therapy is represented by angiogenesis, the formation of new blood vessels from the pre-existing ones. Moreover, tumour angiogenesis is target of several cannabinoids, which not only down-regulate the production of pro-angiogenic factors in cancer cells, but also directly modulate endothelial cell growth [27]. It is hence surprising the lack of any data on CBD ability to influence angiogenesis.

As Solinas et al. recently demonstrated [63], CBD is a potent inhibitor of HUVE cell proliferation, migration and invasion, acting through the induction of endothelial cell cytostasis, but without triggering apoptosis. Interestingly, CBD affected endothelial cell differentiation into tubular capillaries and blocked the outgrowth of capillary-like structures from HUVEC spheroids *in vitro*. Moreover, CBD anti-angiogenic effect was also evident *in vivo* in a matrigel sponge model. The cellular mechanisms elicited seem to involve down-modulation of several molecules associated with angiogenesis, including MMP2 and MMP9, uPA, Endothelin-1, PDGF-AA and CXCL16.

These preliminary data are very promising and demonstrate for the first time that, besides its well known pro-apoptotic anti-proliferative and anti-invasive actions, CBD may also exert anti-angiogenic effects, thus further strengthening its potential application in cancer therapy.

## 11. Conclusion

Much interest has been addressed to CBD since it is a plant-derived cannabinoid devoid of psychoactive properties. Many evidences support its pro-apoptotic and anti-proliferative actions in different types of tumours, as well as its anti-migrative, anti-invasive, anti-metastatic and perhaps anti-angiogenic properties. This wide range of anti-tumour effects indicate that CBD may likely be a potent inhibitor of both cancer growth and spreading.

In this regard, it is worth noting that, at least *in vitro*, this compound seems to exert its anti-cancer effect selectively on cancer cells, without affecting normal cell viability. Moreover, CBD revealed extremely efficient in inhibiting tumour growth: its versatility can be ascribed to the modulation of multiple cellular pathways that control tumourigenesis and consequent altering of different intracellular signalling, depending on the cancer type considered.

In particular, among all, increase in ROS production appears to be one of the most common and crucial mechanisms induced by CBD to exert its effects in all of the considered cancer cell lines. Less obvious is the role of cannabinoid and vanilloid receptors in mediating CBD action. In some cases (lung, leukaemia, colon) exposure of the cells to specific antagonists clearly demonstrated the essential contribution of these receptors. In other kinds of cancer (breast and glioma) their relevance appears only marginal or absent.

Of note, CBD demonstrated to efficiently inhibit cancer development not only *in vitro*, but also in several *in vivo* tests, determining reduction of tumour growth and, in some cases, of metastatization.

Nonetheless, the opportunity to introduce CBD in clinical practice for cancer treatment needs some consideration. A good starting point comes from high tolerability and from the lack of toxic effects. Indeed oral administration of CBD 700 mg/day for 6 weeks did not show any overt toxicity in humans [64] suggesting its possible exploitation for prolonged treatment. On the other hand, CBD oral absorption is slow and unpredictable, making it difficult to realize the optimal route of administration. Previous trials indicated that 6 weeks of oral CBD treatment 10 mg/kg/day induced a mean plasma level of CBD between 6 and 11 ng/ml (about 0.0036 μM) [65] and that this value did not differ significantly over the 6 weeks of administration. Of note, this same range of concentration was effective in inhibiting lung cancer cell invasion [55,56]: for instance in this case, the oral route could be the appropriate choice. Moreover, according to experimental data showing that combined treatment with CBD and $\Delta^9$-THC could be more effective in reducing cancer cell proliferation, the co-administration may represent a better choice for cancer therapy. In line with this, oromucosal treatment with SativexTM 10 mg (a formulation consisting of 1:1 ratio of $\Delta^9$-THC and CBD and recently approved for multiple sclerosis) provoked CBD plasma level of approximately 0.01 μM and up to 0.05 μM in humans, a concentration range effective in reducing lung cell invasion *in vitro*. As reported, the use of different associations of phytocannabinoids in a variable proportion might lead to a better outcome without pharmacokinetic interaction [66]. Another favourable aspect of oromucosal administration is its possible application in presence of nausea and vomiting. In view to overcome the several limitations to the systemic administration of cannabinoids in part derived from their high lipophilicity, a recent work from Hernán Pérez de la Ossa et al. [67] investigated the effects of CBD-and $\Delta^9$THC-loaded poly-ε-caprolactone microparticles as an alternative delivery system for long-term cannabinoid administration in a murine xenograft model of glioma. Local administration of $\Delta^9$-THC-, CBD-or a mixture (1:1 w:w) of Δ9THC- and CBD-loaded microparticles every 5 days to mice bearing glioma xenografts reduced tumour growth with the same efficacy than a daily local administration of the equivalent amount of those cannabinoids in solution. Moreover, treatment with cannabinoid-loaded microparticles enhanced apoptosis and decreased cell proliferation and angiogenesis in these tumours.

Moreover, it would be worth evaluating the possibility to use CBD (or Sativex) in combination with classical chemotherapeutic agents: this would enable to check for the presence of a synergistic effect that might potentially allow clinical chemotherapeutic dose reduction, and consequently reduce toxicity while maintaining efficacy.

Bearing in mind that CBD is already currently used in patients with multiple sclerosis, and in light of the findings here summarized, it can be concluded that CBD might be a good candidate for a future clinical approach and/or for the synthesis of a second generation compound, as suggested by McAllister's group. In view of these opportunities and based on the data here

http://dx.doi.org/10.5772/59193

presented, further research should be addressed to continue exploration of CBD and/or of CBD analogues as alternative agents for cancer therapy.
Nomenclature

The drug/molecular target nomenclature conforms to the BJP's Guide to Receptors and Channels [68].

## Author details

Marta Solinas, Valentina Cinquina and Daniela Parolaro*

*Address all correspondence to: daniela.parolaro@uninsubria.it

Department of Theoretical and Applied Sciences, Centre of Neuroscience, University of Insubria, Busto Arsizio, Italy

## References

[1] Howlett AC. The cannabinoid receptors. Prostaglandins & Other Lipid Mediators 2002;68-69 619-631.

[2] Van Sickle MD, Duncan M, Kingsley PJ, Mouihate A, Urbani P, Mackie K, Stella N, Makriyannis A, Piomelli D, Davison JS, Marnett LJ, Di Marzo V, Pittman QJ, Patel KD, Sharkey KA. Identification and functional characterization of brainstem cannabinoid CB2 receptors. Science 2005;310(5746) 329-332.

[3] Devane WA, Hanus L, Breuer A, Pertwee RG, Stevenson LA, Griffin G, Gibson D, Mandelbaum A, Etinger A, Mechoulam R. Isolation and structure of a brain constituent that binds to the cannabinoid receptor. Science 1992;258(5090) 1946-1949.

[4] Stella N, Schweitzer P, Piomelli D. A second endogenous cannabinoid that modulates long-term potentiation. Nature 1997;388(6644) 773-778.

[5] Sugiura T, Kishimoto S, Oka S, Gokoh M. Biochemistry, pharmacology and physiology of 2-arachidonoylglycerol, an endogenous cannabinoid receptor ligand. Progress in Lipid Research 2006;45(5) 405-446.

[6] Mechoulam R, Ben-Shabat S, Hanus L, Ligumsky M, Kaminski NE, Schatz AR, Gopher A, Almog S, Martin BR, Compton DR, Pertwee RG, Griffin G, Bayewitch M, Barg J, Vogel Z. Identification of an endogenous 2-monoglyceride, present in canine gut, that binds to cannabinoid receptors. Biochemical Pharmacology 1995;50(1) 83-90.

[7] Piomelli D. The molecular logic of endocannabinoid signalling. Nature Reviews. Neuroscience 2003;4(11) 873-884.

[8] De Petrocellis L, Di Marzo V. An introduction to the endocannabinoid system: from the early to the latest concepts. Best Practice & Research. Clinical Endocrinology & Metabolism 2009;23(1) 1-15.

[9] Di Marzo V, Petrosino S. Endocannabinoids and the regulation of their levels in health and disease. Current Opinion in Lipidology 2007;18(2) 129-140.

[10] Ross RA. Anandamide and vanilloid TRPV1 receptors. British Journal of Pharmacology 2003;140(5) 790-801.

[11] Ryberg E, Larsson N, Sjögren S, Hjorth S, Hermansson NO, Leonova J, Elebring T, Nilsson K, Drmota T, Greasley PJ. The orphan receptor GPR55 is a novel cannabinoid receptor. British Journal of Pharmacology 2007;152(7) 1092-1101.

[12] O'Sullivan SE. Cannabinoids go nuclear: evidence for activation of peroxisome proliferator-activated receptors. British Journal of Pharmacology 2007;152(5) 576-582.

[13] Pertwee RG, Howlett AC, Abood ME, Alexander SP, Di Marzo V, Elphick MR, Greasley PJ, Hansen HS, Kunos G, Mackie K, Mechoulam R, Ross RA. International Union of Basic and Clinical Pharmacology. LXXIX. Cannabinoid receptors and their ligands: beyond $CB_1$ and $CB_2$. Pharmacological Reviews 2010;62(4) 588-631.

[14] McPartland JM, Norris RW, Kilpatrick CW. Coevolution between cannabinoid receptors and endocannabinoid ligands. Gene 2007;397(1-2) 126-135.

[15] Pacher P, Bátkai S, Kunos G. The endocannabinoid system as an emerging target of pharmacotherapy. Pharmacological Reviews 2006;58(3) 389-462.

[16] Appendino G, Chianese G, Taglialatela-Scalfati O. Cannabinoids: occurrence and medicinal chemistry. Current Medicinal Chemistry 2011;18(7) 1085-1099.

[17] Munson AE, Harris LS, Friedman MA, Dewey WL, Carchman RA. Antineoplastic activity of cannabinoids. Journal of the National Cancer Institute 1975;55(3) 597-602.

[18] Galve-Roperh I, Sánchez C, Cortés ML, Gómez del Pulgar T, Izquierdo M, Guzmán M. Anti-tumoral action of cannabinoids: involvement of sustained ceramide accumulation and extracellular signal-regulated kinase activation. Nature Medicine 2000;6(3) 313-319.

[19] Sánchez C, de Ceballos ML, Gomez del Pulgar T, Rueda D, Corbacho C, Velasco G, Galve-Roperh I, Huffman JW, Ramón y Cajal S, Guzmán M. Inhibition of glioma growth in vivo by selective activation of the CB(2) cannabinoid receptor. Cancer Research 2001;61(15) 5784-5789.

[20] Casanova ML, Blázquez C, Martínez-Palacio J, Villanueva C, Fernández-Aceñero MJ, Huffman JW, Jorcano JL, Guzmán M. Inhibition of skin tumour growth and angiogenesis in vivo by activation of cannabinoid receptors. The Journal of Clinical Investigation 2003;111(1) 43-50.

[21] Blázquez C, Carracedo A, Barrado L, Real PJ, Fernández-Luna JL, Velasco G, Malumbres M, Guzmán M. Cannabinoid receptors as novel targets for the treatment of melanoma, FASEB Journal 2006;20(14) 2633-2635.

[22] Carracedo A, Gironella M, Lorente M, Garcia S, Guzmán M, Velasco G, Iovanna JL. Cannabinoids induce apoptosis of pancreatic tumor cells via endoplasmic reticulum stress-related genes. Cancer Research 2006;66(13) 6748-6755.

[23] Cianchi F, Papucci L, Schiavone N, Lulli M, Magnelli L, Vinci MC, Messerini L, Manera C, Ronconi E, Romagnani P, Donnini M, Perigli G, Trallori G, Tanganelli E, Capaccioli S, Masini E. Cannabinoid receptor activation induces apoptosis through tumor necrosis factor alpha-mediated ceramide de nono synthesis in colon cancer cells. Clinical Cancer Research 2008;14(23) 7691-7700.

[24] Bifulco M, Di Marzo V. Targeting the endocannabinoid system in cancer therapy: a call for further research. Nature Medicine 2002;8(6) 547-550.

[25] Bifulco M, Laezza C, Pisanti S, Gazzerro P. Cannabinoids and cancer: pros and cons of an antitumour strategy. British Journal of Pharmacology 2006;148(2) 123-135.

[26] Bifulco M, Malfitano AM, Pisanti S, Laezza C. Endocannabinoids in endocrine and related tumours. Endocrine-Related Cancer 2008;15(2) 391-408.

[27] Freimuth N, Ramer R, Hinz B. Antitumorigenic effects of cannabinoids beyond apoptosis. The Journal of Pharmacology and Experimental Therapeutics 2010;332(2) 336-344.

[28] Pertwee RG, Ross RA, Craib SJ, Thomas A. (-)-Cannabidiol antagonizes cannabinoid receptor agonists and noradrenaline in the mouse vas deferens. European Journal of Pharmacology 2002;456(1-3) 99-106.

[29] Thomas A, Baillie GL, Phillips AM, Razdan RK, Ross RA, Pertwee RG. Cannabidiol displays unexpectedly high potency as an antagonist of CB1 and CB2 receptor agonists in vitro. British Journal of Pharmacology 2007;150(5) 613-623.

[30] Massi P, Solinas M, Cinquina V, Parolaro D. Cannabidiol as potential anticancer drug. British Journal of Clinical Pharmacology 2013;75(2) 303-312.

[31] Ligresti A, Moriello AS, Starowicz K, Matias I, Pisanti S, De Petrocellis L, Laezza C, Portella G, Bifulco M, Di Marzo V. Antitumor activity of plant cannabinoids with emphasis on the effect of cannabidiol on human breast carcinoma. The Journal of Pharmacology and Experimental Therapeutics 2006;318(3) 1375-1387.

[32] McAllister SD, Christian RT, Horowitz MP, Garcia A, Desprez PY. Cannabidiol as a novel inhibitor of Id-1 gene expression in aggressive breast cancer cells. Molecular Cancer Therapeutics 2007;6(11) 2921-2927.

[33] McAllister SD, Murase R, Christian RT, Lau D, Zielinski AJ, Allison J, Almanza C, Pakdel A, Lee J, Limbad C, Liu Y, Debs RJ, Moore DH, Desprez PY. Pathways media-

ting the effects of cannabidiol on the reduction of breast cancer cell proliferation, invasion, and metastasis. Breast Cancer Research and Treatment 2011;129(1) 37-47.

[34] Shrivastava A, Kuzontkoski PM, Groopman JE, Prasad A. Cannabidiol induces programmed cell death in breast cancer cells by coordinating the cross-talk between apoptosis and autophagy. Molecular Cancer Therapeutics 2011;10(7) 1161-1172.

[35] Cho DH, Jo YK, Hwang JJ, Lee YM, Roh SA, Kim JC. Caspase-mediated cleavage of ATG6/Beclin-1 links apoptosis to autophagy in HeLa cells. Cancer Letters 2009;274(1) 95-100.

[36] Wirawan E, Vande Walle L, Kersse K, Cornelis S, Claerhout S, Vanoverberghe I, Roelandt R, De Rycke R, Verspurten J, Declercq W, Agostinis P, Vanden Berghe T, Lippens S, Vandenabeele P. Caspase-mediated cleavage of Beclin-1 inactivates Beclin-1-induced autophagy and enhances apoptosis by promoting the release of proapoptotic factors from mitochondria. Cell Death & Disease 2010;1 e18.

[37] Jacobsson SO, Rongård E, Stridh M, Tiger G, Fowler CJ. Serum-dependent effects of tamoxifen and cannabinoids upon C6 glioma cell viability. Biochemical Pharmacology 2000;60(12) 1807-1813.

[38] Massi P, Vaccani A, Ceruti S, Colombo A, Abbracchio MP, Parolaro D. Antitumor effects of cannabidiol, a nonpsychoactive cannabinoid, on human glioma cell lines. The Journal of Pharmacology and Experimental Therapeutics 2004;308(3) 838-845.

[39] Massi P, Vaccani A, Bianchessi S, Costa B, Macchi P, Parolaro D. The non-psychoactive cannabidiol triggers caspase activation and oxidative stress in human glioma cells. Cellular and Molecular Life Sciences 2006;63(17) 2057-2066.

[40] Marcu JP, Christian RT, Lau D, Zielinski AJ, Horowitz MP, Lee J, Pakdel A, Allison J, Limbad C, Moore DH, Yount GL, Desprez PY, McAllister SD. Cannabidiol enhances the inhibitory effects of delta9-tetrahydrocannabinol on human glioblastoma cell proliferation and survival. Molecular Cancer Therapeutics 2010;9(1) 180-189.

[41] Torres S, Lorente M, Rodríguez-Fornés F, Hernández-Tiedra S, Salazar M, García-Taboada E, Barcia J, Guzmán M, Velasco G. A combined preclinical therapy of cannabinoids and temozolomide against glioma. Molecular Cancer Therapeutics 2011;10(1) 90-103.

[42] Solinas M, Massi P, Cinquina V, Valenti M, Bolognini D, Gariboldi M, Monti E, Rubino T, Parolaro D. Cannabidiol, a non-psychoactive cannabinoid compound, inhibits proliferation and invasion in U87-MG and T98G glioma cells through a multitarget effect. PLoS One 2013;8(10) e76918.

[43] Massi P, Valenti M, Vaccani A, Gasperi V, Perletti G, Marras E, Fezza F, Maccarrone M, Parolaro D. 5-Lipoxygenase and anandamide hydrolase (FAAH) mediate the antitumor activity of cannabidiol, a non-psychoactive cannabinoid. Journal of Neurochemistry 2008;104(4) 1091-1100.

[44] Vaccani A, Massi P, Colombo A, Rubino T, Parolaro D. Cannabidiol inhibits human glioma cell migration through a cannabinoid receptor-independent mechanism. British Journal of Pharmacology 2005;144(8) 1032-1036.

[45] Nabissi M, Morelli MB, Santoni M, Santoni G. Triggering of the TRPV2 channel by cannabidiol sensitizes glioblastoma cells to cytotoxic chemotherapeutic agents. Carcinogenesis 2013;34(1) 48-57.

[46] Soroceanu L, Murase R, Limbad C, Singer E, Allison J, Adrados I, Kawamura R, Pakdel A, Fukuyo Y, Nguyen D, Khan S, Arauz R, Yount GL, Moore DH, Desprez PY, McAllister SD. Id-1 is a key transcriptional regulator of glioblastoma aggressiveness and a novel therapeutic target. Cancer Research 2013;73(5) 1559-1569.

[47] Gallily R, Even-Chena T, Katzavian G, Lehmann D, Dagan A, Mechoulam R. Gamma-irradiation enhances apoptosis induced by cannabidiol, a non-psychotropic cannabinoid, in cultured HL-60 myeloblastic leukemia cells. Leukemia & Lymphoma 2003;44(10) 1767-1773.

[48] McKallip RJ, Jia W, Schlomer J, Warren JW, Nagarkatti PS, Nagarkatti M. Cannabidiol-induced apoptosis in human leukemia cells: A novel role of cannabidiol in the regulation of p22phox and Nox4 expression. Molecular Pharmacology 2006;70(3) 897-908.

[49] McKallip RJ, Lombard C, Fisher M, Martin BR, Ryu S, Grant S, Nagarkatti PS, Nagarkatti M. Targeting CB2 cannabinoid receptors as a novel therapy to treat malignant lymphoblastic disease. Blood 2002;100(2) 627-634.

[50] Li R, Wang H, Bekele BN, Yin Z, Caraway NP, Katz RL, Stass SA, Jiang F. Identification of putative oncogenes in lung adenocarcinoma by a comprehensive functional genomic approach. Oncogene 2006;25(18) 2628-2635.

[51] Adjei AA. Novel combinations based on epidermal growth factor receptor inhibition. Clinical Cancer Research 2006;12(14 Pt 2) 4446s–4450s.

[52] Erler JT, Bennewith KL, Nicolau M, Dornhöfer N, Kong C, Le QT, Chi JT, Jeffrey SS, Giaccia AJ. Lysyl oxidase is essential for hypoxia-induced metastasis. Nature 2006;440(7088) 1222-1226.

[53] Molina JR, Adjei AA, Jett JR. Advances in chemotherapy of non-small cell lung cancer. Chest 2006;130(4) 1211-1219.

[54] Ramer R, Merkord J, Rohde H, Hinz B. Cannabidiol inhibits cancer cell invasion via upregulation of tissue inhibitor of matrix metalloproteinases-1. Biochemical Pharmacology 2010;79(7) 955-966.

[55] Ramer R, Rohde A, Merkord J, Rohde H, Hinz B. Decrease of plasminogen activator inhibitor-1 may contribute to the anti-invasive action of cannabidiol on human lung cancer cells. Pharmaceutical Research 2010;27(10) 2162-2174.

[56] Ramer R, Hinz B. Inhibition of cancer cell invasion by cannabinoids via increased expression of tissue inhibitor of matrix metalloproteinases-1. Journal of the National Cancer Institute 2008;100(1) 59-69.

[57] Sativex Product Monograph. Salisbury, Wiltshire U.K.: GW Pharma Ltd.; SP4 0JQ Submission Control No: 091289; April 2003.

[58] Ramer R, Heinemann K, Merkord J, Rohde H, Salamon A, Linnebacher M, Hinz B. COX-2 and PPAR-$\gamma$ confer cannabidiol-induced apoptosis of human lung cancer cells. Molecular Cancer Therapeutics 2013;12(1) 69-82.

[59] Lee CY, Wey SP, Liao MH, Hsu WL, Wu HY, Jan TR. A comparative study on cannabidiol-induced apoptosis in murine thymocytes and EL-4 thymoma cells. International Immunopharmacology 2008;8(5) 732-740.

[60] Wu HY, Chu RM, Wang CC, Lee CY, Lin SH, Jan TR. Cannabidiol-induced apoptosis in primary lymphocytes is associated with oxidative stress-dependent activation of caspase-8. Toxicology and Applied Pharmacology 2008;226(3) 260-270.

[61] Sreevalsan S, Joseph S, Jutooru I, Chadalapaka G, Safe SH. Induction of apoptosis by cannabinoids in prostate and colon cancer cells is phosphatase dependent. Anticancer Research 2011;31(11) 3799-3807.

[62] Aviello G, Romano B, Borrelli F, Capasso R, Gallo L, Piscitelli F, Di Marzo V, Izzo AA. Chemopreventive effect of the non-psychotropic phytocannabinoid cannabidiol on experimental colon cancer. Journal of Molecular Medicine 2012;90(8) 925-934.

[63] Solinas M, Massi P, Cantelmo AR, Cattaneo MG, Cammarota R, Bartolini D, Cinquina V, Valenti M, Vicentini LM, Noonan DM, Albini A, Parolaro D. Cannabidiol inhibits angiogenesis by multiple mechanisms. British Journal of Pharmacology 2012;167(6) 1218-1231.

[64] Consroe P, Laguna J, Allender J, Snider S, Stern L, Sandyk R, Kennedy K, Schram K. Controlled clinical trial of cannabidiol in Huntington's disease. Pharmacology, Biochemistry, and Behavior 1991;40(3) 701-708.

[65] Consroe P, Kennedy K, Schram K. Assay of plasma cannabidiol by capillary gas chromatography/ion trap mass spectroscopy following high-dose repeated daily oral administration in humans. Pharmacology, Biochemistry, and Behavior 1991;40(3) 517-522.

[66] Karschner EL, Darwin WD, Goodwin RS, Wright S, Huestis MA. Plasma cannabinoid pharmacokinetics following controlled oral delta9-tetrahydrocannabinol and oromucosal cannabis extract administration. Clinical Chemistry 2011;57(1) 66-75.

[67] Hernán Pérez de la Ossa D, Lorente M, Gil-Alegre ME, Torres S, García-Taboada E, Aberturas Mdel R, Molpeceres J, Velasco G, Torres-Suárez AI. Local delivery of cannabinoid-loaded microparticles inhibits tumor growth in a murine xenograft model of glioblastoma multiforme. PLoS One 2013;8(1) e54795.

[68] Alexander SPH, Mathie A, Peters JA. Guide to Receptors and Channels (GRAC), 5th edition. British Journal of Pharmacology 2011;164(Suppl. 1) S1-S324.